Sleisenger and Fordtran's

GASTROINTESTINAL AND LIVER DISEASE

REVIEW AND ASSESSMENT

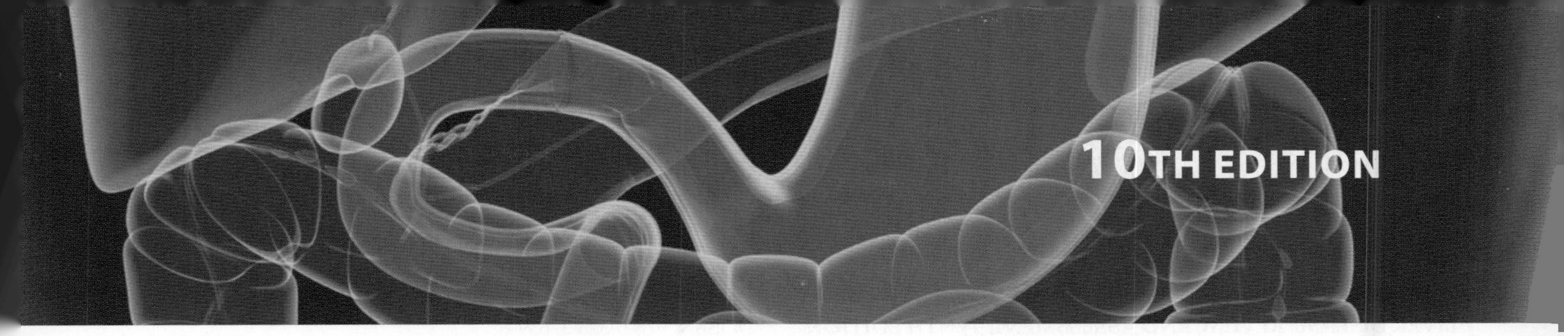

10TH EDITION

Sleisenger and Fordtran's

GASTROINTESTINAL AND LIVER DISEASE

REVIEW AND ASSESSMENT

Emad Qayed, MD
Assistant Professor of Medicine
Division of Digestive Diseases
Emory University School of Medicine
Interim Chief of Gastroenterology
Grady Memorial Hospital
Atlanta, Georgia

Shanthi Srinivasan, MD
Associate Professor of Medicine
Division of Digestive Diseases
Emory University School of Medicine
Chief, Gastroenterology Unit
Atlanta VA Medical Center
Atlanta, Georgia

Nikrad S
Assistan
Divisio
Emor
Atl

Previous e
Library of C
Names: Qay
Nikrad, edi
Title: Sleiseng
and assessm
Shahnavaz.
Other titles: Ga
Review and as
Description: Ten
bibliographical
Identifiers: LCCN
Subjects: | MESH:
Questions
Classification: LCC
available at http://lc

Senior Content Strategist
Senior Content Developme
Publishing Services Manag
Project Manager: Amanda
Book Designer: Brian Salisb

Printed in China

Last digit is the print number:

ELSEVIER

1600 John F. Kennedy Blvd.
Ste 1800
Philadelphia, PA 19103-2899

SLEISENGER AND FORDTRAN'S GASTROINTESTINAL AND LIVER DISEASE: REVIEW AND ASSESSMENT, TENTH EDITION ISBN: 978-0-323-37639-6

Notices

Knowledge and best practice in this field are constantly changing. As new research and experience broaden our understanding, changes in research methods, professional practices, or medical treatment may become necessary.

Practitioners and researchers must always rely on their own experience and knowledge in evaluating and using any information, methods, compounds, or experiments described herein. In using such information or methods they should be mindful of their own safety and the safety of others, including parties for whom they have a professional responsibility.

With respect to any drug or pharmaceutical products identified, readers are advised to check the ost current information provided (i) on procedures featured or (ii) by the manufacturer of each oduct to be administered, to verify the recommended dose or formula, the method and duration administration, and contraindications. It is the responsibility of practitioners, relying on their experience and knowledge of their patients, to make diagnoses, to determine dosages and the treatment for each individual patient, and to take all appropriate safety precautions.

the fullest extent of the law, neither the Publisher nor the authors, contributors, or editors, e any liability for any injury and/or damage to persons or property as a matter of products y, negligence or otherwise, or from any use or operation of any methods, products, tions, or ideas contained in the material herein.

ditions copyrighted 2010, 2007, 1999, and 1996.

ongress Cataloging-in-Publication Data
ed, Emad, editor. | Srinivasan, Shanthi, editor. | Shahnavaz,
tor.
er and Fordtran's gastrointestinal and liver disease. Review
nt / [edited by] Emad Qayed, Shanthi Srinivasan, Nikrad

strointestinal and liver disease. Review and assessment |
sessment
h edition. | Philadelphia, PA : Elsevier, [2017] | Includes
references.
2015045935 | ISBN 9780323376396 (hardcover : alk. paper)
Gastrointestinal Diseases | Liver Diseases | Examination

RC801 | NLM WI 18.2 | DDC 616.3/30076--dc23 LC record
cn.loc.gov/2015045935

Suzanne Toppy
nt Specialist: Anne Snyder
er: Patricia Tannian
Mincher
ury

9 8 7 6 5 4 3 2 1

DEDICATION

To my dear wife, Yara; my children, Bassem and Zaina; and my mother, Nawal.
Emad Qayed

To my parents; my husband, Srini; and my children, Karthik, Arjun, and Anand.
Shanthi Srinivasan

To my wife, Suzanne; my parents, Roya and Shahpoor; and my grandmother, Rafat.
Nikrad Shahnavaz

And to all of our colleagues, contributors, and trainees.

ACKNOWLEDGMENTS

The authors would like to thank Suzanne Toppy, Anne Snyder, and Amanda Mincher for their valuable contributions in publishing this book.

CONTRIBUTORS

Khaled Abdeljawad, MD
Gastroenterology Fellow
Division of Digestive Diseases
Emory University School of Medicine
Atlanta, Georgia

Muhammad Fuad Azrak, MD, MPH
Clinical Assistant Professor
Internal Medicine
Wayne State University
Detroit, Michigan
Attending Physcian
Internal Medicine
Oakwood Hospital and Medical Center
Dearborn, Michigan

Matthew Barnes, MD
Resident, Internal Medicine Residency Program
University of Tennessee Health Science Center
Memphis, Tennessee

Stephen Hans Berger, MD
Gastroenterology Fellow
Division of Digestive Diseases
Emory University School of Medicine
Atlanta, Georgia

Jason M. Brown, MD
Gastroenterology Fellow
Division of Digestive Diseases
Emory University School of Medicine
Atlanta, Georgia

Saurabh Chawla, MD
Director of Endoscopy
Grady Memorial Hospital
Assistant Professor of Medicine
Division of Digestive Diseases
Emory University School of Medicine
Atlanta, Georgia

Jennifer Christie, MD, FASGE
Associate Professor of Medicine
Emory University School of Medicine
Division of Digestive Diseases
Director of Gastrointestinal Motility and Clinical Research
Emory Healthcare
Atlanta, Georgia

Sunil Dacha, MD
Associate in Medicine
Division of Digestive Diseases
Department of Internal Medicine
Emory University School of Medicine
Atlanta, Georgia

Kanak Das, MBBS
Assistant Professor
Division of Gastroenterology and Hepatology
Department of Medicine
University of Tennessee Health Science Center
Memphis, Tennessee

Nader Dbouk, MD
Assistant Professor of Surgery
Methodist University Hospital Transplant Institute
University of Tennessee Health Science Center
Memphis, Tennessee

Tanvi Dhere, MD
Assistant Professor
Director of Inflammatory Bowel Diseases
Digestive Diseases
Emory University School of Medicine
Atlanta, Georgia

Anthony Gamboa, MD
Gastroenterology Fellow
Division of Digestive Diseases
Emory University School of Medicine
Atlanta, Georgia

Stephan U. Goebel, MD
Assistant Professor of Medicine
Division of Digestive Diseases
Emory University School of Medicine
Atlanta VA Medical Center
Atlanta, Georgia

William Joseph Goldkamp, MD
Chief Resident
Department of Medicine
University of Tennessee Health Science Center
Memphis, Tennessee

Hazem Hammad, MD
Assistant Professor of Clinical Medicine
Division of Gastroenterology
University of Missouri Hospital
Columbia, Missouri

Melanie Harrison, MD
Assistant Professor of Medicine
Division of Digestive Diseases
Emory University School of Medicine
Atlanta, Georgia

Heba Iskandar, MD, MSCI
Assistant Professor of Medicine
Division of Digestive Diseases
Emory University School of Medicine
Atlanta, Georgia

Elnaz Jafarimehr, MD
Gastroenterology Fellow
Emory University School of Medicine
Atlanta, Georgia

Steven Keilin, MD, FASGE
Assistant Professor of Medicine
Director of Pancreaticobiliary Service
Associate Director, Advanced Endoscopy Fellowship
Division of Gastroenterology
Emory University Hospital
The Emory Clinic
Atlanta, Georgia

Jan-Michael A. Klapproth, MD
Associate Professor of Medicine
Division of Gastroenterology
University of Pennsylvania
Phildalphia, Pennsylvania

Rahul Maheshwari, MD
Gastroenterology Fellow
Division of Digestive Diseases
Emory University School of Medicine
Atlanta, Georgia

Julia Massaad, MD
Assistant Professor of Medicine
Director, GI Fellowship Program
Director of Education
Division of Digestive Diseases
Emory University School of Medicine
Atlanta, Georgia

Parit Mekaroonkamol, MD
Division of Digestive Diseases
Emory University School of Medicine
Atlanta, Georgia

Brett Mendel, MD
Gastroenterology Fellow
Division of Digestive Diseases
Emory University School of Medicine
Atlanta, Georgia

Fazia Mir, MD
Fellow
Division of Gastroenterology
University of Missouri–Columbia
Columbia, Missouri

Jeffrey Nadelson, MD
Gastroenterology Fellow
Medicine-GI
University of Tennessee Health Sciences Center
Memphis, Tennessee

Behtash Ghazi Nezami, MD
Postdoctoral Research Fellow
Division of Digestive Diseases
Emory University School of Medicine
Atlanta, Georgia

John Paul Norvell, MD
Assistant Professor of Medicine
Division of Digestive Diseases
Emory Transplant Center
Emory University School of Medicine
Atlanta, Georgia

Joshua Novak, MD
Assistant Professor of Medicine
Division of Gastroenterology and Hepatology
Emory University School of Medicine
Atlanta, Georgia

Samir Parekh, MD
Director of Hepatology
Department of Medicine
Emory University School of Medicine
Atlanta, Georgia

Mehul Parikh, MD
Gastroenterologist
Gastroenterology Specialists of Gwinnett
Lawrenceville, Georgia

George M. Philips, MD
Advanced Endoscopy Fellow
Emory University School of Medicine
Atlanta, Georgia

Anjana Pillai, MD
Assistant Professor of Medicine
Division of Digestive Diseases
Emory Transplant Center
Emory University School of Medicine
Atlanta, Georgia

Emad Qayed, MD
Assistant Professor of Medicine
Division of Digestive Diseases
Emory University School of Medicine
Interim Chief of Gastroenterology
Grady Memorial Hospital
Atlanta, Georgia

José Rivera-Acosta, MD, MSc
Assistant Professor
Department of Internal Medicine, GI Division
University of Puerto Rico, School of Medicine
Liver Transplant Hepatology Faculty
Transplant Center
Hospital Auxilio Mutuo
San Juan, Puerto Rico

Sonali Sakaria, MD
Assistant Professor of Internal Medicine
Associate Program Director
Division of Digestive Diseases
The Emory Clinic
Emory University School of Medicine
Grady Memorial Hospital
Atlanta, Georgia

Kavya M. Sebastian, MD
Assistant Professor
Division of Digestive Diseases
Emory University School of Medicine
Atlanta, Georgia

Nikrad Shahnavaz, MD
Assistant Professor of Medicine
Division of Digestive Diseases
Emory University School of Medicine
Atlanta, Georgia

Lauren M. Shea, MD
Gastroenterology
Emory University School of Medicine
Atlanta, Georgia

Sagar Shroff, MD
Fellow
Division of Digestive Diseases
Emory University School of Medicine
Atlanta, Georgia

Shanthi Srinivasan, MD
Associate Professor of Medicine
Division of Digestive Diseases
Emory University School of Medicine
Chief, Gastroenterology Unit
Atlanta VA Medical Center
Atlanta, Georgia

Sahar Taba Taba Vakili, MD, MPH
Lead Research Specialist
Division of Digestive Diseases
Emory University School of Medicine
Atlanta, Georgia

Ravi Vora, MD
Gastroenterology Fellow
Division of Digestive Diseases
Emory University School of Medicine
Atlanta, Georgia

Joel P. Wedd, MD, MPH
Assistant Professor of Medicine
Division of Digestive Diseases
Emory University School of Medicine
Atlanta, Georgia

Field F. Willingham, MD, MPH
Director of Endoscopy
Associate Professor of Medicine
President of the Georgia Gastroenterologic and Endoscopic Society
Division of Digestive Diseases
Emory University School of Medicine
Atlanta, Georgia

PREFACE

In writing this tenth edition of *Sleisenger and Fordtran's Gastrointestinal and Liver Disease Review and Assessment*, we have been fortunate to work with an extremely talented group of faculty and fellows from our own division of digestive diseases at Emory University, and also from prominent institutions nationwide.

In this edition, we compiled all new questions that are board-style, case-based patient vignettes, with a strong focus on clinically relevant information. These questions test medical knowledge, clinical reasoning and interpretation, and problem solving skills. The new edition mimics the contents of the gastroenterology board examinations in content, style, and number of questions for each section, and each question has a single best answer. We avoided questions that have more than one correct answer choice, as well as "all of the above," "none of the above," and "all except" types of questions. In writing and editing the answers, we made sure every answer clearly explained the correct and incorrect answer choices, thereby making this book a stand-alone review tool. However, the reader is encouraged to review the main textbook for further information and to sharpen his or her clinical knowledge.

Another exciting aspect of the new edition is the availability of an online testing mode. An online test component can be taken in an untimed study mode or in a timed assessment mode. We compiled three exams (200 questions each, with four sections of 50 questions) that can be accessed in a timed mode to simulate exam settings. If you are thinking of completing these exams, we recommend that you do that first, as they contain questions taken from throughout this book.

We hope you enjoy testing your gastroenterology knowledge using this book as much as we enjoyed writing and editing these questions.

Emad Qayed
Shanthi Srinivasan
Nikrad Shahnavaz

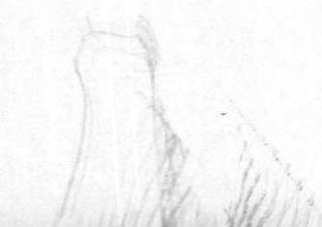

LAB STUDIES REFERENCE RANGES

ABIM Laboratory Reference Ranges - January 2015	
Laboratory Test	**Reference Range**
Albumin, serum	3.5–5.5 g/dL
Alkaline phosphatase, serum	30–120 U/L
Alkaline phosphatase, bone specific	5.6–18.0 ug/L for premenopausal women
Alpha$_1$-antitrypsin (AAT), serum	150–350 mg/dL
Alpha-fetoprotein serum	Less than 10 ng/mL
Aminotransferase, serum alanine (ALT, SGPT)	10–40 U/L
Aminotransferase, serum aspartate (AST, SGOT)	10–40 U/L
Ammonia, blood	40–70 μg/dL
Amylase, serum	25–125 U/L (80–180 [Somogyi] units/dL)
Amylase, urine	1–17 U/hr
Antibodies to double-stranded DNA	0–7 IU/mL
Anti-F-actin antibodies, serum	1:80 or less
Antihistone antibodies	Less than 1:16
Anti-LKM	Less than 1:20
Antimitochondrial antibodies	1:5 or less
Antinuclear antibodies	1:40 or less
Anti–smooth muscle antibodies	1:80 or less
Bicarbonate, serum	23–28 mEq/L
Bilirubin, serum Total Direct Indirect	 0.3–1.0 mg/dL 0.1–0.3 mg/dL 0.2–0.7 mg/dL
Calcium, serum	8.6–10.2 mg/dL
CD4 (T4) lymphocyte count	530–1570/μL
Chloride, serum	98–106 mEq/L
Cholesterol, serum Total Desirable Borderline-high High	 Less than 200 mg/dL 200–239 mg/dL Greater than 239 mg/dL
Copper, serum	100–200 μg/dL
Copper, urine	0–100 μg/24 hr

Continued

ABIM Laboratory Reference Ranges - January 2015—cont'd	
Laboratory Test	**Reference Range**
C-reactive protein	0.8 mg/dL or less
C-reactive protein (high sensitivity), serum	Low risk = less than 1.0 mg/L; Average risk = 1.0–3.0 mg/L; High risk = more than 3.0 mg/L
Creatine kinase, serum Total MB isoenzymes	 Female: 30–135 U/L; male: 55–170 U/L Less than 5% of total
Creatinine clearance, urine	90–140 mL/min
Creatinine, serum	0.7–1.5 mg/dL
D-dimer, plasma	Less than 0.5 μg/mL
Electrolytes, serum Sodium Potassium Chloride Bicarbonate	 136–145 mEq/L 3.5–5.0 mEq/L 98–106 mEq/L 23–28 mEq/L
Erythrocyte sedimentation rate (Westergren)	Female: 0–20 mm/hr; male: 0–15 mm/hr
Fecal fat	Less than 7 g/24 hr
Fecal pH	7.0–7.5
Fecal potassium	Less than 10 mEq/L
Fecal sodium	Less than 10 mEq/L
Ferritin, serum	Female: 11–211 ng/mL; male: 20–235 ng/mL
Folate, red cell	150–450 ng/mL of packed cells
Folate, serum	1.8–9.0 ng/mL
Gamma-glutamyl transpeptidase, serum	Female: 8–40 U/L; male: 9–50 U/L
Gastric secretion Basal acid analysis Basal acid output Maximal output after pentagastrin stimulation	 10–30 units of free acid Female: 2.0 ± 1.8 mEq of HCl/hr; male: 3.0 ± 2.0 mEq of HCl/hr 23 ± 5 mEq of HCl/hr
Gastrin, serum	Less than 100 pg/mL
Haptoglobin, serum	83–267 mg/dL
Hematocrit, blood	Female: 37%–47%; male: 42%–50%
Hemoglobin, A_{1c}	4.0%–5.6%
Hemoglobin, blood	Female: 12–16 g/dL; male: 14–18 g/dL
Immunoglobulins, serum IgA IgE IgG IgM	 90–325 mg/dL Less than 380 IU/mL 800–1500 mg/dL 45–150 mg/dL
Insulin, serum (fasting)	Less than 20 μU/mL
Iron, serum	50–150 μg/dL
Iron-binding capacity, serum (total)	250–310 μg/dL
Lactate dehydrogenase, serum	80–225 U/L
Lactate, arterial blood	Less than 1.3 mmol/L (Less than 1.3 mEq/L)
Lactate, serum	0.7–2.1 mmol/L
Lactate, venous blood	0.6–1.8 mEq/L; 6–16 mg/dL
Lactic acid, serum	6–19 mg/dL (0.7–2.1 mmol/L)

ABIM Laboratory Reference Ranges - January 2015—cont'd	
Laboratory Test	**Reference Range**
Leukocyte count	4000–11,000/ μL
Segmented neutrophils	50%–70%
Band forms	0–5%
Lymphocytes	30%–45%
Monocytes	0–6%
Basophils	0–1%
Eosinophils	0–3%
Lipase, serum	10–140 U/L
Magnesium, serum	1.6–2.6 mEq/L
Magnesium, urine	14–290 mg/24 hr
Mean corpuscular hemoglobin	28–32 pg
Mean corpuscular hemoglobin concentration	33–36 g/dL
Mean corpuscular volume	80–98 fL
Mean platelet volume	7–9 fL
Osmolality, serum	275–295 mOsm/kg H_2O
Osmolality, urine	38–1400 mOsm/kg H_2O
Oxygen saturation, arterial blood	95% or greater
Phosphatase (alkaline), serum	30–120 U/L
Platelet count	150,000–300,000/μL
Potassium, serum	3.5–5.0 mEq/L
Prealbumin, serum	16–30 mg/dL
Total	5.5–9.0 g/dL
Albumin	3.5–5.5 g/dL
Globulin	2.0–3.5 g/dL
Alpha1	0.2–0.4 g/dL
Alpha2	0.5–0.9 g/dL
Beta	0.6–1.1 g/dL
Gamma	0.7–1.7 g/dL
Prothrombin time, plasma	11–13 seconds
Red cell distribution width (RDW)	9.0–14.5
Reticulocyte count	0.5%–1.5% of red cells
Reticulocyte count, absolute	25,000–100,000/uL
Sodium, serum	136–145 mEq/L
Specific gravity, urine	1.002–1.030
Transferrin saturation	20%–50%
Transferrin, serum	200–400 mg/dL
Triglycerides, serum (fasting)	
Optimal	Less than 100 mg/dL
Normal	Less than 150 mg/dL
Borderline high	150–199 mg/dL
High	200–499 mg/dL
Very high	Greater than 499 mg/dL
Urea nitrogen, blood	8–20 mg/dL
Urea nitrogen, urine	12–20 g/24 hr
Uric acid, serum	3.0–7.0 mg/dL
Uric acid, urine	250–750 mg/24 hr
Vitamin B_{12}, serum	200–800 pg/mL
Zinc, serum	75–140 μg/dL

Modified from American Board of Internal Medicine, Philadelphia, Pa.

CONTENTS

CHAPTER

1

Biology of the Gastrointestinal Tract

Emad Qayed and Mehul Parikh

QUESTIONS

1. A 65-year-old man presents to his primary care physician with rectal bleeding for the past several months. His hemoglobin is 9.8 g/dL. He undergoes a colonoscopy that reveals a large, friable mass in the ascending colon and another smaller mass in the transverse colon. Biopsies of both masses confirm the diagnosis of adenocarcinoma. An abdominal computed tomography (CT) scan reveals multiple hypodense liver lesions consistent with metastatic spread. Treatment with chemotherapy combined with cetuximab is considered. Which of the following genetic mutations should be tested prior to initiating therapy with cetuximab?
   A. *APC*
   B. *MSH2*
   C. *SMAD4*
   D. *KRAS*
   E. *MYC*

2. Which of the following terms describes the process by which cells permanently lose their ability to divide?
   A. Apoptosis
   B. Mitosis
   C. Meiosis
   D. Cytokinesis
   E. Senescence

3. Which of the following signaling pathways plays an important role in intestinal epithelial cell proliferation?
   A. Wnt pathway
   B. mTOR pathway
   C. HER2/Neu pathway
   D. NOTCH pathway
   E. Toll-like receptor (TLR) pathway

4. Which of the following genetic events results in sporadic, microsatellite unstable colon cancer?
   A. Germline mutation of *MLH1* gene
   B. CpG island hypermethylation
   C. Mutation of *APC* gene
   D. Mutation of *KRAS* gene
   E. Mutation of *TP53* gene

5. Which of the following hereditary gastrointestinal cancer syndrome is associated with mutation in *PTEN* gene?
   A. Juvenile polyposis
   B. Hereditary diffuse gastric cancer
   C. Peutz-Jeghers syndrome
   D. Cowden syndrome
   E. Multiple endocrine neoplasia (MEN) type 1

6. Which of the following genes is rarely mutated in gastrointestinal (GI) malignancies?
   A. *TP53*
   B. *APC*
   C. *SMAD4*
   D. *VHL*
   E. *MLH1*

7. A 35-year-old man is seen in clinic with nausea, vomiting, and 15-pound weight loss over the past 6 months. An upper endoscopy is performed and shows diffuse ulceration and thickening in the gastric body and antrum. Biopsies show gastric adenocarcinoma. CT scan shows diffuse abdominal lymphadenopathy and liver metastasis. Genetic testing shows a germline mutation in *CDH1*. Loss of which of the following proteins facilitates tumor metastasis in this hereditary syndrome?
   A. E-cadherin
   B. Vascular endothelial growth factor-A (VEGF-A)
   C. Basic fibroblast growth factor (bFGF)
   D. Transforming growth factor-β (TGF-β)
   E. Vascular endothelial growth factor receptor-3 (VEGFR-3)

8. Which of the following terms describes the mutation that results in a premature stop codon?
   A. Missense
   B. Nonsense
   C. Silent
   D. Insertion
   E. Deletion

9. A 37-year-old man presents with rectal bleeding and anemia. A colonoscopy is performed that reveals a large ulcerated mass in the ascending colon and a smaller mass in the transverse colon. Biopsies of both masses are consistent with colonic adenocarcinoma. His mother was diagnosed with endometrial cancer at age 51, and his maternal uncle was diagnosed with colon cancer at age 50. Which of the following mutations is characteristic of his malignancy?
   A. *CDH1*
   B. *MUTYH*
   C. *PTEN*
   D. *APC*
   E. *MSH2*

10. A 62-year-old man is diagnosed with locally advanced pancreatic cancer. The oncologist recommends starting chemotherapy with an agent that predominantly impairs

cell division. Which of the following phases of cellular proliferation is being targeted?
A. G0 phase
B. G1 phase
C. S phase
D. G2 phase
E. M phase

11. A 22-year-old man presents with iron deficiency anemia. Colonoscopy is performed and shows greater than 100 polyps throughout the colon. Some of these polyps are sampled, and histology is consistent with tubular adenomas. Genetic testing will most likely reveal a mutation in which of the following types of genes?
A. Peptide growth factor oncogene
B. DNA mismatch repair gene
C. Tumor suppressor gene
D. Noncoding RNA gene
E. Nuclear oncogene

12. Which of the following is the most abundant antibody in mucosal secretions?
A. Immunoglobulin (Ig)G
B. IgM
C. IgA
D. IgD
E. IgE

13. Which of the following is produced by plasma cells and binds two IgA molecules forming secretory IgA dimer?
A. Secretory component
B. Polymeric Ig receptor
C. J chain
D. Fc fragment
E. Fab fragment

14. Which of the following accurately describes the function of the M (microfold) cells in Peyer's patches?
A. They secrete antibacterial proteins
B. They secrete specialized digestive proteases
C. They specialize in endocytosis of luminal antigens
D. They specialize in absorption of specific luminal nutrients
E. They secrete gastrointestinal hormones

15. The M (microfold) cells are specialized cells found in the Peyer's patches. Which of the following is a structural feature of these cells?
A. They have extensive microvilli on their apical surface
B. They have a thick mucin overlayer
C. They have abundant cytoplasm
D. They contain few lysosomes
E. They have abundant granules containing digestive enzymes

16. Which of the following proteins protects the secretory immunoglobulin in the GI tract from degradation by luminal proteases?
A. J chain
B. Polymeric Ig receptor
C. Light chain
D. Heavy chain
E. CD23

17. Antigen-presenting cells possess the capacity to recognize microbial components called pathogen-associated molecular patterns (PAMPs). Which of the following is an intracellular receptor for PAMPs?
A. Nuclear oligomerization domain (NOD)
B. Toll-like receptor
C. Major histocompatibility complex (MHC)
D. CX3CR1
E. Polymeric Ig receptor

18. A 60-year-old man undergoes a colonoscopy to evaluate for chronic diarrhea. Endoscopic examination reveals normal colonic mucosa. Random biopsies were obtained from the right and left colon. Microscopic examination reveals normal histology. Under normal conditions, which of the following colonic wall layers contains the majority of inflammatory cells?
A. Lamina propria
B. Muscularis mucosa
C. Submucosa
D. Muscularis propria
E. Serosa

19. The enteric microbiota provides trophic, metabolic, and protective effects on the host. Which of the following correctly describes germ-free animals compared to their colonized counterparts?
A. They have lower nitrogen intake
B. They have higher dietary caloric requirements
C. They have a more mature mucosal immune system
D. They have increased gastrointestinal motility
E. They require higher doses of infectious pathogens to cause disease

20. Which of the following bacteria is an example of a pathobiont?
A. Enterohemorrhagic *Escherichia coli*
B. *Shigella*
C. *Clostridium difficile*
D. *Yersinia enterocolitica*
E. *Campylobacter jejuni*

21. Which of the following terms refers to an indigestible food ingredient that selectively promotes the growth of bacteria in the digestive tract in a way that benefits the host?
A. Probiotic
B. Prebiotic
C. Synbiotic
D. Pharmabiotic
E. Antibiotic

22. Which of the following phyla contribute to the majority of bacteria in the distal bowel?
A. *Firmicutes* and *Bacteroidetes*
B. *Firmicutes* and *Proteobacteria*
C. *Bacteroidetes* and *Acintobacteria*
D. *Acintobacteria* and *Proteobacteria*
E. *Bacteroidetes* and *Proteobacteria*

23. Which of the following statements concerning the normal intestinal microbiota is true?
A. The composition of the intestinal microbiota is similar among individuals
B. The intestinal microbiota starts to develop in utero
C. The aerobe/anaerobe ratio is greater within the lumen that at the mucosal surface
D. The intestinal microbiota is more resilient in infancy compared to adulthood
E. The intestinal microbiota changes in response to diet, drugs, physiologic status, and morbidity

24. A 36-year-old woman with irritable bowel syndrome is enrolled in a clinical trial to evaluate the effects of a probiotic containing *Bifidobacterium infantis* on her symptoms and the gut microbiome. DNA extraction methods from fecal samples are used to amplify 16S rRNA sequences and study the bacterial composition of the gut. Which of the following terms is used to characterize a group of microbes that share 16S rRNA sequence homology?

A. Taxonomy
B. HITChip
C. Phylum
D. Genus
E. Operational taxonomic unit

25. Which of the following describes the process of quorum sensing?

A. Regulation of gene expression based on bacterial density and diversity
B. Attachment of bacteriophages to specific bacterial receptors
C. Regulation of bacterial protein synthesis based on the osmolarity of the culture medium
D. The ability of the bacteria to become pathogenic in a susceptible host
E. Sporulation in response to low sodium concentration

26. Somatostatin is produced by gastric antral D cells. Which of the following modes of signaling is the main mechanism by which somatostatin inhibits gastric acid secretion?

A. Endocrine signaling
B. Autocrine signaling
C. Paracrine signaling
D. Synaptic signaling
E. Direct signaling through gap junctions

27. Which of the following accurately describes the location of the myenteric plexus in the GI tract?

A. Between the epithelial basement membrane and the muscularis mucosa
B. Between the mucosa and the submucosa
C. Between the submucosa and the circular muscle layers
D. Between the circular and the longitudinal muscle layers
E. Between the longitudinal muscle layer and the serosal surface

28. Which of the following hormones stimulates pancreatic bicarbonate and fluid secretion?

A. Vasoactive intestinal peptide (VIP)
B. Pancreatic polypeptide (PP)
C. Cholecystokinin (CCK)
D. Somatostatin
E. Secretin

29. A 45-year-old man presents with a 4-month history of chronic voluminous watery diarrhea. The diarrhea is not relieved by fasting and persists despite treatment with loperamide. He also complains of abdominal bloating, epigastric pain, nausea, and a 10-pound unintentional weight loss. He has a history of erosive esophagitis for which he takes omeprazole. On physical examination, his blood pressure is 95/55 mm Hg, and heart rate is 110 bpm. There is mild middle abdominal tenderness to deep palpation. Abdominal CT scan shows a 5.1 x 5.8 x 4 cm pancreatic tail mass. Overproduction of which of the following peptides is the most likely cause of the patient's symptoms?

A. Pancreatic polypeptide
B. Vasoactive intestinal peptide
C. Peptide tyrosine tyrosine (peptide YY)
D. Somatostatin
E. Gastrin

30. Which of the following peptides is secreted periodically and its blood levels correlate with the migratory motor complex (MMC)?

A. Motilin
B. Cholecystokinin
C. Vasoactive intestinal peptide
D. Somatostatin
E. Gastrin

31. Which of the following statements about secretin is true?

A. It is secreted from the gastric antrum
B. It stimulates pancreatic secretion rich in digestive enzymes
C. It stimulates gastric acid secretion
D. It stimulates gallbladder contraction
E. It is secreted as a result of acid in the duodenum

32. Which of the following is the main source of circulating leptin?

A. Brain
B. Adipose tissue
C. Stomach
D. Duodenum
E. Distal ileum

33. A 40-year-old man is seen in clinic for abdominal pain and watery diarrhea for the past 6 months. He also reports weight loss and lower extremity edema. Physical exam reveals abdominal tenderness and symmetric lower extremity edema. Laboratory results include:

Hemoglobin	11 g/dL
Platelets	210,000/μL
WBC	8000/μL
Total bilirubin	1.2 mg/dL
Creatinine	1.1 mg/dL
INR	1.3
Albumin	2.5 g/dL
Total protein	4 g/dL

EGD is performed and reveals severely enlarged gastric folds. Mucosal biopsies show foveolar hyperplasia, cystically dilated gastric glands, and loss of parietal cell mass. Enhanced signaling through which of the following receptors is the underlying pathophysiologic mechanism of this disease?

A. Platelet-derived growth factor (PDGF) receptor
B. Insulin-like growth factor (IGF) receptor
C. Epidermal growth factor (EGF) receptor
D. Fibroblast growth factor (FGF) receptor
E. c-Kit receptor

34. Which of the following peptides suppresses glucagon secretion, delays gastric emptying, and induces satiety?

A. Leptin
B. Amylin
C. Ghrelin
D. Motilin
E. Serotonin

35. A 14-year-old boy is seen in clinic for evaluation of chronic heartburn and obesity. His mother states that he has had multiple medical problems since birth. He was born with neonatal hypotonia and had issues with failure to thrive that resolved by the end of his first year of life. Childhood was complicated by delay in reaching developmental milestones and excessive weight gain. He is now morbidly obese. The mother complains about the boy's obsession with food. He digs through garbage and steals money for food. He sees a psychiatrist for obsessive-compulsive

disorder and frequent temper tantrums. Pertinent findings on physical exam include a body mass index of 35, short stature, almond-shaped eyes with strabismus, and hypogonadism. Which of the following hormones is implicated in obesity associated with this syndrome?
A. Leptin
B. Peptide tyrosine tyrosine (peptide YY)
C. Amylin
D. Glucagon-like peptide-1 (GLP-1)
E. Ghrelin

36. Which of the following gastrointestinal hormones stimulates insulin secretion after carbohydrate ingestion?
A. GLP-1
B. Amylin
C. Cholecystokinin
D. Secretin
E. Ghrelin

37. A 23-year-old woman is admitted to the hospital with intractable nausea and vomiting. Medical history is significant for poorly controlled diabetes mellitus and gastroparesis. She is treated with insulin, intravenous fluids, and erythromycin. She subsequently develops abdominal cramping and diarrhea. Which hormone receptor is most likely responsible for these side effects?
A. Gastrin
B. Cholecystokinin
C. Secretin
D. Motilin
E. Peptide YY

38. A 40-year-old Hispanic woman presents for evaluation of intermittent right upper quadrant abdominal pain of 1-year duration. Her pain is worse after fatty meals. She has no other medical problems. On physical exam, she is obese with a body mass index of 34. Abdominal exam reveals no tenderness. Labs including complete blood count and liver enzymes are unremarkable. Which of the following hormones is associated with increasing her symptoms after meals?
A. Gastrin
B. Cholecystokinin
C. Secretin
D. Peptide YY
E. Vasoactive intestinal polypeptide

ANSWERS

1. **D** (S&F ch1)
Cetuximab is a monoclonal antibody that inhibits epidermal growth factor receptor (EGFR). It improves survival in metastatic colon cancer. The presence of KRAS-activating mutations predicts a poor response to cetuximab therapy. Therefore, cetuximab is restricted to patients with wild-type (nonmutated) KRAS. The other mutations (APC, MSH2, SMAD4, and MYC) do not predict response to cetuximab in metastatic colon cancer.

2. **E** (S&F ch1)
Cellular senescence describes the process in which normal diploid cells lose their ability to divide. This phenomenon prevents excessive proliferation and is lost during carcinogenesis. Apoptosis is the programmed, controlled cell death. Loss of apoptosis can result in carcinogenesis. Mitosis is a type of cell division, with both daughter cells having the same number of chromosomes as the parent cell. In contrast, meiosis results in two daughter cells with half the number of chromosomes as the parent cell. Cytokinesis describes the division of cellular cytoplasm into two daughter cells.

3. **A** (S&F ch1)
The Wnt pathway plays a key role in intestinal cell proliferation. Activating this pathway results in the translocation of β-catenin into the nucleus where it regulates the expression of target genes. The majority of colorectal cancers have impaired Wnt signaling. The other pathways (mTOR, Her2/Neu, NOTCH, toll-like receptor) do not play an important role in intestinal cell proliferation.

4. **B** (S&F ch1)
CpG island hypermethylation results in silencing of the *MLH1* gene, leading to sporadic, microsatellite unstable colon cancer. Germline mutation in *MLH1* results in hereditary nonpolyposis colon cancer (Lynch syndrome). Mutations in APC, K-ras, and TP53 are key steps in the development of colon cancer through the chromosomal instability pathway, but they do not lead to microsatellite instability.

5. **D** (S&F ch1)
Cowden syndrome is associated with a mutation in *PTEN* gene. The other syndromes are associated with other mutations as follows: juvenile polyposis: *SMAD4* and *BMPR1A*; hereditary diffuse gastric cancer: *CDH1*; Peutz-Jeghers syndrome: *LKB1/STK11*; MEN 1: menin.

6. **D** (S&F ch1)
VHL plays an important role in renal cell cancer, but is rarely mutated in GI malignancies. The other genes (*TP53, APC, SMAD4,* and *MLH1*) are the main genes involved in colon cancer carcinogenesis.

7. **A** (S&F ch1)
Germline mutations in *CDH1* are associated with hereditary diffuse gastric cancer. The protein product of this gene is E-cadherin, which plays an important role in cell adhesion. Loss of E-cadherin allows epithelial tumor cells to invade the basement membrane and metastasize to distant sites. VEGF-A, bFGF, TGF-β, and VEGFR-3 are protein growth factors/receptors involved in tumor angiogenesis and lymphangiogenesis.

8. **B** (S&F ch1)
A nonsense mutation is a point mutation in a sequence of DNA that results in a premature stop codon. A missense mutation is a point mutation in which a single nucleotide change results in a change in amino acid encoded by the codon. A silent mutation is a point mutation that results in the production of the same amino acid (or a different amino acid with very similar properties). Insertion and deletion mutations refer to the addition or removal of a nucleotide.

9. **E** (S&F ch1)
This patient has Lynch syndrome. *MSH2* is one of the DNA mismatch repair genes associated with this hereditary colon cancer syndrome. *CDH1* is associated with hereditary diffuse gastric cancer. *MUTYH* is associated with MUTYH polyposis. *PTEN* is associated with Cowden's disease. *SMAD4* is associated with juvenile polyposis.

10. **E** (S&F ch1)
The cell cycle consists of different phases (see figure). In the M phase (mitosis), the cell divides into two daughter cells. G0 is the quiescent phase. The G1 phase is the initial growth phase. Duplication of the genome occurs in the S phase. The G2 phase is the second growth phase in preparation for cell division.

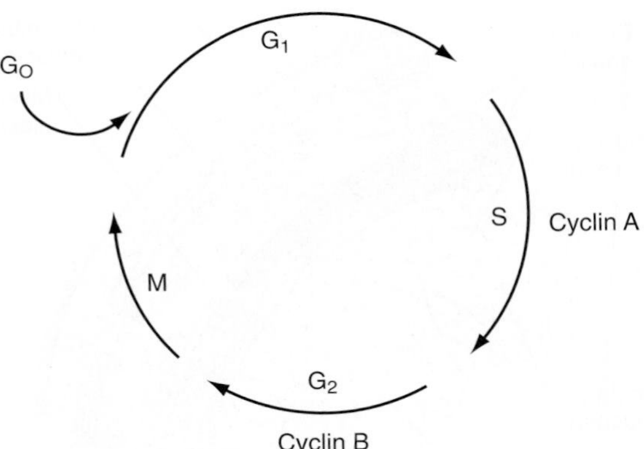

Figure for answer 10.

11. **C** (S&F ch1)
The patient's presentation is consistent with familial adenomatous polyposis (FAP) caused by a germline mutation in the adenomatous polyposis coli *(APC)* gene, which is a tumor suppressor gene. It is the gatekeeper in the multistep progression from a normal epithelium to colon cancer. This gene is associated with FAP and Gardner syndrome. The other types of genes are not associated with FAP.

12. **A** (S&F ch2)
IgA is the most abundant antibody present in mucosal secretions. IgG is the most common isotype in the systemic immune system. IgM is also present in mucosal secretions, but is less common than IgA. IgG, IgD, and IgE are not present in mucosal secretions.

13. **C** (S&F ch2)
The J (joining) chain is a protein produced by plasma cells that links two IgA molecules, forming the secretory IgA dimer. The secretory component (also called polymeric Ig receptor) is a glycoprotein that binds to dimeric IgA and protects it from degradation by luminal proteases. The Fc and Fab portions are parts of the immunoglobulin structure and do not play a role in the formation of the IgA dimer (see figure).

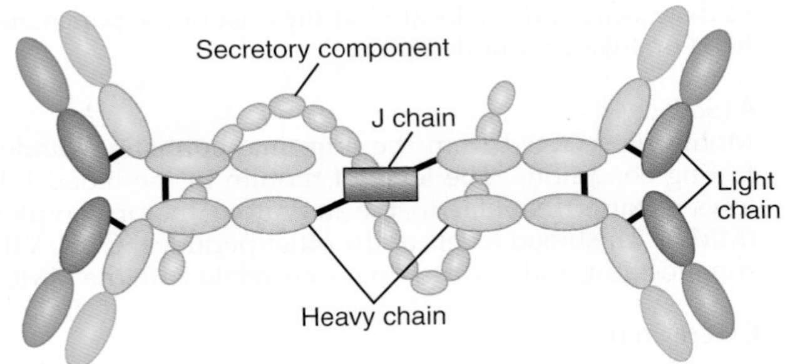

Figure for answer 13.

14. **C** (S&F ch2)
M cells specialize in phagocytosis and endocytosis of luminal antigens. These antigens are transported to the subepithelial spaces where they are presented to lymphocytes and other immune cells, initiating an immune response. They do not secrete antibacterial proteins, digestive enzymes, or hormones. They do not contain microvilli and do not absorb luminal nutrients.

15. **D** (S&F ch2)
M (microfold) cells have few lysosomes, resulting in little or no processing of the antigens following their endocytosis. M cells to do not have microvilli. Instead, their surface has broad "microfolds," hence the name. They have a thin mucin overlayer. Their cytoplasm is thin and forms a pocket that surrounds subepithelial immune cells. M cells do not secrete digestive enzymes.

16. **B** (S&F ch2)
Polymeric Ig receptor (secretory component) is a specialized glycoprotein expressed by the basolateral membrane of intestinal epithelial cells. This glycoprotein binds dimeric IgA or pentameric IgM and is secreted into the lumen. In the lumen, it protects IgA and IgM from luminal proteases and gastric acid. The J (joining) chain links two IgA molecules to form dimers. The light and heavy chains are components of the immunoglobulin structure. CD23 is a low-affinity IgE Fc receptor.

17. **A** (S&F ch2)
NOD is a cytosolic receptor for pathogen associated molecular patterns (PAMP). Another important PAMP receptor is the Toll-like receptor (TLR); however, this is present on the surface of antigen presenting cells. PAMPs are bacterial and viral components recognized by mucosal antigen presenting cells. Their detection leads to cytokine secretion and initiation of an inflammatory reaction to control the infection. PAMPs include a long list of bacterial, viral, and fungal components. Examples include flagellin (flagellated bacteria), lipoteichoic acid (bacterial component), single-stranded RNA (viral component), and mannan (fungal component). MHC is a surface receptor on antigen presenting cells. CX3CR1 is a surface chemokine receptor. Polymeric Ig receptor (also called secretory component) is expressed on the surface of intestinal epithelial cells and binds dimeric IgA or IgM.

18. **A** (S&F ch2)
The lamina propria is a thin layer of connective tissue beneath the epithelium. The majority of lymphocytes in the colon are present within the laminal propria and play an important role in mucosal immunity. The muscularis mucosa and muscularis propria are muscle layers. The submucosa and serosa have minimal inflammatory infiltrate.

19. **B** (S&F ch2)
Results from studies conducted on germ-free animals provide several interesting insights about the role of fecal microbiota. Germ-free animals have higher dietary caloric requirements compared to colonized animals. They also have higher nitrogen intake, a less mature immune system, and reduced gastrointestinal motility. Germ-free animals succumb to infection at a lower pathogen dose compared to colonized animals, probably due to the lack of protective effect of the microbiota.

20. **C** (S&F ch3)
A pathobiont is an organism that has the potential to cause disease under certain circumstances. *Clostridium difficile*

resides in the intestine and causes disease when the microbiota is perturbed. The other bacteria (Enterohemorrhagic *E. coli*, *Shigella*, *Yersinia*, and *Campylobacter*) are considered pathogens, not pathobionts.

21. **B** (S&F ch3)
A prebiotic is an indigestible food that selectively induces the growth of beneficial bacteria. It does not contain live microorganisms. A probiotic contains live microorganisms that, when administered in adequate amount, confers a health benefit on the host. A pharmabiotic is a term given to any biologic product that is obtained from the human microbiota and has biologic activity. It may include bacterial cells (live or dead) or their products (enzymes, metabolites, lipids). A synbiotic is a mixture of prebiotics and probiotics, in which these products have a synergistic health benefit.

22. **A** (S&F ch3)
Firmicutes and *Bacteroidetes* contribute to more than 90% of the species in the distal bowel. The other bacterial phyla (*Proteobacteria*, *Acintobacteria*, and *Spirochaetes*) contribute to less than 10% of the microbiota.

23. **D** (S&F ch3)
The intestinal microbiota is less resilient in infancy compared to adulthood. For example, antibiotics are more likely to permanently change the composition of the microbiota in infants compared to adults. The composition of the intestinal microbiota is variable among individuals. This variation arises primarily at species and strain levels. Rapid colonization of the intestine occurs after birth, and the composition of the microbiota is influenced by mode of delivery (vaginal vs. cesarean). The aerobe/anaerobe ratio is greater at the mucosal surface than within the lumen. While the microbiota reaches relative stability in adulthood, there are constant changes depending on environmental factors and the general well being of the individual.

24. **E** (S&F ch3)
The term "operational taxonomic unit" is used to group microbes according to their 16S rRNA sequence homology. Taxonomy is a general term that refers to the classification of organisms. HITChip (human intestinal tract chip) is a technique used to rapidly identify the microbial populations within the intestinal tract. Phylum and genus are taxonomic terms used to classify organisms.

25. **A** (S&F ch3)
Quorum sensing is a form of communication between related bacteria that senses the bacterial density and diversity in the local environment, leading to regulation of a variety of physiologic activities.

26. **C** (S&F ch4)
Somatostatin is secreted from the antral D cells in response to low intragastric pH. It exerts a paracrine effect on adjacent acid-producing parietal cells to inhibit gastric acid secretion. Endocrine signaling occurs when the transmitters are released into the circulation to exert their hormonal effect. The term "autocrine" signaling is used when the transmitter exerts its effect on the same cell that secreted the transmitter. Synaptic transmission refers to the release of transmitter molecules through nerve-to-nerve synapses. Gap junction signaling allows for small intracellular mediators (e.g., calcium) to diffuse between cells connected by gap junction. Somatostatin does not pass through gap junctions to exert its inhibitory effect.

27. **D** (S&F ch4)
The myenteric (Auerbach) plexus is located between the circular and the longitudinal muscle layers of the GI tract. The submucosal (Meissner) plexus is located in the submucosa (see figure).

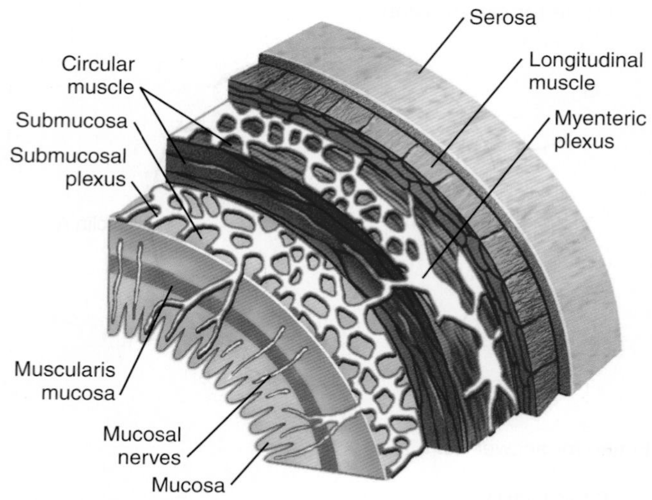

Figure for answer 27.

28. **E** (S&F ch4)
Secretin is secreted in the duodenum in response to acid. It stimulates pancreatic fluid and bicarbonate secretion. VIP is a neuromodulator that leads to vasodilation, smooth muscle relaxation, and increased epithelial secretion. Pancreatic polypeptide (PP) inhibits pancreatic enzyme secretion. CCK stimulates pancreatic enzyme secretion, gallbladder contraction, and sphincter of Oddi relaxation. Somatostatin inhibits gastric acid secretion.

29. **B** (S&F ch4)
This patient is presenting with severe watery diarrhea, which is typical of Verner-Morrison syndrome caused by hypersecretion of VIP from a pancreatic neuroendocrine tumor. Other features are hypokalemia and achlorhydria. The tumor is usually large (>5 cm) at presentation. Overproduction of pancreatic polypeptide or peptide YY does not result in diarrhea. Overproduction of somatostatin results in steatorrhea and cholelithiasis, usually from a duodenal tumor. Overproduction of gastrin can result in diarrhea; however, this is usually mild to moderate in severity. Gastrinomas are usually small (<5 cm) at the time of diagnosis, and are located in the area of the pancreatic head or adjacent duodenum.

30. **A** (S&F ch4)
Motilin is secreted from the intestinal epithelium under fasting conditions. The level of motilin in the blood follows a pattern similar to the migratory motor complex (MMC). The blood levels of the other peptides (CCK, VIP, somatostatin, and gastrin) do not correlate with the MMC.

31. **E** (S&F ch4)
Secretin is secreted from specialized "S" cells in the duodenum in response to acid in the duodenal lumen. It stimulates pancreatic secretion of fluid and bicarbonate. It inhibits gastric acid secretion and does not stimulate gallbladder contraction. CCK stimulates pancreatic enzyme secretion.

32. **B** (S&F ch4)
Leptin is primarily secreted from adipocytes. Its main role is to decrease food intake. Only small amounts of leptin are secreted from the stomach. The other tissues (brain, duodenum, distal ileum) do not secrete leptin.

33. **C** (S&F ch4)
The patient has classic symptoms of Ménétrier's disease. The gastric mucosa demonstrates irregular hypertrophic folds. The main histologic finding is foveolar hyperplasia and dilated cystic glands. Increased production of transforming growth factor alpha, which binds epidermal growth factor receptor, leads to mucosal gland hyperplasia. Enhanced signaling through the c-Kit receptor and the platelet-derived growth factor receptor is responsible for most cases of gastrointestinal stromal tumors.

34. **B** (S&F ch4)
Amylin is a peptide synthesized by the beta cells of the pancreas. It suppresses glucagon secretion, delays gastric emptying, and induces satiety. Leptin induces satiety but does not delay gastric emptying or inhibit glucagon secretion. Motilin stimulates insulin release, but it simulates gastric emptying. Ghrelin is also called the "hunger hormone," and it increases food intake. Serotonin is important in gut motility but plays no role in satiety or glucagon secretion.

35. **E** (S&F ch4)
This boy has features of Prader-Willi syndrome. High serum levels of ghrelin are seen in patients with Prader-Willi syndrome, suggesting that it is responsible for hyperphagia in these patients. Ghrelin is also called the "hunger hormone," and it increases food intake. All the other hormones listed (leptin, peptide YY, amylin, and GLP-1) suppress food intake.

36. **A** (S&F ch4)
GI hormones regulate postprandial glucose levels via insulin secretion, inhibition of hepatic gluconeogenesis, and delaying gastric emptying. GLP-1 stimulates insulin release to regulate postprandial blood glucose levels. The other important hormone that stimulates postprandial insulin release is glucose-dependent insulinotropic polypeptide (GIP). Amylin, cholecystokinin, and secretin delay gastric emptying.

37. **D** (S&F ch4)
Erythromycin is a motilin receptor agonist. Motilin stimulates smooth muscle propulsive activity and may cause side effects of cramping and diarrhea. Cholecystokinin, secretin, and peptide YY delay gastric emptying.

38. **B** (S&F ch4)
High fat-content meals stimulate cholecystokinin release and lead to gallbladder contraction. The patient has multiple risk factors for cholelithiasis, which may lead to biliary pain. Gastrin causes gastric acid secretion and elevated levels may lead to peptic ulcer disease. Secretin induces pancreatic and bicarbonate fluid secretion from the pancreas. Peptide YY inhibits vagally induced gastric acid secretion and other motor and secretory functions. Vasoactive intestinal polypeptide is a vasodilator and stimulates epithelial cell secretion.

CHAPTER

2

Nutrition in Gastroenterology

Nikrad Shahnavaz and Jason M. Brown

QUESTIONS

1. You are evaluating a 58-year-old man who was admitted in the hospital 7 days ago with severe alcoholic hepatitis. He was drinking on average 12 beers daily in the last 6 months before admission. Currently, he is afebrile and normotensive. Significant jaundice and moderate ascites are noted in the physical exam. He is lethargic and moderately confused. He has been started on prednisolone 40 mg daily since admission. You correctly emphasize the effect of optimized nutrition in the patient's outcome. Which of the following measures would have the best value in the assessment of his nutritional status?
   A. Body mass index
   B. Midarm muscle circumference
   C. Fist-grip dynamometry
   D. Creatinine-height index
   E. Serum transferrin level

2. Chronic use of which of these medications can potentially contribute to B_{12} deficiency?
   A. Cholestyramine
   B. Sulfasalazine
   C. Omeprazole
   D. Penicillamine
   E. Isoniazid

3. A 29-year-old woman with fistulizing Crohn's disease who had multiple resections of small bowel in the past has been on total parenteral nutrition (TPN) for the last 2 months. She continues to have watery diarrhea and some discharge from an enterocutaneous fistula despite not taking anything by mouth. She presented to your clinic and complains of impaired taste, hair loss, skin rash, and difficult vision at night in the last 2 weeks. In the physical exam you note several erythematous and vesicular lesions on her elbows and hands. Basic blood tests are as follows:

WBC	9000/μL
Hemoglobin	11g/dL
MCV	88 fL
Electrolytes normal	
Albumin	3.2 g/dL

What would be your next step in the management of her recent manifestations?
   A. Check plasma zinc level
   B. Empiric zinc supplementation
   C. Check blood niacin level
   D. Empiric niacin supplementation
   E. Empiric copper supplementation

4. A 61-year-old homeless man with history of chronic heavy alcohol use presented to your clinic with complaint of chronic loose, greasy foul smelling stool in the last 9 months. He has not had any doctor's visit in the last 20 years. He also mentions fatigue and moderate dyspnea with minimal exertion in the last 2 weeks. On the physical exam, he is afebrile and normotensive but the exam is positive for mild pallor and 2/6 systolic murmur at the left sternal border. Neurological exam shows hyporeflexia and loss of proprioceptive sensation in the extremities. Basic blood studies include:

Hemoglobin	9 g/dL
MCV	84 fL
WBC	6000/μL
Platelet count	140,000/μL
Glucose	190 mg/dL (fasting)
Creatinine	0.7 mg/dL
AST	104 U/L
ALT	55 U/L
Total bilirubin	4 mg/dL
Direct bilirubin	0.7 mg/dL
LDH	600 IU/L
Haptoglobin	10 mg/dL
Iron panel is normal	

Which of the following tests would be more likely to detect the vitamin deficiency in this patient?
   A. Serum α-tocopherol level
   B. Serum cobalamin level
   C. Plasma retinol level
   D. Serum riboflavin level
   E. Plasma pyridoxine level

5. A 41-year-old woman with short-gut syndrome secondary to extensive small bowel resection after trauma has been on total parenteral nutrition for the last 6 months without any complication. Several attempts to initiate enteral feeding have been unsuccessful. Her only other medical history includes diabetes, which had been appropriately controlled with a stable dosage of insulin until 4 weeks ago. Since then, despite a stable total parenteral nutrition regimen, her insulin requirement has increased significantly, and she had episodes of hyperglycemia with blood glucose levels up to 250 mg/dL almost every day. Her recent blood study was also significant for elevated free fatty acid concentrations. Which of the following trace minerals deficiency can explain these new metabolic disorders in this patient?
   A. Selenium
   B. Copper
   C. Chromium
   D. Molybdenum
   E. Manganese

6. A 78-year-old woman with Alzheimer's disease presents to your clinic for the management of acid reflux. On further questioning, she complains of nausea, mild headache,

bone and muscle pain, and hair loss. When you ask about her medications, she mentions that she does not take any medicine except multiple vitamins every day. Physical exam is remarkable for ataxia, alopecia, and erythematous patches on her earlobes and neck. The blood tests from yesterday showed the following:

Creatinine	0.9 mg/dL
AST	82 U/L
ALT	73 U/L
ALP	103 U/L
Total bilirubin	1.3 mg/dL
Direct bilirubin	0.7 mg/dL
Total cholesterol	244 mg/dL
LDL	170 mg/dL
Triglyceride	265 mg/dL

Chronic toxicity with which of these vitamins is the most likely cause of her presentation?

A. Vitamin A
B. Vitamin B_6 (pyridoxine)
C. Vitamin C
D. Vitamin D
E. Vitamin E

7. A 29-year-old previously healthy woman was admitted in the critical care unit 48 hours ago with septic shock after appendiceal perforation and severe peritonitis. She underwent emergent laparotomy with peritoneal irrigation on the day of admission. However, she is still intubated, febrile, and hemodynamically unstable, requiring high doses of vasopressor agents in addition to broad-spectrum antibiotics. You are consulted by the ICU team regarding the best strategy for nutritional support in this patient. What would be the most appropriate recommendation?

A. Insert a post-pyloric feeding tube and initiate small bowel feeding as soon as possible with provision of 120% of energy requirements
B. Initiate parenteral nutrition with provision of 80% of energy requirement as soon as possible
C. Initiate parenteral nutrition with provision of 120% of energy requirement as soon as possible
D. Initiate parenteral nutrition with provision of 80% of energy requirement on day 8 of hospitalization
E. Initiate parenteral nutrition with provision of 120% of energy requirement on day 8 of hospitalization

8. Which of the following statements is correct regarding diet and Crohn's disease?

A. Vitamin D deficiency is seen in about 10% of patients
B. Vitamin D may upregulate tumor necrosis factor (TNF)-α–related genes
C. In children with Crohn's disease, enteric nutrition has been shown to be just as effective as glucocorticoids in inducing clinical remission during flare-up
D. Bowel rest has been proved necessary to achieve remission in hospitalized patients with active Crohn's disease
E. Studies have confirmed the benefit of routine total parenteral nutrition in patients with Crohn's disease who undergo surgery

9. You successfully placed a nasojejunal (NJ) tube during endoscopy for a patient with gastroparesis and confirmed the proper position of the tube with a plain film. Before discharging the patient, you discuss with him and his family the proper use of the tube. Which of the following instructions is correct?

A. Check the tube for residual content at least once a day
B. Flush the tube at the end of each day
C. Crush the tablets to use via the tube
D. Avoid mixing tube feeding with potassium chloride
E. The NJ tube needs to be exchanged every 3 months with a new tube

10. A 67-year-old man is seen in clinic 6 weeks after successful placement of a gastrostomy feeding tube for stroke-related dysphagia. He has been on stable rate and formula of tube feed with caloric density of 1.5 kcal/mL since the beginning. However, in the last 2 weeks, he has been experiencing symptoms of abdominal pain, bloating, nausea and diarrhea in addition to flushing and sweating about 30 minutes after receiving of his tube feedings by bolus. On physical exam, he is afebrile and normotensive. Abdomen is soft, nontender, nondistended, and bowel sounds are present (see figure of the gastrostomy tube). Which of the following complications is the most likely cause of his recent symptoms?

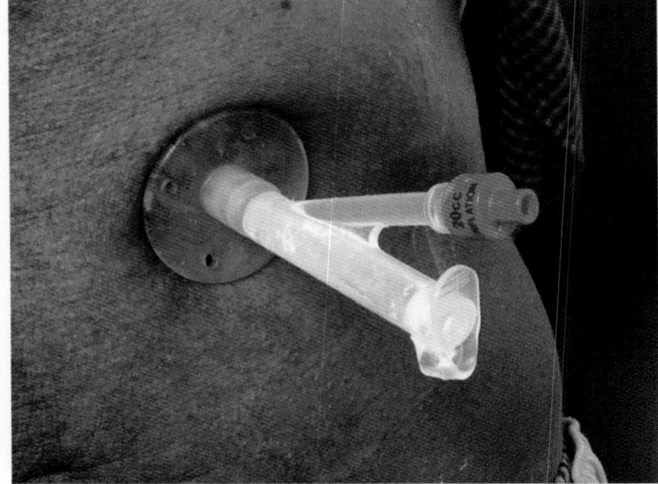

Figure for question 10.

A. Gastric outlet obstruction
B. Migrated gastrostomy tube
C. Buried bumper syndrome
D. Obstructed gastrostomy tube
E. Colocutaneous fistula

11. Which of the following measures has been shown to reduce the risk of aspiration during enteral feeding in intubated ICU patients?

A. Head of bed elevation to 15 degrees
B. Bolus feeding instead of continuous infusion
C. Monitoring gastric residual volume and withholding of enteral feeding if it is 300 mL or more
D. Start tube feeding at least 24 hours after gastrostomy tube placement
E. Narcotic antagonists

12. A 50-year-old man with hepatitis C–related cirrhosis is seen in your clinic for routine follow-up. His only complaint is mild alteration in his sense of taste, which has been bothering him in the last 3 months. Despite that, his appetite is good and he tries to keep a balanced diet. He does not have history of heavy alcohol use in his life. Hepatitis C infection was successfully treated with triple therapy last year. Within the last 12 months, he had 2 episodes of mild hepatic encephalopathy, but he denies any sign of gastrointestinal (GI) bleeding. His ascites is well controlled with furosemide 40 mg and spironolactone 100 mg daily by mouth. On physical exam, he is alert and oriented. Mild icterus is noted. Abdominal exam shows minimal ascites without any tenderness. No asterixis is noted. His model of end stage liver disease score has been stable at 8. Which of the following nutritional statements is correct in this patient?

A. Reducing daily protein intake by 25% decreases the chance of hepatic encephalopathy
B. There is no role for thiamine supplementation for this patient
C. He should use branched-chain amino acids as the only source of protein
D. Hypermagnesemia may be the cause of the change in his taste
E. Vitamin A deficiency may increase the chance of hepatocellular carcinoma in this patient

13. A 47-year-old man with history of Crohn's disease has had multiple resections of the small bowel, including the last surgery around 6 months ago, which resected most of the terminal ileum secondary to stricture. Currently, he has about 90 cm of intact small intestine remaining, and his colon is present without any disease involvement. In the last month, you have attempted to wean parenteral nutrition for him and introduce oral feeding, but severe diarrhea has been the main limiting factor to reach this goal. Which of the following therapeutic measures could potentially cause worsening of the diarrhea in this patient?

A. Bile-binding resins
B. Fat restriction
C. Atropine
D. Pantoprazole
E. Teduglutide

14. A 53-year-old woman presents to your clinic for consultation regarding weight loss. She has tried lifestyle modification, including appropriate diet and exercise in the last year with minimal effect in her weight. She has been suffering from anxiety, which is under control with paroxetine. She has history of narcotic abuse about 4 years ago and had to go to rehabilitation. Currently, she denies any drug abuse. On the physical exam, her body mass index (BMI) today is 29 kg/m^2. Blood pressure is 130/80 mm Hg and heart rate is 80 bpm. Abdominal exam shows central obesity. Recent blood tests showed ALT 20 U/L, AST 19 U/L, alkaline phosphatase 82 U/L, total bilirubin 1.1 mg/dL, creatinine 1.1 mg/dL, thyroid-stimulating hormone 1.5 mIU/L, fasting glucose 100 mg/dL, low-density lipoprotein (LDL) 190 mg/dL, HDL 338 mg/dL, and triglycerides 220 mg/dL. You have a long discussion with her and the final decision is to consider pharmacotherapy for 1 year in addition to continuing lifestyle modifications. Which of the following drugs would you recommend for her?

A. Orlistat
B. Lorcaserin
C. Phentermine-topiramate ER
D. Phendimetrazine
E. Diethylpropion

15. Which of the following cancers has been shown to be significantly more common in obese compared to nonobese women?

A. Lung cancer
B. Rectal cancer
C. Colon cancer
D. Gallbladder cancer
E. Glioblastoma multiform

16. Which of the following statements is correct regarding the new antidiabetic drug pramlintide?

A. It is a U.S. Food and Drug Administration (FDA)-approved drug for obesity treatment
B. It is a glucagon-like peptide-1 agonist
C. It has more weight loss effect on African Americans compared to Caucasians
D. It is usually not tolerated for a long-term use secondary to severe gastroparesis
E. The FDA has issued a notice about potential risks of pancreatitis

17. A 45-year-old woman comes to you in the outpatient gastroenterology clinic for "weight problems." She has struggled with "being on the heavier side" since childhood, and review of her primary care physician records reveals a body mass index consistently between 36 kg/m^2 and 39 kg/m^2 for the past decade, despite multiple self-driven attempts at weight loss through diet and exercise. She currently has no other comorbid conditions and takes no medications, prescribed or otherwise. Her blood pressure in the office today is 115/72 mm Hg. She has read about bariatric surgery, and after watching some online videos and reading multiple blogs about it, she has decided she is ready to try it. What is the most appropriate next step in management?

A. Schedule the patient for an endoscopic transoral outlet reduction procedure
B. Refer to a bariatric surgeon
C. Recommend pharmacologic management of obesity
D. Continue self-driven attempts at diet and exercise
E. Continue attempts at diet and exercise with the support of a nutritionist

18. A 39-year-old woman with insulin-controlled diabetes and body mass index of 42 kg/m^2 is referred to you for evaluation of candidacy for bariatric surgery. The patient has worked with her primary care physician repeatedly to lose weight, cycling through multiple exercise and diet programs. She has even been under the care of a psychiatrist, who directs her in cognitive-behavioral therapy for weight loss. In reviewing the psychiatrist's notes, you discover that the patient is also being treated for major depression, having just been discharged a month ago for a short stay at an inpatient psychiatric unit. This was not on her primary care physician's problem list at time of referral. When you ask the patient about this, she becomes tearful and says, "There are so many things in my life that are off track, maybe I could jumpstart things with this surgery." What is the most appropriate next step in management?

A. Schedule the patient for an endoscopic transoral outlet reduction procedure
B. Refer to a bariatric surgeon for a laparoscopic gastric band surgery
C. Refer to a bariatric surgeon for a laparoscopic Roux-en-Y surgery
D. Decline to refer the patient, informing her that she will never be a candidate for the surgery
E. Decline to refer the patient, informing her that she could potentially be a candidate for the surgery in the future, if her depressive episode resolves and she remains in the care of a psychiatrist who endorses her candidacy

19. A 56-year-old man with a body mass index of 42 kg/m^2 and a past medical history of coronary artery disease with prior drug-eluting stent placement in the left main coronary (taking aspirin 325 g daily and clopidogrel 75 mg daily), hypertension, and insulin-controlled diabetes is referred to you for evaluation of candidacy for bariatric surgery. He had an episode of major depression that lasted 3 years in his early 40s, though he has had no symptoms of depression since. On review of systems, he has no GI complaints. His wife helpfully offers that he routinely snores in his sleep and seems excessively tired during the day, even during periods of vacation from work. What is the next best step in management?

A. Immediate referral to a bariatric surgeon
B. Psychiatric and anesthesia evaluation prior to referral
C. Psychiatric evaluation, anesthesia evaluation, and cardiology evaluation prior to referral
D. Psychiatric evaluation, anesthesia evaluation, cardiology evaluation, and polysomnography prior to referral
E. Psychiatric evaluation, anesthesia evaluation, cardiology evaluation, polysomnography, and esophagogastroduodenoscopy prior to referral

20. A 35-year-old woman undergoes a laparoscopic Roux-en-Y gastric bypass. On day 2 after surgery, the patient develops 10 out of 10 abdominal pain and begins to display hematochezia. On examination, her abdomen is rigid and exquisitely tender. Which of the following is the most likely diagnosis?

A. Anastomotic leak
B. Anastomotic ulcer
C. Bowel ischemia
D. Diverticular bleed with intestinal wall rupture
E. Bowel obstruction

21. A 32-year-old woman underwent laparoscopic Roux-en-Y gastric bypass 8 weeks ago. She calls you, the on-call gastroenterologist, from home complaining of intractable nausea and vomiting with abdominal pain. She notes initially having trouble digesting solids 2 weeks ago, but this has progressed such that she cannot keep any solid or liquid down and has not been able to do so for 48 hours. Her husband and child are sick with nausea, vomiting, abdominal cramping, and diarrhea. What is the next best step in management?

A. Call in a trial of metoclopromide to the pharmacy
B. Oral rehydration as tolerated and antiemetics
C. Reassurance of the patient and asking her to call back if symptoms worsen
D. Referral to the nearest emergency department for admission, intravenous fluids, observation, and endoscopic or surgical management
E. Call in a short course of ciprofloxacin and metronidazole to the pharmacy

22. A 33-year-old woman with a preoperative body mass index of 42 kg/m^2 underwent laparoscopic Roux-en-Y gastric bypass. Her medicine reconciliation form is being completed prior to discharge, and her hospitalist calls you to review it. What is the best regimen to recommend?

A. Vitamin supplementation
B. Vitamin supplementation, cessation of nonsteroidal antiinflammatory drugs (NSAIDs)
C. Vitamin supplementation, cessation of NSAIDs, proton pump inhibitor (PPI)
D. Vitamin supplementation, cessation of NSAIDs, PPI, 6 months of cholestyramine
E. Vitamin supplementation, cessation of NSAIDs, PPI, 6 months of ursodiol

23. A 34-year-old woman with a body mass index of 42 kg/m^2 visits your outpatient clinic for advice on which bariatric surgery to pursue. She wants to know which type of weight loss operation will most minimize postoperative complications and maximize weight loss. Of all the techniques currently practiced, the techniques she is most interested in are Roux-en-Y gastric bypass (RYGB) and laparoscopic adjustable gastric banding (LAGB). Which of the following statements best characterizes the risk-benefit profile of these two techniques?

A. RYBG patients have less mortality but less weight loss than LAGB
B. LAGB patients have a higher complication rate but more weight loss than RYBG
C. LAGB patients suffer more postoperative GI bleeding than RYGB
D. RYBG patients lose more weight but have a higher overall mortality and complication rate
E. RYGB patients have a higher postoperative leak rate but less overall mortality

24. A 46-year-old man with a history of irritable bowel syndrome with diarrhea predominance underwent Roux-en-Y gastric bypass 3 weeks ago and is in your office for follow-up. Although he felt well in the hospital, he has been feeling poorly since transitioning home. Approximately 20 minutes after eating, he notes a severe, cramping abdominal pain. He feels bloated for a short time and shortly thereafter has voluminous diarrhea. Lately, he has noted symptoms of dizziness, nausea, and flushing surrounding the events. Which of the following diagnoses do you suspect?

A. Peptic ulcer
B. Biliary colic
C. Irritable bowel syndrome
D. Early dumping syndrome
E. Late dumping syndrome

25. A 28-year-old man with a history of irritable bowel syndrome and a body mass index of 43 kg/m^2 undergoes laparoscopic Roux-en-Y gastric bypass. His postoperative course was uncomplicated. He comes to see you in clinic for a postoperative check 4 weeks after discharge. Lately, he's been noticing that approximately 2 hours after a meal, he feels dizzy, sweaty, weak, and fatigued. The symptoms gradually resolve on their own. These episodes are affecting his job performance, and his wife has noticed an impact in his engagement at home. What is the next best step in management?

A. Order an abdominal magnetic resonance angiography
B. Prescribe a tricyclic antidepressant
C. Refer to a pain specialist for nonnarcotic therapy
D. Attempt dietary modifications
E. Refer to the surgery clinic

26. A 62-year-old man presents to your office 3 months after Roux-en-Y gastric bypass. He is brought in by his wife, who has to help him transfer from the car and the waiting room because he is having trouble walking. He appears sluggish and does not participate in the conversation. She relates that ever since discharge from his surgery he has been vomiting nearly every day, and over the past couple of weeks he has become more sluggish, more forgetful, and has begun to act bizarrely (e.g., putting his shoes in the freezer). He has not been taking any of his prescribed medications. On physical exam, you note nystagmus. In addition to intravenous (IV) fluids, which of the following is the most appropriate management?

A. Urgent computed tomography scan of head
B. Upper endoscopy
C. IV chromium
D. IV thiamine
E. IV selenium

27. A 52-year-old man presents 3 years after Roux-en-Y gastric bypass surgery to your office for a continuity visit. His body mass index has gone from 41 kg/m^2 to 28 kg/m^2, and he reports feeling quite well. He is compliant with all medications, including a multivitamin. He incidentally jokes that "this whole surgery has aged me," noting a rapid progression of graying hair on his scalp and mild memory problems as well as "losing half a step on the tennis court." Otherwise, review of systems is negative. The only serologic abnormality noted is a hemoglobin level of 11 g/dL. What is the most likely diagnosis?
A. Vitamin D deficiency
B. Dementia
C. B_{12} deficiency
D. Iron deficiency anemia
E. Vitamin A deficiency

28. A 32-year-old woman with a body mass index of 40 kg/m^2 and no other past medical or surgical history comes to you for advice about whether to pursue gastric bypass for weight loss. In discussing the risks and benefits, you attempt to counsel the patient on how much weight loss to expect. Which of the follow most accurately reflects how much weight the patient could be expected to lose?
A. 10% of total weight
B. 30% of excess weight
C. 60% of total weight
D. 60% of excess weight
E. 100% of excess weight

29. A 29-year-old man presents to the emergency department 3 weeks after Roux-en-Y bypass surgery with hematemesis. He is stabilized and admitted to the ICU, where you undertake an esophagogastroduodenoscopy and find an anastomotic ulcer. In addition to executing an endoscopic intervention to stop the bleeding, what discharge medications would be best to recommend for treatment of his ulcer?
A. Oral proton pump inhibitor (PPI) capsules ingested twice daily
B. Oral PPI capsules broken open and ingested twice daily
C. Oral PPI capsules ingested twice daily and 1 g sucralfate solution 4 times daily
D. Oral PPI capsules broken open and ingested twice daily and 1 g sucralfate tablets 4 times daily
E. Oral PPI capsules broken open and ingested twice daily, 1 g sucralfate solution 4 times daily

30. A 55-year-old woman underwent Roux-en-Y gastric bypass approximately a year ago. She has had intermittent, epigastric abdominal pain that has gradually become more frequent and more intense over the past few months. You decide to perform an esophagogastroduodenoscopy, and during your exam you find a surgical suture with a small (5 mm), white-based ulcer approximating it. What is the next best step in management?
A. Proton pump inhibitor therapy
B. Surgical revision
C. Low dose imipramine
D. *Helicobacter pylori* triple therapy
E. Endoscopic removal of the suture

31. Jeff, a 32-year-old male cardiologist, is brought to you by Mike, his brother, for evaluation. Jeff was a male model in his late teens and early 20s, and Mike describes Jeff as "always in shape, almost obsessive about how he looks and how much he weighs." Lately, Mike has noticed that his brother's weight loss appears excessive. Although Jeff will typically "diet" to restrict his caloric intake to 1200 kcal/day, he notes that he does so to "cut loose on the weekends," often dining out three times a day, eating excessive amounts at each meal. Mike brings pill bottles for furosemide, which Jeff has prescribed himself, even though he has no medical conditions that would require this therapy. In reviewing Jeff's diet, you find that Jeff drinks nearly 5 cups of coffee a day, less to stay alert and more "to help keep my appetite in check." Jeff's body mass index is 17 kg/m^2 today in your office. What diagnosis do you suspect?
A. Avoidant/restrictive food intake disorder
B. Anorexia nervosa
C. Bulemia nervosa
D. Binge eating disorder
E. Rumination disorder

32. A 19-year-old woman is admitted to the hospital with diarrhea of 3-week duration. She passes loose stools multiple times daily with occasional rectal bleeding. You note severe dehydration with orthostasis as well as a body mass index of 16.5 kg/m^2. On physical exam, the patient's parotid glands are enlarged. Laboratory values are as follows:

Hemoglobin	12 g/dL
WBC	10,000/μL
Total bilirubin	1.5 g/dL
Alkaline phosphatase	148 U/L
ALT	98 U/L
AST	105 U/L
Creatinine	0.5 mg/dL
BUN	10 mg/dL

Which diagnosis do you suspect?
A. Prolonged viral gastroenteritis
B. Microscopic colitis
C. Irritable bowel syndrome with diarrhea predominance
D. Anorexia nervosa
E. Ulcerative colitis

33. A 24-year-old female graduate student is brought to you by her parents for evaluation. They are concerned that she has "anorexia," and they request your opinion on further management. After obtaining a history with the parents present, you ask them to leave the room to obtain a history from the patient herself. In discussing her eating habits, she typically eats 1600 kcal/day; however, during periods of the spring and summer, she will limit herself to 1000 kcal/day for a few months. Since she enrolled in college at age 18, she would go to a different fast food chain and eat over 2500 kcal at a time at least twice a week. After doing so, she feels ashamed and employs an over-the-counter laxative to help prevent weight gain. You ask what she thinks of her weight, and she confesses she feels "chubby" and far too overweight for her personal goals. You note a body mass index of 21 kg/m^2. Which pharmacologic agent is best suited to treat this condition?
A. Fluoxetine 20 mg daily
B. Fluoxetine 60 mg daily
C. Olanzapine 2.5 mg daily
D. Olanzapine 10 mg daily
E. Topiramate 25 mg daily

34. A 28-year-old man was admitted to the hospital 7 days ago for "failure to thrive." He has a history of anorexia nervosa, and the nurse recorded a body mass index of

16.8 kg/m^2 on admission. A Dobhoff tube was placed, and the patient has been receiving enteral feeding at a rate of 2200 kcal/day. Over the past few days, the patient has been less alert and poorly oriented. He has rapidly developed peripheral edema. Which of the following lab values would have been most important to closely monitor for prevention of this condition?
A. Thiamine
B. Magnesium
C. Potassium
D. Sodium
E. Phosphorus

35. A 45-year-old woman with a body mass index of 32 kg/m^2 comes to your office for evaluation of obesity. She is very distressed about her weight, and she wants to discuss options for bariatric surgery. Upon taking a careful history, you note that she has tried caloric restriction diets numerous times over the past 10 years, but they have all been unsuccessful. When tracking food diaries over the past few months, you note meticulous counts of caloric intake revealing multiple days during the week in which she has ingested well over 2500 kcal/day. On these days, she feels out of control with respect to her food intake. The next day she would "punish" herself at the gym by working out for twice as long, even doing so if injured. She drinks caffeinated beverages to manage her appetite, and for a time, even tried smoking cigarettes. Which diagnosis do you suspect?
A. Binge eating disorder
B. Anorexia nervosa
C. Bulimia nervosa
D. Obesity, no eating disorder
E. Hypothyroidism

36. A 19-year-old male student is referred to your clinic from his university health center for multiple episodes of pruritus, mild swelling of the lips, and sensation of throat swelling after eating certain fruits. You take a detailed history and realize that in each of the episodes, his symptoms started within 2 minutes of ingesting fruits (in particular watermelon, honeydew, or cantaloupe) and then completely resolved within 30 minutes. He denies any other medical history except seasonal allergic rhinitis. Physical exam, including the exam of the oral cavity, is unremarkable. Which of the following statements is correct regarding his condition?
A. It is a mixed IgE- and non-IgE–mediated disorder
B. He may also become symptomatic after eating certain cooked fruits or vegetables
C. His hay fever is most likely associated with ragweed pollens
D. Fifty percent of affected individuals may have systemic reactions
E. Eosinophilia is found in up to 50% of the cases

37. A 6-week-old infant is being evaluated for presence of small amount of blood in his stool noted in the last 2 weeks. He is solely breast-fed. He appears healthy and has been gaining weight as expected. The exam of the perineal area is unremarkable. The routine blood tests are within normal limits. What is the best next step in the management of this infant?
A. Reassurance of the parents
B. Perform skin prick testing
C. Elimination of dairy products from mother's diet
D. Stop breast-feeding and start hypoallergenic formula
E. Sigmoidoscopy

38. An 11-month-old infant has been evaluated by pediatric gastroenterology service for vomiting, failure to thrive, and generalized edema. Serologic studies are notable for peripheral eosinophilia and hypoalbuminemia. Upper endoscopy with biopsy was performed, which showed prominent eosinophilic infiltration in the stomach and small bowel. Which of the following statements is correct regarding the underlying disorder in this infant?
A. Children usually outgrow the disease in less than 1 year
B. It is an IgE-mediated disorder
C. Glucocorticoid therapy is the first line of treatment
D. It may present with gastric outlet obstruction
E. It is strongly associated with HLA-DQ2

39. Which of the following childhood food allergies tend to be lifelong?
A. Tree nut
B. Soy
C. Egg
D. Wheat
E. Cow's milk

ANSWERS

1. B (S&F ch5)
Mid-arm muscle circumference (MAMC) is a measurement of skeletal muscle mass. It has a particular value in the assessment and management of nutritional status in patients with cirrhosis or severe alcoholic hepatitis. A low value of MAMC has been shown to be an independent poor prognostic factor in these patients. Body mass index can be misleading in the setting of ascites and volume overload. Fist-grip dynamometry uses maximal handgrip strength as a surrogate of total body protein. It has shown considerable promise for rapid and convenient assessment of protein-calorie status in both inpatients and outpatients, but its use is limited in patients with altered mental status or encephalopathy. Creatinine-height index measures the amount of creatinine excreted in the urine over a 24-hour period, corrected for the patient's height. Although it is an excellent tool for assessment of total skeletal muscle mass, glucocorticoid administration can alter this index independently of muscle mass. The serum levels of prealbumin, transferrin, or retinol-binding protein are used as indicators of nutritional status; however, all these proteins act as negative acute-phase reactants, and their synthesis by the liver drops in the acutely ill patient with severe alcoholic hepatitis.

2. C (S&F ch5)
Chronic proton pump inhibitors use can potentially impair B_{12} absorption by causing small intestinal bacterial overgrowth or decreased gastric acid/pepsin secretion. Cholestyramine can adsorb folate and vitamin D in the small bowel and decrease their absorption. Sulfasalazine inhibits folate-dependent enzymes and impairs its absorption. Penicillamine is known to increase renal excretion of zinc. Isoniazid can impair uptake of pyridoxine.

3. **B** (S&F ch5)
Zinc depletion is a particularly important issue to remember in patients with chronic diarrhea or fistula in inflammatory bowel disease. It can be seen in patients on total parenteral nutrition solutions lacking appropriate amount of zinc supplementation to compensate for ongoing GI loss. Dysgeusia (impaired taste), alopecia, glossitis, dermatitis on the extremities, and loss of dark adaptation are commonly seen in marked zinc deficiency. Plasma or other body fluid zinc levels are not accurate indicators of zinc status because it can shift from serum into the liver in acute illness. For this reason, it is usually recommended to proceed with zinc supplementation in patients with high risk of zinc deficiency based on the clinical scenario. Copper or niacin deficiency is not completely consistent with the clinical scenario mentioned in the question. Although copper deficiency can be seen in individuals on long-term total parenteral nutrition without copper, it usually manifests with skin or hair depigmentation, leukopenia, microcytic anemia, and neurologic abnormalities. Marked deficiency can be detected by low serum copper and ceruloplasmin level. Niacin deficiency (pellagra) is often seen in carcinoid syndrome or individuals in which corn is the major source of nutrition. Blood concentration is not reliable to detect deficiency. Measurement of urinary excretion of the niacin metabolites is the most reliable tests of assessment.

4. **A** (S&F ch5)
Based on the history of heavy alcohol use, steatorrhea, and hyperglycemia, the patient has developed chronic pancreatitis with possible malabsorption of fat-soluble vitamins (A, D, E, and K vitamins). This patient shows manifestations of vitamin E deficiency, including hemolytic anemia and neurologic abnormalities from posterior column spinal disease or peripheral neuropathy. Serum levels of α-tocopherol (the most biologically active form of vitamin E) is used to measure vitamin E status.

Although it is water soluble, vitamin B_{12} deficiency is also seen in pancreatic insufficiency (secondary to lack of pancreatic proteases to free cobalamin from R protein in the proximal small bowel). It takes several years to deplete the entire B_{12} storage in the liver, and this patient has shown clinical signs of pancreatic insufficiency only in the past year. On the other hand, anemia from B_{12} deficiency is characteristically megaloblastic with macrocytosis and hypersegmented neutrophils (not hemolytic anemia). Neurologic diseases like posterior column spinal disease is also seen in B_{12} deficiency.

Retinol concentration in the plasma, is an accurate measures of vitamin A status. Clinical features of vitamin A deficiency include follicular hyperkeratosis and night blindness in the early stages. Conjunctival xerosis (dryness), degeneration of the cornea (keratomalacia), and blindness are seen in late stage of severe deficiency.

Riboflavin (vitamin B_2) and pyridoxine (vitamin B_6) are water-soluble vitamins and are not part of the pancreatic insufficiency syndrome. Deficiency of riboflavin may result in angular stomatitis, glossitis, cheilosis, seborrheic dermatitis, and normocytic anemia. Vitamin B_6 deficiency may produce angular cheilosis, stomatitis, glossitis, depression, irritability, and confusion in moderate depletion and normochromic, normocytic anemia in severe cases.

5. **C** (S&F ch5)
Chromium deficiency in humans has only been seen in patients on long-term total parenteral nutrition with inadequate chromium supplementation. Hyperglycemia or impaired glucose tolerance are commonly seen in these cases. Less commonly reported abnormalities include elevated plasma free fatty acid concentrations, neuropathy, or encephalopathy. Copper, selenium, or molybdenum deficiency can also occur in patients on long-term total parenteral nutrition lacking these trace minerals. Clinical features of copper deficiency include dermatologic abnormalities (skin or hair depigmentation), hematologic disorders (leukopenia or microcytic anemia), neurologic disturbances, and skeletal abnormalities. The anemia is secondary to impaired uptake of iron and therefore iron deficiency anemia. Selenium deficiency is known to cause cardiomyopathy and/or myalgias. Molybdenum deficiency may result in hyperoxypurinemia, hypouricemia, and central nervous system disturbances. Manganese deficiency syndrome has not been conclusively defined in humans. On the other hand, there are reports of manganese toxicity from total parenteral nutrition causing deposition of the mineral in the basal ganglia that resulted in extrapyramidal symptoms or seizures.

6. **A** (S&F ch5)
Chronic vitamin A toxicity may manifest as alopecia, bone and muscle pain, dermatitis, cheilitis, conjunctivitis, pseudotumor cerebri (headache and nausea), ataxia, transaminitis, hyperlipidemia, and hyperostosis. Toxicity with water-soluble vitamins like B or C is less common. However, habitual daily intake of large dose of vitamin B_6 may cause photosensitivity or peripheral neuropathy. High doses of vitamin C may result in nausea or diarrhea. Moreover, in theory, acidification of urine with high doses of vitamin C may increase the risk of oxalate nephrolithiasis. Toxicity with vitamin D can give rise to very high serum concentrations of calcium and phosphate with metastatic calcifications, kidney injury, and altered mental status.

High doses of vitamin E intake (1000 mg) has been reported to be associated with reduced levels of vitamin K–dependent pro-coagulants and mildly increased risk in the incidence of hemorrhagic stroke. Also, impaired leukocyte function has been reported with vitamin E toxicity.

7. **D** (S&F, ch6)
Enteric nutrition is generally preferred over parenteral nutrition in critically ill patients; however, in this particular case with high demand of vasopressor agents and hemodynamic instability from septic shock and peritonitis, small bowel feeding is not feasible. On the other hand, in previously healthy individuals without evidence of malnutrition, parenteral nutrition should be started after 7 days of hospitalization. The evidence to support this recommendation has come from a large clinical trial of early (within 48 hours of ICU admission) versus late (8 days or later after ICU admission) initiation of parenteral nutrition, which showed less complications with infection and cholestasis as well as earlier discharge from ICU and hospital in the late group. Moreover, in all critically ill individuals who are on total parenteral nutrition, permissive underfeeding with provision of 80% of caloric requirement (25 kcal/kg actual body weight) at the beginning is recommended to reduce the incidence of hyperglycemia and infection and also shorten the length of mechanical ventilation or hospital stay.

8. **C** (S&F ch6)
Enteric nutrition has been proved to be an important part of inflammatory bowel disease therapy. Although in

adults, glucocorticoid therapy is more effective than enteric nutrition alone for inducing clinical remission of Crohn's disease, enteric nutrition in children has been shown to be just as effective as steroid therapy in achieving clinical remission.

Vitamin D deficiency is very common in patients with Crohn's disease and can be seen in about 50% of these individuals. Moreover, it has been implicated in the pathogenesis of Crohn's disease because vitamin D may downregulate tumor necrosis factor-α–related genes.

In hospitalized patients with Crohn's flare-up, no significant differences in response have been found in patients randomized to receive enteric or parenteral nutrition. After 3 weeks and after 1 year of treatment, 60% to 71% and 42% to 56%, respectively, of patients will be in remission and will remain in remission with either therapy. These findings confirmed that bowel rest is not necessary to achieve remission in Crohn's disease.

Although malnutrition is an independent risk factor for postoperative complications, routine preoperative total parenteral nutrition therapy in patients with Crohn's disease has not demonstrated a benefit in postsurgical outcomes.

9. D (S&F ch6)
Certain medications like potassium chloride or theophylline are known to coagulate the tube feeding material and should not be mixed with tube feed to avoid obstruction of the NJ tube. Jejunal feeding tubes should never be checked for residual content as it has poor correlation with actual residual content in the small bowel. More importantly, these are small-bore tubes and aspirating the residuals through them increases the chance of clogging. Nasoenteric tubes should be flushed after every use, including feeding or medication instillation. To minimize the risk of tube clogging, only liquid or completely dissolved medications should be placed in the tube. Due to potential long-term complications of nasoenteric tubes, including nasal mucosal ulcerations, pharyngitis, sinusitis, tube migration, or obstruction, they are indicated to be used for less than 1 month and more permanent access like jejunostomy or gastrojejunostomy may need to be considered in this patient with gastroparesis if he tolerates post-pyloric feeding.

10. B (S&F ch6)
This patient has been experiencing the symptoms of early dumping syndrome in the last 2 weeks. The likely cause of developing dumping syndrome is migration of the feeding tube into the duodenum and bolus delivery of the moderately hyperosmolar tube feed in the small bowel. The picture shows migrated gastrostomy tube with only short segment of the tube visible and external bumper against the abdominal wall. Migration of the gastrostomy tube can also cause gastric outlet obstruction; however, the symptoms that this patient has been experiencing are not consistent with obstruction. Buried bumper syndrome is a consequence of excessive pressure between internal and external bumpers of the tube and occurs when the internal bumper slowly erodes into the gastric mucosa. Its manifestations include peristomal inflammation, inability to rotate or mobilize the tube, leakage, or pain with enteral feeding. The presentation in this case is not consistent with obstructed gastrostomy tube. Colocutaneous fistula usually manifests after the original tube is removed and a replacement gastrostomy tube is passed through the tract into a part of colon that has been interpositioned between the stomach and the wall of the abdomen. These cases present with diarrhea and malnutrition secondary to delivery of the tube feeds straight into the colon.

11. E (S&F ch6)
Measures to reduce the risk of aspiration include converting bolus feedings to continuous infusion, keeping the head of the bed elevated 30 to 45 degrees, administering prokinetics (metoclopramide or erythromycin) or narcotic antagonists (naloxone or alvimopan), and changing to post-pyloric feeding. Unless there are obvious signs of intolerance, tube feeding should not be withheld for gastric residual volumes less than 500 mL. Based on available data, tube feeding via gastrostomy tube can be initiated within 2 hours of placement in adults.

12. E (S&F ch6)
Vitamin A deficiency can be seen in cirrhosis and has been shown to be a risk factor for hepatocellular carcinoma. It has been found that diet with a normal protein intake does not worsen hepatic encephalopathy and limiting protein intake can lead to protein-calorie malnutrition in this group of individuals with increased protein needs. Branched-chain amino acids (leucine, isoleucine, and valine) are not metabolized in the liver and could be used in patients with "liver failure." Also, some clinical trials have found a significant decline in hepatic encephalopathy or refractory ascites in patients with "advanced cirrhosis" who were only on branched-chain amino acids. However, due to their high cost and poor tastiness, they are not routinely recommended. Thiamine deficiency is not only seen in alcoholics but also in patients with hepatitis C–related cirrhosis. For this reason, thiamine supplementation is recommended in all patients with cirrhosis to prevent Wernicke's encephalopathy and Korsakoff's dementia. Hypomagnesemia (not hypermagnesemia) could be seen in this cirrhotic patient on diuretics and potentially could be associated with dysgeusia (alteration in the sense of taste).

13. A (S&F ch6)
In patients with short bowel syndrome who only have a limited length of ileum remaining and an intact colon, bile-binding resins like cholestyramine, can cause relative bile salt deficiency and fat malabsorption, which will lead to worsening of the diarrhea. Fat restriction in the oral diet may be useful in these patients for reducing the diarrhea. On the other hand, in a patient with less extensive ileal resection and an intact colon, diarrhea could be the result of the colonic irritation by unabsorbed bile salts and, for that reason, bile-binding resins can be used to reduce bile salt–induced diarrhea. Anticholinergic agents like atropine are used to slow intestinal transit. However, larger doses of anticholinergics are generally required because absorption of the oral medication may be limited in patients with short bowel syndrome. Proton pump inhibitors are also used to reduce gastric secretions and can help with diarrhea. Glucagon-like peptide-2 (GLP-2) is a small intestine mucosal stimulator for improved absorption. Teduglutide binds and activates GLP-2 receptors and was shown in a randomized placebo-controlled study to significantly decrease the volume and number of days of parenteral support required by patients with intestinal failure.

14. A (S&F ch7)
Currently, there are only three FDA-approved drugs for long-term (12 months) treatment of obesity. They include orlistat, lorcaserin, and phentermine-topiramate (extended release). Orlistat inhibits pancreatic lipase and reduces fat absorption. For this reason, it has beneficial effects on low-density lipoprotein cholesterol that make it a better option for this patient with dyslipidemia. Lorcaserin is a potent

selective serotonin 5-HT2C agonist and results in weight loss with promoting satiety and regulating food intake. Its use is contraindicated in patients who take selective serotonin reuptake inhibitors (SSRI) like paroxetine. Phentermine is a sympathomimetic drug with risk for addiction. Its combination with topiramate (an anticonvulsant drug) has been proved in at least 2 clinical trials to be effective and safe for weight loss. Although this combination drug has less prominent behavioral side effects, it is not recommended in individuals with history of drug abuse. Phendimetrazine and diethylpropion are 2 noradrenergic agents, which are only approved for short-term use (less than 3 months).

15. **D** (S&F ch7)
Multiple studies have shown increased risk of colon cancer, prostate cancer, and, to a lesser extent, rectal cancer in obese men. In obese women, however, cancers of gallbladder, reproductive system, and breast cancer (not rectal cancer) are more common than in nonobese women.

16. **C** (S&F ch7)
Pramlintide is one of the new antidiabetic drugs that is associated with weight loss, especially in African American diabetics, although it is not an FDA-approved medicine for obesity. Pramlintide is a synthetic amylin analog with a prolonged half-life. Amylin is a peptide found in the pancreatic beta cells that is deficient in type 1 diabetes. Although nausea is the most common side effect with this drug, it is usually mild and improves after the first month. Exenatide and liraglutide are other medications approved for type 2 diabetes that also have weight loss effects. These medications are glucagon-like peptide-1 (GLP-1) agonists. GLP-1 increases insulin secretion, inhibits glucagon secretion and also delays gastric emptying. The increased level of GLP-1 after gastric bypass may be responsible for the additional weight loss and improvement in diabetes seen after these procedures. Gastroparesis is a common side effect of these drugs. Pancreatitis is a potential adverse event seen in patients on exenatide.

17. **C** (S&F ch8)
According to National Institutes of Health consensus criteria, to qualify for bariatric surgery, patients must have a body mass index of either over 40 kg/m^2 or greater than 35 kg/m^2 with obesity-related comorbidities (hypertension, diabetes mellitus, hyperlipidemia, gastroesophageal reflux disease, irritable bowel syndrome, obstructive sleep apnea, or non-alcoholic steatohepatitis). Therefore, nonsurgical management of obesity is recommended. Pharmacologic therapy is the best option in this patient who has been unsuccessful in losing weight by diet and exercise alone. Option "A" is incorrect; endoscopic treatments have the same entry criteria as bariatric surgery. Additionally, the patient has undergone only self-driven attempts at weight loss. She has never been engaged in serious, physician-driven dietary or lifestyle modification plans. Option "D" alone has not worked for the patient thus far. Option "E" introduces a nutritionist, who has a role in patient and physician-led efforts for weight loss, but this alone is unlikely to be effective without pharmacotherapy.

18. **E** (S&F ch8)
While the patient meets body mass index criteria for an endoscopic weight loss procedure or bariatric surgery referral, she also has active major depression. Schizophrenia, developmental delay, recent major depression with hospitalization or suicide attempts, and severe bipolar disease are all contraindications to referral for bariatric surgery. Other contraindications include severe cardiac disease, severe coagulopathy, and inability to comply with postoperative nutritional requirements. Of note, Roux-en-Y in patients older than 65 and younger than 18 are controversial but not absolute contraindications.

19. **E** (S&F ch8)
Preoperative evaluation of candidates for bariatric surgery requires a multidisciplinary approach. The patient in this question has multiple potentially high-risk comorbid cardiac and psychiatric conditions, and his wife's ancillary history suggests possible obstructive sleep apnea. These should be further investigated and fully defined with the help of relevant specialists. Additionally, an esophagogastroduodenoscopy (EGD) is recommended as part of the routine preoperative workup to detect any upper GI lesions that may affect postoperative outcome or surgical approach. No other choice but E includes both an EGD and all relevant specialty referral required for proper preoperative patient evaluation.

20. **C** (S&F ch8)
Bowel ischemia, in this case due to a twisted Roux limb, presents with the cardinal symptoms of severe abdominal pain, hematochezia, and an acute abdomen. The patient presented above displays all three. Anastomotic leaks would not present with hematochezia. An anastomotic ulcer could theoretically perforate; however, that is less likely in this scenario (early postoperative) than bowel ischemia. A diverticular bleed with wall rupture could also present like this, though the likelihood of this occurring during the postoperative period is unlikely as well. Frank bowel obstruction would present with nausea, vomiting, abdominal pain, and distension as well as lack of flatus or bowel movements.

21. **D** (S&F ch8)
Stenosis of the gastrojejunostomy is a late complication of Roux-en-Y gastric bypass present in 2% to 14% of patients. It presents as vomiting and progressive dysphagia initially to solids and subsequently to liquids. Appropriate treatment calls for endoscopic dilation with balloon or Savary dilators; alternatively, electrosurgical revision can be employed. Balloon dilation can be performed 4 weeks postoperatively, is successful in 90% of cases, and can be repeated every 2 to 3 weeks for 2 to 3 sessions. Vagal injury should present very early postoperatively, making choice A incorrect. Although the patient has sick contacts, her symptoms are more alarming than typical viral gastroenteritis and require immediate attention. Even viral gastroenteritis should not be treated empirically with antibiotics.

22. **E** (S&F ch8)
Cholelithiasis develops in up to 38% of patients undergoing Roux-en-Y gastric bypass. In some cases, the surgeon will perform a concurrent cholecystectomy during a Roux-en-Y surgery; however, this is less common with a laparoscopic approach. Gallstones form secondary to a combination of vagus nerve injury as well as altered enteric nerve stimulation, decreased gallbladder emptying, and changes in the calcium concentration and the bile salt to cholesterol ratio. Daily ursodiol for the first 6 months postoperatively can reduce the incidence of gallstone formation to 2%; the same effect is not seen with cholestyramine. Vitamin supplementation, cessation of NSAIDs, and proton pump inhibitor therapy are all recommended following Roux-en-Y surgery.

23. **D** (S&F ch8)
Roux-en-Y gastric bypass (RYGB) carries a 0.2% mortality rate, a 17% overall complication rate, a 2.2% anastomotic

leak rate, and a 2.0% GI bleed rate; RYGB attain an estimated 61% excess weight loss. By contrast, laparoscopic adjustable gastric banding patients have a 0.02% mortality rate, a 7% overall complication rate, no anastomotic leaks (no anastomosis created), and a 0.3% GI bleed rate; they are estimated to lose 47% of excess weight.

24. **D** (S&F ch8)
Either early or late dumping syndrome can occur in as many as 20% of patients following Roux-en-Y gastric bypass. Symptoms of cramping, abdominal pain, voluminous diarrhea, bloating, dizziness, nausea, flushing, and tachycardia within 15 to 20 minutes of a meal is a hallmark of early dumping syndrome and distinguishes this condition from late dumping syndrome. These symptoms are caused by hypovolemia and a subsequent sympathetic response. Such rapid onset of symptoms is thought to be related to hyperosmotic food entering quickly into the jejunum. A peptic ulcer would cause abdominal pain and possible GI bleeding, but generally not the other symptoms mentioned. Although biliary colic is also postprandial in nature, it generally presents as episodic right upper quadrant pain devoid of the other symptoms mentioned. The patient's symptoms do not match Rome III criteria for an irritable bowel syndrome diagnosis.

25. **D** (S&F ch8)
Late dumping syndrome occurs 2 to 3 hours after a meal (compared to early dumping syndrome, which occurs 15 to 20 minutes after a meal). Late dumping syndrome occurs because of rapid glucose absorption, which releases glucagon-like peptide 1 and gastric inhibitory peptide, triggering an exaggerated insulin response, leading to hypoglycemia and hypokalemia. It is best treated with dietary modification, such as avoiding simple sugars, acidic foods, and nutrient rich drinks. High protein and high fiber foods are the best diet for these patients. Additionally recommended are lifestyle modifications, such as smaller, more frequent meals; avoidance of hot and cold foods; and avoidance of lying down after meals. Although the patient's symptoms are reminiscent of mesenteric ischemia, this is typically of more rapid onset, and the patient above lacks classic risk factors for embolic phenomena. The symptoms in this vignette do not meet Rome III criteria for irritable bowel syndrome. The patient has no history of chronic pain syndrome, and his symptoms have been occurring for only 4 weeks.

26. **D** (S&F ch8)
Thiamine (vitamin B_1) deficiency can arise from prolonged vomiting. This patient is presenting with classic symptoms of Wernicke's encephalopathy: confusion, ataxia, ophthalmoplegia, and impaired short-term memory. Intravenous or intramuscular thiamine is the treatment of choice with acute presentations. A CT scan of the head is not required at this time because the patient's presentation is more consistent with Wernicke's encephalopathy than an acute transient ischemic attack or cerebral vascular accident. An upper endoscopy should be considered to investigate the cause of persistent vomiting but is not the appropriate next step in this patient with severe symptoms. Chromium deficiency may result in peripheral neuropathy and hyperglycemia, while selenium deficiency results in cardiomyopathy and ataxia.

27. **C** (S&F ch8)
Parietal cells in the stomach produce intrinsic factor, necessary for vitamin B_{12} absorption in the terminal ileum. In a Roux-en-Y procedure, the gastric pouch is separated from parietal cells, which often cease to produce intrinsic factor given their lack of contact with food after surgery. This patient presents with graying hair, mild memory disturbance, mild ataxia ("losing half a step"), and anemia (likely macrocytic); these are all symptoms of vitamin B_{12} deficiency. B is incorrect because the patient is not presenting with new, acute-onset dementia. Choices A, D, and E are also incorrect because although variable deficiencies in these vitamins and elements may occur, the patient's presentation is not consistent with those deficiencies.

28. **D** (S&F ch8)
Presurgical counseling is critical prior to referring patients for gastric bypass. Patients deserve to know and must be educated on the risks and benefits of such an invasive, potentially life-changing, and even life-threatening procedure. All other answers but D reflect incorrect representations of the amount of weight lost after gastric bypass.

29. **E** (S&F ch8)
For the best efficacy after gastric bypass, nonsoluble proton pump inhibitor capsules should be broken open; this should be done twice daily. Additionally, sucralfate solution (not tablets) is recommended four times daily.

30. **E** (S&F ch8)
Surgical sutures are foreign bodies and often provoke inflammatory responses, resulting in pain, ulceration, or obstruction. Foreign bodies can be associated with pain even in the absence of visible inflammation on endoscopy. As many as 71% of patients have experienced immediate symptomatic improvement with endoscopic removal of foreign bodies. Choice A may treat inflammation but will not remove the foreign body, which is provoking pain. *H. pylori* testing should be performed if not already checked prior to surgery, but empiric treatment is not appropriate. Tricyclics would be inappropriate because the pain is not functional. Surgery is usually not indicated to remove the suture.

31. **B** (S&F ch9)
Anorexia nervosa (AN) is a disorder in which a patient has excessive concerns about body weight or image while being significantly underweight. Patients with AN typically engage restrictive eating patterns; however, binging patterns may occur as well. Purging or other efforts to control weight or neutralize caloric intake (in Jeff's case, furosemide usage) may be exhibited in up to 50% of patients with AN. Binge eating and purging do not occur with avoidant/restrictive food intake disorder. Patients with bulemia are normal weight or overweight. Patients with binge eating disorder are similarly normal weight or overweight; moreover, they do not engage in restrictive eating patterns. Rumination syndrome patients voluntarily vomit but not as a method to control weight (see table at end of chapter).

32. **D** (S&F ch9)
Clinical features of anorexia nervosa (AN) are wide-ranging, but they can be grouped along either the restriction/binge eating or purging/refeeding behaviors. Often, without appropriate historical information, the signs can be subtle; clinicians with suspicion for eating disorders must take careful histories, and even then, the patient may attempt to obfuscate critical details. In this patient, the combination of low body mass index (BMI) and parotid gland enlargement are strong suggestions of AN with purging/refeeding characteristics. Diarrhea, rectal

bleeding, and elevated liver function tests are also supportive of this diagnosis. A prolonged viral gastroenteritis would not be expected to reduce the patient's BMI so drastically. Microscopic colitis typically does not present this young, and rectal bleeding is rarely a feature of this disease. Irritable bowel syndrome with diarrhea predominance would also not be expected to so drastically lower BMI. Although ulcerative colitis may present with bloody diarrhea and low BMI, the patient's parotid gland enlargement does not fit.

33. B (S&F ch9)
The patient meets diagnostic criteria for bulimia nervosa (BN) (normal weight/overweight, restrictive eating pattern can occur, binge eating pattern at least once a week for 3 months, purging once a week, and excess concern with body weight). The management of eating disorders is multidisciplinary and challenging. It begins with an evaluation and education of the patient and any caregivers. Primary care providers, dieticians, and mental health providers must all work closely together to monitor symptoms and progress. Various forms of psychotherapy can be employed. For BN, fluoxetine 60 mg daily is the only FDA-approved pharmacotherapy. Studies on the efficacy of Olanzapine in anorexia nervosa show conflicting results. Topiramate has shown efficacy in reducing binge and purge symptoms in two randomized controlled trials, but more evidence is needed.

34. E (S&F ch9)
The patient has developed refeeding syndrome, a constellation of hypophosphatemia, hypokalemia, assorted vitamin deficiencies, delirium, and heart failure. Hypophosphatemia is the main electrolyte abnormality, and it is central to the development of all the other associated symptoms.

35. C (S&F ch9)
This patient is suspected to have bulimia nervosa. Anorexia nervosa and bulimia nervosa can be challenging to distinguish. Both disorders have patients who may exhibit restrictive feeding patterns and binge eating patterns, as well as purging behavior. Both disorders have patients with excess concern about their body image. The principle difference is that patients with anorexia nervosa will be underweight; bulimic patients are normal weight or overweight. Patients with binge eating disorder do not exhibit restrictive eating or purging behavior. Choice "D" is incorrect because although there can be a fine clinical line between "normal" dieting behavior, exercise, and criticalness of body image, this patient exhibits extreme examples of behavior. Choice "E" is not supported by typical features of hypothyroidism.

36. C (S&F ch10)
The clinical presentations are typical for "pollen-food allergy syndrome," which is a form of IgE-mediated food hypersensitivity. The symptoms results from immediate hypersensitivity to proteins that are similar to plant pollens. In about half of patients with ragweed-induced allergic rhinitis, ingestion of banana or melons will cause oral allergic reactions, including swelling of the lips, tongue, or throat. These proteins are heat labile and destroyed after cooking, so the allergic reactions are only seen with ingestion of uncooked fruits or vegetables. The symptoms in pollen-food allergy syndrome are limited to oropharyngeal area, and systemic reactions are very rare. Systemic eosinophilia is not a common feature in these patients.

37. C (S&F ch10)
This infant has the typical presentation of allergic eosinophilic proctocolitis (AEP). It usually presents in the first 1 or 2 months of life and is the result of cow's milk or soy protein hypersensitivity. Because of food antigens passed in mother's breast milk, it is commonly seen in breast-fed infants. The manifestations are limited to blood in the stool. Diarrhea, nausea, vomiting, or even anemia are not common features for this condition. The first step in management is the elimination of the responsible allergens (commonly cow's milk) from the maternal diet. IgE antibodies have no role in this disease, and skin prick testing is not helpful in the diagnosis. Mothers are encouraged to continue with breast-feeding after elimination of the allergens in their diet. In most cases, significant improvement is seen within 3 days, and there is no need to pursue further tests, including sigmoidoscopy. However, endoscopic findings may vary from patchy mucosal injection to small aphthoid ulcerations and bleeding. Biopsies show prominent eosinophilic infiltrate in the crypt epithelia and lamina propria.

38. D (S&F ch10)
The clinical presentations and findings in this infant are consistent with eosinophilic gastroenteritis. In young children, it may present with protein-losing enteropathy. Also, it can result in pyloric stenosis and gastric outlet obstruction in this group. The long-term natural history of eosinophilic gastroenteritis is not well studied, but available data have shown persistence of this condition for 2.5 to 5.5 years, especially in patients with protein-losing enteropathy. The exact pathogenesis of this disease is not known, but is believed to primarily involve cell-mediated (not IgE-mediated) mechanisms. The initial treatment in children includes an empiric elimination diet or an elemental diet. If dietary therapy does not result in clinical improvement, a trial of glucocorticoids is recommended. HLA-DQ2 is strongly associated with celiac disease, not eosinophilic gastroenteritis.

39. A (S&F ch10)
Peanut, tree nut, sesame, and seafood allergies tend to be lifelong, but about one fifth of children with peanut allergy develop "clinical tolerance" later in their life. In young children, the most common food allergens include milk (2.5%), egg (1.5%), peanut (1.4%), tree nuts (1.0%), wheat (≈0.4%), and soy (≈0.4%). However, the most common food allergens in adults include shellfish (2%), peanut (0.6%), tree nuts (0.4%), and fish (0.4%).

TABLE FOR ANSWER 31 Distinguishing Features of Feeding and Eating Disorders

Feeding or Eating Disorder	Physical Signs Included in Diagnostic Criteria	Restrictive-Pattern Eating	Binge-Pattern Eating	Purging and Other Behaviors to Control Weight or Neutralize Effects of Caloric Intake	Excess Concern with Body Image or Weight
ARFID	Significantly underweight or other nutritional deficiency	Typically; may include avoidance of certain kinds of food	No	No	No
AN	Significantly underweight	Typically	May occur	Purging may occur in up to one half of patients	Yes
BN	None (patients are generally normal weight or overweight)	May occur as behavior to control weight	Must occur an average of once per week for at least 3 mo	Must occur an average of once per week to meet diagnostic criteria	Yes
BED	None (patients are frequently overweight or obese)	No	Must occur an average of once per week for at least 3 mo	No	Yes
Rumination disorder	No	No	No	Voluntary regurgitation occurs but is not intended to purge calories	No
Pica	No	No	No	No	No

AN, Anorexia nervosa; ARFID, avoidant/restrictive food intake disorder; BED, binge eating disorder; BN, bulimia nervosa.
Data from American Psychiatric Association. *Diagnostic and statistical manual of mental disorders.* 5th ed. (DSM-5.) Arlington, Va.: American Psychiatric Association; 2013.

CHAPTER

3

Symptoms, Signs, and Biopsychosocial Issues

Heba Iskandar, Sunil Dacha, Sahar Taba Taba Vakili, Emad Qayed, and Shanthi Srinivasan

QUESTIONS

1. A 64-year-old man presents to the emergency department with complaints of constant, dull left lower quadrant abdominal pain for the past 2 days. He reports a temperature of 102° F at home with associated chills. He has not had a bowel movement in three days. On examination, his temperature is 101° F, respiratory rate is 94 breaths/min, blood pressure is 150/70 mm Hg. Physical exam is significant for tenderness in the left lower quadrant. Laboratory exam was significant for leukocytosis. A computed tomography (CT) scan of abdomen was obtained, which showed evidence of diverticulitis of the sigmoid colon with a localized pericolic abscess (Hinchey grade I). What is the next best step in the management of this patient?
   A. Discharge with oral antibiotics
   B. Admit to the hospital for intravenous (IV) antibiotics and hydration
   C. Emergent surgery
   D. Call interventional radiology for CT-guided drain placement
   E. Perform colonoscopy

2. A 56-year-old man with past medical history of hypertension and atrial fibrillation presents to the emergency department with complaints of sudden onset severe abdominal pain in the periumbilical area for the past 2 hours. He had an episode of black tarry stools also at that time. His medications include aspirin and losartan. Vital signs were as follows:

Temperature	100° F
Respiratory rate	20 breaths/min
Heart rate	100 bpm
Blood pressure	90/60 mm Hg

He rates his abdominal pain as 10/10. On physical examination, he appears acutely ill. His abdominal exam shows mild tenderness in the midabdomen. Rectal exam shows melena. What is the next best step in diagnosing this condition?
   A. CT scan of the abdomen
   B. Esophagogastroduodenoscopy (EGD)
   C. Emergency laparotomy
   D. Admit to hospital for observation
   E. Obtain abdominal x-ray

3. A 20-year-old woman presents to the hospital with severe lower abdominal pain that started abruptly an hour ago. She was treated for vaginal *Chlamydia* infection in the past 3 weeks. Her last menstrual period was 2 months ago. Vital signs were as follows:

Blood pressure	90/60 mm Hg
Heart rate	110 bpm
Respiratory rate	16 breaths/min

On physical examination, she appears in moderate distress. Physical exam revealed tenderness in the lower abdomen. Laboratory exam was significant for hemoglobin of 9 g/dL. Urine pregnancy test is positive. Pelvic ultrasound suggests a tubal pregnancy. The patient's nurse goes to talk to her about the results and witnesses that she turns pale and collapses suddenly. What is the most likely diagnosis?
   A. Ruptured ectopic pregnancy
   B. Acute appendicitis
   C. Acute pancreatitis
   D. Acute cholecystitis
   E. Tubo-ovarian abscess

4. A 32-year-old woman is seen in the clinic as a referral for chronic abdominal pain, from which she has been suffering for the past 8 years. She can point to an exact location where the pain is located immediately left of the umbilicus. The pain is not associated with eating. She has no nausea, vomiting, constipation, diarrhea, rectal bleeding, melena, or bloating. She has tried a gluten-free diet with no benefit. She does not take nonsteroidal antiinflammatory drugs (NSAIDs). Omeprazole and hyoscyamine have not provided any benefit. She had an extensive workup including EGD, colonoscopy, magnetic resonance imaging (MRI) of the abdomen, small bowel follow through, and a capsule endoscopy, which were normal. Her routine laboratory testing was normal. She has missed her work frequently due to the pain. On physical examination, tenderness is only present in a one-inch area to the left of the umbilicus. Tenderness increases when the patient is asked to raise her head from the exam table while supine. What is the next best step in the management?
   A. Endoscopic retrograde cholangiopancreatography (ERCP) with biliary manometery
   B. Diagnostic laparoscopy
   C. Inject the site of pain with a combination of local anesthetic with or without glucocorticoid
   D. Obtain CT scan of the abdomen
   E. Tell the patient she has irritable bowel syndrome and not to worry about it

5. A 28-year-old woman patient is seen in the clinic for evaluation of chronic abdominal pain for the past 2 years.

She has a history of chronic back pain for which she was taking oxycodone on a regular basis. She was admitted to a hospital 1 year ago for severe abdominal pain, nausea, vomiting, and constipation. Workup during that hospitalization included EGD, colonoscopy, routine laboratory studies (CBC, complete metabolic panel, lipase) and CT of the abdomen and pelvis, which were normal. She had a normal anorectal manometry as well. Since then she uses methyl naltrexone for constipation as needed with some benefit. More recently she has noticed worsening of her abdominal pain despite taking increased doses of oxycodone. She does not report weight loss, diarrhea, hematochezia, or melena. What is the most likely diagnosis?

A. Irritable bowel syndrome
B. Narcotic bowel syndrome
C. Crohn's disease
D. Hirschsprung's disease
E. Celiac disease

6. A 42-year-old man is seen in the clinic for evaluation of abdominal pain, of which he has been suffering for the past 7 years. He is otherwise healthy with no known medical issues and has never had any surgeries. The pain is located in the right lower chest and right upper quadrant. The pain may vary between a sudden lancinating pain in the right subcostal region and a dull achy pain. Pain worsens with inspiration. He tried NSAIDS with some benefit. He subsequently had an EGD, which was normal, and proton pump inhibitor (PPI) therapy did not help. CT of the abdomen was normal. Physical examination revealed tenderness along lower chest with anterior movement of right lower ribs and a popping sound was heard. He is concerned, as the pain has significantly affected his quality of life. What is the next best step in the management of his condition?

A. Perform a hepatobiliary (hydroxy iminodiacetic acid [HIDA]) scan
B. Costochondral nerve block
C. ERCP with biliary manometry
D. Colonoscopy
E. Laparoscopic exploration

7. A 51-year-old man with history of gastroesophageal reflux disease and hypertension presents to the clinic for evaluation of chest pain for the past 4 weeks. Currently he takes antacids as needed and amlodipine. He is otherwise healthy. He describes the chest pain as squeezing or burning substernal sensation that radiates to the back, neck, and sometimes to his jaw and arms. He has awakened from sleep a few times with severe chest pain that resolved spontaneously in 1 or 2 hours, or with antacid ingestion. His vital signs are within normal limits. Physical exam is unremarkable. What is the best next step in evaluation of his chest pain?

A. Perform EGD to assess for reflux esophagitis
B. CT scan of the abdomen
C. Refer for cardiac evaluation
D. No further testing suggested
E. Esophageal manometry

8. A 19-year-old college student is seen for evaluation of painful swallowing. She has a history of acne and has been taking doxycycline for this issue as needed. She is sexually active with her boyfriend but is monogamous and uses protection. She has no other medical issues and is otherwise feeling well. She mentions that her grandfather died of esophageal cancer at the age of 75 years. She has severe pain with eating and has been avoiding eating due to fear of pain. Her vital signs and physical exam are within normal limits. What is the most likely diagnosis?

A. Pill-induced esophagitis
B. Esophageal cancer
C. Peptic esophagitis
D. *Candida* esophagitis
E. Herpes simlex virus (HSV) esophagitis

9. A 72-year-old man is admitted to the hospital with complaints of epigastric abdominal discomfort and early satiety for the past 10 weeks. He has no appetite and reports a 20-pound weight loss in past 3 months. He reports black tarry stools on and off. He has a history of osteoarthritis, coronary artery disease, and hyperlipidemia. His grandfather died of colon cancer at the age of 67 years. He has been taking ibuprofen for his knee pain daily for the past few months and is taking aspirin and clopidrogel daily for coronary artery disease. Physical examination is significant for epigastric tenderness. His vital signs included a blood pressure of 110/70 mm Hg, heart rate of 110 bpm, oxygen saturation of 99%, and respiratory rate of 14 breaths/min. His laboratory testing is significant for hemoglobin of 9 g/dL. What is the next best step?

A. Obtain CT scan of the chest, abdomen, and pelvis
B. Perform an EGD
C. Perform a colonoscopy
D. Test for *Helicobacter pylori* stool antigen and treat
E. No further work up needed.

10. A 28-year-old man from Mexico presents with complaints of abdominal pain for 2 months. He has some benefit by taking famotidine. He has no black stools or blood in the stool. His weight has been stable. He reports no known medical issues. Lab work from his primary care physician's office shows normal blood counts and chemistry. He is anxious and concerned that he has a cancer. What is the next best step?

A. Reassure and suggest to continue famotidine
B. Test for *H. pylori* and treat accordingly
C. Suggest upper endoscopy
D. Diagnose him with functional dyspepsia
E. Order a CT scan of abdomen

11. A 45-year-old woman presents with complaints of epigastric burning for the past 3 years that has been significantly affecting her quality of life. She has seen two other gastroenterologists in the past for the same complaints. Her reports show two normal upper endoscopies, with biopsies excluding *H. pylori* and a normal CT scan of the abdomen and pelvis. She has early satiety and epigastric burning with meals most of the days. She has no weight loss, hematemesis, melena, or hematochezia. Laboratory studies performed 2 weeks prior are as follows:

Hemoglobin	12.8 g/dL
WBC	7000/μL
Alkaline phosphatase	130 U/L
AST	25 U/L
ALT	26 U/L
Total bilirubin	1.8 mg/dL
Direct bilirubin	0.8 mg/dL
Albumin	3.6 gm/dL

She has been on three different types of PPIs with no benefit. She has avoided fast food, which has provided some benefit. She has no other medical issues. There is no family history of cancers. What is the next step in treatment?

A. Suggest avoiding spicy food and trial of nortryptiline
B. Repeat EGD with biopsies
C. Perform colonoscopy
D. Perform ERCP with sphincter of Oddi manometry
E. Tell the patient she has no medical issue and stop worrying

12. What is the frequency of delayed gastric emptying in patients with functional dyspepsia?
A. <5%
B. 5%-10%
C. 20%-50%
D. 60%-75%
E. >75%

13. A 32-year-old woman presents with early satiety and postprandial fullness for the past 2 months. She has associated epigastric pain and bloating. Antacids provide minimal benefit. She has a history of hypothyroidism, well-controlled with levothyroxine. An ultrasound of the right upper quadrant shows multiple small gallbladder stones. Her grandfather died of colon cancer at the age of 76 years. A 4-week course of proton pump inhibitor therapy has provided no benefit. Upper endoscopy is normal, including gastric and duodenal biopsies. What is the most likely diagnosis?
A. Celiac disease
B. Irritable bowel syndrome
C. Functional dyspepsia
D. Chronic pancreatitis
E. Cholelithiasis

14. A 28-year-old man presents for evaluation of nausea and vomiting. He had episodes of nausea and vomiting that begin abruptly and subside in a week. These episodes have occurred every 2 to 3 months for the past 2 years. He has a past medical history of migraine. His mother had history of migraines. During these episodes he is confined to home. He remains asymptomatic between these episodes. He has no psychiatric issues. All prior workup has been normal, including EGD, CT of abdomen, gastric emptying study, video capsule endoscopy, small bowel follow through, and MRI of brain. He has derived some benefit from antiemetics and smokes marijuana regularly to prevent these episodes. What is the most likely diagnosis?
A. Bulimia nervosa
B. Cyclical vomiting syndrome
C. Malingering
D. Crohn's disease
E. Functional vomiting

15. A 42-year-old woman presents with a history of persistent nausea and vomiting. She had the symptoms for more than 2 years after she intentionally lost 30 lb, decreasing her body mass index to 18 kg/m^2 from 23 kg/m^2. Her symptoms include middle abdominal pain, nausea, and bilious vomiting after she eats. Symptoms improve by adopting a prone or knee-chest position. She was hospitalized multiple times for dehydration in the past year. Recent tests including EGD, *H. pylori* testing, colonoscopy, 4-hour gastric emptying study, capsule endoscopy, and MRI of brain have been normal. A nasojejunal tube was placed for nutrition and completely relieved her symptoms. Which of the following is the best test to confirm the diagnosis?
A. Single balloon enteroscopy (SBE)
B. No further workup needed
C. Refer to psychiatry
D. Upper gastrointestinal (GI) barium contrast study
E. Repeat gastric emptying study

16. A 23-year-old G2P1 woman was seen in consultation for severe nausea and vomited during her eleventh week of gestation. Her pregnancy has been associated with severe nausea and vomiting, necessitating hospitalization twice for IV hydration. Streaks of blood were noticed in the vomitus at times. She had similar complaints during her prior pregnancy that subsided in her second trimester. On physical examination, her BMI was 34 kg/m^2; her vital signs and physical exam are within normal limits. Her symptoms are controlled well with antiemetics and rest. Which of the following is true about this condition?
A. Associated with increased risk of toxemia of pregnancy
B. High risk of spontaneous abortion
C. This condition is not associated with low birth weight
D. Small and frequent protein-rich, low-fat meals are recommended
E. Malnutrition is not a risk with this condition

17. A 53-year-old woman with a history of hypothyroidism and celiac disease is seen in the outpatient clinic for diarrhea of 1-year duration. She is having 10 liquid stools per day with occasional episodes of incontinence. She was seen 2 years ago for bloating and occasional diarrhea, when upper endoscopy revealed flattening of villi in duodenum and biopsies confirmed a diagnosis of celiac disease. Her bloating improved with a gluten-free diet and there was improvement in diarrhea as well. Repeat EGD last month showed normal villi and biopsies were normal, but she continues to have diarrhea on a gluten-free diet. Her tissue-transglutaminase is now normal. She feels well otherwise. Her stool studies are normal. Colonoscopy was performed revealing normal colonic mucosa and terminal ileum. Biopsies were obtained. Her only medication is levothyroxine. What is the most likely cause of her diarrhea?
A. Ulcerative colitis
B. Celiac disease
C. Microscopic colitis
D. Irritable bowel syndrome with diarrhea predominance
E. Laxative abuse

18. A 36-year-old man with no known medical issues is seen in the clinic for evaluation of chronic diarrhea for the past year. He does not take any medications. He has six to eight watery stools per day and has excessive foul smelling gas. He feels well otherwise. Stool studies were negative for any infectious causes. Stool sodium was 45 mEq/L, potassium was 30 mEq/L, and stool pH was 5. Which of the following is the likely cause of diarrhea?
A. Carbohydrate malabsorption
B. Carcinoid tumor
C. Irritable bowel syndrome
D. Giardiasis
E. Congenital chloridorrhea

19. A 22-year-old African-American man with fibrostenotic Crohn's disease maintained on infliximab is seen for follow-up for chronic diarrhea, which has been affecting his job for the past 2 years. He has no other symptoms and feels well. He had a resection of 60 cm of his ileum along with cecum 2 years ago when he presented with intestinal obstruction. He was started on infliximab after his surgery. His recent colonoscopy and EGD with biopsies are normal. A magnetic resonance enterography is normal. His stool infectious studies are negative. He did not have diarrhea prior to his surgery. What is the next best step in his management?
A. Empirical trial of cholestyramine
B. Add 6-mercaptopurine

C. Obtain endoscopic ultrasound to rule out pancreatic neuroendocrine tumor
D. Repeat colonoscopy
E. No further treatment is needed.

20. A 52-year-old man is seen in the clinic for evaluation of chronic diarrhea. He has a history of psoriasis and ankylosing spondylosis. He was admitted to a local hospital last year for exertional dyspnea and was found to have restrictive cardiomyopathy. A cardiac biopsy was performed and the histology revealed apple green birefringence with Congo red stain under polarized light. He has complaints of early satiety and excessive bloating along with excessive diarrhea. On physical examination, he has macroglossia, pinch purpura, and hepatomegaly. Which of the following is the most likely mechanism of diarrhea in this condition?
A. Acute bacterial Infection
B. Smooth muscle hyperactivity
C. Intestinal dysmotility and small intestinal bacterial overgrowth
D. Central nervous system neuropathy
E. Activation of cyclic guanosine monophosphate (cGMP)

21. Which of the following gas diffuses the fastest across the mucosa of GI tract?
A. O_2
B. CO_2
C. H_2
D. CH_4
E. N_2

22. A 50-year-old male with no known medical issues is seen in the office for excessive flatulence for the past year. He is a real estate agent, and mentions that he has excessive foul smelling gas every day and has to excuse himself to avoid embarrassment when he is with clients. He has tried a gluten-free diet and yogurt without benefit. He mentions that his diet consists of a bowl of cereal with milk in the morning and eats only lean meats for lunch and dinner. His colonoscopy performed last year was reportedly normal. What is the most likely cause of his symptoms?
A. Lactose intolerance
B. Celiac disease
C. Functional flatulence
D. Air swallowing
E. Sorbitol

23. A 75-year-old woman with poorly controlled diabetes who resides in a nursing home presents to the outpatient clinic with episodes of fecal soiling approximately twice weekly for the last 2 months. She does not have a strong urge to defecate, and the nursing staff provided her with adult diapers. Furthermore, she has chronic low back pain requiring narcotics. She feels like she has great difficulty having a regular bowel movement due to hard stools. She does not have any blood in her stool, diarrhea, abdominal pain, or weight loss. She has a history of three vaginal deliveries. Which of the following is the least likely contributing factor for her incontinence?
A. Diabetes mellitus
B. Impaired rectal sensation
C. Hard stool
D. Irritable bowel syndrome
E. Sphincter trauma

24. A 60-year-old woman with a past medical history of depression on fluoxetine presents to the clinic with fecal incontinence for the last 3 months. She feels the urge to defecate and has to run to the bathroom, but frequently does not make it. Her stools are liquid in consistency. This causes her great embarrassment and limits her ability to go out to locations without a bathroom. Her primary care physician has performed stool studies that were negative for infectious etiologies of diarrhea. Her physical exam shows no abdominal tenderness. She has lost 5 lbs. When her stools were formed, prior to the last 3 months, she did not have incontinence. What is the most appropriate next step in evaluation?
A. Anorectal manometry
B. MRI
C. Colonoscopy
D. Anal endosonography
E. Defecography

25. A 50-year-old woman presents to the clinic with fecal incontinence. She has had 2 previous vaginal deliveries at ages 28 and 33; one required a forceps for delivery with some injury requiring suturing. She also had a history of hemorrhoids requiring a hemorrhoidectomy. Which of the following is the least helpful test for the evaluation of incontinence in this patient?
A. Anorectal manometry
B. MRI
C. Defecography
D. Anal endosonography
E. Barium enema

26. A 55-year-old woman with stool incontinence is found to have a weak anal sphincter on anorectal manometry. Further testing reveals no sensory abnormalities. Which of the following is the most appropriate next step in treatment?
A. Surgical sphincter repair
B. Injection of a sphincter bulking agent
C. Biofeedback therapy
D. Sacral nerve stimulation
E. Colostomy

27. An 80-year-old woman presents with complaints of semi-formed stools and fecal incontinence. She underwent colonoscopy with biopsies, breath testing for lactose intolerance and small intestinal bacterial overgrowth, and routine blood work and stool studies, which were all normal. Which of the following pharmacologic therapies is the most appropriate first therapeutic step in the management of her fecal incontinence before she undergoes further workup?
A. Tincture of opium
B. Loperamide
C. Docusate
D. Magnesium citrate
E. Alosetron

28. Which of the following is a risk factor for constipation?
A. Advanced age
B. Male gender
C. High level of education
D. High socioeconomic status
E. White ethnicity

29. Which of the following best describes normal transit constipation?
A. Incomplete evacuation; abdominal pain may be present but not a predominant feature
B. Infrequent bowel movements (<3/week), lack of urge to defecate, poor response to fiber and laxatives, generalized symptoms

C. Frequent straining, incomplete evacuation, need for manual maneuvers to facilitate defecation
D. Normal evacuation without straining
E. Incomplete evacuation with abdominal pain that gets better with a bowel movement and worse with constipation

30. A 32-year-old woman with no known medical issues is seen in the clinic for complaints of constipation for the past 6 months. She mentions having a bowel movement every 2 to 3 weeks and needs to strain to have a bowel movement. She feels bloated and mentions that constipation has been having a negative impact on her quality of life. She has modified her diet and includes more than 30 g of soluble fiber per day, drinks at least 2 liters of water per day, and exercises regularly. She has no other complaints. She does not take any other medications. Her father died of colon cancer at 70 years. Rectal examination is normal, and the rest of her physical exam is unremarkable. Colonoscopy was normal a year ago. What is the next best step in management?
A. Polyethylene glycol
B. Perform colonic transit study
C. Anorectal manometry/balloon expulsion test
D. Magnetic resonance (MR) defecography
E. Tell patient to increase fiber to 50 g per day

31. A 17-year-old man is seen for constipation for the past 3 years. He has no other medical issues. He has a bowel movement once or twice per week. He has to strain at defecation and sometimes performs digital evacuation. He has tried multiple classes of medications for constipation from two other gastroenterologists. He had a normal colonoscopy 1 year ago. You suspect Hirschsprung's disease and order a balloon expulsion testing and anorectal manometry. Which of the following findings is suggestive of Hirschsprung's disease?
A. Absence of rectoanal inhibitory reflex
B. A high resting anal pressure
C. Rectal hyposensitivity
D. Inappropriate contraction of external anal sphincter
E. Inability to expel a 50 mL water-filled balloon during attempted defecation

32. A 55-year-old woman is seen with complaints of "hard, rock-like" stool. She mentions difficulty with bowel movements for 5 years. She has to strain for a long time and perform digital evacuation of stool every time she has bowel movement, and has sensation of incomplete evacuation. She had a normal colonoscopy; blood counts and chemistry are normal. Thyroid stimulating hormone is normal. She has tried multiple prescription medications with no benefit. During a balloon expulsion test, she could not expel the balloon at 2 minutes. Anorectal manometry tracing during balloon expulsion revealed simultaneous increase in rectal pressure and anal pressure. Which of the following is the next step in management of this condition?
A. Perform subtotal colectomy
B. Perform chest x-ray
C. Biofeedback therapy
D. Perform colonoscopy
E. Continue current medications

33. A 38-year-old man is seen in the clinic with complaints of blood and mucus in the stool for the past 2 months. He has no other known medical issues. He has a bowel movement once or twice a week and has to strain during defecation. He is a heterosexual male and currently sexually active with single partner. Rectal exam revealed small external hemorrhoids and he was exquisitely tender to rectal exam. A colonoscopy was performed, which revealed erythema, hyperemia, a 1 cm rectal ulcer, and small polypoid lesions over the anterior rectal wall. Biopsies were performed, which revealed collagen infiltration of lamina propria. Which of the following is the most likely cause for the rectal ulcer?
A. Crohn's disease
B. Malignancy
C. Rectal prolapse
D. Physical trauma
E. Syphilis

34. A 62-year-old man with metastatic prostate cancer to bones is seen in consultation in the hospital for constipation. He has been failing all treatment regimens for prostate cancer and is being treated for his terminal illness symptomatically. He is currently on morphine and fentanyl for pain control from bone metastases. He reports having a bowel movement with straining once a week now. He has nausea, abdominal discomfort, and bloating due to constipation. He had not had constipation before he was hospitalized. Stool softeners, polyethylene glycol, and enemas have not been helpful. Which if the following is the best treatment option for constipation in this patient?
A. Methylnaltrexone
B. Linaclotide
C. Alvimopan
D. Lubiprostone
E. Tegaserod

35. What is the mechanism of action of linaclotide?
A. Activates intestinal chloride-2 channels
B. Activates the guanylate cyclase C receptor
C. μ-opioid receptor antagonist
D. 5-HT_4 agonist
E. Ileal bile acid transporter inhibitor

36. According to the American College of Gastroenterology Chronic Constipation Task Force, which of the following medications has grade A evidence (i.e., based on two or more randomized controlled trials (RCTs) with adequate sample sizes and appropriate methodology) for treatment of chronic constipation?
A. Polyethylene glycol (PEG)
B. Lubiprostone
C. Stool softeners
D. Stimulant laxatives
E. Calcium polycarbophil

37. A 48-year-old woman is seen in the clinic for chronic constipation. She has been suffering from constipation for the past 6 years. She has to strain for prolonged periods of time and has to assume unusual postures on the toilet to facilitate stool expulsion. She had to digitally evacuate stool on many occasions. She has learned to apply pressure to the posterior vaginal wall every time she has rectal emptying now. In addition, she suffers from urinary incontinence. She has tried many laxatives and enemas with no benefit. She has three children, all of whom were born by normal vaginal delivery. She underwent a surgery for uterine prolapse 5 years ago. Rectal exam revealed a "defect" in the anterior wall of rectum. The patient was unable to empty the contrast during barium defecography. Which of the following is the best option in the management of this patient?
A. Kegel exercises
B. Surgical repair

C. Endoscopic ultrasound
D. Linaclotide
E. Biofeedback therapy

38. A 69-year-old woman presents to the emergency department with 1 day history of melena. She has a history of rheumatoid arthritis, diabetes mellitus, and hypertension. Her medications include methotrexate, metformin, aspirin 81 mg, and ibuprofen 400 mg three times daily. On physical examination, her vital signs are as follows:

Temperature	37° C
Blood pressure	80/55 mm Hg
Heart rate	120 bpm
Respiratory rate	12 breaths/min

Her abdominal exam is soft and non-tender. Laboratory values are as follows:

Hemoglobin	8 g/dL
WBC	7000/μL
Platelet count	190,000/μL
Total bilirubin	1.8 mg/dL
Creatinine	1.5 mg/dL
INR	1.3

She is adequately resuscitated with IV normal saline, and her blood pressure increases to 105/85 mm Hg and heart rate drops to 92 bpm. The emergency department physician starts an omeprazole drip. An endoscopy is planned in the morning. Which of the following is a proven benefit of PPI drip in this patient?
A. Decrease in mortality
B. Decrease in the need for surgery
C. Decrease in the rebleeding rate after endoscopy
D. Decrease in the need for endoscopic therapy
E. Decrease in the blood transfusion requirement

39. A 60-year-old man presents to the emergency department with 1 day history of hematemesis and melena. He has a history of osteoarthritis, diabetes mellitus, and hypertension. He has a remote history of hepatitis C, which was treated successfully in the 1990s. His medications include metformin, glimepiride, aspirin 81 mg, and ibuprofen 400 mg three times daily. On physical examination, his vital signs are as follows:

Temperature	36° C
Blood pressure	90/55 mm Hg
Heart rate	110 bpm
Respiratory rate	12 breaths/min

His abdominal exam is soft and nontender. Laboratory studies are as follows:

Hemoglobin	7.5 g/dL
WBC	6000/μL
Platelet count	290,000/μL
Total bilirubin	1.4 mg/dL
Creatinine	1.2 mg/dL
INR	1.8

Which of the following recommendations is correct for this patient's management?
A. IV octreotide should be started in the emergency department
B. Blood transfusion is indicated to a hemoglobin of at least 9 g/dL
C. Endoscopy should be delayed until the INR is corrected to <1.5
D. IV erythromycin is recommended prior to endoscopy
E. IV proton pump inhibitor drip is superior to IV PPI twice daily dosing in this patient

40. What percentage of GI bleed admissions in the United States have a source of bleeding from the small intestine?
A. 10%
B. 20%
C. 25%
D. 30%
E. 35%

41. A 50-year-old woman with chronic NSAID use for osteoarthritis of her knees is admitted to the hospital for hematemesis. She reports a history of epigastric burning sensation with regurgitation worse with spicy foods. On physical examination, her vital signs are as follows:

Temperature	37° C
Blood pressure	90/50 mm Hg
Heart rate	130 bpm
Respiratory rate	12 breaths/min

Her abdominal exam is soft and with mild epigastric tenderness. Laboratory studies are as follows:

Hemoglobin	7 g/dL
WBC	8000/μL
Platelet count	190,000/μL
Total bilirubin	1.9 mg/dL
Creatinine	1.4 mg/dL
INR	1.2

She is given IV fluids and an EGD is performed. A large 4 cm gastric ulcer is noted in the antrum with an adherent clot. There is some oozing of blood around the clot. Which of the following is the most appropriate next step in management?
A. No further endoscopic therapy, start proton pump inhibitor drip
B. Dual endoscopic therapy and proton pump inhibitor drip for 72 hours
C. Remove clot with a snare and treat underlying lesion and start IV proton pump inhibitor
D. Send the patient to interventional radiology for further therapy
E. Inject epinephrine around the clot to stop oozing and give patient IV proton pump inhibitor

42. Which statement is true about endoscopic thermal electrocoagulation?
A. High power (>50 W) is essential for good coaptive coagulation
B. Therapy is optimum if applied for moderate amount of time (8 to 10 sec)
C. Current is generated at the base of the probe
D. Heater probes can coagulate arteries up to 1 mm in diameter
E. Heater probes can deliver a variable amount of energy depending on the tissue resistance.

43. A 55-year-old man with past medical history of gastroesophageal reflux disease (GERD), tobacco abuse, and obesity presents to the emergency department after an episode of syncope. He had a 2-day history of melena prior to his syncope. He is fluid resuscitated and receives a blood transfusion. During an urgent EGD, he is found to have a single 3 cm gastric ulcer with a nonbleeding visible vessel in the antrum. The ulcer is treated with dual therapy (epinephrine injection and endoclips) and hemostasis is achieved. Which of the following is the most appropriate management for this patient?
A. IV proton pump inhibitor (PPI) therapy for 72 hours and then switch to oral PPI
B. Empiric therapy for *H. pylori*

C. Repeat upper endoscopy prior to discharge to obtain biopsies from the ulcer
D. Oral PPI therapy for 4 weeks and repeat endoscopy to check for healing
E. Start IV PPI therapy for 72 hours, and octreotide IV infusion for 48 hours

44. An 81-year-old female presents to the emergency department for several episodes of bright red blood per rectum that started last night. Her medical history includes coronary disease, diabetes mellitus, peripheral artery disease. She takes metoprolol, aspirin, and metformin daily. She denies any abdominal pain. On arrival, she was tachycardic with heart rate of 115 bpm and blood pressure of 98/64 mm Hg. On exam, she had a nontender abdomen and blood in the rectal vault. Her hemoglobin is 7 g/dL. She is medically resuscitated and stabilized. Colonoscopy is performed and the following is noted in the sigmoid colon (see figure). What is the next step in the management?

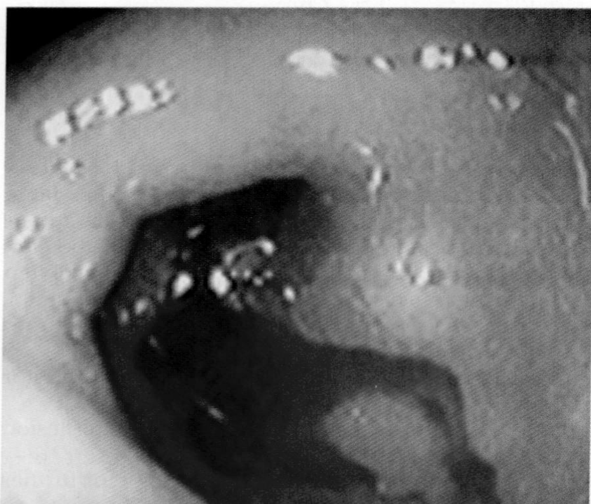

Figure for question 44.

A. Endoscopic therapy with epinephrine and hemoclip
B. Send patient to interventional radiology for embolization
C. Tattoo the bleeding area for future localization
D. Refer the patient to surgery
E. Transfuse the patient and watch as the bleeding will stop spontaneously

45. A 50-year-old male undergoes polypectomy for two polyps found during a screening colonoscopy. Three days later, he has three episodes of painless rectal bleeding and is seen in the emergency department. He receives fluid resuscitation and is admitted for repeat colonoscopy. Which of the following is a reported risk factor for postpolypectomy bleeding?
A. Polyp size of 1.5 cm
B. Pedunculated polyp
C. Polyp in the right colon
D. Ulcerated polyp
E. Previous history of postpolypectomy bleed

46. A 65-year-old woman presents to the hospital for a 3-day history of coffee-ground emesis. She usually takes ranitidine for chronic reflux symptoms and aspirin for peripheral vascular disease. After she is medically stabilized, endoscopy is performed and the following is noted in the antrum of the stomach (see figure). Which of the following is the most appropriate management?

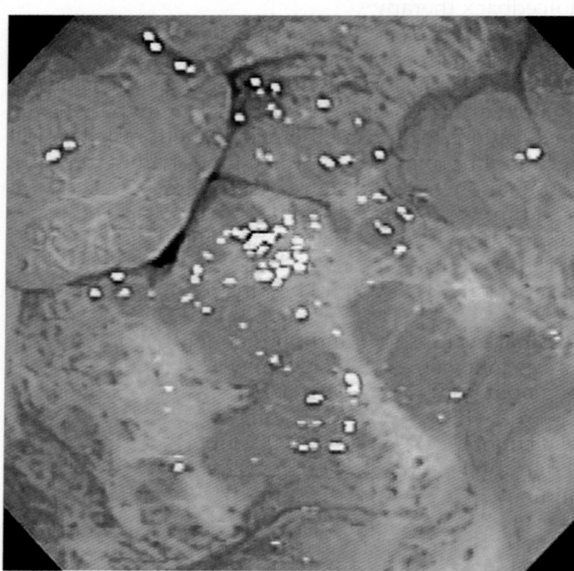

Figure for question 46.

A. Biopsy for *H. pylori* and check serum gastrin level
B. Endoscopic hemostasis with bipolar electrocautery
C. Endoscopic thermal therapy with argon plasma coagulator
D. Transjugular intrahepatic portovenous shunt (TIPS)
E. IV octreotide and start β-blockers at discharge

47. A 58-year-old woman presents with painless hematemesis and melena. She has the history of chronic knee pain and hypertension. Among her chronic medications are ibuprofen for knee pain and aspirin for coronary prophylaxis. The endoscopy findings are a gastric ulcer with a flat red spot. Of the following, the appropriate management is:
A. Triple therapy for *H. pylori* eradication and treatment with a proton pump inhibitor
B. Dual therapy endoscopic coagulation and observation in a monitored bed setting
C. Epinephrine injection and biopsy for malignancy
D. Stopping NSAIDs, biopsy for *H. pylori,* and early feeding
E. Discontinuation of ibuprofen and aspirin and discharge home

48. A 68-year-old woman comes to the emergency department with one episode of hematemesis and melena. Past history includes coronary artery disease, hypertension, and abdominal aortic aneurysm repair. She is on aspirin 81 mg once daily. On physical examination, her vital signs are as follows:

Temperature	37° C
Blood pressure	80/50 mm Hg
Heart rate	125 bpm
Respiratory rate	12 breaths/min

Her abdominal exam is soft and nontender. Laboratory values are as follows:

Hemoglobin	7.5 g/dL
WBC	8000/μL
Platelet count	200,000/μL
Total bilirubin	1.8 mg/dL
Creatinine	1.5 mg/dL
INR	1.4

An urgent EGD is performed and does not reveal a source of bleeding. What is the most appropriate next step?

A. Colonoscopy
B. Red blood cell tagged technetium scan
C. Angiography
D. Upper GI series with small bowel follow-through
E. Abdominal CT scan with IV contrast

49. A 55-year-old man comes to you with hematemesis and melena. He also complains of lightheadedness and nausea. A few weeks ago he presented to his gastroenterologist for evaluation of elevated liver enzymes, and a liver biopsy was performed 2 days prior to presentation. His past medical history is negative except lower back pain after a work-related lifting injury for which he had to take ibuprofen 800 mg three times daily. On physical examination, his vital signs are as follows:

Temperature	37° C
Blood pressure	95/55 mm Hg
Heart rate	110 bpm
Respiratory rate	12 breaths/min

His abdomen is soft with moderate tenderness in the epigastrium. Laboratory values are as follows:

Hemoglobin	8.5 g/dL
WBC	7000/μL
Platelet count	240,000/μL
Total bilirubin	3.3 mg/dL
ALT	60 U/L
AST	89 U/L
Creatinine	1.2 mg/dL
INR	1.2

You perform an upper endoscopy and note the following finding in the duodenum (see figure). What is the next best step in the management?

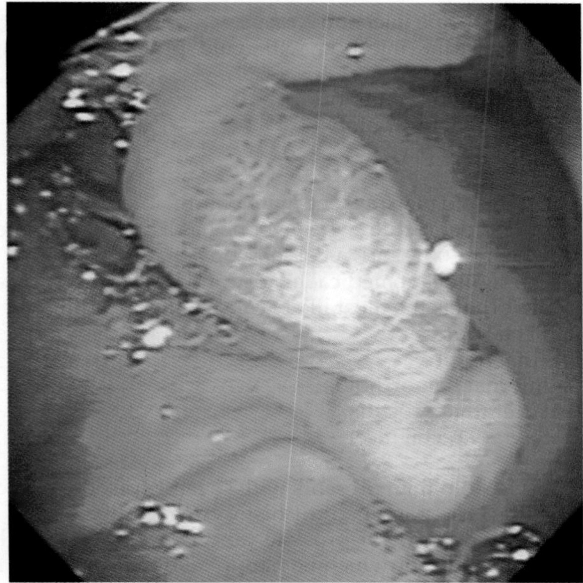

Figure for question 49.

A. Injection with epinephrine
B. Arterial embolization
C. Endoscopic thermal ablation monotherapy
D. Dual endoscopic thermal ablation therapy
E. Refer the patient to surgery

50. A 58-year-old woman presents to the emergency department with light-headedness and a history of several bloody bowel movements over the past 24 hours. She denies any abdominal pain. She is hypotensive and anemic. Resuscitative measures are instituted. Both the upper endoscopy and colonoscopy are not diagnostic, but she continues to pass clots per rectum. Her hematocrit is 33%. What is the most effective management strategy?

A. Capsule endoscopy
B. Abdominal CT scan with contrast
C. Scintigraphy and angiography
D. MRI
E. Emergency surgery

51. A 70-year-old healthy woman with a history of duodenal ulcer is placed on low-dose aspirin for coronary prophylaxis. Two weeks later, she presents to the emergency department with one episode of melena and lightheadedness. On physical examination, she has a normal blood pressure and resting heart rate of 90 bpm without orthostatic changes. Melena is confirmed on rectal exam. Her admission hematocrit is 36%. She is placed on high-dose proton pump inhibitor therapy (omeprazole 40 mg twice daily). Because of other complications, endoscopy is not performed until the tenth hospital day, and it shows a small (5 mm) duodenal ulcer with a clean base. Serum antibody test is negative for *H. pylori*. Which of the following should be performed now?

A. Stop proton pump inhibitor therapy and switch to an H_2 receptor antagonist
B. Treat with IV proton pump inhibitor for 72 hours
C. Treat empirically with antibiotics for *H. pylori*
D. Continue high-dose proton pump inhibitor and perform another test to exclude *H. pylori*
E. Obtain serum gastrin level to exclude Zollinger-Ellison syndrome

52. An 87-year-old, debilitated woman presents with severe hematochezia requiring 4 units of blood. Colonoscopy demonstrates fresh blood in the left colon with marked diverticulosis. The right colon is normal without blood in the lumen. Upon withdrawal of the colonoscope, there was active oozing of blood from the neck of a diverticulum in the distal sigmoid colon. The most appropriate management now is:

A. Supportive care with transfusion requirements as necessary
B. Technetium-labeled red blood cell scan
C. Angiography
D. Endoscopic clipping of the bleeding diverticulum
E. Immediate surgical therapy

53. A 51-year-old woman undergoes index screening colonoscopy with removal of two, 2 cm polyps. Ten days later she has rectal bleeding with dizziness. Colonoscopy reveals what is pictured in the figure. What is the next step?

A. Epinephrine injection
B. Endoclip with or without epinephrine injection
C. Thermal coagulation
D. Refer to surgery
E. Conservative management

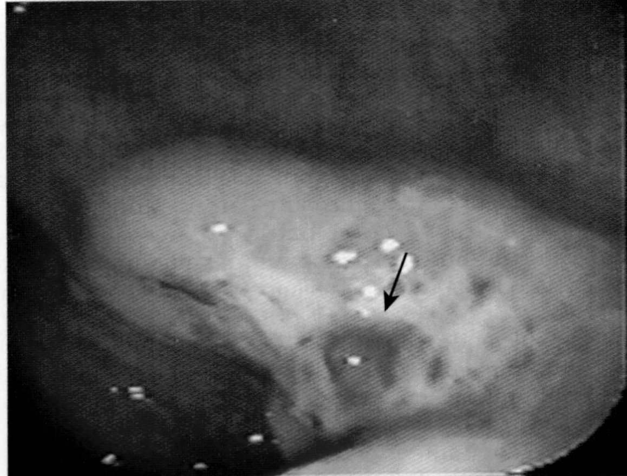

Figure for question 53.

54. A 71-year-old woman presents to the emergency department with abdominal pain and three episodes of rectal bleeding. Her past medical history is positive for diabetes and 2 weeks ago she was admitted to the hospital with pneumonia and septic shock. She reports that 6 months ago she had a screening colonoscopy, which did not reveal any polyps, and was told to repeat the test in 5 years. Her medications include methotrexate, metformin, aspirin 81 mg daily, and ibuprofen 400 mg three times daily. On physical examination, her vital signs are as follows:

Temperature	37° C
Blood pressure	80/55 mm Hg
Heart rate	118 bpm
Respiratory rate	14 breaths/min

Her abdominal exam is soft and nontender. Laboratory values are as follows:

Hemoglobin	8 g/dL
WBC	9000/μL
Platelet count	195,000/μL
Total bilirubin	1.9 mg/dL
Creatinine	1.8 mg/dL
INR	1.3

She is resuscitated and prepared for colonoscopy. Which of the following is the most likely endoscopic finding?

A. Large, friable mass in the ascending colon
B. Left-sided ulcerative colitis to the splenic flexure
C. Isolated visible vessel in the transverse colon
D. Pandiverticulosis
E. Focal colitis at the splenic flexure

55. A 30-year-old man with a 6-year history of pancolitis secondary to ulcerative colitis presents to you with 2 weeks of increasing rectal bleeding and diarrhea. The blood is red and mixed with the stool. His disease had previously been in steroid-free remission for 3 years on maintenance dose of oral mesalamine. He is hemodynamically stable at this visit. In addition to evaluating for progression of disease, what is the most important test to perform?

A. Stool testing for *Clostridium difficile*
B. Stool testing for *H. pylori*
C. CT scan of the abdomen
D. Stool testing for occult blood
E. Upper endoscopy

56. A 55-year-old man presents to the emergency department with hematemesis and melena. He takes ibuprofen 400 mg three times daily as needed for lower back pain. On physical examination, his blood pressure is 100/50 mm Hg and heart rate is 105 bpm. His abdomen is soft with tenderness in the epigastric area. Laboratory values are as follows:

Hemoglobin	6.8 g/dL
WBC	8000/μL
Total bilirubin	2.0 g/dL
Platelet count	150,000/μL

The patient is placed on omeprazole IV drip and receives 2 units of packed red blood cells. His vital signs stabilize and repeat hemoglobin is 8.8 g/dL. An upper endoscopy is performed and an ulcer is seen in the duodenal bulb (see figure). Which of the following is the most appropriate endoscopic management?

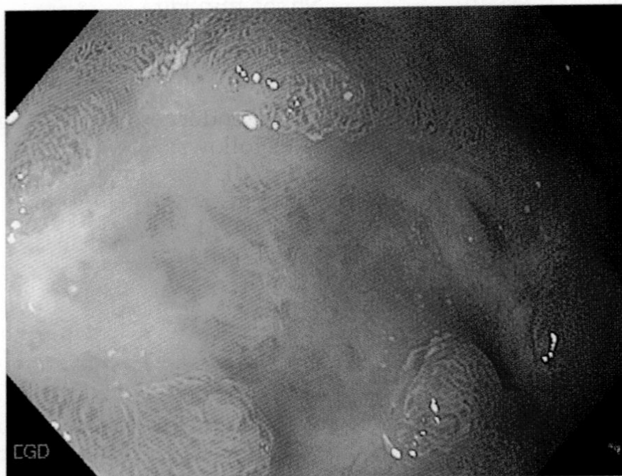

Figure for question 56.

A. Epinephrine injection
B. Epinephrine injection with gold probe thermocoagulation
C. Endoclip placement
D. Duodenal ulcer biopsy
E. Gastric biopsy

57. A 55-year-old man presents with painful intermittent bright red blood per rectum whenever he has a bowel movement. One year ago he had a colonoscopy that was normal. He has no significant medical history and his hemoglobin is 14 g/dL. What is the most likely cause of his bleeding?

A. Rectal varices
B. Anal fissure
C. Internal hemorrhoids
D. Ulcerative proctitis
E. Solitary rectal ulcer

58. A 70-year-old man presents with several episodes of rectal bleeding. His past medical history is negative except for radiation therapy for prostate cancer 2 years ago. He has low back pain for which he had to take ibuprofen 800 mg three times daily. A flexible sigmoidoscopy is performed and the following is noted in the rectum (see figure). What is the most likely etiology of the suspected lower gastrointestinal hemorrhage?

A. Ulcerative colitis
B. Radiation proctitis
C. Rectal varices

D. Solitary rectal ulcer
E. Rectal ischemia

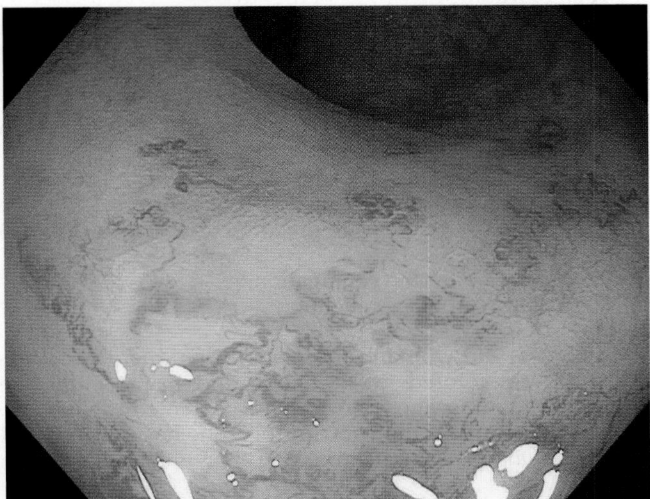

Figure for question 58.

59. Which of the following statements is true about gastric antral vascular ectasia (GAVE)?
A. GAVE is reversed with *H. pylori* treatment
B. Mucosal biopsies can differentiate between portal hypertensive gastropathy and GAVE
C. The majority of cases of GAVE are associated with cirrhosis
D. Bleeding from GAVE can be treated with transjugular intrahepatic portosystemic shunt (TIPS)
E. Bleeding from GAVE can be treated by β-blockers

60. A 75-year-old man presents to the emergency department with multiple episodes of bright red blood per rectum. He reports being constipated for the past 3 months and having to use suppositories and enemas to have bowel movements. He has a history of Parkinson's disease and hypertension. One week prior to presentation he was admitted to the hospital for treatment of pneumonia. His medications are aspirin 81 mg and carbidopa/levodopa. On physical examination, his vital signs are as follows:

Temperature	37° C
Blood pressure	90/60 mm Hg
Heart rate	130 bpm
Respiratory rate	12 breaths/min

His abdominal exam is soft and nontender. Laboratory values are as follows:

Hemoglobin	10 g/dL
WBC	7000/μL
Platelet count	190,000/μL
Total bilirubin	1.8 mg/dL
Creatinine	1.5 mg/dL
INR	1.3

The patient is admitted and a colonoscopy is performed the next day. What is the most likely finding on colonoscopy?
A. Rectal varices
B. Anal fissure
C. Internal hemorrhoids
D. Colonic angiectasia
E. Rectal ulcer

61. A 61-year-old woman presents to the emergency department with a 1-day history of retching and hematemesis. She has a history of chronic alcohol intake abuse. On physical examination, her vital signs are as follows:

Temperature	37° C
Blood pressure	110/65 mm Hg
Heart rate	90 bpm
Respiratory rate	14 breaths/min

Her abdominal exam is soft and nontender. Laboratory values are as follows:

Hemoglobin	8 g/dL
WBC	7000/μL
Platelet count	90,000/μL
Bilirubin	3 mg/dL
INR	1.4

She is started on omeprazole drip, octreotide drip, and antibiotics. An endoscopy is performed and a lesion is found in the distal esophagus (see figure). Which of the following is the most appropriate management?

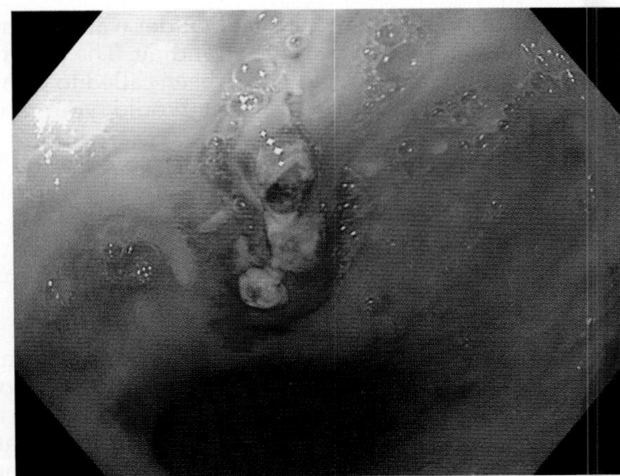

Figure for question 61.

A. Epinephrine injection
B. Epinephrine injection and endoclips placement
C. Epinephrine injection and gold probe thermocoagulation
D. Band ligation
E. Mucosal biopsy

62. A 35-year-old woman presents to the emergency department with intermittent melena for the past 4 months. She reports that she has a history of hematochezia for which she was admitted to another hospital 2 months ago. During that hospitalization, she received blood transfusions and underwent colonoscopy and upper endoscopy without finding a cause of bleeding. She denies abdominal pain, weight loss, diarrhea, or fevers. Today, on physical examination, her vital signs are as follows:

Temperature	37° C
Blood pressure	110/55 mm Hg
Heart rate	90 bpm
Respiratory rate	14 breaths/min

Her abdominal exam is soft. Laboratory values are as follows:

Hemoglobin	9 g/dL
WBC	16,000/μL
Total bilirubin	3.0 mg/dL

A repeat upper endoscopy and colonoscopy do not reveal a cause of bleeding. Which of the following is the most common cause of GI bleeding in this patient?
- **A.** Small bowel tumor
- **B.** Angiectasia
- **C.** Meckel's diverticulum
- **D.** Peptic ulcer disease
- **E.** Small bowel Crohn's disease

63. A 67-year-old woman in the intensive care unit has been intubated for 10 days with a multifocal pneumonia. She requires multiple vasopressors to maintain her blood pressure at 80/50 mm Hg. She is febrile with a temperature of 39° C. Her abdominal exam reveals tenderness to palpation in the right upper quadrant. Laboratory values are as follows:

WBC	19,000 cells/μL
Neutrophils—bands	10%
Bilirubin	1.6 mg/dL
Alkaline phosphatase	176 U/L
AST	73 U/L
ALT	72 U/L

Abdominal ultrasound showed the gallbladder wall was thickened with noted pericholecystic stranding. The patient is started on antibiotics and you have been called to provide additional recommendations. What would you recommend for the patient at this point?
- **A.** CT scan with contrast of the abdomen/pelvis
- **B.** Emergent laparoscopic cholecystectomy
- **C.** Cholecystostomy tube placement
- **D.** Open cholecystectomy
- **E.** Continued conservative management with IV fluids and antibiotics

64. A 45-year-old obese woman presents with jaundice, intermittent right upper quadrant pain and low-grade fever over the past few months. Her symptoms began 4 days ago and are progressing gradually. Her pain begins approximately 30 minutes after eating and then subsides over a few hours. However, the pain has been constant over the last 4 days. She has a temperature of 39.4° C, scleral icterus, and right upper quadrant pain. Laboratory studies are as follows:

WBC	16,000/μL
AST	120 U/L
Alkaline phosphatase	400 U/L
Total bilirubin	4 mg/dL

Abdominal ultrasonography reveals cholelithiasis with a large stone in the cystic duct and a dilated common hepatic duct to 12 mm. The common bile duct has normal caliber. IV antibiotics are initiated and the endoscopic retrograde cholangiopancreatography (ERCP) reveals a smooth extrinsic compression of the common hepatic duct resulting in up-stream ductal dilation. The gallbladder did not fill with contrast. A bile duct stent is placed. Brushings of the stricture were negative. What is the next appropriate step in the management of this patient?
- **A.** Repeat ERCP in 3 months for stent
- **B.** Cholecystectomy
- **C.** Perform magnetic resonance cholangiopancreatography (MRCP)
- **D.** Perform an endoscopic ultrasound
- **E.** Perform a hepatobiliary (HIDA) scan

65. A 24-year-old man comes to his primary care physician for a routine physical exam. He has no past medical history and no recent illnesses. Physical exam is normal. Laboratory studies are as follows:

Total bilirubin	4 mg/dL
Direct bilirubin	0.7 mg/dL
ALT	35 U/L
AST	30 U/L

Which of the following is the pathophysiologic abnormality in this syndrome?
- **A.** Impaired canalicular export of conjugated bilirubin
- **B.** Mutation in the coding region of *UGT1A1*
- **C.** Increased bilirubin UDP-glucuronyltransferase (B-UGT) activity
- **D.** Impaired bilirubin conjugation
- **E.** Absent bilirubin conjugation

66. A 55-year-old woman presents with fatigue, icteric feature, light-colored greasy stool, and pruritus for the past 3 months ago. She has no past medical history. Family history is noncontributory. She has normal vital signs. On physical examination, her vital signs are as follows:

Temperature	37° C
Blood pressure	100/60 mm Hg
Heart rate	72 bpm
Respiratory rate	12/min

Physical exam shows mild hepatomegaly but no splenomegaly. Rectal examination shows guaiac-negative stool. Laboratory values are as follows:

Hemoglobin	9 g/dL
WBC	8000/μL
Platelet count	180,000/μL
Total bilirubin	1.7 mg/dL
Creatinine	1.5 mg/dL
INR	1.3

Serum IgM is elevated and additional studies show the presence of antimitochondrial antibodies. Which of the following is associated with this disease?
- **A.** Cholangiocarcinoma
- **B.** Cholangitis
- **C.** Hepatocellular cancer
- **D.** Acute hepatitis
- **E.** Markedly increased serum cholesterol

67. Which of the following areas in the brain is affected in irritable bowel syndrome?
- **A.** Post cingulate cortex
- **B.** Ventromedial prefrontal cortex
- **C.** Oribitofrontal cortex
- **D.** Dorsal anterior cingulate cortex (ACC)
- **E.** Hippocampus

68. Which of the following is appropriate in verbal and nonverbal behaviors that facilitate physician-patient communication?
- **A.** Using open-ended questions to test the hypothesis and close-ended to generate them
- **B.** Summarizing the patient's statements in a judgmental fashion
- **C.** Eliciting psychosocial information in a sensitive and nonthreatening way
- **D.** Avoid echoing and affirmative gestures
- **E.** Use of leading questions

69. Brain-gut communication involves several ascending and descending pathways. Which ascending tract

projects as third-order neurons to the primary somatosensory cortex thereby helping in the location and intensity of pain?
A. Spinomesencephalic tract
B. Spinothalamic tract
C. Spinoreticular tract
D. Reticulothalamic tract
E. Fibers from the perigenual anterior cingulate cortex (pACC)

70. Which statement can explain the effects of stress on gastrointestinal function?
A. Stress affects the mucosa to enhance proinflammatory cytokine production and mast cell activation and degranulation, particularly near enteric neurons, thereby leading to visceral sensitization
B. Stress reduces mucosal permeability due to strengthening of tight junctions, with an increase in bacterial translocation into the intestinal wall
C. Acute stress triggers the hypothalamic-pituitary axis, leading to increases in cortisol levels and activation of the autonomic nervous system, with increases in interleukin (IL)-5 and interferon (IFN)-γ
D. Stress cannot change the intestinal microflora composition
E. Decreased gastric motility and secretion were linked to feelings of anger, intense pleasure, or aggressive behavior toward others

71. Which statement is true regarding the factitious disorders and malingering illness?
A. They both are DSM-5 disorders *(Diagnostic and Statistical Manual of Mental Disorders-5)*
B. Factitious disorder has internal incentive but malingering illness has external incentives and the assumption of playing the sick role
C. They both need to be referred to health care provider
D. Malingering illness is associated with antisocial personality disorders
E. Factitious disorders have unintentional falsification but malingering has intentional production of symptoms and signs

72. Which of the following patients has the highest likelihood of having a subtle form of factitious disorder?
A. A 27-year-old male complaining of acute abdominal pain for 12-hour duration, no past medical history, no previous surgeries
B. A 40-year-old male nurse who complains of sharp radiating leg pain, this is his fourth admission with this type of pain
C. A 15-year-old boy with history of cocaine abuse complaining of chest pain, he has an abnormal electrogardiogram and cardiac markers
D. A 34-year-old nurse complaining of fatigue and vertigo with serum blood glucose of 45 mg/dL. She has had similar episodes before
E. A 40-year-old woman who is admitted with acute abdominal pain, she has a history of multiple abdominal surgeries, this is her fourth admission

73. Which of the following strategies is useful regarding confirmation of self-induced or factitious disease?
A. Referral to a tertiary center
B. Review previous biopsy slides, looking for foreign body material in wounds, melanosis coli, and other clues
C. Have patient's family observe the patient to detect tampering behavior
D. Search the patient's home
E. Ask the patient's colleagues and boss whether he/she has a personality disorder or psychiatric disease

74. A 34-year-old woman with a history significant for major depression presents to the emergency department for evaluation of anemia. This is her fifth visit to the emergency department in the past year. Each time she is evaluated for a sudden drop in hemoglobin by 1 to 2 g/dL. GI work-up with EGD, colonoscopy, and capsule endoscopy was previously performed and was unremarkable. Other work-up for anemia is also negative. On physical examination in the emergency department her vital signs are as follows:

Temperature	37° C
Heart rate	110 bpm
Blood pressure	110/60 mm Hg

She is well appearing but has a lot of scars on her hands and legs. Rectal exam reveals brown stool without blood. Laboratory testing reveals a hemoglobin of 11 g/dL. Which of the following is the most likely diagnosis?
A. Factitious disease
B. Anemia of chronic disease
C. Malingering disorder
D. Missed ulcer on EGD
E. Porphyria

ANSWERS

1. B (S&F ch11)
This patient has an acute sigmoid diverticulitis. Approximately 80% of affected patients are older than 50 years of age. Hinchey grading is used to grade the severity of diverticulitis on CT scan. Hinchey grade I diverticulitis (localized inflammation or pericolic abscess) necessitates admission to hospital with IV antibiotics. Outpatient management is suggested in patients with mild disease having no comorbid conditions, and with no CT findings of perforation. Patients with Hinchey grade II diverticulitis (pelvic, intraabdominal, or retroperitoneal abscess) should undergo CT-guided drainage of the abscess and receive a course of broad-spectrum intravenous antibiotics. Patients with Hinchey grade III (generalized purulent peritonitis) and grade IV (generalized fecal peritonitis) diverticulitis frequently require emergency surgery. Colonoscopy is contraindicated with acute diverticulitis.

2. A (S&F ch11)
This patient has an acute mesenteric ischemia (AMI). AMI can develop from embolic occlusion of mesenteric vessels or a thrombosis of mesenteric vessels. Acute mesenteric embolism, mesenteric thrombosis, and nonocclusive mesenteric ischemia each account for approximately one third of cases of acute mesenteric ischemia and have a combined mortality rate of 60% to 100%. The hallmark for the diagnosis is abrupt onset, cramping

pain in the epigastrium or periumbilical region and symptoms out of proportion to abdominal exam findings. CT scan of abdomen is the best initial diagnostic test of suspected AMI. Mesenteric angiography may be useful for determining the cause of intestinal ischemia and defining the extent of vascular disease. Patients with AMI can have melena from intestinal ischemia and an EGD is not indicated as a first step in this situation. Admission for observation is incorrect given high mortality with delayed diagnosis of AMI. An abdominal x-ray will not provide significant additional information to diagnose this condition.

3. **A** (S&F ch11)
This patient has a ruptured ectopic pregnancy. The patient's last menstrual period was 2 months ago and has a positive pregnancy test, which is confirmed by pelvic ultrasound findings. She has a history of chlamydia that puts her at risk for pelvic inflammatory disease and increased risk for ectopic pregnancy from tubal scarring. Patients with ruptured ectopic pregnancy have severe abdominal pain and a hemorrhagic shock from massive bleeding, with a rapid deterioration of clinical status as in this patient. Prompt resuscitation and surgery is indicated. All the other options provided do not have such a dramatic presentation. Acute cholecystitis presents with a right upper quadrant or epigastric pain. A right upper quadrant ultrasound or hepatobiliary (HIDA) scan provides accurate diagnosis. Acute pancreatitis usually presents with upper abdominal pain with radiation to the back. Acute hemorrhagic pancreatitis can present with hemodynamic instability but is not as dramatic as seen in ruptured ectopic pregnancy. Appendicitis and tubo-ovarian abscess can present with a similar pain pattern but this patient has a confirmed tubal pregnancy.

4. **C** (S&F ch12)
This patient's chronic abdominal pain is likely from anterior cutaneous nerve entrapment syndrome (ACNES). In ACNES, entrapment of a cutaneous branch of a sensory nerve from spinal levels T7 to T12 is the cause for abdominal wall pain. The nerve entrapment can occur from pressure of an intraabdominal or extraabdominal lesion or to another localized process like fibrosis or edema. Moreover, pain originating from the abdominal wall is discrete and localized, in contrast to pain originating from an intraabdominal source, which is diffuse and poorly localized. Patients are usually able to point out the site of pain. The Carnett sign is present (clinician will note increased localized tenderness to palpation when the patient tenses the abdominal muscles). For mild cases, nonsteroidal antiinflammatory drugs, heat therapy, and physiotherapy may be considered. In severe cases trigger point injection therapy with a local anesthetic, with or without a glucocorticoid, is recommended.

This patient's pain is not typical of biliary etiology and, moreover, she has no abnormality on imaging and her lab work is normal. ERCP with biliary manometry is not recommended. While laparoscopy is not a first step, in carefully selected patients with symptoms refractory to injection therapy, diagnostic laparoscopy with open exploration of abdominal trigger points may be beneficial. In one study, lysis of intraabdominal adhesions in close proximity to trigger points and subcutaneous nerve resection provided benefit. CT scan will not provide any further information. This patient does not meet the Rome III criteria for irritable bowel syndrome, and trigger point injection therapy may be helpful; therefore, not performing any further treatment is incorrect.

5. **B** (S&F ch12)
This patient has narcotic bowel syndrome, which is a clinical condition characterized by paradoxical increasing abdominal pain with escalating doses of narcotics. In one large case series, this condition was seen in well-educated young females. Patients usually have anxiety or depression and seek medical care frequently. Current understanding suggests that opioid-induced activation of central nervous system glial cells leads to production of inflammatory cytokines, which leads to a reduction in analgesia, tolerance to narcotics, and eventually unwanted hyperalgesia. Managing this patient population is a challenge for clinicians and enrollment in opioid detoxification is recommended. Irritable bowel syndrome is not the correct answer as the patient does not meet Rome III criteria and has worsening pain with narcotics. The patient's history and workup is not suggestive of Crohn's disease or celiac disease. Hirschsprung's disease is unlikely given the etiology of constipation likely related to narcotics.

6. **B** (S&F ch12)
This patient has a slipping rib syndrome, which is characterized by hypermobility of the costal cartilage at the anterior end of a false rib (rib 8, 9, or 10), with slipping of the affected rib behind the superior adjacent rib during contraction of the abdominal musculature, such as with inspiration. The mechanism of pain includes nerve entrapment or soft tissue inflammation. Hooking maneuver is positive, when the physician slides fingers beneath the lower ribs and moves the ribs anteriorly, eliciting pain. Initial treatment includes conservative measures. Costochondral nerve block or surgical rib resection may be required. HIDA scan, ERCP, and colonoscopy are not the correct answers as the patient's pain appears to be arising from the ribs. Laparoscopy with lysis of adhesions for chronic abdominal pain is a debated topic with conflicting results in patients with chronic abdominal pain, and it is not indicated for this patient with no history of surgery in the past.

7. **C** (S&F ch13)
This patient needs cardiac evaluation first to rule out cardiac etiology of chest pain. It is not uncommon, for patients as well as their health care providers, to have difficulty distinguishing chest pain of esophageal origin from angina pectoris. The esophagus and heart are anatomically adjacent and share innervation. In fact, once cardiac disease is excluded, esophageal disorders are probably the most common causes of chest pain. Clinical history alone does not suggest chest pain originating from esophagus. Indeed exercise can exacerbate gastroesophageal reflux disease (GERD) causing exertional dyspnea similar to angina pectoris. Moreover, nitroglycerin may help alleviate chest pain from either cause. Once cardiac causes of chest pain are ruled out, an EGD may be considered. There is no role for a CT of the abdomen in this scenario. Esophageal manometry along with ambulatory pH testing is indicated if the patient derives no benefit from appropriate proton pump inhibitor (PPI) therapy and neuromodulator medications. Chest pain may respond to PPI therapy even in patients with motility disorder.

8. **A** (S&F ch13)
This patient likely has pill-induced esophagitis from doxycycline. Tetracycline and its derivatives are some of the most commonly implicated medications. Odynophagia can cause a dull retrosternal ache on swallowing or a stabbing

pain with radiation to the back so severe the patient cannot eat or even swallow his or her own saliva. Infectious esophagitis is more likely in immunocompromised host and this patient does not have any known immunosuppressed state. History of gastroesophageal reflux disease (GERD) is seen in patients with peptic esophagitis. Esophageal cancer is very rare in this age group. However an EGD with biopsies is usually indicated to assess the cause of odynophagia and to rule out any esophageal mass.

9. B (S&F ch14)
This patient needs a prompt EGD. He has been taking NSAIDs, aspirin, and clopidrogel that put him at risk for peptic ulcer disease. In addition, new onset abdominal pain in an elderly patient, associated with early satiety, weight loss, and anemia is concerning for a cancer. A colonoscopy is indicated if EGD were normal. A CT scan will be indicated in the workup for identifying a cancer and for staging purposes if a cancer is found, but is not the next best step. Although *Helicobacter pylori (H. pylori)* is an important cause for peptic ulcer disease, testing antigen alone is incorrect. Doing no further workup is incorrect with many alarm features. Based on the American College of Gastroenterology guidelines, a prompt EGD for dyspepsia is indicated in patients more than 55 years of age, or those with alarm features like bleeding, anemia, early satiety, unexplained weight loss (>10% body weight), progressive dysphagia, odynophagia, persistent vomiting, a family history of gastrointestinal cancer, previous gastrointestinal malignancy, previous documented peptic ulcer, lymphadenopathy, or an abdominal mass.

10. B (S&F ch14)
This is a young patient with no alarm features. Based on Rome III criteria for dyspepsia, testing for *H. pylori* and treating accordingly would be the next step. Famotidine has been providing only partial benefit and is not the recommended treatment. An EGD is indicated if *H. pylori* is negative and the patient derived no benefit from acid suppressive therapy. Functional dyspepsia is a diagnosis of exclusion when no cause for abdominal pain in found after appropriate testing. A CT scan is not the first step in the work up of young patient with no alarm features.

11. A (S&F ch14)
This is a patient with functional dyspepsia. She had a normal EGD, including biopsies and normal abdominal imaging. Her symptoms have not subsided with acid suppressive therapy. In these cases, tricyclic antidepressants are commonly used if conventional approaches fail. The effects on dyspepsia appear to be independent of the presence of depression. Although antidepressants have been thought to decrease visceral sensitivity, no significant effects of antidepressants on visceral sensitivity have been established in functional dyspepsia. Some patients benefit by avoiding a high fat diet, spicy foods, and coffee (if causing symptoms). This patient has two normal EGDs and will not benefit from repeat endoscopy. Colonoscopy is not indicated with patient's symptoms. There is no indication for ERCP in this patient. This patient has long-standing, lifestyle-limiting symptoms and asking the patient not to worry about her symptoms is not the correct approach.

12. C (S&F ch14)
The presence of delayed gastric emptying in functional dyspepsia ranges from 20% to 50%. In a meta-analysis of 17 studies involving 868 dyspeptic patients and 397 controls, a significant delay in solid gastric emptying was present in almost 40% of patients with functional dyspepsia. However, studies failed to find a convincing relationship between delayed gastric emptying and the pattern of symptoms.

13. C (S&F ch14)
This patient has functional dyspepsia. Rome III criteria include one or more of the following:
1. Bothersome postprandial fullness
2. Early satiation
3. Epigastric pain
4. Epigastric burning

In addition, there should be no evidence of structural disease (including at EGD) that is likely to explain the symptoms. Patient has a history of hypothyroidism and bloating; however, duodenal biopsies are normal. The patient did not benefit from gluten-free diet. Celiac disease is unlikely to be the cause of her symptoms. Epidemiologic studies have shown no association between dyspeptic symptoms and gallstones. The clinical presentation of biliary colic is easily distinguishable from that of dyspepsia. A cholecystectomy should not be suggested for dyspepsia alone. This patient does not meet criteria for irritable bowel syndrome with no bowel issues. Chronic pancreatitis is unlikely the underlying diagnosis with this clinical presentation.

14. B (S&F ch15)
This patient has cyclical vomiting syndrome (CVS). The Rome III Consensus Committee's definition of cyclic vomiting syndrome requires three or more discrete episodes of vomiting (with no apparent explanation) during the preceding year. CVS can occur at any age, but it is more common in children. There is no gender predilection. A personal or family history of migraine is supportive of CVS. There is an association between marijuana use and CVS, and there are reports of improvement with discontinuing marijuana. Treatment is conservative during the episodes, consisting of avoiding dehydration and electrolyte disturbances. Antiemetics have some benefit. There is no specific medication approved for CVS, and this condition may spontaneously subside after many years. The patient does not have a history suggestive of eating disorder or psychiatric illness; thus, bulimia nervosa is not the correct answer. He had an extensive work up to rule out Crohn's disease; specifically no small bowel disease was seen. Consensus criteria for functional vomiting by the Rome III Consensus Committee on Functional Gastrointestinal Disorders include one or more episodes of vomiting per week for 3 months, with the onset of symptoms at least 6 months prior to diagnosis. Eating disorders, rumination, self-induced vomiting, major psychiatric disorders, chronic cannabinoid use, and organic causes of vomiting (i.e., with a definable structural or physiologic basis) should be excluded.

15. D (S&F ch15)
This patient has superior mesenteric artery (SMA) syndrome, which is a rare condition caused by increased acute angulation between the aorta and SMA causing partial duodenal obstruction. Patients with functional or cyclical vomiting syndrome are often inappropriately labeled with SMA syndrome. Precipitating factors include weight loss, lordosis, loss of abdominal muscle tone, and surgery with prolonged bed rest. Symptoms

include middle abdominal discomfort, postprandial nausea and bilious vomiting as obstruction is distal to ampulla of Vater. Some patients adapt a knee-chest or prone position for relief. Diagnosis is usually made with upper GI barium contrast study or CT of the abdomen showing dilation and stasis proximal to the duodenum where the SMA crosses it. A nasojejunal tube placed distal to the obstruction provides symptomatic relief. Laparoscopic proximal duodenal jejunostomy is the preferred treatment.

SBE is not the preferred test. This patient has needed multiple hospitalizations; thus, not performing appropriate work-up is incorrect. Work-up for structural causes is not complete; thus, referral for psychological assessment is not appropriate. Patient had a normal 4-hour gastric emptying study; repetitive testing is of no further benefit.

16. D (S&F ch15)
This patient has hyperemesis gravidarum, which is a condition associated with unusually severe nausea and vomiting, which can lead to complications like malnutrition, dehydration, Mallory-Weiss tears, and electrolyte disturbances. Multiparous and obese women are at increased risk. It represents an exaggerated form of nausea and vomiting associated with pregnancy. Hormonal, psychological factors, and hyperthyroidism are thought to contribute to this condition. Symptoms usually develop in first trimester and may continue to other trimesters. Some patients will require hospitalization for fluid and electrolyte management along with antiemetics. Small frequent meals with low fat and high protein are suggested. This condition is not associated with an increased risk of toxemia of pregnancy or spontaneous abortion, and may be associated with low fetal weight at term.

17. C (S&F ch16)
Microscopic colitis is frequently seen in middle-aged women. They often have a history of nonsteroidal anti-inflammatory drug use, associated autoimmune diseases like arthritis, and hypothyroidism. Both celiac disease and microscopic colitis are linked with human leukocyte antigen (HLA)-DQ2 and HLA-DQ1,3 (including the HLA-DQ1,3 subtypes HLA-DQ1,7, HLADQ1,8, and HLA-DQ1,9) suggesting the possibility that the immune mechanisms involved in the pathogenesis of microscopic colitis and celiac disease are similar. In addition, microscopic colitis has been associated with celiac disease and may be a cause of persistent diarrhea in patients with celiac disease who are treated with a gluten-free diet. A colonoscopy with biopsies is the next step in evaluating such cases.

This patient is on a gluten-free diet and has negative serology, endoscopy, and biopsies for celiac disease. She had a normal colonoscopy; thus, ulcerative colitis is not the correct answer. The patient does not meet Rome III criteria for irritable bowel syndrome, with no abdominal discomfort. Laxative abuse is not the correct option prior to work-up ruling out organic causes.

18. A (S&F ch16)
This patient has osmotic diarrhea from carbohydrate malabsorption. Stool osmotic gap is calculated by subtracting twice the sum of sodium and potassium concentration from 290 mOsm/kg. Small osmotic gap (<50 mOsm/kg) is suggestive of secretory diarrhea, whereas a large (>100 mOsm/kg) osmotic gap is suggestive of osmotic diarrhea. In this patient, the osmotic gap is high at 140 mOsm/kg and the pH is low at 5 pointing to carbohydrate malabsorption. Sugars and sugar alcohols are the other major category of substances that cause osmotic diarrhea, which results from either malabsorption or lack of nutrient transporter. The most common clinical syndrome of disaccharidase deficiency is acquired lactase deficiency, which accounts for lactose intolerance in many adults. All the other answer options provided cause secretory diarrhea.

19. A (S&F ch16)
Conjugated bile acids reaching the colon inhibit electrolyte absorption and stimulate secretion of water by the colonic mucosa. Malabsorption of bile salts is seen with ileal disease or resection, allowing excessive amounts of conjugated bile acid to enter the colon. In patients with suspected bile acid diarrhea, a trial of bile acid binding resins should be considered. This patient has well-controlled Crohn's disease on infliximab. Neuroendocrine tumor is unlikely; however, bile acid diarrhea should be considered and treated first. The patient's diarrhea has been affecting his lifestyle; thus, not treating further is not the correct option.

20. C (S&F ch16)
This patient has features suggestive of reactive amyloidosis based on his cardiac biopsy. He has all the classic physical findings of amyloidosis, including macroglossia, pinch purpura, and hepatomegaly. Reactive amyloidosis is seen in patients with rheumatoid arthritis, psoriasis/ankylosing spondylosis, inflammatory bowel disease, and familial Mediterranean fever. Patients with gastrointestinal amyloidosis have diarrhea from many causes, including malabsorption caused by mucosal infiltration by amyloid, gastrointestinal dysmotility caused by amyloid protein infiltrating neuromuscular tissue, and stasis from dysmotility leading to small intestinal bacterial overgrowth. Patients have bloating, diarrhea, excessive gas, and early satiety as associated symptoms. Diagnosis of GI amyloidosis is made by duodenal or rectal biopsies. Acute bacterial infections and smooth muscle hyperactivity are not causes of diarrhea specific to amyloidosis. Activation of cyclic GMP is a cause of secretory diarrhea from various causes; for example, *Escherichia coli* heat-stable enterotoxin interacts with the guanylate cyclase C receptor on the luminal side of the enterocyte.

21. B (S&F ch17)
The diffusivity of a gas across the mucosa of the GI tract depends on its solubility in water. For a given partial pressure, carbon dioxide diffuses faster than other gases in the GI tract. H_2 and CH_4 absorbed from the GI tract are not metabolized by humans and are excreted in the expired air. This forms the basis for end alveolar testing of H_2 and CH_4 levels in breath testing for bacterial overgrowth.

22. A (S&F ch17)
Lactose intolerance is the most likely cause of this patient's foul smelling gas. Most adults malabsorb lactose because of a genetically programmed reduction in lactase synthesis. Diagnosis is established by avoiding milk products to observe the difference. Celiac disease is less likely given no response to gluten-free diet and can be considered if avoiding lactose does not improve symptoms. Severe flatulence secondary to air swallowing has been reported, but it is very rare. Belching is more often seen with excess air swallowing. Sorbitol is a low calorie sugar substitute with poor absorption and bacteria in the colon ferment this compound causing flatulence. In patients with functional

flatulence (i.e., no demonstrable intestinal absorptive defect), gas production can be effectively reduced by a low-flatulogenic diet.

23. D (S&F ch18)
Elderly patients are at risk for fecal incontinence. This patient may have impaired rectal sensation due to neurologic damage from poorly controlled diabetes. This could lead to accumulation of stool in the rectum and fecal impaction. Similarly, hard stools due to narcotic use can worsen constipation and fecal impaction. She does not have abdominal pain, which makes irritable bowel syndrome unlikely.

24. C (S&F ch18)
Colonoscopy with colonic biopsies is warranted as a first next step in evaluation of this patient with incontinence as a result of severe diarrhea. She is at risk for microscopic colitis given her age and selective serotonin reuptake inhibitor (SSRI) use. Inflammatory bowel disease is also a possibility. Anorectal manometry, endosonography, defecography testing, and MRI for pelvic anatomy would investigate anal and pelvic floor abnormalities; however, this would be premature at this stage because her incontinence is related to a change in stool consistency or diarrhea.

25. E (S&F ch18)
This patient most likely has a sphincter defect or weakness due to injury from prior vaginal deliveries and/or surgical hemorrhoidectomy. In order to diagnose this condition, anorectal manometry and anal endosonography are indicated. The quality of evidence for the usefulness of both of these tests is good. MRI and defecography are also useful as adjuncts to other tests as the quality of evidence for the usefulness of these tests is fair. Barium enema can provide evidence of structural lesion but its utility in evaluating ano-rectal dysfuction is limited.

26. C (S&F ch18)
Neuromuscular training, most commonly performed with biofeedback therapy and Kegel exercises, is the most appropriate next step in management (see figure). This has been shown to improve fecal incontinence using a repeated training and feedback to reinforce learning of improved coordination, anorectal perception, and to strengthen the anal sphincter. All the other therapies, including surgical repair, injection of a sphincter-bulking agent, and sacral nerve stimulation, may be effective therapies, but can be reserved as second line treatment due to their more invasive nature. Colostomy is a last resort in patients with incontinence.

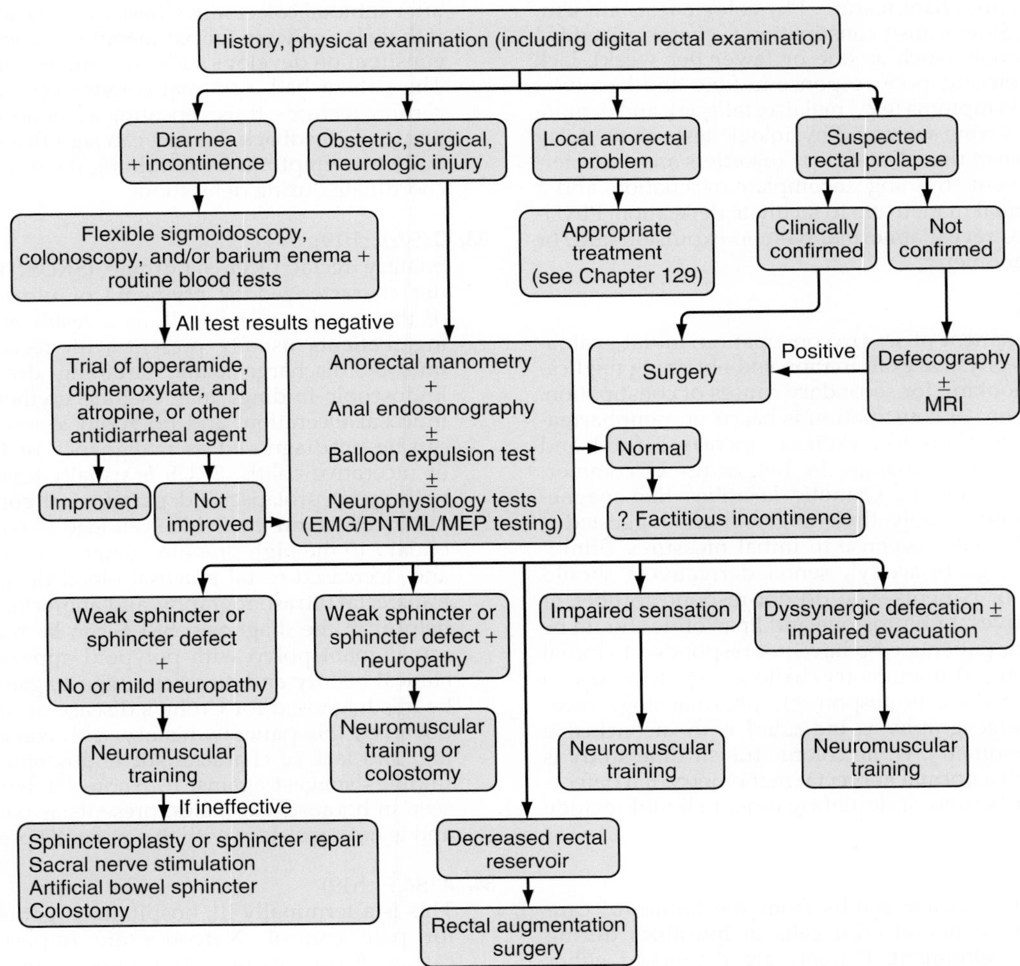

Figure for answer 26.

27. B (S&F ch18)
The correct answer is loperamide. There is evidence in controlled trials that this therapy, as well as diphenoxylate and atropine sulfate, is effective for reducing incontinence. Due to the side effect profile, sedation in the case of tincture of opium, and ischemic colitis and severe constipation in the case of alosetron, these two medications are not good choices for first-line therapy. Docusate and magnesium citrate are laxatives, and since there is no suggestion of fecal impaction in this case, these would not be appropriate therapies and would likely make her condition worse.

28. A (S&F ch19)
Advanced age is a known risk factor for constipation. Female gender, low levels of income and education, nonwhite ethnicity, and a low level of physical activity are risk factors for constipation in the United States. Diet, life style, medications (e.g., nonsteroidal antiinflammatory drugs, acetaminophen), and some medical disorders also play a role in development of constipation.

29. A (S&F ch19)
Constipation can be functional (primary disorder of colon or rectum) or secondary to a systemic illness or medication. Functional constipation is divided into normal transit constipation, slow transit constipation, and defecatory disorder. Normal transit constipation is characterized by incomplete evacuation; abdominal pain may be present but not a predominant feature. Physiologic tests are usually normal. Slow transit constipation is characterized by: Infrequent stools (such as one or fewer per week), lack of urge to defecate, poor response to fiber and laxatives, generalized symptoms (e.g., malaise, fatigue), and is more prevalent in young women. Physiologic tests show delay in colonic transit time. Defecatory disorders are characterized by frequent straining, incomplete evacuation, and a need for manual maneuvers to facilitate defecation. Physiologic studies reveal abnormal balloon expulsion and/or anorectal manometry.

30. A (S&F ch19)
In the management of severe constipation, initial evaluation includes physical examination and obtaining medication history looking for secondary causes of constipation. Initial treatment of constipation is based on nonpharmacologic interventions like exercise, increased fluid and fiber intake through changes in diet, or use of commercial fiber supplements. Osmotic laxatives like magnesium hydroxide or polyethylene glycol are suggested if there is inadequate response to initial measures. Stimulant agents (e.g., bisacodyl, senna derivatives) should be reserved for patients who do not respond to fiber or osmotic laxatives. Lubiprostone and linaclotide should be considered for patients who have not responded to initial therapy. Anorectal manometry/balloon expulsion test is performed if there is no response to pharmacologic measures. MR defecography is indicated with inconclusive anorectal manometry, while colonic transit time study is indicated with a normal anorectal manometry. If a defecatory disorder is present, initial treatment should include biofeedback.

31. A (S&F ch19)
Hirschsprung's disease results from the failure of caudal migration of neural crest cells in intestines during embryonic development. Patients are diagnosed either early in life with delayed passage of meconium, or later in life with constipation that develops due to a short segment of involved colon. Absence of rectoanal inhibitory reflex on anorectal manometry raises the possibility of Hirschsprung's disease. A high resting anal pressure is seen in the presence of an anal fissure or anismus (paradoxical contraction of the external anal sphincter in response to straining or pressure within the anal canal). Rectal hyposensitivity suggests a neurologic disorder. Inappropriate contraction of the anal sphincter while bearing down is seen in patients with defecatory disorder. Inability to expel the balloon in nonspecific but suggests a defecatory disorder.

32. C (S&F ch19)
This patient has pelvic dyssynergia or functional anorectal outlet obstruction. During normal defecation there is an increase in rectal pressure accompanied by contraction of puborectalis sling, which narrows the anorectal angle; subsequent relaxation of anal sphincter muscles allows evacuation of bowels. In pelvic dyssynergia there is paradoxical contraction of the anal sphincter when patients bear down, which leads to difficulty in evacuation of bowels. If a defecatory disorder is present, initial treatment should include biofeedback; up to 75% of patients with disordered evacuation respond to biofeedback, and many do not respond well to fiber supplementation or oral laxatives.

A subtotal colectomy is usually the last resort in patients with slow transit constipation and not with pelvic dyssynergia. Indeed some patients with pelvic dyssynergia, having a wrong diagnosis, end up with constipation after subtotal colectomy. Chest x-ray should be considered if there is a concern for paraneoplastic constipation, where constipation develops suddenly and is not a chronic issue. The patient had a normal colonoscopy and has no concerning features; thus, repeating a colonoscopy is inappropriate. Biofeedback therapy can significantly improve the patient's symptoms by retraining the muscles to properly coordinate during defecation.

33. C (S&F ch19)
Solitary rectal ulcer syndrome (SRUS) is a rare disorder characterized by erythema or ulceration, generally of the anterior rectal wall, as a result of chronic straining. Patients usually present with rectal bleeding and mucous discharge while straining during defecation. Endoscopic findings may include erythema, hyperemia, mucosal ulceration, and polypoid lesions. These lesions can be misdiagnosed as malignancy or Crohn's disease or ulcerative colitis. SRUS is usually seen in association with rectal prolapse and paradoxical contraction of the puborectalis muscle, which can lead to rectal trauma secondary to the high pressure generated within the rectum and decreased rectal mucosal blood flow. Defecography, transrectal ultrasonography, and anorectal manometry are helpful in the diagnosis. SRUS can be misdiagnosed for a malignant polyp with polypoid appearance; however, clinical history and biopsies suggest against it. SRUS can be misdiagnosed for Crohn's disease or ulcerative colitis; however, this patient's history with constipation, straining, and lack of characteristic endoscopic and histologic findings suggest against it. Anorectal syphilis is usually seen in homosexual males, presents as painless chancres, and is not consistent with this patient's presentation.

34. A (S&F ch19)
This is a terminally ill, hospitalized patient on narcotics for pain control. Narcotics are important secondary causes of constipation. Methylnaltrexone is a peripherally acting μ-opioid receptor antagonist approved by the FDA in 2008 for the treatment of opioid-induced

constipation in patients with a late-stage advanced illness. The FDA approved linaclotide in 2012 for the treatment of men and women with chronic constipation. Lubiprostone was approved for the treatment of chronic idiopathic constipation for men and women in the United States and women with irritable bowel sydrome with constipation predominance. Alvimopan is another μ-opioid receptor antagonist approved by the FDA to accelerate bowel recovery following surgery, but not for opioid-induced constipation. Tegaserod has been withdrawn from market due to cardiovascular safety concerns. It was approved for chronic constipation and had also been used in women with irritable bowel syndrome with constipation predominance.

35. B (S&F ch19)
Linaclotide is a minimally absorbed 14–amino acid peptide that activates the guanylate cyclase C receptor on the luminal surface of the intestinal epithelium, resulting in increased levels of cyclic guanosine monophosphate (cGMP) and increased secretion of chloride and bicarbonate into the intestinal lumen. Lubiprostone activates the intestinal chloride 2 channels, thereby increasing intestinal fluid secretion and transit. Peripherally acting opioid antagonists like methylnaltrexone have been shown to reverse opioid-induced bowel dysfunction without reversing analgesia or precipitating central nervous system withdrawal signs. 5-Hydroxytryptamine-4 (5-HT-4) receptor agonists like tegaserod stimulate afferent nerves in the wall of the GI tract, inducing peristaltic contraction of the intestine. Elobixibat (A3309) is a novel investigational, minimally absorbed, ileal bile acid-transporter inhibitor that increases the flow of bile into the colon.

36. A (S&F ch19)
According to the American College of Gastroenterology Chronic Constipation Task Force, PEG and lactulose have grade A evidence for treatment of chronic constipation. Stool softeners, stimulant laxatives, and bulking agents (psyllium and calcium polycarbophil) have grade B evidence for treatment of chronic constipation (i.e., based on evidence from a single RCT of high quality or conflicting results from high-quality RCTs or two or more RCTs of lesser quality). Lubiprostone and linaclotide are not yet graded.

37. B (S&F ch19)
This patient has a rectocele that has been causing severe constipation. A rectocele is the bulging or displacement of the rectum through a defect in the anterior rectal wall. Damage to the rectovaginal septum or its supporting structures during vaginal childbirth have been implicated in the pathogenesis of rectocele. Rectoceles can cause inability to complete fecal evacuation, perineal pain, sensation of local pressure, and appearance of a bulge at the vaginal opening on straining. Affected patients report the need to apply pressure to the posterior vaginal wall to complete defecation. Women may also report the need to use a finger to digitally evacuate the rectum. Kegel exercises are suggested for asymptomatic women, and instructions to avoid repetitive increases in intraabdominal pressure may help prevent progression of the rectocele. Surgery should be considered only for patients in whom contrast is retained during defecography and patients in whom constipation is relieved with digital vaginal pressure to facilitate defecation. Endoscopic ultrasound is used for evaluation of anal sphincters with incontinence and not for constipation. Biofeedback is suggested for pelvic dyssynergia and not for rectocele. This patient has a defecatory disorder and will not benefit from linaclotide.

38. D (S&F ch20)
The patient is likely bleeding from peptic ulcer disease secondary to her risk factors, including age, nonsteroidal antiinflammatory drugs, and aspirin. Treatment with PPI prior to endoscopy accelerates the healing of ulcers and reduces the need for endoscopic therapy. None of the other benefits listed in the question are proven benefits of PPI prior to endoscopy.

39. D (S&F ch20)
The patient is likely bleeding from peptic ulcer disease secondary to his risk factors, including nonsteroidal antiinflammatory drugs and aspirin. IV erythromycin has been shown to improve visualization and decrease the need for a second endoscopy, and is recommended in the most recent American College of Gastroenterology guideline on upper GI bleeding. Alternatives that could also improve visualization are IV metoclopramide or nasogastric suction. There is no suspicion of cirrhosis in this patient despite history of hepatitis C, which was successfully treated. Therefore, octreotide is not appropriate at this time. While it is appropriate to correct the elevated INR, there is no proof that this improves outcomes. As long as the INR is <2.5, endoscopy should not be delayed solely for the purpose of correcting the INR. Treatment with a PPI prior to endoscopy accelerates the healing of ulcers and reduces the need for endoscopic therapy, but is not proven to decrease re-bleeding rates, need for surgery, or mortality. There is no proof that an IV PPI drip is superior to IV twice daily dosing. Studies have shown that a restrictive transfusion strategy (with transfusion only if hemoglobin <7 g/dL) improves outcomes of rebleeding and mortality, compared to a liberal transfusion strategy. Therefore, in patients without massive bleeding or cardiac disease, the recommended transfusion threshold is 7 g/dL.

40. A (S&F ch20)
About 50% of the admissions for GI bleed are for upper GI bleeding, 40% for lower GI bleeding, and 10% for bleeding from the small intestine (obscure bleeding).

41. C (S&F ch20)
This patient is presenting with upper GI bleed secondary to gastric ulcer. Because the ulcer has an adherent clot, the most appropriate course of action is to attempt removal of the clot with rigorous irrigation and/or a snare, and treat the underling lesion. If the clot cannot be removed, then epinephrine injection can be considered, particularly in high-risk patients. In addition, IV PPI therapy should be given following endoscopic therapy. Dual therapy (epinephrine injection plus thermocoagulation/clips) is indicated for an actively bleeding lesion or a non-bleeding visible vessel.

42. B (S&F ch20)
The most commonly used probe is the bipolar electrocoagulation probe in which heat is generated through current flowing between wires intertwined at the tip of the probe. Ideal settings are low power (12-16 W) and moderate time (8-10 sec). The heater probe can coagulate vessels up to 2 mm in diameter. Heater probes provide a fixed amount of joules of energy that does not vary with the tissue resistance.

43. A (S&F ch20)
This patient has a single gastric ulcer that underwent endoscopic hemostasis. It is the standard of care to give IV PPI therapy for 72 hours following endoscopic hemostasis. Repeat EGD with possible biopsy should be done

in patients with a gastric ulcer after 6 weeks of acid suppression. This is to confirm healing of the ulcer and obtain biopsies if needed. *H. pylori* therapy should be initiated if the patient is positive for *H. pylori.* IV octreotide is given in cases of variceal bleeding and has no role in the management of peptic ulcer disease bleeding.

44. A (S&F ch20)
This patient has an active diverticular bleed. The next step in management is endoscopic hemostasis with injection of epinephrine and hemoclip. If this fails then the patient can be referred to interventional radiology or surgery. Tattooing the area after endoscopic hemostasis is reasonable for future endoscopic or surgical localization.

45. C (S&F ch20)
The location in the right colon has been reported as a risk factor for the postpolypectomy bleeding. Other risk factors for postpolypectomy bleed are large polyp (>2 cm), thick stalk, sessile polyp, and use of anticoagulation or aspirin.

46. C (S&F ch20)
This patient has the endoscopic appearance of gastric antral vascular ectasia (GAVE). The presentation here is classic with rows of ectatic mucosal blood vessels in the pylorus. Endoscopic therapy with argon plasma coagulation decreases oozing rates and improves hematocrit levels. Usually several sessions about 4 to 8 weeks apart are required. Biopsy for *H. pylori* and checking serum gastrin level is indicated in patients with peptic ulcer disease. Bipolar cautery is used in patients with active hemorrhage or a visible vessel in a bleeding ulcer, but is not appropriate for widespread applications, such as treatment of GAVE. TIPS, IV octreotide, and β-blockers are indicated in upper GI bleeding secondary to portal hypertension such as variceal bleeding.

47. D (S&F ch20)
Stopping NSAIDs, doing a biopsy for *H. pylori*, and early feeding is the best management for this gastric ulcer with a flat spot. Endoscopic therapy is not indicated because rebleeding rates on medical therapy are 5% to 7%. *H. pylori* may be a risk factor for patients ingesting NSAIDs and biopsies are indicated for diagnosis of infection, before empiric treatment. Recognition of the stigmata, early feeding, and consideration for early discharge are recommended. Discontinuation of all NSAIDs and aspirin, substitution of non-NSAID analgesia, and education of the patient about the long-term risk of NSAIDs without cotherapy are also recommended. Epinephrine injection is not indicated and biopsy for malignancy can be deferred until a follow-up endoscopy is performed to document endoscopic healing. Malignancy occurs in less than 3% of all benign-appearing gastric ulcers, and would be very uncommon in this prepyloric gastric ulcer.

48. E (S&F ch20)
In this setting, bleeding from an aortoenteric fistula is the most important consideration and the patient's initial presentation may be the "herald" bleed. After an EGD has failed to show other potential causes of upper GI hemorrhage, an abdominal CT series should be done urgently to rule out an aortoenteric fistula. A colonoscopy would be appropriate with a history of hematochezia, but is unlikely to be of help in this patient with hematemesis. In the absence of acute bleeding, neither scintigraphy nor angiography is likely to have a high diagnostic yield. A push enteroscopy could also be considered for diagnosis and localization if the CT scan is negative in this patient.

49. B (S&F ch20)
This patient had a recent liver biopsy and is now presenting with hemobilia. The best way to manage this is by arterial embolization. Injection with epinephrine, mono or dual endoscopic therapy will not be able to stop the bleeding source. Surgery is not indicated at this time if bleeding control can be achieved by arterial embolization.

50. C (S&F ch20)
In a patient with continuing lower GI hemorrhage and EGD and colonoscopy that are nondiagnostic, scintigraphy and angiography should be the next tests. Scintigraphy may be especially useful in small bowel and colonic sites of active bleeding; however, surgery should not be performed based on scintigraphy localization alone. Angiography may be useful for both diagnosis and treatment of upper GI, small intestine, or colonic lesions. Abdominal CT or MRI imaging studies are important tests in patients with suspected aortoenteric fistula; however, in the absence of a prior abdominal aneurysm repair, large abdominal aneurysm, or severe peripheral vascular disease on exam, these imaging tests are not required in the evaluation of severe hematochezia. A barium enema should not be done because it cannot detect active bleeding and will delay and obscure angiography.

51. D (S&F ch20)
The patient has recently been started on aspirin, which can precipitate bleeding from a preexisting ulceration. Given her past history of duodenal ulcer, one would clearly need to exclude *H. pylori.* This patient has a high likelihood of *H. pylori*, and given that the serologic test for *H. pylori* is negative, this result should be confirmed with another active test (e.g., stool antigen, urea breath test) later as an outpatient. In addition, the repeat test should ideally be performed off proton pump inhibitors for at least 2 weeks. Although *H. pylori* is likely present given the history of duodenal ulcer, additional tests would be best to exclude this infection rather than treating with antibiotics empirically. There is no indication to start an IV proton pump inhibitor in this setting or to switch to a H_2 receptor antagonist. There is no indication to rule out Zollinger-Ellison syndrome, such as recurrent peptic ulcer disease, *H. pylori*- and NSAID-negative ulcers, and thick gastric folds.

52. D (S&F ch20)
Recent studies suggest that endoscopy is both effective and safe for the therapy of a bleeding diverticulum. After endoscopic hemostasis of a bleeding diverticulum is completed, a permanent submucosal tattoo should be placed around the lesion to allow identification of the site in case colonoscopy is repeated or surgery is performed for recurrent bleeding. After colonoscopic hemostasis, patients should be told to avoid aspirin and other nonsteroidal antiinflammatory drugs and take a daily fiber supplement on a long-term basis. Given this woman's overall medical condition, endoscopic therapy is appropriate. Because the site of bleeding has been localized by colonoscopy, technetium-labeled red blood cell scan would only likely confirm the bleeding segment of the colon. Angiography would be reasonable in this woman to identify and possibly treat the bleeding diverticulum; however, there is morbidity from this procedure, particularly in an elderly woman with known vascular disease.

53. B. (S&F ch20)
On colonoscopy a nonbleeding visible vessel is noted with ulceration at the site of the polypectomy. Most major

stigmata of recent hemorrhage in postpolypectomy ulcers are better treated with endoclips (with or without epinephrine injection) because hemoclips do not cause tissue damage, as is seen with thermal coagulation.

54. E (S&F ch20)
Ischemic colitis is the most common type of bowel ischemia, accounting for about 75% of intestinal ischemia. It is a common cause of significant lower GI bleeding, along with diverticular and hemorrhoidal bleeding. Ischemic colitis classically occurs in the elderly with risk factors for a low-flow state, as in those with atherosclerosis. It commonly presents with abdominal pain and hemodynamic disturbances, and affects watershed areas, such as the splenic flexure. Treatment is usually supportive. New onset inflammatory bowel disease or a missed lesion (either a large mass or innumerable polyps) is very unlikely with a recent normal colonoscopy, and generally does not present with a large amount of bleeding. While diverticulosis is possible, it typically presents with painless bleeding. Isolated visible vessel represents a Dieulafoy lesion, which can cause massive bleeding; however, it is a rare cause of lower GI bleeding, and would not result in abdominal pain.

55. A (S&F ch20)
In patients with known ulcerative colitis (UC) who present with symptoms suggesting a flare of disease, often manifested as bloody diarrhea, it is critical to exclude *C. difficile* (and oftentimes cytomegalovirus) as the cause because this affects management and more broadly the risk of needing surgery. Infectious colitis should be excluded in any patient with severe lower GI bleeding and colitis. Lower GI bleeding can occur with infection caused by *Campylobacter jejuni*, *Salmonella*, *Shigella*, enterohemorrhagic *E. coli* (O157:H7), cytomegalovirus, or *C. difficile*. Significant blood loss is rare except in patients with severe coagulopathy. The diagnosis is made by stool cultures and flexible sigmoidoscopy or colonoscopy. Treatment is with medical management; the use of antibiotics depends on the causative organism.

56. E (S&F ch20)
This patient has a white-based duodenal ulcer for which no endoscopic therapy is required. Gastric biopsy to rule out *H. pylori* is indicated. Duodenal ulcer biopsy is not required unless a tumor is seen or a malignant duodenal ulcer is suspected.

57. B (S&F ch20)
Painful rectal bleeding particularly when having a bowel movement is characteristic of an anal fissure. Ulcerative proctitis is unlikely with a recent negative colonoscopy. All other choices are associated with painless rectal bleeding.

58. B (S&F ch20)
This patient has a history of radiation for prostate cancer. Endoscopic appearance is consistent with radiation proctitis with diffuse telengectasias and oozing. The changes in the rectum usually occur 6 to 18 months after radiation therapy. There is no presence of ulceration or dilated veins, which makes the other choices less likely.

59. B (S&F ch20)
Mucosal biopsies can differentiate between portal hypertensive gastropathy and GAVE. In GAVE there are dilated mucosal capillaries and spindle cell proliferation. Bleeding from GAVE is not related to portal hypertension and therefore TIPS and β-blockers are not helpful. GAVE is associated with cirrhosis; however, most GAVE is not seen in patients with cirrhosis. GAVE is not related to *H. pylori* infection.

60. E (S&F ch20)
This patient has significant rectal bleeding. In the setting of constipation, one of the most likely causes for this can be a rectal ulcer. This usually happens in the setting of a patient being hospitalized. The pathophysiology of this seems to be similar to a stress ulcer. The treatment is a combination of thermal therapy, injection therapy, and suture ligation if needed. The other causes listed are less likely in the given setting of presentation.

61. B (S&F ch20)
This patient has significant upper GI bleeding from a Mallory-Weiss tear (MWT). There is a large visible vessel. The most appropriate therapy for this lesion is epinephrine injection with endoclip placement because this would reduce the high risk of rebleeding and result in the least tissue damage, while actually closing the ulcer (see figure). Epinephrine alone is not sufficient for this high-risk lesion. Gold probe thermocoagulation is less preferred because it leads to increased tissue damage in this ulcer at the gastroesophageal junction. Band ligation is appropriate for variceal bleeding, not MWT. Mucosal biopsy is not required for MWT.

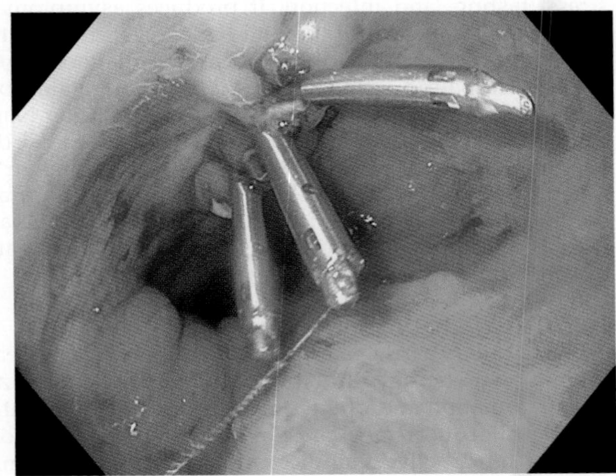

Figure for answer 61.

62. A (S&F ch20)
This young patient has obscure overt GI bleeding. The most common cause of obscure GI bleeding in patients younger than 50 years is small bowel tumors, while small bowel angiectasias are the most common cause in those older than 50 years. Missed peptic ulcer disease on two upper endoscopic examinations is unlikely. The other etiologies all can result in obscure GI bleeding, but are less likely than small bowel tumors in this patient.

63. C (S&F ch21)
In unstable patients who cannot tolerate anesthesia, any form of surgical intervention may be contraindicated. In these patients, drainage of the gallbladder may be performed under radiologic guidance via percutaneous cholecystostomy. The ultrasound imaging is adequate to diagnose acalculous cholecystitis and CT would not be necessary. There is high risk for perforation and abscess formation, and thus antibiotics alone is not adequate treatment.

64. B (S&F ch21)
The patient presents with Charcot triad of fever, right upper quadrant pain, and jaundice suggestive of cholangitis. Initial management should consist of IV antibiotics and ERCP for bile duct clearance and/or decompression with a stent. The clinical picture as well as the cholangiogram findings is suggestive of Mirizzi syndrome. Mirizzi syndrome is a common hepatic duct obstruction caused by a gallstone impaction in the gallbladder neck or cystic duct. Jaundice and biliary obstruction can result. After decompression of the bile duct with a stent, the next most appropriate step in management is to perform a cholecystectomy for definitive treatment. The clinical history and cholangiogram findings alone are enough to raise the suspicion of this diagnosis. Therefore, further radiographic testing with MRCP, endoscopic ultrasound, and HIDA scan are not likely to be beneficial. A repeat ERCP for stent removal can be performed once the gallbladder is removed. Leaving the stent in for surgery is beneficial because it can help the surgeon identify the common bile duct in order to help avoid ductal injury.

65. D (S&F ch21)
Gilbert syndrome is a relatively common hereditary condition. It occurs due to a genetic defect in the enzyme system, bilirubin UDP-glucuronyltransferase leading to reduced activity of *UGT1A1*. The jaundice is related to stress, fasting, and infection. It produces asymptomatic unconjugated hyperbilirubinemia and it is important to know the disease to avoid unnecessary diagnostic procedures. Impaired canalicular export of conjugated bilirubin is seen in Dubin-Johnson syndrome. Crigler-Najjar syndrome represents several hereditary diseases due to mutation in the coding region of *UGT1A1* known by severe rise in unconjugated bilirubin. The type 1 is a fatal one in which conjugation is absent. Rotor syndrome and Dubin-Johnson syndrome are relatively mild conjugated hyperbilirubinemias.

66. E (S&F ch21)
Primary biliary cirrhosis (PBC) is a chronic liver disease of unknown etiology (autoimmune) that is characterized by inflammation and granulomatous destruction of intrahepatic bile ducts. The presentation of biliary cirrhosis includes obstructive jaundice and pruritus; xanthomas, xanthelasmas, and elevated serum cholesterol; fatigue; and cirrhosis (late complication). The other conditions listed are not associated with primary biliary cirrhosis. Hepatocellular carcinoma risk is increased in patients with cirrhosis secondary to PBC.

67. D (S&F ch22)
Based on functional MRI studies the dorsal ACC is affected in irritable bowel syndrome; the hippocampus is affected and can undergo neurodegeneration in posttraumatic stress disorder and sexual abuse patients; the posterior cingulate cortex and ventromedial prefrontal cortex is affected in chronic somatic pain disorders; and the ACC and oribitofrontal cortex is affected in major depression and bipolar disorder.

68. C (S&F ch22)
Eliciting psychosocial information in a sensitive and nonthreatening way. Physicians should use open-ended questions to generate the hypothesis and close-ended to test them. Patient statements should be summarized in a nonjudgmental fashion. The use of echoing and affirmative gestures facilitates communication. Leading or multiple choice questions do not facilitate good communication.

69. B (S&F ch22)
The spinothalamic tract terminates in the medial thalamus and projects as third order neurons to the primary somatosensory cortex (see figure). This is important for sensory discrimination and localization of visceral versus sensory pain. The spinoreticular tract is involved in the emotional component of pain. The perigenual anterior cingulate cortex (pACC) is involved in affect modification and the midcingulate cortex (MCC) is involved with behavioral response. The cingulate cortex, therefore, is important in multicomponent integration of nociceptive information, and this results in variability of experience and reporting of pain.

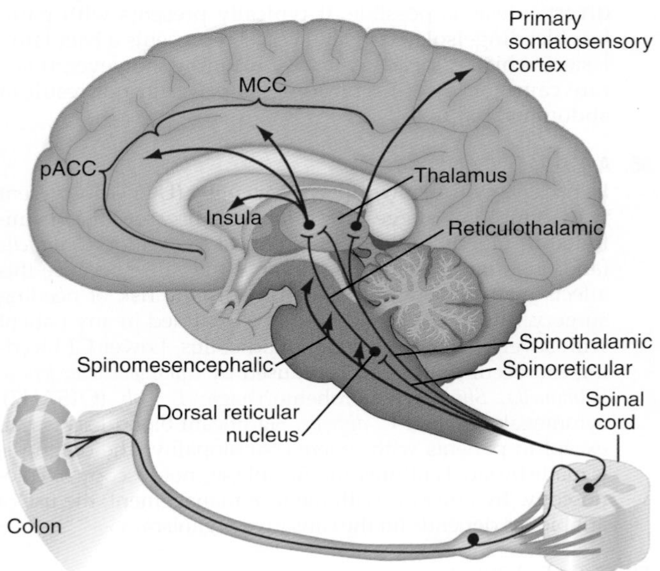

Figure for answer 69.

70. A (S&F ch22)
In both animal models and human studies stress affects the mucosa to enhance proinflammatory cytokine production and mast cell activation and degranulation, particularly near enteric neurons, thereby leading to visceral sensitization. Stress also enhances mucosal permeability due to weakening of tight junctions, with an increase in bacterial translocation into the intestinal wall. Acute stress triggers the hypothalamic-pituitary axis, leading to increases in cortisol levels and activation of the autonomic nervous system, with increases in proinflammatory cytokines like tumor necrosis factor (TNF)-α, interleukin (IL)-6, and interferon (IFN)-γ. Stress can lead to a change in intestinal microflora composition, with a shift from "good" to "bad" bacteria. These changes, along with an altered immune response, can result in inflammation and susceptibility to both irritable bowel syndrome (particularly postinfection irritable bowel syndrome) and inflammatory bowel disease. Gastric hyperemia and increased motility and secretion were linked to feelings of anger, intense pleasure, or aggressive behavior toward others.

71. D (S&F ch23)
People with factitious disease take action to cause or simulate disease in the absence of external rewards, which often leads to excessive intervention. Malingering is motivated by acquisition of external rewards like financial compensation or opiates. Malingering illness is associated with antisocial personality disorders. Factitious disease is a DSM-5 disorder while malingering illness is not. Factitious illness requires referral to a health care provider while malingering illness may require referral to a court system. The motivation is internal incentive for factitious disease and external incentive for malingering illness. Assumption of the sick role is generally seen in factitious disease. Both factitious disorders and malingering illness have intentional falsification.

72. E (S&F ch23)
Clues to subtle forms of factitious disease include: predominantly seen in women, previous experience in the medical field, multiple procedures/surgeries, visits to referral centers, history of substance abuse, and inconsistency of certain aspects of history.

73. B (S&F ch23)
Methods that have been used to confirm a suspicion of factitious disease are reviewing old biopsy slides looking for foreign body material, obtaining a psychiatric evaluation, and testing biological fluids. In addition, having nursing staff (not the patient's family) observe the patient to detect tampering behavior can help with the diagnosis. Searching the patient's belongings and not their home can also give clues toward the diagnosis. It is not appropriate to ask the patient's supervisor regarding their medical condition.

74. A (S&F ch23)
This patient has a psychiatric background and multiple emergency department visits with a lack of diagnosis despite a complete work-up. In such a situation one should consider factitious disease where there is internal incentive to assume a sick role as is seen in this patient.

CHAPTER

4

Topics Involving Multiple Organs

Jan-Michael A. Klapproth, Stephan U. Goebel, Melanie Harrison, Elnaz Jafarimehr, and Shanthi Srinivasan

QUESTIONS

1. A 55-year-old woman is referred to the GI clinic for management of anemia and occasional melena. On physical examination, she appears pale but in no acute distress. Examination of the lips is shown in the figure. Labs show a hemoglobin of 6.9 g/dL; ferritin of 6 ng/mL; and serum iron of 34 μg/dL. Which of the following is most likely found on examination of the gastrointestinal tract?

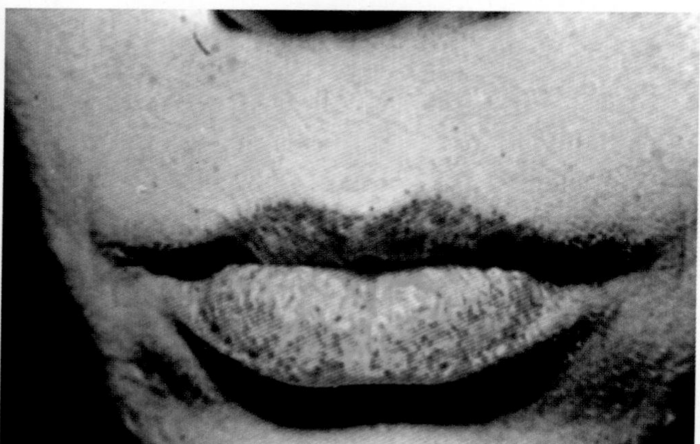

Figure for question 1.

   - **A.** Hamartomatous polyps
   - **B.** Adenomatous polyps
   - **C.** Telangiectasias
   - **D.** Carcinoid tumor
   - **E.** Gastrointestinal stromal tumor (GIST)

2. An 18-year-old man referred by his dentist is seen for mandibular bone loss, identified on a panoramic x-ray of the upper and lower jaw imaging, and recurrent angular chilitis. The patient denies any abdominal symptoms, except occasional painless rectal discharge of mucus, occurring once a week after a regular bowel movement for the past 6 months, without hematochezia or melena. His past medical history is negative, as are family and social history, and physical exam is unremarkable. Laboratory values are as follows:

Hemoglobin	13 g/dL
WBC	7000/μL
MCV	79 fL
Total bilirubin	1.0 g/dL
Alkaline phosphatase	118 U/L
ALT	18 U/L
AST	25 U/L

What is the most important next step in the management of this patient?

   - **A.** Perform a diagnostic flexible sigmoidoscopy
   - **B.** Perform a diagnostic colonoscopy
   - **C.** Perform a diagnostic flexible sigmoidoscopy with random biopsies
   - **D.** Perform a diagnostic colonoscopy with random biopsies of the terminal ileum and colon
   - **E.** Recommend a bone density study, vitamin D 800 IU, and calcium 1.5 g, both per day now, and repeat bone density study in 1 year

3. A 52-year-old man with therapy-refractory chronic hepatitis C infection, genotype 1, diagnosed 13 years ago, presents with a complaint of small skin lesions on his neck and both dorsal aspects of his hands. These lesions have been present for the past month. He admits to moderate alcohol consumption, drinking a beer at night. On physical exam you find vesicular, faintly erythematous lesions limited to the dorsum of his hands and neck, which are not pruritic. The remainder of his history and physical exam is unremarkable. Which of the following is the most appropriate next step in management?
   - **A.** Prescribe a course of topical steroids 0.5% for the next 2 months
   - **B.** Check serologies for celiac disease
   - **C.** Refer to dermatology for punch biopsy
   - **D.** Perform a colonoscopy to rule out concurrent Crohn's disease
   - **E.** 24-hour urine collection for uroporphyrin

4. A 57-year-old man with isolated, moderately active, small bowel Crohn's disease presents to clinic with complaints of malaise and gum bleeding. The patient is status post total colectomy, 26 cm terminal ileum resection, and creation of a right lower quadrant ileostomy for intractable disease. This was complicated by perforation with abscess formation, requiring repeat courses of antibiotics. Currently, the patient is managed with intravenous infliximab 10 mg/kg every 4 weeks and azathioprine 150 mg by mouth every day. Laboratory values are as follows:

Hematocrit	27%
MCV	100 fL
Erythrocyte sedimentation rate	45 mm/hr
C-reactive protein	52 mg/L

On physical exam you note a midline scar, soft abdomen, and intact right lower quadrant ileostomy. In addition, you find areas of focal alopecia with fine scalp papules and skin that shows punctuate hemorrhage. Oral mucosa is remarkable for severely erythematous gums. What is the next intervention?

A. Replace vitamin B_{12} parenterally
B. Ascorbic acid 800 mg per day
C. Reduce azathioprine to 150 mg by mouth per day and check metabolites
D. Check antiinfliximab antibodies
E. Add zinc 1 mg/kg

5. A 56-year-old woman is referred to your clinic for a 6-month history of nonprogressive and intermittent dysphagia to solids. Despite chewing her food thoroughly, she still experiences a foreign body sensation with large boluses. She denies odynophagia, regurgitation, halitosis, and weight loss. The patient admits to a 3-year history of reflux disease, presenting as dyspepsia, initially treated with ranitidine 150 mg by mouth per day. One month ago she switched to over-the-counter omeprazole 40 mg daily to control her symptoms. Her past medical history was otherwise negative. The patient does not smoke and drinks a maximum of one glass of wine with dinner. Her physical exam is unremarkable, except the macular skin lesions at both of her wrists (see figure). The skin lesions developed about 2 months ago; they are not pruritic and have not increased in size. Besides scheduling an EGD, what other serology tests would be indicated and most likely be positive?

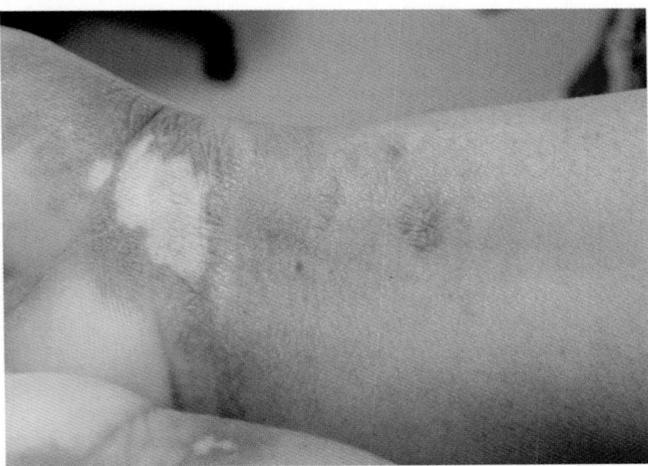

Figure for question 5.

A. Hepatitis C and antimitochondrial antibody
B. Anti–*Sacchoaromyces cerevisiae* antibodies (ASCA) and perinuclear antineutrophil cytoplasmic antibody (p-ANCA)
C. Tissue transglutaminase (tTG) antibody and antiendomysial antibody
D. C-reactive protein and erythrocyte sedimentation rate
E. Immunoglobulin (Ig)G4 and liver function tests

6. A 62-year-old man presents to clinic with a 2-week history of a metallic taste in his mouth and oropharyngeal dysphagia for 3 months duration. He denies lymph node swelling, weight loss, regurgitation, halitosis, and odynophagia. His sleep is irregular with frequent awakenings at night, and his wife complains about her husband snoring excessively, in particular when lying on his back. His past medical history is remarkable for long-standing rheumatoid arthritis (RA) treated with methotrexate 25 mg intramuscularly once a week and ibuprofen 400 mg twice a day as needed. Last year the patient underwent a colonoscopy that was consistent with a sessile serrated adenoma at the hepatic flexure, measuring 1.5 cm in diameter, which was completely excised. An upper gastroenterological series ordered by his primary care physician was reported as normal. Previously ordered laboratory exams revealed a hematocrit of 38%, mean corpuscular volume of 79 fL, creatinine 2.5 mg/dL, and alanine aminotransferase 67 IU. Examination of his oropharynx revealed the following physical finding (see figure). What is the next step in the workup of this patient?

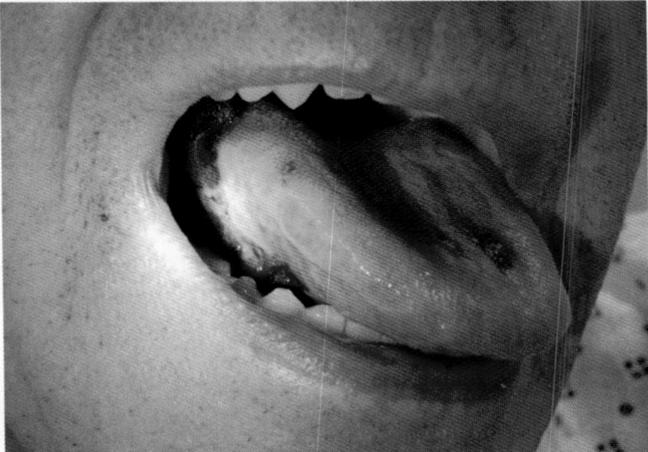

Figure for question 6.

A. Liver biopsy with trichrome and reticulin connective tissue stains
B. EGD with biopsies from esophagus and stomach
C. Biopsy of tongue with stains for Congo red
D. Immediate referral to otolaryngology for fiberoptic exam of oropharynx with biopsies
E. Computed tomography (CT) of the head, neck, and chest for staging purposes

7. A 49-year-old woman, initially presented to her dermatologist with a single macular papular lesion on the posterior aspect of her right leg, close to the knee joint (see figure). The solitary lesion appeared 10 days ago and has increased in size from 2 mm to now greater than 1.5 cm in diameter. She admits to intermittent fever to 39°C lasting for hours, fatigue, and diffuse arthralgias. Her dermatologist has requested your help as the patient has developed progressive epigastric, sharp pain, which is radiating to her back. The pain is not related to eating or bowel movements but can result in nausea, vomiting, and lose stools. She initially treated the pain by taking calcium carbonate twice a day, then ranitidine 150 mg by mouth twice a day, and was finally prescribed esomeprazole 40 mg per day. None of these measures have made a difference. Her past medical history is significant for breast cancer with recurrence 5 years ago, treated with high-dose alkylating chemotherapy and radiation. According to her oncologist, who saw her last 11 months ago, she is in full remission. Her laboratory exam has been unremarkable, including a blood smear, a hemoglobin of 39%, and white blood count 2400/μm^3, which has been stable for years. Having examined the image of the skin lesion, what is your most important differential diagnosis?

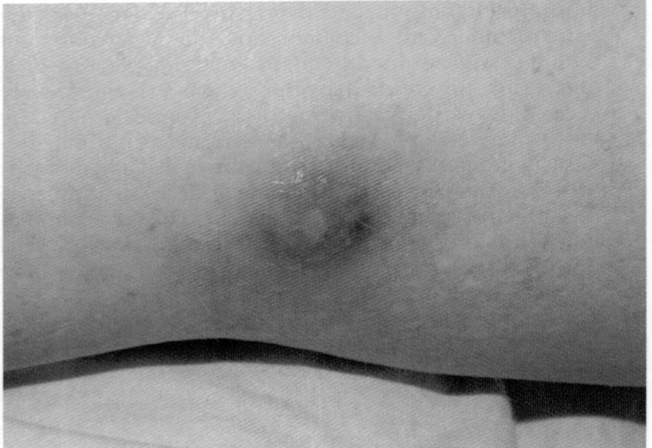

Figure for question 7.

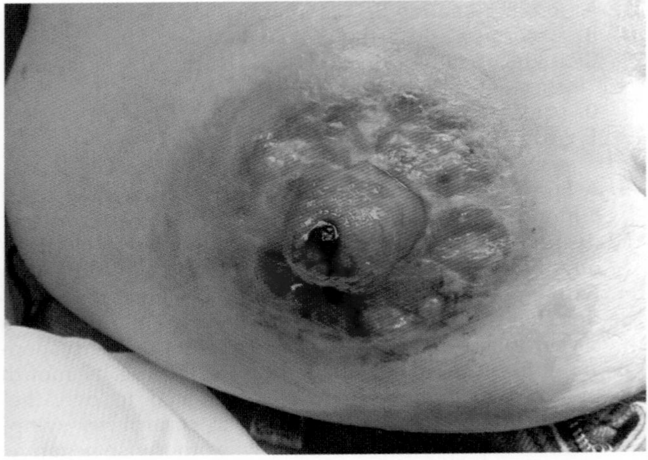

Figure for question 8.

A. Breast cancer recurrence with metastasis to skin and abdomen
B. Local abscess with sepsis in a patient with chemotherapy-induced decreased white and red blood cell count
C. Acute pancreatitis with skin necrosis
D. Necrolytic migratory erythema in a patient with glucagonoma
E. Gastric non-Hodgkin's lymphoma

8. A 64-year-old man presents to your clinic after being referred by a private practice colleague, requesting assistance with the patient's ileostomy. The patient was diagnosed 36 years ago with ileocolonic Crohn's disease and, in the first year of diagnosis, underwent an ileocolonic resection due to complicated, therapy-refractory disease. Postoperatively, he was treated with mesalamine 400 mg tablets, three tablets, three times a day. Within 3 years of the first surgically-induced remission, the patient had a second operation for an anastomotic stricture with obstruction, treated with resection and primary anastomosis. The postoperative course was complicated by dehiscence and abscess formation, resulting in creation of an ileostomy, mucus fistula, and colonic stump of about 60 cm in length. The patient recovered and was treated during the ensuing years with azathioprine 175 mg by mouth, once a day, with metabolites in the therapeutic range. However, 10 months prior to his visit with you, azathioprine had to be stopped due to severe neutropenia with a WBC count of 1100/μL. The patient's regimen was adjusted to ciprofloxacin 500 mg by mouth per day, plus budesonide 9 mg by mouth per day, when he developed a peristomal rash that progressed to a circumferential open, painless lesion (see figure). A short course of prednisone 40 mg taper for 50 days had little effect controlling the lesion. What is your next step in management for the peristomal lesion?
A. Surgery consultation for revision of the ileostomy to control the inflammation
B. Quantiferone test, hepatitis B serologies, chest x-ray
C. Prednisone 60 mg by mouth per day taper and reintroduction of azathioprine at a lower dose to prevent neutropenia
D. Topical therapy with cromolyn sodium
E. Change ileostomy bag brand after consultation with the stoma nurse

9. A 37-year-old man presents to your clinic for further workup of sudden onset of secretory diarrhea with ten to twelve watery bowel movements day and night. With a job as an executive, he finds himself increasingly fatigued, with occasional lapses in focus and confusion; he finds he is unable to follow conversations. Current medications are ibuprofen 400 mg as needed for joint pain or headaches. His past medical, social, and family history are negative. On physical exam he appears dehydrated with normal vital signs. Physical exam is remarkable for two light purple, macular and scaling lesions on his forehead and left forearm. You order a stool culture and osmolytes; *Clostridium difficile* polymerase chain reaction (PCR); ova and parasites, and stool stain; sedimentation rate; C-reactive protein; complete blood count; comprehensive metabolic panel; and 24-hour urine collection. What additional blood test would support your suspicion?
A. Niacin
B. Thiamine
C. Riboflavin
D. Pyridoxine
E. Folic acid

10. A 78-year-old man presents to gastroenterology outpatient clinic for a 4-month history of progressive globus sensation, cough, and halitosis. The patient's symptoms are aggravated by large food boluses. He feels that food gets stuck in the throat during swallowing and has intermittent nocturnal regurgitation of food. He has lost 8 pounds over the past 3 months. His past medical history is significant for long-standing hypertension, coronary artery disease with ischemic heart failure, and prostate cancer stage III. The patient's current medical regimen consists of nifedipine, metoprolol, aspirin, nitroglycerine, warfarin, and goserelin. On physical exam you note that the patient is edentulous. In the left submandibular triangle you discover a soft, mobile nodule that is tender to palpation and indistinguishable from an enlarged left thyroid lobe. The rest of his exam is relevant for a 3/6 systolic murmur, bilateral decreased breath sounds, and a normal abdominal exam. The patient had a colonoscopy 6 years ago that was consistent with three hyperplastic polyps in the rectum and left colonic diverticulosis. His laboratory exam showed anemia with a hematocrit of

36%, normal MCV, and creatinine of 2.5 mg/dL. Which of the following is the most appropriate next diagnostic step?

A. Noncontrast CT of chest and neck
B. EGD
C. Referral to otolaryngology for endoscopic exam of pharynx with visualization of vocal cords and swallowing study
D. Upper gastrointestinal (GI) series
E. Thyroid ultrasound with thyroid-stimulating hormone serum concentration

11. A 24-year-old female graduate student presents to your outpatient clinic with a 3-year history of irritable bowel syndrome with daytime diarrhea and diffuse, cramping abdominal pain, predominantly located in the left lower quadrant. Her pain is consistently precipitated by food with a delay of 2 hours, followed by two episodes of massive diarrhea. She was managed with a combination of simethicone as needed, omeprazole 20 mg per day, imodium 2 mg by mouth twice a day, and oral hyoscyamine 0.125 mg as needed. Her past medical history is negative. She smokes a cigarette on occasion and has a glass of wine on weekends only. Initially, laboratory exams were normal for complete blood count and comprehensive metabolic panel. Celiac serologies, stool studies for pathogenic bacteria, fecal fat, and white cells all were negative. Due to persistent symptoms, you schedule a lactulose breath test, which is reported positive with 146 ppm after 2 hours. Treatment with sulfamethoxazole and trimethoprim (Bactrim DS) twice daily lead to complete resolution of her symptoms. However, within 2 months her symptoms recurred with increased severity, now including a 6-pound weight loss, nausea, severe abdominal distention, and borborygmi. You repeat the breath test, which is again positive with 234 ppm. The decision is made to treat with rifaximin 550 mg three times a day for 14 days. Laboratory results show an albumin at 3.5 g/dL, microcytic anemia with a hematocrit 35%, and vitamin B_{12} of 108 ng/L. The patient is tearful and frustrated with her course of disease and care, which interfers with her studies. What is your next step?

A. Stop omeprazole
B. Increase imodium 2 mg by mouth to three times a day.
C. Magnetic resonance enterography
D. EGD with biopsies and duodenal aspirate
E. Small bowel follow-through

12. You are called to the emergency department to help evaluate a 58-year-old woman with syncope after complaining of sudden onset of left lower quadrant sharp abdominal pain at home. Her physical exam is remarkable for a heart rate of 110 bpm, a markedly distended abdomen with minimally active bowel sounds, and left upper quadrant tenderness to palpation, but no rebound or guarding. Her vital signs normalize with intravenous normal saline. The patient is known to have long-standing systemic sclerosis complicated by numerous small bowel diverticuli, ranging in size from 3 cm to 3.6 cm. Laboratory evaluation reveals a WBC of 12,800/μL, hematocrit of 38%, and normal liver function tests. An abdominal x-ray is consistent with massively dilated loops of small bowel. What is the next step in the management of this patient?

A. Nasogastric (NG) and small bowel decompression, nothing by mouth, correction of electrolytes
B. Endoscopic decompression with EGD
C. Surgical consultation for exploratory laparotomy
D. Endoscopic decompression with colonoscopy
E. Metoclopramide 10 mg intravenously

13. An 88-year-old man with a known asymptomatic and stable 2 cm Zenker diverticulum diagnosed 4 years ago presents to your clinic with sensation of progressive left-sided neck fullness and blood in expectorant. At that time, diagnosis was made by upper gastroenterologic series, followed up with an EGD. The endoscopy revealed a second lumen proximal to the upper esophageal sphincter, and the proximal esophagus was intubated without difficulties. At the time of diagnosis the patient decided to not have the diverticulum surgically removed, given that he was asymptomatic. His past medical history is significant for pulmonary emphysema, deep venous thrombosis, and recent onset of arthritis of his left wrist after a fall 6 years ago, treated with ibuprofen 400 mg by mouth, three times a day. The patient denies dysphagia, odynophagia, halitosis, and regurgitation. He is worried about the change in symptoms. What is the main concern in this patient?

A. Increased risk of adenocarcinoma of the esophagus
B. Increased risk of squamous carcinoma of the esophagus
C. Increased risk of tonsillar carcinoma
D. Increased risk of squamous carcinoma in the diverticulum
E. Increased risk of infection due to entrapped food residue

14. A 23-year-old man from India presents to your clinic with the complaint of intermittent, sharp, nonradiating 9 out of 10 abdominal pain, lasting up to an hour, for the past year. He recently arrived in the United States to fill a postdoctoral position at your university for the next 2 years. Upon review of systems he admits to a temperature of 39.8° C, chills, 15-pound weight loss, productive cough, and malaise. On physical exam you find a thin man, clearly uncomfortable with a fever, pronounced bilateral breath sounds, tachycardia, and a tender left lower quadrant to palpation. Laboratory investigation shows a hematocrit of 29%, microcytosis, WBC of 29,000/μL, and positive quantiferone test. His chest x-ray reveals a cavitary lesion in the right upper lung lobe. His enhanced computer enterography is consistent with left lower quadrant massive lymphadenopathy, inflamed terminal ileum with marked narrowing of the lumen, and numerous distinct, prestenotic, round, loose 1 cm filling defects. Besides admission to the hospital and isolation, what has to be done about the terminal ileum filling defects?

A. Polyethyline glycol/electrolytes (GoLYTELY) prep for dissolution of filling defects and passage
B. Endoscopic intervention with retrieval of foreign bodies
C. Repeat CT prior to discharge
D. Single balloon enteroscopy with biopsies
E. Surgery consultation for resection of terminal ileum

15. A 56-year-old man is seen in clinic for abdominal pain for the last 3 months. His pain is sharp, located around the umbilicus, and nonradiating. The pain is related to food intake, delayed by 2 hours after eating, most severe during daytime, and associated with nausea but without vomiting. Since the onset of his symptoms, the patient has decreased the frequency of his meals and has lost approximately 17 pounds of weight. Pain is not relieved by bowel movements or position. He has been to the emergency department twice during that time and discharged with pain medications after a CT did not reveal any masses or obstruction. His past medical history is remarkable for a gunshot wound to the abdomen with exploratory laparotomy at the age of 21, hypertension, and chronic renal insufficiency. Social history revealed him to be an active smoker with a 35-year history of tobacco use. The only medication he is taking right now is lisinopril. On physical exam the patient is in mild distress; his weight is 278 lb. He has a midline abdominal scar, which is well-healed. He has localized periumbilical tenderness to deep palpation and a negative rectal exam for blood. Repeated blood work showed a creatinine of 2.3 mg/dL but was otherwise unremarkable. Which of the following is the most appropriate next step?

A. Small bowel follow-through
B. CT with intravenous contrast
C. Magnetic resonance enterography
D. Abdominal ultrasound in an upright position
E. Referral to pain clinic for trigger point injection

16. A 57-year-old man is being brought to the emergency department for acute onset of retching, abdominal distention, and a small amount of blood in his expectorant. The patient complained since earlier that morning of sharp, nonradiating, 6 out of 10 abdominal pain, awakening him from sleep. He also developed intractable retching, and eventually fresh blood was present in his sputum. The patient's nurse informs you that she has been unable to pass an NG tube for decompression. His past medical history is relevant for vascular dementia, after sustaining a stroke 4 years ago. Current medications include aspirin and Crestor. On physical exam he is in mild distress, constantly retching, with tense tympanic abdomen and absent bowel sounds. Rectal exam did not reveal any blood, but formed brown stool. Laboratory exam was consistent with a WBC of 11,000/μL, potassium 3.5 mEq/L, and lactic acid 0.7 mEq/L. A chest x-ray reveals a gas bubble above the diaphragm, obscuring the left cardiac margin. What is the next step in management of this patient?

A. Careful attempt of endoscopic decompression under fluoroscopic guidance
B. Surgical consult for immediate laparoscopic laparotomy
C. Repeat attempt of NG tube placement
D. CT of the chest and abdomen
E. Magnetic resonance enterography

17. A 55-year-old woman presents to your clinic after being referred by her primary care provider for further workup of iron deficiency anemia. Approximately 1 month ago, the patient noted the onset of dyspnea on exertion after climbing two flights of stairs. She was found to be anemic with a hemoglobin of 8 g/dL, MCV of 75 fL, and ferritin of 6 ng/mL. The remainder of her laboratory exam was negative, including a urine analysis. She was found to be heme-positive on rectal exam. The patient has a long-standing history of coronary artery disease, currently treated with aspirin, atorvastatin, furosemide, and metoprolol. She received 2 units of packed red blood cells, and she had an appropriate response. EGD shows a large hiatal hernia with small erosions at the diaphragmatic impression on the proximal stomach, non-erosive gastritis and duodenitis, and 5 diminutive gastric polyps. Colonoscopy shows multiple diverticula in the sigmoid colon, but it is otherwise a normal exam. Which of the following explains this patient's anemia?

A. Duodenitis
B. Gastritis
C. Erosions at the hiatal hernia
D. Gastric polyps
E. Diverticulosis

18. A 55-year-old man with alcoholic cirrhosis presents to the endoscopy suite for massive diuretic refractory ascites. For the past year, the patient required paracentesis every 6 weeks, completed without complication. He was evaluated by the transplant committee but was rejected because of noncompliance regarding smoking cessation, alcohol consumption, and medication management. On physical exam, you note caput medusae, hypoactive bowel sounds, tenderness, ascites with tachypnea, and an umbilical hernia. Following successful insertion of a draining catheter in the right lower quadrant, a total of 7 L of clear yellow fluid is drained. The patient developed periumbilical severe abdominal pain. On physical exam you note the now deflated umbilical hernia, which is extremely tender to palpation and is increased in size. Which of the following is the most appropriate next step in management?

A. Admit the patient for observation and intravenous antibiotics
B. Manually reduce the hernia after achieving adequate moderate sedation
C. Surgical consult, laparoscopic repair, repeat postoperative paracentesis if necessary
D. Replace paracentesis catheter and drain additional residual fluid
E. Scheduled the patient for transjugular intrahepatic portosystemic shunt

19. A 24-year-old man is brought to the emergency department by his girlfriend after having swallowed a large number of razor blades of various size and glass fragments in an attempt to commit suicide. The patient is intoxicated with incoherent and slurred speech. He is complaining of epigastric abdominal pain and sore throat with specks of blood staining his sputum. On physical exam, he has a heart rate of 90 bpm and blood pressure of 90/52 mm Hg. Abdominal exam shows a tender epigastrium with hyperactive bowel sounds. An abdominal x-ray shows numerous square radiodense foreign bodies in the right upper quadrant without free air. Laboratory investigations show a normal INR, WBC, and basic metabolic panel. Which of the following is the most appropriate management?

A. Do not attempt endoscopic retrieval as foreign bodies are no longer within reach of the standard endoscope
B. Attempt endoscopic retrieval with the standard endoscope
C. Attempt endoscopic retrieval with endotracheal intubation and a standard endoscope
D. Attempt endoscopic retrieval after patient recovers from intoxication
E. Place a NG tube and give polyethylene glycol solution

20. A 24-year-old man is being brought from the airport directly to the emergency department on the suspicion of being a body packer, as identified by a service dog. Upon his arrival, you are requested for advice regarding further management. The patient is anxious, tremulous, and diaphoretic but has normal vital signs, complete blood count, and metabolic panel. His abdominal exam is unremarkable. An abdominal x-ray reveals a large, 4 x 15 cm foreign body in the rectum. The emergency department attending physician requests removal of the item by flexible sigmoidoscopy because of concern that the patient is diaphoretic and the package might be leaking its content. What are your recommendations regarding the management of this patient?

A. Give two mineral oil enemas and await spontaneous passage of the foreign body
B. Flexible sigmoidoscopy and retrieval of the foreign body with forceps and Roth Net retrieval device
C. Give polyethylene glycol solution and await spontaneous passage of the foreign body
D. Avoid manipulation of the package and await spontaneous passage
E. Surgical consultation for surgical removal

21. A 45-year-old man presents to the emergency department after drinking brake fluid by accident, which was stored in an unlabeled lemonade bottle. The patient immediately noticed the error after swallowing a significant amount of battery fluid and spat out the rest. He drank several cups of water, which did not prevent the onset of severe chest pain, increased salivation, cough, and regurgitation of a small amount of blood. Upon admission his vital signs show tachycardia of 115 bpm, blood pressure of 130/92 mm Hg, but an otherwise negative physical exam. Laboratory investigations revealed and increased WBC of 16.4/μL, a hemoglobin of 14 g/dL, and normal electrolytes. A chest x-ray is negative for free air. By the time you see the patient, his vital signs have normalized with a heart rate of 64 bpm, but he complains of persistent chest pain, salivation, and hoarseness. You performed an EGD in the emergency room, identifying damage to the esophagus in the form of deep and serpiginous ulcerations with exudate involving the entire esophagus. The stomach contains a significant amount of fluid, which reveals moderate antral erythema after aspiration but no ulcers or perforation. What is the most appropriate management approach?

A. Clear liquid diet, acid suppression, and eventually advance diet as tolerated, and if asymptomatic, discharge in the morning
B. Admission to the intensive care unit (ICU) for observation, intravenous fluids, and otolaryngology consultation
C. Place NG tube and gastric lavage, followed by a regular diet
D. Surgical consultation for esophagectomy
E. Clear liquid diet, acid suppression, and esophageal stent placement to prevent future complications of stricturing

22. A 50-year-old prisoner swallowed several objects, including pencil fragments, small razor blades, and plastic fragments, with suicidal intent. The patient complains of severe abdominal pain, 9 out of 10, sharp, radiating to his back, associated with nausea but no vomiting. Vital signs are stable, and his physical exam is benign, with mild tenderness in the epigastrium. The abdominal x-ray taken upon admission to the emergency department reveals three objects, measuring 1.2 cm x 2.1 cm in the right upper quadrant. While preparing the patient for an upper endoscopy, you review the likelihood of spontaneous passage of foreign bodies within the GI tract, depending on size. What are the maximum dimensions for a long foreign body to pass through the GI tract being expelled spontaneously?

A. Diameter < 2.5 cm, length < 5 cm
B. Diameter < 3 cm, length < 5.5 cm
C. Diameter < 3.5 cm, length < 6 cm
D. Diameter < 4 cm, length < 6.5 cm
E. Passage is independent of diameter and length

23. A 45-year-old man is being brought to the emergency department from a nursing home, where he resides because of mental retardation from cerebral palsy after perinatal asphyxia. Witnessed by one of his caregivers, the patient ingested two magnets from a kitchen cabinet door. The magnets were round and smooth and approximately 1.5 cm in diameter. However, the incident was not reported until the following day. The patient initially appeared fine but overnight developed malaise and appeared uncomfortable in the emergency department. His abdominal exam was unremarkable, except the neurologic sequelae from the perinatal asphyxia. Laboratory exam was unremarkable, and an abdominal x-ray showed two objects in close proximity in the left upper quadrant. What is the most appropriate management approach for this patient?

A. No further workup or interventions are required, given the high likelihood of spontaneous passage
B. Admit the patient for observation
C. EGD for foreign body retrieval
D. Surgical consultation
E. Polyethylene glycol solution rapid purge and await passage of the foreign body

24. A 27-year-old man presents to the emergency department complaining of acute onset esophageal dysphagia. He was eating a steak dinner when he started to have dysphagia. He is unable to swallow his own saliva, with retrosternal pain, hiccup, and hoarseness. He is barely able to speak, giving the large amount of oral secretions that he cannot swallow. He denies any past medical history but reports a 20–pack/year history of tobacco and alcohol consumption every day. On physical exam, the patient is clearly uncomfortable, constantly spitting into a basin. An EGD is performed that shows a foreign body at 24 cm from the gums that completely occludes the distal lumen of the esophagus. Initial attempts to bypass the obstacle to ensure patency of the distal esophagus, allowing the foreign body to be advanced into the stomach, are met with resistance and were terminated. What is your next intervention to complete the procedure?

A. Terminate the procedure, give glucagon 1 mg intravenously, and reattempt endoscopy in 12 hours
B. Withdraw endoscope, insert an overtube and attempt piecemeal foreign body removal
C. Terminate procedure, give carbonated drink, and reattempt endoscopy in few hours
D. Continue current procedure, using increased force to dislodge foreign body
E. Terminate procedure and use a colonoscope to push the foreign body into the stomach

25. A 37-year-old woman with known severe fistulizing perianal and ileocolonic Crohn's disease presents to your clinic with a complaint of right lower quadrant sharp abdominal pain. Initially her disease was diagnosed approximately 2 years ago, and she was maintained on azathioprine 50 mg by mouth per day and intravenous infliximab 5 mg/kg every 6 weeks. Despite immunomodulators and biologic therapy, she continued to develop intermittent flares of her disease, presenting with right lower quadrant dull discomfort and loose bowel movements. The patient now states that her symptoms from earlier this week are different, as her pain is now sharp and progressive. The pain has developed over the past 3 days, with a temperature of 38.9° C earlier this morning. On physical exam, her temperature is 38.8° C, tender in the right lower quadrant, with hypoactive bowel sounds. Her WBC is elevated to 15,900/µL, hemoglobin of 8 g/dL. Laboratory studies are otherwise unremarkable. CT scan performed in the emergency department with and without contrast reveals a large, 3.4 x 6.2 cm fluid collection. Following the initiation of intravenous normal saline, antibiotics, and admission, the intraabdominal abscess is drained percutaneously under radiographic guidance. A total of 35 mL of pus is aspirated, leaving the percutaneous catheter in place. The following day, the patient denies any pain, her white cell count has normalized, and she feels markedly improved. Over the next 3 days catheter output decreases to 15 mL of clear liquid per day. A repeat CT scan shows resolution of the intraabdominal abscess but no improvement of the ileocolonic fistulizing Crohn's disease. In anticipation of surgical and medical intervention, the question of when to discontinue the percutaneous catheter arises. What is your recommendation as to when discontinue the percutaneous catheter?

A. Decrease in output from the percutaneous catheter to less than 50 mL per day
B. Decrease in output from the percutaneous catheter to less then 20 mL per day
C. No output from the percutaneous catheter per day
D. Discontinuation of percutaneous catheter after complete cessation of drainage and an additional 3 days of antibiotics
E. Discontinuation of percutaneous catheter after complete cessation of drainage and an additional 5 days of antibiotics

26. You are taking care of an 18-year-old college student from the local university. The patient was diagnosed with fistulizing Crohn's disease with an enterocutaneous fistula that was draining fluid and undigested food. The fistulous tract extends from the proximal jejunum to the periumbilical area, confirmed by fistulogram and small bowel follow-through. Management of the fistulous tract has been difficult, as the output decreased by only 25% in response to intravenous infliximab 5 mg/kg every 6 weeks. You increase the frequency of infliximab to every 4 weeks, added weight-adjusted azathioprine at 75 mg by mouth per day, which resulted in further reduction of output from the fistula, estimated at 50%. Determination of 6 MMP and 6-TG show that azathioprine is dosed correctly. However, the patient is worried about the residual persistent output. Physical exam revealed the fistula, but in otherwise soft, nontender abdominal exam, with a normal-sized liver and no palpable spleen tip. His WBC is 7200/µL, hemoglobin of 11 g/dL, antiinfliximab antibodies 16 µg/mL, and a normal renal function. The patient is eager to get the symptoms under control, considering interference of the disease with his social and professional life. What are your recommendations to control output from the fistulous tract?

A. Change to adalimumab
B. Change methotrexate for azathioprine
C. Refer for surgical resection
D. Consider vedolizumab
E. Increase azathioprine to 100 mg by mouth per day

27. A 24-year-old man with a gunshot wound to the abdomen 3 months ago and exploratory laparotomy, presents to the emergency department, complaining of massive fluid output from an opening on his abdominal wall in the left upper quadrant. The patient is status postresection of 20 cm proximal jejunum, complicated by postoperative infection due to partial dehiscence without free air that required a prolonged hospital course and conservative management with antibiotics. Initially, he noted an erythematous nodular lesion in his left upper quadrant that eventually started draining clear fluid but developed into discharge of solid food and a large amount of fluid. This morning after waking up, he noted massive discharge from the opening in his left upper quadrant, soiling his bed and clothes, as well as a syncopal episode. The patient is being admitted for dehydration and was started on intravenous fluids. Physical exam is remarkable for a left upper quadrant fistulous tract that is draining continuously, containing food residue and bile. The patient's laboratory evaluation revealed a potassium of 2.4 mEq/L, hemoglobin of 12 g/dL, and creatinine of 3.2 mg/dL. A CT scan confirms the suspicion of a postoperative enterocutaneous fistula. As a consultant for immediate management of the fistulous tract, what are your recommendations?

A. Surgical consultation for resection and revision of the fistulous tract and anastomosis
B. Fibrin plug of the fistulous track
C. Intravenous normal saline at half the rate of the fistulous tract output
D. Intravenous normal saline supplemented with potassium to match the output from the fistulous tract
E. Octreotide subcutaneously to control the output from the fistulous tract

28. An 18-year-old college student returns for follow-up after successful resection of an enterocutaneous high output fistula due to Crohn's disease. The patient had an uneventful postoperative recovery, has resumed his daily activities, denies any pain, nausea, or vomiting, and maintains a normal appetite, regaining three pounds of weight over the past 2 weeks since being discharged from the hospital. His abdominal exam is remarkable for left upper quadrant, well-healed incision, without evidence of inflammation or infection. His abdomen is soft and nontender with normoactive bowel sounds. His medical regimen includes adalimumab with the addition recent of azathioprine. The patient inquires about infectious complications, being on two medications to control his disease and is concerned about the recurrence of fistulae. Which of the following statements is true regarding fistulae recurrence after surgical resection?

A. Chances of developing recurrent fistula is estimated at 5%
B. Chances of developing recurrent fistula is estimated at 10% to 20%
C. Surgical resection decreases the likelihood of recurrent fistula
D. Surgical resection increases the likelihood of recurrent fistula
E. Medical therapy has little effect on the development of recurrent fistula

29. Your review an abdominal CT scan of a 74-year-old man with diverticulosis, complicated by diverticulitis and formation of a new left lower quadrant fluid collection, measuring 7 cm x 3 cm. What are the two most specific findings indicating an intraabdominal abscess on contrast-enhanced CT scan?

A. Extraluminal gas, fluid collection less then 20 Hounsfield units
B. Extraluminal gas, fluid collection greater than 20 Hounsfield units
C. Contrast-enhanced rim, tissue reaction surrounding the fluid collection
D. Ill-defined heterogeneous collection, tissue reaction surrounding the fluid collection
E. Hypodense fluid collection, tissue reaction surrounding the fluid collection

30. A 18-year-old man presents to the emergency department after an argument that escalated into a knife flight, receiving a stab wound to the left upper quadrant. The patient arrives at your local hospital with stable vital signs, 2 out of 10 sharp pain in the left upper quadrant, and a small, nonbleeding incision close to the tenth rib. A peritoneal lavage was negative for blood, and a laparoscopic laparotomy did not reveal perforated viscus. Postoperatively, the patient is admitted for observation and was discharged 3 days later. Within 10 days, the patient returns for follow-up to surgery clinic with the complaint of left upper quadrant pain, nausea, vomiting, and a temperature to 40° C. On physical exam, the patient is in mild distress with a heart rate of 102 bpm, blood pressure of 90/50 mm Hg, and a WBC of 15,000/μL. The CT obtained the same day reveals a large, contained infradiaphragmatic 5.6 cm x 7.2 cm abscess with displacement and compression of the fundus. Which of the following is true regarding endoscopic drainage of intraabdominal abscesses?
A. Given the proximity of the abscess to the diaphragm, an endoscopic approach is not warranted
B. An abscess in the left infradiaphragmatic location should always be drained surgically
C. The abscess would be amenable for endoscopic drainage, independent of anatomic location but dependent on distance of lumen to abscesses wall being less than 2.5 cm
D. Endoscopic drainage is possible for the infradiaphragmatic location, with a lumen to abscesses wall distance of 1 cm or less
E. Endoscopic drainage should only be considered after unsuccessful attempts by interventional radiology

31. A 36-year-old man is seen in clinic for follow-up of eosinophilic esophagitis (EoE). Six months ago, he had an episode of esophageal food bolus impaction. Endoscopy was performed to disimpact the food bolus, and biopsies from the mid and distal esophagus showed eosinophilic infiltration of the mucosa. The patient wished to avoid steroid treatment and was treated using the six-food elimination diet (SFED). He has been symptom free for 6 months. He is now inquiring about reintroducing food groups. What is the recommended sequence for food reintroduction?
A. Milk, nuts/soy, wheat, seafood, eggs
B. Eggs, wheat, seafood, nuts/soy, milk
C. Wheat, eggs, milk, seafood, nuts/soy
D. Seafood, eggs, nuts/soy, milk, wheat
E. Nuts/soy, wheat, milk, seafood, eggs

32. A 35-year-old man presents to his local physician. He reports increasing difficulty swallowing meat and intermittent chest pain. He denies significant weight loss. Over the last 12 months, he had three episodes of esophageal food bolus obstruction. An upper endoscopy is performed, and biopsies from the mid and distal esophagus showed eosinophilic infiltration of the mucosa, compatible with EoE. His symptoms persisted despite treatment with twice daily omeprazole. However, he improves symptomatically after starting swallowed topical fluticasone. Which of the following is the recommended duration of treatment?
A. 2 weeks
B. 2 months
C. 6 months
D. 12 months
E. Indefinitely

33. A 63-year-old woman presents to her primary care physician for weight loss and abdominal discomfort for the past 6 months. She reports persistent watery diarrhea that occasionally wakes her up at night. An upper endoscopy is performed, which shows gastric erythema and edema. Colonoscopy reveals normal mucosa. Biopsy specimens from the stomach, duodenum, and colon reveal dense eosinophilic infiltration, suggestive of eosinophilic gastroenteritis. Due to her persistent symptoms, you are considering oral prednisone treatment. Which of the following infections have to be ruled out prior to beginning therapy?
A. *Giardia lamblia*
B. *Helicobacter pylori*
C. Methicillin-resistant *Staphylococcus aureus* (MRSA)
D. *Strongyloides stercoralis*
E. *Escherichia coli*

34. A 25-year-old man is seen in clinic for evaluation of intermittent dysphagia for the past 6 months. He feels that solid food gets stuck in the middle of his chest but has no problems with liquids. He denies heartburn, sour taste in his mouth, or weight loss. His past medical history is otherwise unremarkable. An upper endoscopy is performed, which reveals normal esophagus with no strictures. Biopsies from the esophagus show eosinophilic infiltration of the mucosa with eosinophils at 5 to 7 eosinophils (eos) per high-powered field (HPF). Which of the following is the most appropriate next step in management?
A. Omeprazole twice a day
B. Oral prednisone
C. Start elemental diet
D. Swallowed fluticasone
E. SFED

35. A 12-year-old girl presents to her gastroenterologist complaining of intermittent midepigastric pain, diarrhea, and occasional nausea and vomiting. She has previously underwent an upper and lower endoscopy. Her esophageal biopsies are normal. The pathologist has commented on the presence of eosinophils in the duodenal and terminal ileal biopsies. Which of the following describes the distribution of eosinophils in the normal GI tract in children?
A. Eosinophils are present in decreasing density from the proximal to the distal GI tract
B. Eosinophils are present in increasing density from the proximal to the distal GI tract
C. Eosinophils are present in a constant density throughout the GI tract
D. Eosinophils are absent in the normal GI tract
E. There is not particular pattern of eosinophil distribution in the GI tract

36. A 48-year-old woman has repeated episodes of vomiting, abdominal, pain, and diarrhea. She has gradually developed iron deficiency anemia after her hysterectomy

5 years ago. Her physical exam is unremarkable. She has upper and lower endoscopies performed that are normal. A capsule endoscopy shows thickened folds in the jejunum. A push enteroscopy is performed, and biopsies show mucosal infiltration with eosinophils (30 eos/HPF). There is no villous atrophy, and granulomas are not seen. Deficiency of which immunoglobulin is associated with this disorder?

A. IgG
B. IgD
C. IgM
D. IgE
E. IgA

37. A 28-year-old man is seen in clinic with complaints of dysphagia and occasional chest pain. He reports that sometimes food gets stuck in the midchest, and he needs to drink water to make it pass. Upper endoscopy is normal, and several biopsies are obtained, and a representative one is shown in the figure. The patient is interested in dietary and lifestyle therapies rather than medications. Which of the following would you recommend to this patient?

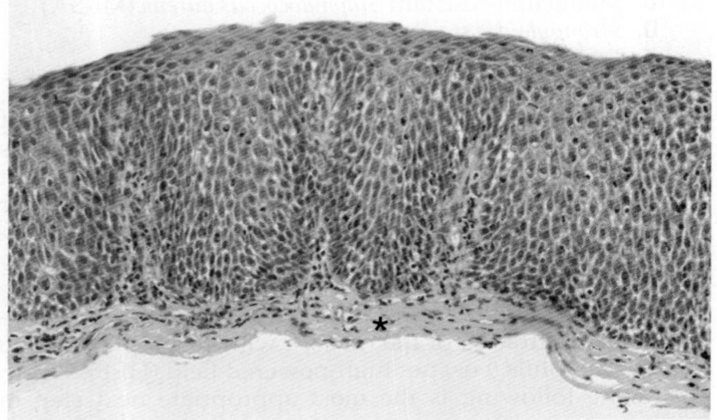

Figure for question 37.

A. Head-of-bed elevation; avoid fatty food, chocolate, and coffee
B. Low FODMAP (Fermentable Oligo-Di-Monosaccharides and Polyols) diet
C. Avoid cow's milk, wheat, seafood, nuts, soy, eggs (SFED)
D. Avoid milk and milk products (lactose free)
E. No dietary modification

38. A 31-year-old woman is seen in clinic with intermittent dysphagia to solids. She reports that sometimes food gets stuck in the midchest, and she needs to drink water to make it pass. Last month, she had an episode of food impaction that resolved when she arrived to the emergency department. You consider the differential diagnosis in this patient. Which of the following is a feature of EoE?

A. More common in females
B. Mucosal furrows
C. Esophageal webs
D. Eosinophils 7 to 10 eos/HPF
E. Clinical response to inhaled fluticasone

39. A 55-year-old man presents for worsening diarrhea and increasing swelling of his lower extremities over the past 2 months. Physical exam is remarkable for 3+ pitting edema in his legs. His laboratory values are as follows:

Hemoglobin	8 g/dL
Platelet count	150 000/μL
WBC	11,000/μL
Albumin	1.3 g/dL
INR	1.3

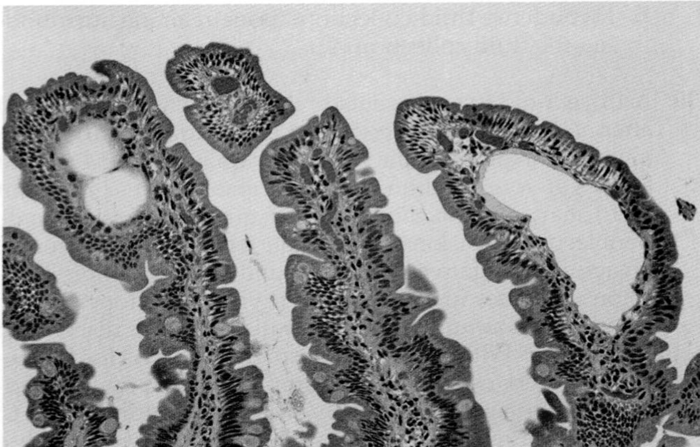

Figure for question 39.

Upper endoscopy is performed and a representative image of the small bowel biopsy is shown in the figure. What is the underlying cause of his clinical symptoms?

A. Eosinophilic gastroenteritis
B. Sarcoidosis
C. Constrictive pericarditis
D. Amyloidosis
E. Celiac disease

40. A 63-year-old woman presents for evaluation of chronic diarrhea. For the last 3 years she has 10 bowel movements/day, without any visible blood. During the last year she has developed peripheral edema not responsive to diuretics. Symptoms started 6 months after returning from a family vacation in Mexico. Her past medical history includes diabetes, hypertension, and systemic lupus erythematosus (SLE). Laboratory studies are as follows:

Hemoglobin	12 g/dL
Platelet count	250,000/μL
WBC	9000/μL
Total bilirubin	1.3 mg/dL
Creatinine	1.1 mg/dL
Total protein	4 g/dL
Albumin	1.6 g/dL
INR	1.2

Which of the following tests best explains the patient's symptoms?

A. 72-hour stool for fecal fat
B. α_1-Antitrypsin (α_1-AT) plasma clearance
C. 24-hour urine protein collection
D. Stool studies for ova and parasite (O&P)
E. Stool electrolytes (sodium, potassium)

41. A 23-year-old man presents to his primary care physician for evaluation of chronic lower extremity edema for several years. He also reports recurrent bouts of prolonged diarrhea. As a child he had open heart surgery but cannot recall the exact defect. Laboratory results are significant for persistent hypoalbuminemia. A recent echocardiogram shows normal cardiac function

and pressures. A colonoscopy with random biopsies was normal. What would be the best treatment for this patient?
A. High-dose diuretics
B. Oral steroids
C. Gastrectomy
D. High protein, low fat diet enriched with medium-chain triglycerides (MCT)
E. Trial of metronidazole

42. A 73-year-old man is seen for worsening diarrhea and increasing peripheral edema. He recently started treatment for a B-cell lymphoma located in his mediastinal lymph nodes. His cardiac function is normal, and a urine dipstick is negative for proteinuria. He has no evidence of cirrhosis. Stool studies for O&P as well as a colonoscopy are normal; a human immunodeficiency virus (HIV) test is negative. Which serum protein level would remain normal in this condition?
A. Transferrin
B. Albumin
C. Clotting factors
D. IgG
E. Fibrinogen

43. A 60-year-old woman presents with dyspepsia, a weight loss of 10 pounds and postprandial nausea for 3 months. Her past medical history is significant for hypertension and breast cancer, treated with surgery and adjuvant chemotherapy 5 years ago. Her physical exam reveals normal vital signs, cardiac, pulmonary, and abdominal exams. She has peripheral edema. She is referred to a gastroenterologist and undergoes an EGD. This shows hypertrophic gastric folds with ample secretions. Antral biopsy shows a few *H. pylori* organisms. Which of the following is the most appropriate treatment?
A. Proton pump inhibitor (PPI)
B. Gastrectomy
C. Octreotide
D. Antiemetics
E. *H. pylori* eradication

44. A 58-year-old woman presents with persistent burning epigastric discomfort not resolved with empiric PPI therapy for the past 4 weeks. She has repeated episodes of diarrhea but denies nausea and vomiting. On physical exam she has normal vital signs, is thin and pale but not acutely ill appearing. The remainder of her exam is normal. Her serum tTG level is equivocal, and you decide to perform an upper endoscopy. On endoscopy you see a 1.8-cm mucosal mass in the fundus. Biopsies of the mass show proliferating nests of lymphocytes; duodenal biopsies are normal. What is the next diagnostic step in the workup of this neoplastic lesion?
A. No further workup necessary
B. PCR for gene rearrangements
C. Repeat biopsies for flow cytometry
D. Bone marrow biopsy
E. CT of the chest, abdomen, and pelvis

45. A 65-year-old woman presents with dyspepsia. She reports a 6-month history of epigastric burning and occasional nausea. She denies any weight loss. A trial of PPI therapy twice daily has not improved her symptoms. Her past medical history is significant for longstanding RA and a history of a bleeding gastric ulcer 3 years ago. Her physical exam is normal. An EGD is performed that shows multiple antral erosions, mucosal erythema, and thickened folds. Biopsies show atypical lymphocytes infiltrating the mucosa, consistent with mucosa-associated lymphoid tissue (MALT) lymphoma. *H. pylori* organisms are present. Her subsequent staging exams are negative for invasive or advanced disease. What is the best treatment regimen for this patient?
A. Referral for endoscopic ultrasound (EUS) and annual surveillance
B. Referral for surgical excision
C. Radiation therapy
D. *H. pylori* eradication
E. Systemic chemotherapy

46. A 65-year-old woman with MALT lymphoma and *H. pylori* organisms was treated successfully. Her subsequent staging exams are negative for invasive or advanced disease. What is the most appropriate surveillance regimen?
A. EGD and EUS every 3 months for 3 years
B. EGD every 6 months for 2 years, then annually
C. Annual EGD for 5 years
D. No follow-up needed
E. CT scans every 3 months for 3 years

47. A 35-year-old man presents to his local emergency department with a 1-day history of melena and rectal bleeding. His past medical history is significant for a small bowel MALT lymphoma treated medically 2 years earlier. He has been taking nonsteroidal antiinflammatory drugs (NSAIDs) for a nagging headache for 1 week. His blood pressure is 110/70 mm Hg and his heart rate is 108 bpm. He is pale and apprehensive; his cardiac and lung exams are normal. His abdomen is soft, non-tender, without organomegaly, and his rectal exam shows frank blood. His laboratory studies are remarkable for a hematocrit of 27%, platelet count 257,000/μL, and an INR of 0.9. You perform an urgent EGD, which is normal. The colonoscopy is normal except for blood entering the colon at the ileoceal (IC) valve. What is the most likely underlying cause of his clinical symptoms?
A. Arteriovenous malformation (AVM)
B. GIST
C. Carcinoid tumor
D. Diffuse large B-cell lymphoma (DLBCL)
E. NSAID enteropathy

48. A 68-year-old woman presents with epigastric discomfort and occasional nausea for the past 2 months. Physical exam is normal. She is started on a trial of PPI, and a serum test for *H. pylori* is positive. She is treated with a course of antibiotics (triple regimen for 14 days); her symptoms subside. She returns with similar complaints and undergoes an EGD. This shows inflammed mucosa and erosions in the distal gastric body. Biopsies from this area are compatible with MALT lymphoma. Further staging evaluation is negative for invasive disease or spread. What is the best treatment for this patient?
A. Chemotherapy
B. Oral imatinib therapy (Gleevec)
C. Surgery
D. Radiation therapy
E. Retreatment with *H. pylori* eradication therapy

49. A 73-year-old man is evaluated for iron-deficiency anemia. His most recent colonoscopy was 7 years ago and was normal. The gastroenterologist decides to repeat the colonoscopy and encounters multiple polyps in the colon and distal terminal ileum. Biopsies are obtained, and the

preliminary diagnosis of lymphoma is made. What is the most likely type of lymphoma?
A. Follicular lymphoma
B. Burkitt's lymphoma
C. Mantle cell lymphoma
D. DLBCL
E. MALT lymphoma

50. A 28-year-old refugee from Syria presents complaining of weight loss and chronic diarrhea for the past 6 months. The patient's physical exam is unremarkable. Laboratory studies reveal a hemoglobin of 8 g/dL. Stool studies reveal *G. lamblia,* but treatment with antibiotics does not improve his symptoms. An upper endoscopy and colonoscopy are normal; biopsies of the duodenum do not show villous atrophy. A video capsule endoscopy (VCE) is performed and shows multiple thickened folds throughout the small bowel. An enteroscopy is performed, and multiple biopsies are taken. What is the most likely diagnosis of the small bowel lesion?
A. Immunoproliferative small intestinal disease
B. Carcinoid tumor
C. Whipple disease
D. Enteropathy-associated T-cell lymphoma (EATL)
E. MALT lymphoma

51. A 55-year-old man with longstanding celiac disease presents to his gastroenterologist. The patient has been adhering to a gluten-free diet. However, he has lost considerable weight and has developed worsening anemia. In addition, he complains of epigastric tenderness, diarrhea, and occasional vomiting. Small bowel endoscopy shows jejunal ulcers and biopsies are obtained. What characteristic feature would suggest enteropathy-associated T cell lymphoma?
A. Monoclonal T-lymphocytes
B. T-cell receptor gene rearrangements
C. Large, pleomorphic, irregular T-lymphocytes
D. Villous atrophy
E. Large, irregular B-lymphocytes

52. A 56-year-old woman with known hepatitis C presents with complains of right upper quadrant pain and mild weight loss for the past 3 months. Her physical exam shows an enlarged liver but is otherwise normal. A CT scan shows a homogeneous low-attenuation mass with a thin enhancing rim in the right hepatic lobe. Her α-fetoprotein is within normal limits. Imaging characteristics on MRI are not indicative of hepatocellular carcinoma (HCC). A biopsy of the mass is performed. What is the most likely finding in this patient?
A. HCC
B. Marginal zone lymphoma
C. Diffuse large B cell lymphoma
D. Hemangioma
E. Focal nodular hyperplasia

53. A 71-year-old woman presents to her gastroenterologist for evaluation of persistent dyspepsia for the past year. She has been on PPI therapy for 1 year without much relief. She denies weight loss or nausea and vomiting. Her physical exam is normal. She has an upper endoscopy performed, and a 3 cm mucosal mass is seen in the antrum. Biopsies are consistent with a diffuse large B cell lymphoma. Staging evaluation reveals stage II disease. What treatment would you recommend this patient?
A. *H. pylori* eradication therapy.
B. Chemotherapy + rituximab
C. Surgery
D. Radiation therapy alone
E. Palliative care

54. A 38-year-old Caucasian woman is referred to her gastroenterologist for persistent burning epigastric discomfort not resolved with empiric PPI therapy. She has occasional watery diarrhea but denies nausea and vomiting. On physical exam she has normal vital signs, is thin and pale, but not acutely ill appearing. The remainder of her exam is normal. Her serum tTG level is equivocal, and you decide to perform an upper endoscopy. On endoscopy you see a 1.8 cm submucosal mass in the antrum. Deep biopsies of the overlying mucosa are normal; duodenal biopsies are also normal. What is the most common molecular aberration found in this neoplastic antral lesion?
A. Smooth muscle actin (SMA) mutation
B. CDH1-mutation
C. Platelet-derived growth factor receptor-α (PDGFRA)
D. p53 mutation
E. c-KIT mutation

55. A 42-year-old Caucasian man is referred for epigastric discomfort not resolved with empiric PPI therapy. He has denies nausea and vomiting. On physical exam he has normal vital signs and is thin and pale. The remainder of his exam is normal. An endoscopy is performed, and you see a 1.5 cm submucosal mass in the antrum. Deep biopsies of the overlying mucosa are normal. An EUS-guided biopsy of the mass demonstrates this histology as shown in the figure. The cells show strong immunoreactivity for c-KIT. What is the most appropriate management?

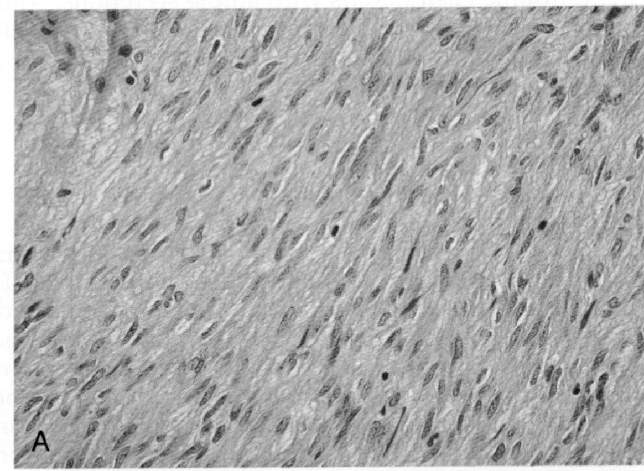

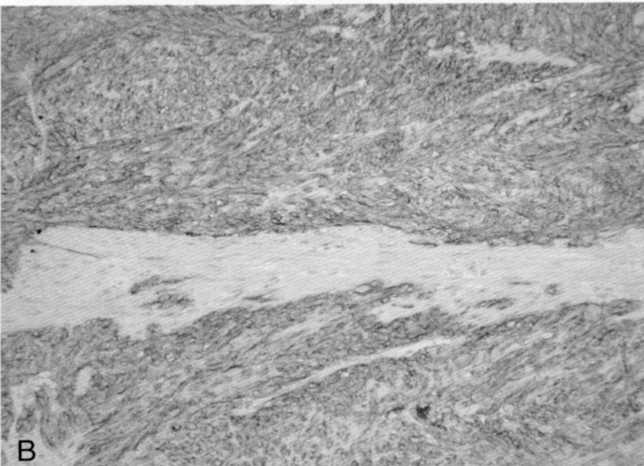

Figure for question 55.

A. Annual surveillance with endoscopic ultrasound
B. Referral for surgical excision
C. No follow-up needed
D. Systemic chemotherapy
E. Attempt an endoscopic removal

56. A 70-year-old man presents to his primary care physician for worsening abdominal pain and weight loss. His physical exam shows normal vital signs and a large hard palpable mass in the epigastrium. He is referred for upper endoscopy, and a large submucosal mass is visualized. The endoscopic ultrasound portion shows a 7 cm heterogeneous hypodense mass in the wall of the gastric body originating from the muscularis propria. A fine-needle aspiration (FNA) cytology is compatible with a gastrointestinal stromal tumor. A PET-CT scan confirms your endoscopic ultrasound findings and does not show any metastatic lesions. What is the most appropriate first treatment?
A. Palliative chemotherapy
B. Surgery
C. Neoadjuvant imatinib therapy
D. Hospice care
E. Radiation therapy

57. A 35-year-old man presents to his local emergency department with a 1-day history of melena and rectal bleeding. His past medical history is significant for neurofibromatosis type I. He has been taking NSAIDs for a nagging headache for 1 week. His blood pressure is 110/70 mm Hg, and his heart rate is 108 bpm. He is pale and apprehensive; his cardiac and lung exams are normal. His abdomen is soft, nontender, with no organomegaly, and his rectal exam shows frank blood. His laboratory studies are remarkable for a hematocrit of 27%, a platelet count of 257,000/μL, and INR of 0.9. You perform an urgent EGD, which is normal. The colonoscopy is normal except for blood entering the colon at the ileocecal valve. What is the most likely source of bleeding?
A. AVM
B. Small bowel lymphoma
C. Carcinoid tumor
D. Small bowel stromal tumor
E. NSAID enteropathy

58. A 63-year-old woman presents to her primary care physician for weight loss and abdominal discomfort. Physical exam shows normal vital signs and a large palpable mass in the epigastrium. A CT scan confirms a 15 cm mass adjacent to the stomach and several hypodense liver lesions. CT-guided biopsy of a liver lesion reveals spindle cells with CD117-positive staining. What is the best treatment for this patient?
A. Palliative chemotherapy
B. Oral imatinib therapy
C. Surgery
D. Hospice care
E. Radiation therapy

59. A 48-year-old woman presents to her oncologist for routine follow-up. She had been diagnosed 8 months earlier with a large GIST (8 cm). Her surgeon suggested neoadjuvant imatinib therapy. She has completed 6 months of oral imatinib 400 mg. You are wondering if she should be referred back to the surgeon for resection. What is the best test to assess the patient's response to therapy?
A. MRI
B. EGD
C. Endoscopic ultrasound (EUS)
D. Somatostatin receptor scintigraphy
E. PET-CT

60. A 73-year-old man presents to his primary care physician for dyspeptic symptoms. He denies weight loss or emesis. He is placed on a PPI without improvement in his symptoms. He is referred to you for EGD. His physical exam is normal. Because his brother died of gastric cancer, you decide to perform an upper endoscopy. The EGD shows a small duodenal ulcer and biopsies are positive for *H. pylori.* On retroflex exam in the stomach you see a 2 cm submucosal mass in the fundus of the stomach, a mucosal biopsy of which comes back showing normal gastric mucosa. What is the most likely diagnosis of the fundal lesion?
A. Gastrointestinal stromal tumor
B. Carcinoid tumor
C. Duplication cyst
D. Pancreatic rest
E. MALT lymphoma

61. A 55-year-old man presents to you for a routine screening colonoscopy. You find two small polyps in the sigmoid colon, which you remove with a cold snare. On retroflex exam in the rectum, 1.5 cm above the dentate line, you see a 1 cm submucosal mass. A mucosal biopsy overlying the mass comes back as normal rectal mucosa. What is the next diagnostic step?
A. Repeat colonoscopy in 5 years
B. MRI of the pelvis
C. Rectal EUS
D. PET-CT
E. Anoscopy and transanal removal

62. A 78-year-old woman is diagnosed with a 6 cm gastrointestinal stromal tumor of the stomach. She undergoes surgical resection and has an uneventful recovery form her surgery. She presents 6 weeks after her surgery to your office to inquire about her further course. You review the pathology report with her. What findings would prompt you to suggest adjuvant imatinib therapy for this patient?
A. CD117 immunostaining
B. 5 mitoses/50 HPFs
C. Epitheloid cell predominance
D. c-KIT mutation
E. PDGFRA mutation

63. A 67-year-old man presents to his oncologist for follow-up care. One year ago he was diagnosed with a large small bowel gastrointestinal stromal tumor. He was referred to a surgeon, but because he had biopsy-proven liver metastases, no surgery was performed. Instead, he was started on imatinib 800 mg orally 6 months ago. After initial response to therapy, as seen on follow-up imaging, his most recent PET-CT shows an increase in the primary tumor size. He comes in today to discuss treatment options. What would you recommend this patient?
A. Continue imatinib 800 mg orally
B. Switch to sunitinib
C. Palliative chemotherapy
D. Surgery
E. Radiation therapy

64. A 58-year-old woman is seen in clinic with the complaints of episodic confusion, dizziness, and fatigue. She also describes recurrent hunger episodes, particularly in the early morning hours. During one of these episodes, her blood glucose was noted to be 28 mg/dL. On physical exam, she is well nourished and in no distress. Her temperature is 99° F, heart rate 85 bpm, respiratory rate is 14 breaths/minute, and her blood pressure is 155/65 mm Hg. Her abdomen is soft and nontender. There is no organomegaly. She is admitted to the hospital for observation and kept nothing by mouth. The next day, she becomes confused and tremulous. Blood glucose level is 40 mg/dL, and serum insulin level is 20 μU/mL. She is now referred for imaging of a possible lesion. Which of the following is the best test for detecting the primary lesion responsible for her symptoms?

A. CT scan
B. Transabdominal ultrasound
C. MRI
D. EUS
E. Somatostatin receptor scintigraphy (SRS)

65. A 28-year-old man comes to his primary care physician's office complaining of severe heartburn for 6 months. He is started on a double dose of PPI and asked to modify his lifestyle. He returns to the office 3 months later with some improvement in his symptoms. After 3 more months his primary care physician requests an EGD. His EGD shows Los Angeles (LA) class D reflux esophagitis. The gastroenterologist requests a serum gastrin level, which comes back at 700 pg/mL (normal <100 pg/mL).What is the most likely reason for the elevated serum gastrin level?

A. Atrophic gastritis
B. Zollinger-Ellison syndrome (ZES)
C. Secondary to PPI dosing
D. Renal failure
E. *H. pylori* infection

66. A 30-year-old man presents with severe epigastric pain for 5 months. He is started on a double dose of PPI and asked to modify his lifestyle. He returns to the office 3 months later with some improvement in his symptoms. After 3 more months his primary care physician requests an EGD. His EGD shows several 1 cm gastric antral ulcers. Serum gastrin is 950 pg/mL (normal <100 pg/mL). What test would make the diagnosis of ZES likely in this patient?

A. Repeat fasting serum gastrin level
B. Measurement of gastric pH
C. Serum PPI level
D. Antiparietal cell antibody test
E. SRS

67. A 67-year-old woman undergoes a routine surveillance colonoscopy for previous colon polyps. On retroflex exam in the rectum, a 1 cm smooth submucosal lesion is noticed. The lesion is biopsied, and pathology reports normal colonic mucosa. An EUS is ordered and shows a 1 cm homogeneous hypoechoic lesion in the submucosa; no lymph nodes are seen. A CT scan of the abdomen is normal. What is the appropriate treatment for this lesion?

A. Surgical resection
B. Chemotherapy
C. Endoscopic resection
D. Yearly surveillance colonoscopies
E. Watchful waiting

68. A 53-year-old man is admitted to the hospital for abdominal pain. On admission, he has an abdominal CT performed that shows several hypodense lesions in the liver. He also complains of epigastric pain, and he undergoes an upper endoscopy. This reveals a 3 cm ulcerated mass in the duodenal bulb. Biopsies report the mass is as compatible with neuroendocrine carcinoma. What is the best treatment for this patient?

A. Palliative chemotherapy
B. Long-acting somatostatin analog (lanreotide)
C. Surgery
D. Hospice care
E. Radiation therapy

69. A 72-year-old woman presents to her primary care physician with epigastric discomfort. She has been treated with empiric PPIs without response. She is referred to a gastroenterologist and undergoes an upper endoscopy. A 1.3 cm nodule is noted in the antrum, which is biopsied. The pathologist reports a neuroendocrine tumor. Her serum gastrin level is 750 pg/mL (normal <100 pg/mL).What is the best treatment for this patient?

A. Endoscopic resection
B. Continue PPI
C. Somatostatin analog injection
D. Surgery
E. Watchful waiting

70. A 57-year-old woman is complaining of left lower abdominal fullness and pain for the last 18 months. She denies diarrhea, rectal bleeding, or weight loss. She has a colonoscopy performed. In the terminal ileum, 10 cm proximal to the iliocecal valve, a 1.5 cm polypoid mass is seen and biopsied. The pathology report indicates a neuroendocrine tumor, (i.e., low-grade carcinoid). In addition to imaging studies, which of the following factors is important in determining the prognosis?

A. Smoking
B. Serum serotonin
C. Serum histamine
D. Serum chromogranin-A
E. Tumor size

71. A 45-year-old man is sent to a gastroenterologist for evaluation of persistent abdominal pain. He reports a burning sensation in the midepigastrium for the last 9 months. He has not lost any weight. He denies nausea or vomiting. He was treated for peptic ulcer disease 5 years ago. His past medical history is significant for kidney stones, hypertension, and parathyroidectomy, years ago. His physical exam is unremarkable. He has an upper endoscopy performed that reveals thickened gastric folds and a several small gastric mucosa nodules. The biopsies are compatible with neuroendocrine tumor. His fasting serum gastrin level is 550 pg/mL (normal <100 pg/mL), and gastric pH is less than 2. What is the next diagnostic step?

A. MRI
B. EUS
C. Somatostatin receptor scintigraphy
D. PET-CT
E. Genetic testing

72. A 50-year-old man presents for evaluation of persistent abdominal pain. He reports a burning sensation in the midepigastrium for the last 7 months. He has not lost any weight. He was treated for peptic ulcer disease 5 years ago. His past medical history is significant for hypertension, diabetes, and parathyroidectomy. His physical exam is unremarkable. He has an upper endoscopy performed that reveals thickened gastric folds and a several small gastric mucosal nodules. The biopsies are compatible with a neuroendocrine tumor. His fasting serum gastrin level is 600 pg/mL (normal <100 pg/mL),

and gastric pH <2. What would be appropriate therapy for this patient?
A. Gastrectomy
B. Pancreatectomy
C. High dose PPI therapy
D. Chemotherapy
E. Endoscopic resection

73. A 50-year-old woman is admitted to the hospital for right lower quadrant abdominal pain. She is seen by a surgeon in the emergency department and taken to the operating room. She undergoes an appendectomy and has an uneventful recovery. She is discharged home and told to follow up with a gastroenterologist for a screening colonoscopy. She comes in today to discuss the pathology report that was sent to her which stated: "inflamed appendix with an 8 mm well-differentiated carcinoid in the tip of the appendix involving the entire wall but not the mesoappendix." No lymph nodes are submitted in the specimen. What would you recommend for this patient?
A. Abdominal CT scan
B. Somatostatin receptor scintigraphy
C. Right completion hemicolectomy
D. 24-hour urine test for 5-hydroxyindoleacetic acid (5-HIAA)
E. Screening colonoscopy

74. A 38-year-old man with a history of HIV (CD4 184/μL) food allergies, and asthma, presents with dysphagia to solid food for 1 week, accompanied by mild substernal discomfort. He denies fevers, chills, or a history of gastroesophageal reflux symptoms. An EGD is performed, which shows diffuse white plaques in the esophagus with associated mucosal hyperemia and friability. Which of the following is the most likely diagnosis?
A. Herpes simplex virus (HSV) esophagitis
B. Cytomegalovirus (CMV) esophagitis
C. Esophageal candidiasis
D. Eosinophilic esophagitis
E. Idiopathic esophageal ulcerations

75. A 24-year-old woman with HIV (CD4 130/μL) presents to the infectious disease clinic with midsternal dysphagia to solids and liquids. A physical exam reveals oral thrush. Which of the following is the most appropriate next step in management?
A. Oral fluconazole
B. EGD
C. Upper GI series
D. Prednisone 40 mg daily, tapered over 4 weeks
E. Initiate treatment with intravenous ganciclovir

76. A 50-year-old African-American man with HIV (CD4 8/μL) complains of substernal chest pain and severe pain with swallowing. An EGD is performed, which shows extensive large and deep ulcerations in the esophagus. Which of the following is most likely to establish a definitive diagnosis?
A. Biopsy from the margins of the ulcer
B. Esophageal brushings and cytology
C. Viral culture
D. Biopsy of granulation tissue from the base of the ulcers
E. Midesophageal random biopsies

77. A 32-year-old man presents to the emergency department with 3 weeks of large volume watery diarrhea, occurring 8 to 10 times per day. He also reports nausea and a 7-lb weight loss. He has a history of gastroesophageal reflux disease (GERD) on a PPI, and HIV, not on highly active antiretroviral therapy (HAART). In the emergency department, vital signs are as follows:

Blood pressure	105/65 mm Hg
Heart rate	118 bpm
Respiratory rate	18 breaths/min
Temperature	36.2° C

A physical exam shows dry mucous membranes, and abdominal exam was benign. Laboratory values are as follows:

Hemoglobin	10 gm/dL
Hematocrit	30%
Platelet count	448,000/μL
WBC	24,000/μL
Potassium	2.8 mEq/L

Stool studies are performed, and an acid-fast stain shows bright red spherules. What is the diagnosis?
A. *Cryptosporidium* infection
B. *C. difficile* infection
C. *G. lamblia* infection
D. *Enterocytozoon bieuneusi* infection
E. *Ascaris lumbricoides* infection

78. What is the current most effective therapy for *Cryptosporidium* infection in patients with HIV?
A. Trimethoprim-sulfamethoxazole
B. Metronidazole
C. Highly active antiretroviral therapy (HAART)
D. Amphotericin B, then fluconazole
E. Nitazoxamide

79. A 48-year-old man with HIV and alcohol abuse, who has been noncompliant with his antiretroviral therapy, comes in with a 3-month history of weight loss, greasy, foul smelling diarrhea, intermittent fevers, and generalized abdominal pain. His CD4 count is 41/μL. Stool studies are negative for fecal leukocytes, *C. difficile* toxin, culture, and ova and parasites. Fecal fat is positive, however. A colonoscopy with random biopsies is normal. An upper endoscopy is performed, and yellow mucosal nodules are identified in the second and third portions of the duodenum. Biopsies are taken from the first and second portions of the duodenum, and histology shows blunted villi, acid-fast stain is positive for extensive macrophages filled with acid-fast bacilli. Which of the following is true?
A. Granulomas are usually present in this clinical scenario
B. Blood cultures can be helpful in establishing the diagnosis
C. Eradication of this organism is often achieved with multidrug antibiotic therapy
D. Fecal acid-fast smear if more sensitive than culture
E. A large majority of patients with this disease are symptomatic

80. A 33-year-old man with HIV presents with recurrent rectal bleeding and painful bowel movements. He has not yet initiated antiretroviral therapy. A colonoscopy reveals an irregular mass in the anorectal area. Biopsies show squamous cell carcinoma. Which of the following is associated with this disease?
A. Human papilloma virus (HPV) types 6 and 11
B. HPV types 16 and 18
C. Human herpes virus-8 (HHV-8)
D. Epstein-Barr virus (EBV)
E. Herpes simplex virus-2 (HSV-2)

81. A 42-year-old woman presents with with right upper quadrant pain, intermittent fevers, nausea, and vomiting for several months. She has a history of acquired immunodeficiency syndrome (AIDS) with a CD4 count of 80/μL and noncompliance with HAART. Laboratory values are as follows:

Alkaline phosphatase	700 IU/L
AST	68U/L
ALT	72U/L
Total bilirubin	1.8 mg/dL
WBC	5000 cells/μL

A CT scan shows extrahepatic biliary ductal dilation. An endoscopic retrograde cholangiopancreatography (ERCP) is performed, which demonstrates extrahepatic ductal dilation, papillary stenosis, and no obvious filling defects. Which of the following statements is *true* about this condition?

A. Sphincterotomy is associated with increased risk of complications
B. The most common inciting infections include cryptosporidia, CMV, microsporidia, and *Isospora*
C. Patients typically present with jaundice
D. A risk factor for this disease is a CD4 count less than 500/μL
E. Antibiotic therapy is effective in reversing this condition

82. Which of the following is the most likely cause of liver test abnormalities in patients with HIV?

A. *Mycobacterium avium* complex (MAC)
B. Fungal infections
C. Non-Hodgkin's lymphoma
D. Antiretroviral therapy
E. CMV hepatitis

83. Which of the following statements is *true* concerning HIV and coinfection with viral hepatitis?

A. HBV and HCV patients co-infected with HIV tend to progress less rapidly to cirrhosis
B. HIV patients are less likely to develop a chronic carrier state when exposed to HBV
C. HBV and HCV lead to progression of HIV disease
D. AIDS patients have a much lower risk of hepatocellular carcinoma (HCC) when co-infected with HBV and HCV compared to those who are HIV negative
E. In HIV patients without evidence of prior infection with HBV or HAV, vaccination is most effective when performed while immune function is preserved

84. Infectious complications after a solid organ transplant are a major cause of morbidity and mortality in the first year. What is the most common viral pathogen occurring within the first year?

A. HSV
B. HHV-6
C. CMV
D. Varicella-zoster virus (VZV)
E. EBV

85. A 52-year-old woman with a history of recent kidney transplant for longstanding uncontrolled hypertension, presents with nausea, vomiting, and diarrhea. She is currently taking mycophenolate mofetil 500 mg twice daily. Vital signs and physical exam are normal. Laboratory values are normal, and stool studies are negative. A CT scan of the abdomen is performed, which shows no acute process. An EGD and colonoscopy with biopsies are normal. What is the next best step in management?

A. Switch to mycophenolic acid delayed release tablets
B. Start empiric metoclopromide
C. Intravenous ganciclovir
D. Treat empirically for *H. pylori*
E. Supportive care with intravenous fluids and nothing by mouth until symptoms improve

86. A 40-year-old man presents to the emergency department with fever and bloody diarrhea. He has a history of a liver transplant 4 months ago for acute liver failure from acetaminophen overdose. He is currently taking tacrolimus and mycophenolic acid. His vital signs are as follows:

Blood pressure	110/72 mm Hg
Heart rate	112 bpm
Respiratory rate	18 breaths/min
Temperature	101.4° F

A physical exam reveals mild diffuse abdominal tenderness to palpation. Laboratory values are as follows:

WBC	2200/μL
Hemoglobin	11 g/dL
Hematocrit	33%
Platelet count	156,000/μL
ALT	66 U/L
AST	74 U/L

A CT abdomen and pelvis is normal. Stool studies are unremarkable except for positive fecal leukocytes. A colonoscopy is performed, which shows friable mucosa with deep ulcers in the distal colon and rectum. Biopsies show large nuclear inclusions with a surrounding halo appearance and small cytoplasmic inclusions. Which of the following is the most likely diagnosis?

A. *C. difficile* colitis
B. Ulcerative colitis
C. Eosinophilic colitis
D. CMV colitis
E. HSV colitis

87. The risk of malignancy is increased in transplant recipients. Which of the following malignancies is increased in this patient population?

A. Lymphoma
B. Hepatocellular cancer
C. Meningioma
D. Prostate cancer
E. Sarcoma

88. A patient undergoes an allogenic bone marrow transplantation for aplastic anemia. A few days after transplant, he develops mucositis, nausea, vomiting, anorexia, and early satiety. Which of the following is the most likely etiology of his symptoms?

A. Upper gut acute graft-versus-host disease (GVHD)
B. Myeloablative conditioning prior to transplant
C. CMV infection
D. *Candida* esophagitis
E. Norovirus

89. A 29-year-old woman is 35 days out from an allogenic bone marrow transplant for leukemia. She develops the acute onset of nausea, vomiting, and diarrhea. The diarrhea is large volume, watery, with ropy strands of mucoid material. Stool studies are negative. You are asked by the hematologist to perform an EGD and flexible

sigmoidoscopy. On exam, you note that the mucosa is diffusely edematous and erythematous throughout the stomach and colon. Histologic exam shows epithelial cell apoptosis, localized lymphocytic infiltrates, and intestinal crypt necrosis. What is the best management option?
A. Supportive care
B. Intravenous ganciclovir
C. Intravenous metronidazole
D. Immunosuppressive therapy
E. Intravenous octreotide with oral loperamide

90. A 52-year-old man with acute lymphoblastic leukemia undergoes an allogenic hematopoietic cell transplant. At day 22 he develops a diffuse rash, abdominal pain, and diarrhea. You are consulted to perform endoscopy. Which of the following biopsy sites is preferred for the diagnosis of GVHD?
A. Esophagus
B. Duodenum
C. Jejunum
D. Gastroesophageal junction
E. Rectosigmoid region and stomach

91. A 28-year-old man who underwent a peripheral blood stem cell transplant for acute myeloid leukemia 2 months ago, presents with retrosternal chest pain, hematemesis, and pain with swallowing, which began after several days of nausea and vomiting. Laboratory analysis reveals a hemoglobin of 10 g/dL, hematocrit 30%, and platelet count of 22,000/μL. A CT scan of the chest is performed, which showed a thickened esophagus and intramucosal mass with narrowed lumen. Which of the following is the most likely diagnosis?
A. Esophageal adenocarcinoma
B. Pill esophagitis
C. Intramural esophageal hematoma
D. HSV esophagitis
E. GERD with erosive esophagitis

92. Which of the following statements is *true* concerning hepatobiliary complications of liver transplant?
A. Biliary complications can occur in up to 50% of patients after liver transplantation
B. The most common biliary abnormalities to occur after liver transplantation are bile strictures and leaks, usually at the anastomosis
C. Recurrence of hepatitis C in the liver allograft is rare
D. CMV hepatitis is rare in patients who have undergone orthotopic liver transplant
E. Invasive fungal infections, such as *Candida* species, occur less commonly in liver transplants than other solid organ transplants

93. A 23-year-old woman with leukemia is in need of a bone marrow transplant and has a sibling who is human leukocyte antigen (HLA) matched. On further testing, it is discovered that her sibling is anti-HBc positive and HBsAg negative. Which of the following statements is *true* concerning hepatitis B and allogeneic hematopoietic cell transplant donors?
A. Donors who have prior exposure to hepatitis B as evidenced by anti-HBc positive and HBsAg negative serologies cannot be used if peripheral blood stem cells and serum are HBV DNA negative
B. Donors who are HBsAg positive and serum HBV DNA negative can donate to patients with no prior history of HBV; no antiviral therapy is required after transplant
C. If both donor and recipient are HBV DNA positive, the recipient should be given antiviral therapy before conditioning
D. Treatment of chronic hepatitis B with entecavir or tenofovir in the donor is not indicated to prevent passage of the virus
E. A recipient who is HBsAg positive or anti-HBc positive will not benefit from an anti-HBc positive donor, as adoptive transfer of immunity does not occur

94. A 68-year-old man with a history of RA, hypertension, and diet-controlled diabetes mellitus presents to his primary care physician complaining of epigastric abdominal pain. His medications include naproxen 500 mg twice daily, amlodipine 5 mg daily, and lisinopril 20 mg daily. His vital signs are normal, and physical exam reveals epigastric tenderness with no rebound or guarding. He has a normal skin exam and no neurologic findings. Laboratory studies are also normal, including a lipase. What is the most likely etiology for his abdominal pain?
A. Rheumatoid vasculitis
B. Pancreatitis
C. Esophageal stricture
D. Peptic ulcer disease
E. Bowel infarction

95. A 48-year-old man visiting from Japan presents to your office with several months of diarrhea and right lower quadrant abdominal pain. On further questioning, he reports a history of clusters of oral ulcers, arthritis, and uveitis. Physical exam is remarkable for mild right lower quadrant tenderness and multiple erythematous nodules on his shins. Ulcerations are also found on the glans penis. A colonoscopy is performed, which shows multiple deep ulcers in the terminal ileum and cecum. Which of the following is true about this disease?
A. GI involvement is not common
B. Recurrences rarely occur after surgery
C. It primarily affects small veins and venules, leading to ulcer formation
D. It frequently causes bowel strictures and perianal disease
E. The vasculitis mainly affects the gastric region

96. A 32-year-old woman with progressive systemic sclerosis presents with dysphagia, reflux, nausea, and weight loss. An EGD is performed which shows LA class C esophagitis in the distal third of the esophagus. She continues to have symptoms despite PPI use, and therefore, esophageal manometry is performed. What the most likely finding on manometry?
A. Aperistalsis of the entire esophagus and incomplete relaxation of the lower esophageal sphincter (LES)
B. Normal LES pressure
C. Aperistalsis in the lower two thirds of the esophagus and low LES pressure
D. Abnormally low pharyngeal contraction and upper esophageal sphincter pressure
E. Simultaneous contractions throughout the esophagus

97. A 23-year-old African-American woman with a past medical history significant for sickle cell anemia, presents to the emergency department with intermittent right upper quadrant pain, occurring several hours after eating and then slowly resolving. Vital signs are normal. An abdominal exam is performed, which shows mild right upper quadrant tenderness but no guarding. Labs are as

follows: total bilirubin of 3.3 g/dL, direct bilirubin of 0.5 g/dL, alkaline phosphatase of 128 U/L, ALT of 18 U/L, AST of 15 U/L, and lipase of 40 IU/L. A right upper quadrant ultrasound is performed, which reveals cholelithiasis and a normal common bile duct. What is the next best step in her management?
A. MRCP (magnetic resonance cholangiopancreatography)
B. ERCP
C. Elective cholecystectomy
D. Observation
E. Gastric emptying study

98. A 48-year-old man presents to your office with abdominal pain, nausea, and vomiting. He was recently diagnosed with systemic mastocytosis, which was first suspected after the presence of urticarial pigmentosa. All of his laboratory values are normal. An EGD is performed, which shows thickened gastric folds, multiple shallow gastric ulcerations, and diffuse nodularity. Mucosal biopsies show a mixed infiltrate, including mast cells, few plasma cells, and eosinophils. What would the next best step in management would be?
A. Histamine receptor antagonists
B. Cytoreductive therapy
C. Treat empirically for *H. pylori*
D. Metoclopramide
E. Treat for eosinophilic gastroenteritis

99. A 72-year-old man with a history of alcoholism is admitted to the ICU with left lower lobe pneumonia. *Streptococcus pneumoniae* is isolated from blood cultures and sputum cultures. The patient is requiring 15 L oxygen face mask and pressor support with norepinephrine. A few days after his hospital admission, his laboratory values are as follows:

Total bilirubin	6.8 mg/dL
Direct bilirubin	4.5 mg/dL
Alkaline phosphatase	180 U/L
ALT	75 U/L
AST	60 U/L
INR	1.3

An abdominal exam reveals mild hepatomegaly but no tenderness to palpation. A right upper quadrant ultrasound of the biliary tract shows a common bile duct (CBD) of 4 mm. The gallbladder wall measures 2 mm, without pericholecystic fluid. There is mild hepatomegaly without focal lesions. What is the most likely etiology for the jaundice?
A. Gilbert syndrome
B. Acute cholecystitis
C. Sepsis
D. Acute liver failure
E. Ischemic hepatitis

100. A 75-year-old man with Parkinson's disease, diabetes mellitus, and a history of prior cerebrovascular accident presents to your GI clinic with multiple abdominal complaints, including early satiety, bloating, and constipation. A workup, including CT of the abdomen and pelvis, EGD, and colonoscopy, are performed, which are negative. Which of the following GI findings are increased in Parkinson's disease?
A. Pancreatitis
B. Constipation
C. GI bleeding
D. Cholelithiasis
E. Diarrhea

101. A 63-year-old man with no past medical history presents with diarrhea and greasy and foul-smelling stools for the past 2 months. He also reports difficulty with chewing and speaking. He has had a 20-pound weight loss during this time period. On physical exam, his vital signs are normal. He is cachectic with temporal wasting. An oropharyngeal exam reveals macroglossia with a dry, fissured tongue. An abdominal exam shows diffuse abdominal tenderness and distention. Which of the following is the most likely diagnosis?
A. Celiac disease
B. Chronic pancreatitis
C. Sarcoidosis
D. Small bowel bacterial overgrowth
E. Amyloidosis

102. A 23-year-old woman presents to her primary care physician complaining of nausea, vomiting, anorexia, and diffuse abdominal pain for several months' duration. She reports a 15-pound weight loss. She has a long history of intermittent oral ulcers and arthralgias. Her vital signs are as follows:

Blood pressure	110/70 mm Hg
Heart rate	105 bpm
Respiratory rate	18 breaths/min
Temperature	37.6° C

Abdominal exam shows diffuse abdominal tenderness with some voluntary guarding. Laboratory studies are significant for a WBC of 2900 cells/μL and albumin of 2.3 g/dL. A CT scan shows intermittent small bowel wall thickening and dilation of the intestinal segments, as well as ascites. Additional laboratory studies, including an antinuclear antibody and double-stranded DNA are positive, and complement levels are low. Which of the following is true about this condition?
A. It usually affects large arteries
B. Segmental areas of the duodenum are most commonly affected
C. Glucocorticoids are the first line therapy
D. Endoscopy may show AVMs
E. Bleeding is not associated with lupus vasculitis

103. A 31-year-old patient recently diagnosed with acute myelogenous leukemia undergoing chemotherapy, presents to the emergency department with fever, nausea, vomiting, right lower quadrant pain, and bloody diarrhea. Vital signs show a blood pressure of 90/60 mm Hg, heart rate of 115 bpm, and abdominal exam reveals right lower quadrant tenderness to palpation with guarding. Laboratory studies are significant for the following:

WBC	800 cells/μL
Absolute neutrophil count	420
Hemoglobin	10 g/dL
Hematocrit	30%

A CT scan of the abdomen with oral contrast is performed and shows wall thickening of the cecum with surrounding inflammatory changes. Which of the following is the most likely diagnosis?
A. Crohn's disease
B. Acute appendicitis
C. Neutropenic enterocolitis
D. Colon adenocarcinoma
E. Ischemic colitis

104. A 72-year-old woman undergoes a routine surveillance colonoscopy for a history of polyps. She denies any melena or hematochezia. Her hemoglobin is 14 g/dL, and her hematocrit is 42%. During the colonoscopy, a 9 mm angioectasia is noted in the ascending colon. What is the most important intervention?
A. Argon plasma coagulation
B. Bipolar electrocoagulation
C. Hormonal therapy
D. Biopsy the lesion
E. Observation

105. A 79-year-old man with a history of hypertension, diabetes mellitus, and a cecal angioectasia presents to the emergency department with multiple episodes of bright red blood per rectum. His abdominal exam is normal, and rectal exam reveals bright red blood in the vault. His vital signs are as follows:

Blood pressure	130/90 mm Hg
Heart rate	100 bpm
Respiratory rate	16 breaths/min
Temperature	36.8° C

His initial laboratory studies reveal the following:

Hemoglobin	12 g/dL
Hematocrit	36%
Platelet count	196,000/μL
INR	1.1

A colonoscopy shows blood throughout the colon, obscuring a complete mucosal exam. The terminal ileum is intubated, and no blood is noted. An EGD is also performed, which is normal. What is the next best step in management?
A. Capsule endoscopy
B. Radionuclide scintigraphy followed by angiography
C. Right hemicolectomy
D. Thalidomide therapy
E. Repeat colonoscopy

106. A 5-year-old girl is diagnosed with hereditary hemorrhagic telangiectasias (HHT; also known as Osler-Weber-Rendu disease). The diagnosis of HHT includes three of four relevant clinical criteria. Which of the following is a criterion for this diagnosis?
A. First degree relative with HHT
B. Caput medusae
C. Aphthous ulcers
D. Visceral lesions of the kidney
E. Onset of bleeding in childhood

107. A 56-year-old man with hepatitis C cirrhosis presents to the GI clinic with severe iron deficiency anemia (IDA). A colonoscopy is normal, and therefore, an EGD is performed. No esophageal or gastric varices are identified, but there is evidence of moderate to severe portal hypertensive gastropathy with no bleeding. What is the initial management?
A. Somatostatin analogs
B. Transjuglar intrahepatic portosystemic shunt (TIPS)
C. Iron supplementation and a nonselective β-blocker
D. Observation
E. Test and treat for *H. pylori*

108. A 54-year-old man is admitted to the ICU with melena and anemia with hemodynamic instability. An EGD is performed, and old blood is found in the stomach, but no lesions are identified. He is maintained on a PPI drip in the ICU. Two days later, he develops recurrent melena, and an EGD is repeated. An isolated protruding vessel surrounded by normal mucosa is noted in the body of the stomach and is treated. Which of the following is true of a Dieulafoy lesion?
A. It is more common in women
B. The most common site of bleeding is from the small bowel
C. Therapeutic techniques include injection therapy, heater probe, band ligation, and hemoclip
D. Rebleeding rates are up to 80%
E. In most cases surgery is required to control bleeding

109. A 68-year-old man with a history of hypertension, arthritis, an abdominal aortic aneurysm (AAA) repair 3 years ago, and prior transient ischemic attack presents to the emergency department with multiple episodes of melena. His medications include aspirin, lisinopril, amlodipine, and ibuprofen, the latter of which he takes twice daily. His vitals are as follows:

Blood pressure	100/68 mm Hg
Heart rate	112 bpm
Respiratory rate	16 breaths/min
Oxygen saturation	98%

Abdominal exam is unremarkable. Laboratories values are as follows:

Hemoglobin	11 g/dL
Hematocrit	33%
Platelet count	188,000/μL
INR	1.1

An emergent EGD is performed, which is negative. What is the next most appropriate step in management?
A. CT angiography
B. Capsule endoscopy
C. Colonoscopy
D. Surgical consult
E. Tagged red blood cell scan

110. A 23-year-old woman is referred to your clinic for severe epigastric pain, vomiting, and early satiety. She reports losing 30 lb in the past 3 months. An EGD is normal. An upper GI series and small bowel follow-through exam are performed, which show a markedly dilated second and third portion of the duodenum. What is the best test to order?
A. Colonoscopy
B. Gastric emptying study
C. Magnetic resonance angiography
D. Sitz Marker study
E. EUS

111. A 21-year-old man presents to his primary care physician with hypertrophy of his right lower leg, varicose veins only on the right side, and intermittent hematochezia. He reports that his leg abnormalities have been present since childhood. Which of the following is the most likely diagnosis?
A. Blue rubber bleb nevus
B. Klippel-Trenaunay syndrome
C. Osler-Weber-Rendu disease
D. Congenital AVMs
E. Diffuse intestinal hemangiomatosis

112. A 78-year-old Caucasian man presents to the emergency department with a several-week history of abdominal pain that has significantly worsened over the past 12 hours. He describes the pain as severe, midabdominal in location, and accompanied by back pain, which is worse lying down and improved somewhat by leaning forward. He has a past medical history of alcohol abuse, smoking, and hypertension. Vital signs show a blood pressure of 100/68 mm Hg and a heart rate of 110 bpm. On physical exam, a pulsatile mass is noted left of the umbilicus, and he has tenderness to palpation and mild guarding diffusely. Laboratory values are as follows:

Hemoglobin	10 g/dL
Hematocrit	30%
Platelet count	220,000/μL
WBC	8000/μL

Chemistries are normal, including a lipase. A CT scan is most likely to show which of the following:

A. Pancreatic edema and stranding
B. Normal exam
C. Ruptured abdominal aortic aneurysm with hemorrhage in the retroperitoneal space
D. Colonic wall thickening at the splenic flexure with associated pericolic fluid
E. Small bowel protruding through an abdominal wall defect with a narrowed neck of the hernia sac

113. A 68-year-old woman with a history of systemic sclerosis and arthritis presents with lightheadedness and fatigue and reports several days of dark tarry stools. She denies abdominal pain or other symptoms. She takes meloxicam for her arthritis. Her vital signs are as follows:

Blood pressure	108/68 mm Hg
Heart rate	95 bpm
Respiratory rate	16 breaths/min
Oxygen saturation	99%

Her conjunctiva and mucous membranes are pale, and abdominal exam is unremarkable. Laboratory values are significant for the following:

Hemoglobin	8 g/dL
Hematocrit	24%
Platelet count	558,000/μL
INR	1.1

An EGD is performed, which shows tortuous dilated vessels in the antrum radiating out from the pylorus. What is the best step in management?

A. PPI therapy
B. Octreotide
C. Epinephrine injection
D. Argon plasma coagulation
E. Antrectomy

114. A 50-year-old woman with no past medical history presented with abdominal pain and distention. She complains of a 6-lb weight loss over the past 2 months. Her abdominal pain is diffuse, persistent, and 5 out of 10 in intensity. Physical exam shows a temperature of 37.5° C, blood pressure of 110/60 mm Hg, and a heart rate of 80 bpm. She is cachectic appearing with a distended abdomen. There is diffuse tenderness to palpation but no distinct mass palpable. Abdominal CT scan shows low attenuation, often loculated fluid throughout the peritoneum, omentum, and mesentery, which is suspicious for pseudomyxoma peritonei. On laparoscopy, jelly-like material is noted. Which one of the following site is the origin of primary tumor?

A. Liver
B. Kidney
C. Appendix
D. Uterus
E. Cervix

115. A 36-year-old man presented to emergency department after trauma to his abdomen during playing basketball. He described pain in midabdomen where the ball hit him. On physical exam his vital signs are as follows:

Temperature	37.5° C
Blood pressure	110/70 mm Hg
Heart rate	80 bpm

Abdominal CT scan was performed and incidentally showed a large well-circumscribed mass in the abdomen. CT-guided biopsy revealed Castleman's disease. Which virus is the most likely etiology for this disease?

A. HIV
B. CMV
C. HHV-8
D. EBV
E. Mumps

116. A 63-year-old man presented with nausea, periumbilical pain, and a 15-pound weight loss in the past 3 months ago. The pain is in the midabdomen and is persistent, 5 out of 10 in intensity. Physical exam shows the following:

Temperature	37.5° C
Blood pressure	110/60 mm Hg
Heart rate	80 bpm

His abdomen is distended with mild tenderness around the umbilicus, but no rebound tenderness, and a diffuse mass in the midabdomen. Abdominal CT scan showed a soft tissue mass in the retroperitoneum. Open biopsy of the mass showed inflammation and fibrosis with no evidence of tumor. Glucocorticoid treatment was started, and the mass regressed dramatically. What is the most likely diagnosis?

A. Retroperitoneal fibrosis
B. Mesenteric hemangiopericytomas
C. Mesentery cyst
D. Castleman's disease
E. Multifocal leiomyomas

117. A 55-year-old man underwent laparotomy and partial small bowel resection following bowel perforation. He started having persistent hiccups 3 days after the procedure. Abdominal exam revealed midline scar with mild erythema and edema. He has mild tenderness at the site of laparotomy. Which of the following is the most appropriate next step in management?

A. Perform abdominal CT scan
B. Start chlorpromazine
C. Advise patient to rebreathe from paper bag
D. Consider pacing of diaphragmatic pacemaker
E. This condition is self-limited; no intervention needed

118. What is the most common organism associated with peritonitis secondary to continuous peritoneal dialysis?

A. *Staphylococcus epidermidis*
B. *Pseudomonas aeruginosa*
C. Fungal infection
D. *Mycobacterium tuberculosis*
E. *E. coli*

119. A 35-year-old woman with past medical history of pelvic inflammatory disease and diabetes mellitus presented with fever and right upper quadrant abdominal pain. Abdominal exam showed right upper quadrant tenderness without guarding or rebound tenderness. Abdominal ultrasound was performed, which showed small amount of ascites, normal gall bladder, and normal liver size and counter. Paracentesis showed elevated WBC of 500 cells/μL with 60% neutrophils, and protein content of 9.0 g/dL. Cytology showed no malignant cells, and culture of ascites fluid was negative for any bacterial infection. Laparoscopy shows extensive adhesions around the liver (see figure). What is the most likely diagnosis?

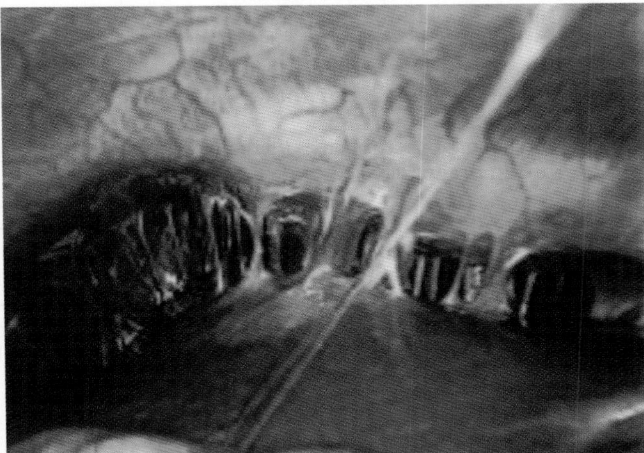

Figure for question 119.

- **A.** Fungal peritonitis
- **B.** Secondary bacterial peritonitis
- **C.** Spontaneous bacterial peritonitis
- **D.** *Chlamydia* peritonitis
- **E.** Starch peritonitis

120. A 53-year-old woman with history of HIV, diabetes mellitus, and chronic kidney disease on peritoneal dialysis presented with abdominal distention and mild fever. Abdominal ultrasound revealed normal size and contour of the liver, normal gallbladder, and moderate sized ascites. Abdominal paracentesis was performed, which showed low serum to ascites albumin gradient (<1.1 g/dL) and high protein concentration. WBC count in ascites fluid was 500 cells/μL, with a lymphocytic predominance. Cytology did not reveal any malignant cells. Furthermore, serum CA-125 as well as ascites-fluid adenosine deaminase levels were elevated. What is the most likely diagnosis?

- **A.** Tuberculosis peritonitis
- **B.** Spontaneous bacterial peritonitis
- **C.** Metastatic ovarian cancer
- **D.** Fungal peritonitis
- **E.** Secondary bacterial peritonitis

121. A 35-year-old woman with history of Wilson's disease on treatment with penicillamine and zinc presented to the clinic for follow-up. She is planning to become pregnant in the next couple of months. How would you advise this patient?

- **A.** She would need to stop penicillamine during pregnancy, as this medication is teratogenic. She can continue zinc supplementation
- **B.** She can start taking penicillamine in the second trimester and can continue taking zinc during pregnancy
- **C.** She should continue at a low dose of penicillamine necessary for chelation and zinc during pregnancy
- **D.** Both medications should be stopped during pregnancy
- **E.** She should increase the dose of penicillamine and stop zinc

122. A 25-year-old woman G1P0, 36 weeks pregnant without any past medical history of liver disease presented to the emergency department with nausea, vomiting, abdominal pain, jaundice, and confusion. Vital signs are as follows:

Temperature	99° F
Blood pressure	95/65 mm Hg
Heart rate	102 bpm

The patient has evidence of asterixis and is disoriented to time, place, and person. Laboratory blood work revealed the following:

AST	200 U/L
ALT	150 U/L
Bilirubin	14 mg/dL
INR	2.3
WBC	16,000 cells/μL
Serum creatinine	2.0 mg/dL
Mildly elevated uric acid	

What is the most likely diagnosis?

- **A.** Acute viral hepatitis
- **B.** Acute fatty liver of pregnancy
- **C.** Cholestasis of pregnancy
- **D.** Gallstone disease
- **E.** Eclampsia

123. Which of the following options are expected to be seen in acute fatty liver of pregnancy (AFLP)?

- **A.** The hallmark of liver biopsy is periportal hemorrhage and intrasinusoidal fibrin deposition
- **B.** Affected individuals have a greater than expected number of female fetuses
- **C.** The fetus usually has long-chain 3-hydroxyacyl coenzyme dehydrogenase (LCHAD) deficiency
- **D.** The disease will be seen in early pregnancy
- **E.** Affected patients most often will require liver transplantation

124. Which of the following is a normal physiologic change during pregnancy?

- **A.** Increased velocity of distal esophageal peristalsis
- **B.** Increased lower esophageal resting pressure
- **C.** Decreased intestinal transit time
- **D.** Increased gastric acid secretion
- **E.** Increased bile acid pool size and gallbladder residual volume

125. A 38-year-old pregnant woman, 35 weeks pregnant presented with complaint of heartburn, regurgitation, nausea, and vomiting. Taking liquid antacids and sucralfate does not control her symptoms. Which of the following options are correct regarding management, physiology, and risk factors of GERD during pregnancy?

- **A.** PPI remains first choice for patients with persistent heartburn despite liquid antacid therapy
- **B.** EGD is required for assessment of persistent GERD
- **C.** Multiparity and older maternal age are risk factors for GERD during pregnancy
- **D.** Resting LES tone progressively increases during pregnancy
- **E.** Omeprazole is pregnancy U.S. Food and Drug Administration (FDA) class B, whereas all other PPIs are class C

126. A 28-year-old Asian woman, 8 weeks pregnant G1P0, is seen in clinic for evaluation of her hepatitis B infection. She was found to have positive HBsAg, negative hepatitis E antigen, and hepatitis B DNA level of 4000 copies/mL. Liver function tests are within normal range. She also has positive hepatitis C antibody. Which is the following is true regarding this patient?
- **A.** The newborn should receive hepatitis B immunoglobulin and vaccine at birth
- **B.** Breast-feeding by the mother is not recommended as there is a risk of viral transmission in infants who received appropriate immunoprophylaxis
- **C.** Treatment with tenofovir appears to be teratogenic during pregnancy
- **D.** Vertical transmission of HCV is common
- **E.** Perinatal HCV infection appears to be higher if baby is delivered vaginally

127. A 28-year-old woman G1P0, 10 weeks pregnant presented to your office with severe nausea, vomiting, and a 5-pound weight loss. There is evidence of ketonuria in her urinalysis. Which of the following options is correct regarding this condition?
- **A.** Prescribing vitamin B_6 is not beneficial in her treatment regimen
- **B.** This condition is usually associated with very high levels of AST, ALT, and total bilirubin
- **C.** Multiple small meals and consumption of a high protein diet is recommended
- **D.** Hormonal change during pregnancy, GI dysmotility, and psychosocial factors do not contribute in developing this condition
- **E.** Phenothiazines are beneficial if antiemetic, and antireflux therapies fail to treat nausea

128. Which of the following medications should be discontinued during pregnancy as part of treatment regimen for inflammatory bowel disease (IBD)?
- **A.** Prednisolone
- **B.** Azathioprine
- **C.** 5-Aminosalicylic acid
- **D.** Methotrexate
- **E.** Budesonide

129. A 35-year-old woman, 35 weeks pregnant G2P1 presented with nausea, vomiting, headache, and blurred vision. Her blood pressure is 160/85 mm Hg, and urine dipstick is positive for protein. Initial laboratory values are as follows:

AST	95 U/L
ALT	150 U/L
Total bilirubin	3.0 mg/dL
Prothrombin time	16 sec
Platelet count	95,000 cells/μL
LDH	600 IU/L

Based on your diagnosis, which of the following statements is correct?
- **A.** Abdominal CT scan is usually normal
- **B.** Liver biopsy should be performed for diagnosis of this condition
- **C.** Preeclampsia is a risk factor for this condition
- **D.** Diagnosis based on assessment of clinical circumstances and the time of presentation is usually not accurate
- **E.** She needs to be monitored in the ICU, and management is primarily supportive

130. Which of the following conditions can be complicated by hepatic rupture during pregnancy?
- **A.** HELLP (hemolysis, elevated liver enzymes, low platelet count) syndrome
- **B.** Autoimmune hepatitis
- **C.** Viral hepatitis
- **D.** Cholestasis of pregnancy
- **E.** Hyperemesis gravidarum

131. Which of the following is true about the effect of pregnancy on GI and hepatic function?
- **A.** Small bowel transit time will be shortened
- **B.** Resting LES tone will be increased
- **C.** Gastric emptying will be delayed
- **D.** Pregnancy does not have any effect on liver enzymes
- **E.** The absorptive capacity of small bowel will decrease during pregnancy

132. A 56-year-old man with history of gastric adenocarcinoma presented with diarrhea with four to five loose, nonbloody bowel movements per day and abdominal bloating for the past 3 months. He received chemoradiotherapy therapy as part of the treatment for gastric adenocarcinoma 2 years ago. On physical exam his vital signs are as follows:

Temperature	37° C
Blood pressure	110/60 mm Hg
Heart rate	80 bpm
Respiratory rate	12 breaths/min

His abdominal exam is mildly distended and nontender. Laboratory values are as follows:

Hemoglobin	10g/dL
WBC	7000/μL
Platelet count	190,000/μL
Creatinine	1.5 mg/dL

Small bowel follow-through (SBFT) shows moderate dilation of a portion of small bowel with a short segment stricture. Initial laboratory blood work revealed low vitamin B_{12} level and high folic acid level. What is the best treatment strategy for his chronic diarrhea?
- **A.** Hyperbaric oxygen therapy
- **B.** Diphenoxylate atropine as needed to control diarrhea
- **C.** Start trial of ciprofloxacin for 2 weeks
- **D.** Subcutaneus octreotide therapy
- **E.** Conservative management with low residue diet

133. A 50-year-old man with past medical history of peripheral vascular disease, hypertension, and Crohn's disease was recently diagnosed with prostate cancer. Over the past 5 years, he has been on infliximab for treatment of his Crohn's disease. He also has history of a partial small bowel resection 2 years ago. He was advised to receive chemoradiotherapy for prostate cancer and wants to know if he has any risk factors for radiation-induced colitis. Which of the following increases the risk of radiation induced injury?
- **A.** Male gender
- **B.** Quiescent IBD
- **C.** Radiation treatment in the prone position
- **D.** Combining chemotherapy with radiation
- **E.** Obese patients

134. A 70-year-old man with history of prostate cancer treated with radiation therapy 2 years ago present with hematochezia and diarrhea. He has four to five small loose bowel movements per day for the past 4 months, with occasional bright red blood. On physical exam his vital signs are as follows:

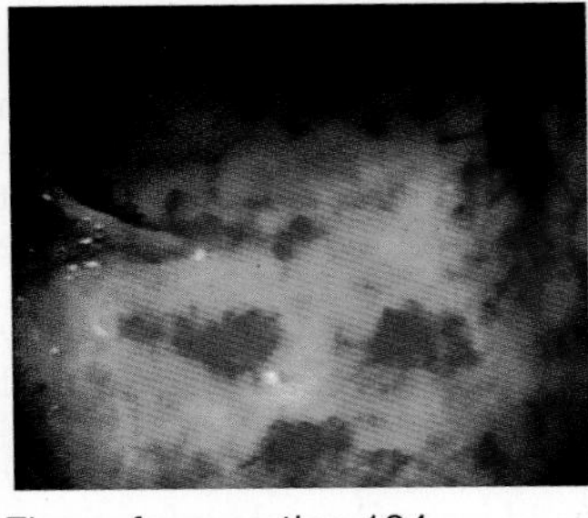
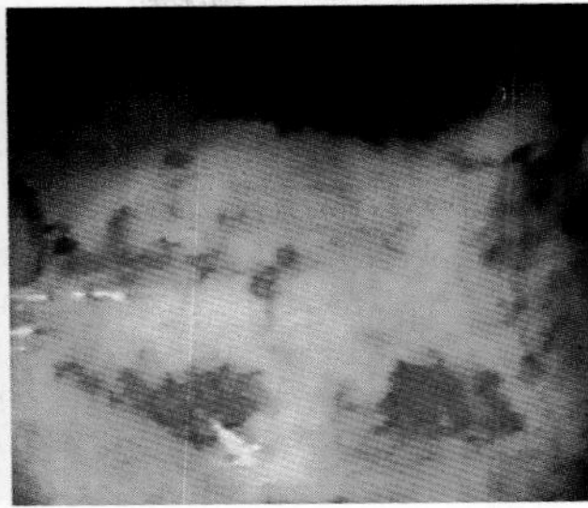

Figure for question 134.

Temperature	37° C
Blood pressure	110/60 mm Hg
Heart rate	80 bpm
Respiratory rate	12 breaths/min

His abdominal exam is soft and nontender. Laboratory values are as follows:

Hemoglobin	8 g/dL
WBC	7000/µL
Platelet count	190,000/µL
Creatinine	1.5 mg/dL

A flexible sigmoidoscopy is performed (see figure). What is the best treatment option?

A. Topical steroids
B. Short-chain fatty acid enemas
C. 5-Aminosalicylate enemas
D. Argon plasma coagulation
E. Surgical resection

135. A 64-year-old man with history of non–small cell carcinoma of the lung underwent lobar resection. He underwent radiation therapy for recurrence of the tumor. Three weeks following initiation of the radiation therapy, he developed sharp sudden onset of chest pain. An EGD was performed, which revealed severe esophagitis, mucositis, and ulceration in mid to distal esophagus. Biopsies of the esophagus show the following (see figure). Which of the following strategies could be used to prevent this condition?

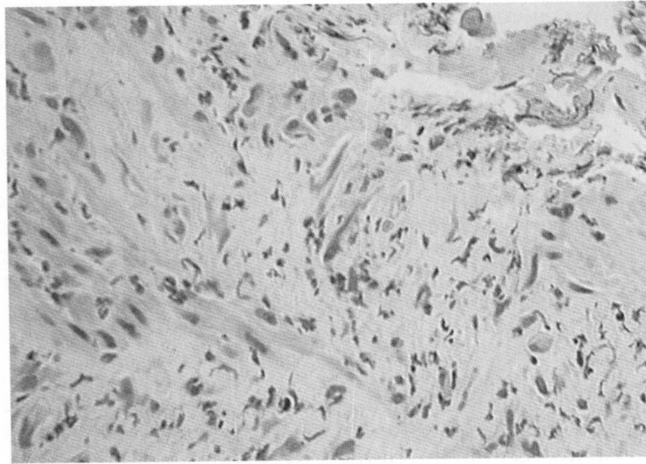

Figure for question 135.

A. Dietary modification, including bland foods, pureed foods, and soft diet
B. Topical anesthetics, including viscous lidocaine
C. High-dose PPI therapy
D. Glutamine/amifostine supplementation during radiation therapy
E. Combination of chemotherapy and radiation therapy

136. A 45-year-old woman with history of lupus, diabetes mellitus, with BMI of 35 kg/m^2 is undergoing radiation therapy of new diagnosis of endometrial cancer. She has history of complicated cholecystitis and underwent open cholecystectomy 3 years ago. Two weeks into the radiation therapy she developed watery diarrhea and nausea. Which intestinal cell damage primarily contributes to the pathophysiology of acute radiation-induced proctitis?

A. Stem cell
B. Foam cells
C. Smooth muscle cell
D. Macrophages
E. Neuronal cells

137. In which of the following situations is prophylactic antibiotics indicated?

A. A 55-year-old man with hepatitis C who presents with hematemesis who is planning to undergo EGD
B. A 65-year-old woman with history of pancreatitis complicated with pseudocyst who presents for EGD for evaluation of nausea
C. A 43-year-old man with history of pancreatitis complicated with pseudocyst who presents for EUS and transgastric aspiration of the cyst
D. A 65-year-old man with history of knee replacement surgery 1 year ago who presents for a colonoscopy with random biopsies for evaluation of diarrhea
E. A 44-year-old man with new finding of pancreatic head solid lesion who presents for EUS and FNA of solid tumor

138. A 60-year-old woman with past medical history of diabetes mellitus and hypertension presented for screening colonoscopy. Colonoscopy was performed, which revealed normal colonic mucosa and scattered diverticulosis. Three hours after the procedure, the patient started having progressive abdominal pain and nausea. On presentation to the emergency department, her vital signs included the following:

Temperature	37.7° C
Blood pressure	110/60 mm Hg
Heart rate	110 bpm

On physical exam, generalized abdominal tenderness with guarding was elicited. Abdominal CT scan was performed, which showed bowel perforation. Which segment of the colon is most likely to perforate after colonoscopy?

A. Sigmoid colon
B. Cecum
C. Transverse colon
D. Ascending colon
E. Descending colon

139. A 60-year-old African-American man with history of diabetes mellitus and symptomatic cholelithiasis presented to the clinic with complaint of persistent right upper quadrant abdominal pain. Laboratory evaluation shows the following:

AST	190 U/L
ALT	150 U/L
Alkaline phosphatase	120 U/L
Total bilirubin	1.1 mg/dL

He underwent cholecystectomy 6 months ago, and his recent abdominal imaging showed moderate intrahepatic and extrahepatic duct dilation. Three years ago, he also had a history of pancreatitis after his last ERCP, which was performed to remove a distal CBD stone. You are planning to perform ERCP. Which combination of risk factors will most increase the risk of post-ERCP pancreatitis?

A. Age, gender, and history of previous post-ERCP pancreatitis
B. Normal bilirubin, age, and gender
C. Normal bilirubin, suspected sphincter of Oddi dysfunction, and prior post-ERCP pancreatitis
D. Age, normal bilirubin, and moderate dilation of biliary tract
E. History of previous PEP, gender, and elevation of transaminase

140. Which one of the following strategies would prevent post-ERCP pancreatitis?

A. Rectal indomethacin
B. Hydration before procedure
C. Prophylactic antibiotic therapy
D. Use of nonionic contrast
E. Avoiding manipulation of CBD

141. Which of the following pathogens persist after disinfection of the endoscopes using proper sterile techniques?

A. Hepatitis C
B. HIV
C. Hepatitis B
D. *C. difficile*
E. Creutzfeldt-Jakob disease

142. A 65-year-old man with history of diabetes mellitus, gastroparesis, congestive heart failure status postautomatic implantable cardioverter defibrillator placement, extensive Crohn's disease with multiple prior abdominal and pelvic surgeries was referred to you for evaluation of occult GI bleeding and iron deficiency anemia. He reports taking ibuprofen for his chronic abdominal pain during the last 3 months. What part of his previous medical history is an absolute contraindication for considering capsule endoscopy for evaluation of obscure GI bleeding?

A. History of gastroparesis
B. Previous abdominal and pelvic surgery
C. Chronic heart failure (CHF) and presence of AICD
D. History of extensive Crohn's disease
E. Previous use of NSAIDs

143. A 55-year-old man presented for screening colonoscopy and was found to have a 3 cm pedunculated polyp in transverse colon, which was removed by hot snare polypectomy. He presented to your office with severe abdominal pain and fever 3 days after the procedure. On physical exam, his vital signs are as follows:

Temperature	38.5° C
Blood pressure	100/60 mm Hg
Heart rate	110 bpm

He has rebound tenderness on abdominal exam. Upon admission, laboratory tests revealed marked leukocytosis (WBC 25,000/μL). Abdominal CT scan did not show any free air. Which of the following choices is the best first step in managing this patient?

A. Bowel rest followed by a consultation to general surgery
B. Bowel rest, broad spectrum antibiotics, and serial abdominal exam
C. This condition is self-limited, and the patient can be safely discharged if there is no evidence of bowel perforation
D. Intravenous fluids, serial abdominal exam, and consultation to general surgery for urgent laparotomy
E. Repeat abdominal CT scan and consultation to general surgery to perform laparotomy as the patient has rebound tenderness

144. A 34-year-old woman with a history of alcoholic cirrhosis presented to the hospital with complaints of dizziness and hematemesis. She was found to be hypotensive and anemic and was admitted to the ICU for resuscitation. You are consulted to manage her upper GI bleeding and decide to perform an EGD. Which of the following is true regarding the complications of EGD?

A. Perforation of the upper GI tract during EGD most commonly happens at the gastroesophageal junction
B. Ulceration following variceal sclerotherapy can occur in up to 30% of patients
C. Topical anesthetic agents such as lidocaine have no associated complications
D. Hypotension during endoscopy is usually due to medication-induced venodilatation in patients who are volume depleted
E. Endoscopic approaches to managing perforations are not recommended

145. A 56-year-old man with history of diabetes mellitus, hypertension, and recent myocardial infarction was referred to you for screening colonoscopy. He underwent percutaneous coronary intervention 3 months ago, with placement of a drug-eluting stent in the midleft anterior descending artery. Currently, his antiplatelet regimen includes aspirin and clopidogrel. How do you advise this patient regarding the plan for screening colonoscopy?

A. Delay the procedure for 1 year until it is safe to stop clopidogrel
B. The patient should stop clopidogrel 5 days before the procedure but can continue aspirin
C. Aspirin and clopidogrel should be stopped 1 week before the procedure
D. Colonoscopy with removal of polyps can be safely performed if indicated
E. Explain to the patient that he is at increased risk of bleeding with polypectomy, document this in your informed consent, and proceed with colonoscopy

ANSWERS

1. C (S&F ch24)
The patient has recurrent GI bleeding and multiple telangiectasias of the lip and vermillion border, consistent with hereditary hemorrhagic telangiectasia (Osler Weber-Rendu disease). Vascular malformations occur in the GI tract, liver, lungs, central nervous system, and genitourinary tract. Patients with Peutz-Jeghers syndrome have multiple mucocutaneous

melanocytic macules that can appear on the lips, but they do not have telangiectasias as shown in the figure. These patients have multiple hamartomatous polyps throughout the GI tract. There is no reason for this patient to have an increased risk of adenomatous polyps, carcinoid tumors, or GIST.

2. **D** (S&F ch24)
Bone loss, angular chilitis, and microcytosis require an explanation in a young and otherwise healthy 18-year-old man. Colonoscopy with surveillance biopsies from terminal ileum to rectum is needed to rule out Crohn's disease or ulcerative colitis. Delay in diagnosing IBD has been shown to range from 3 to 24 months and is associated with complications, such as strictures and surgery. Expert opinion even suggests repeating imaging and laboratory exams for IBD 6 months after an initial study was negative.

3. **E** (S&F ch24)
Porphyria cutanea tarda manifests itself in sun-exposed skin, including dorsum of the hands and neck. The skin manifestations include skin fragility, erosions, scarring, hypertrichosis of the face, alopecia, hyperpigmentation, and sclerodermoid changes. It has been shown that damage to the skin is due to hepatitis C–induced decreased activity of the hepatic enzyme uroporphyrinogen decarboxylase, leading to an increased deposition in the liver and secretion of uroporphyrin in the kidneys. The use of steroid is not indicated in the treatment of porphyria cutanea tarda. The diagnosis is made based on urine collection; there is no indication for punch biopsy or for checking serologies for celiac disease. A colonoscopy is not indicated because there is no increased concurrence of Crohn's disease in this setting.

4. **B** (S&F ch24)
Up to 73% decrease of total and reduced vitamin C has been found in patients with active Crohn's disease. The lack of vitamin C has been shown to hinder recovery of inflammation, resulting in skin manifestations of petechial bleeding, nosebleed, and damaged gums.

5. **A** (S&F ch24)
The image shows the finding of lichen planus. A recent meta-analysis from 2010 has shown that patients with lichen planus are five times more likely to be infected with hepatitis C in comparison to control subjects. In addition to skin, lichen planus can affect mucous membranes, hair, and nails. Thus, it is pertinent to thoroughly examine the patient for additional foci of this skin manifestation. ASCA and p-ANCA are used for the workup of IBD. tTG antibody and antiendomysial antibody make the diagnosis of celiac disease. C-reactive protein and erythrocyte sedimentation rate are nonspecific acute phase markers. IgG4 and liver function tests are used in diagnosing autoimmune pancreatitis.

6. **C** (S&F ch 24)
The image shows tongue nodules suspicious for isolated tongue amyloidosis, and therefore, a biopsy with Congo red staining is appropriate in this setting. In a recent case series of six patients, it was shown that isolated tongue amyloidosis is a rare disorder, usually not associated with systemic disease. However, it still requires extensive workup to exclude systemic manifestations of amyloidosis. Recommended tests are bone marrow biopsy, fat aspiration, and serum and urine protein immunoelectrophoresis. The other tests, including liver biopsy, EGD, exam of the oropharynx, and CT of the head, neck, and chest, will not be useful in this setting of tongue amyloidosis.

7. **E** (S&F ch24)
The presence of neutrophilic dermatitis, like Sweet syndrome, should raise the suspicion for a hematologic malignancy, in particular non-Hodgkin's lymphoma. Non-Hodgkin's lymphoma of the stomach has been associated with chronic *H. pylori* infection. Confirmation of non-Hodgkin's lymphoma and workup includes endoscopy with biopsies, EUS, and abdominal CT scan. If confirmed, further tests for non-Hodgkin's lymphoma include staging with EUS, abdominal and chest CT, right upper quadrant and cervical ultrasound, and bone marrow biopsy.

8. **B** (S&F ch24)
Peristomal pyoderma gangrenosum is a complication of IBD and ileostomy, as shown in the case above. Pyoderma gangrenosum is a neutrophilic dermatitis, similar to Sweet syndrome. Treatment options for peristomal pyoderma gangrenosum include cyclosporine and steroids. Increasing evidence suggest the use of biologics, like anti–TNF-α antibodies, to be superior to conventional therapy. Prior to initiation of biologic therapy, it is mandatory to exclude hepatitis B and tuberculosis infection. Systemic steroids are much more effectual than topical steroids for the treatment of pyoderma gangrenosum. Changing the ileostomy bag brand is not a good treatment option for peristomal pyoderma gangrenosum. Surgery is not the next best management in this setting and should be avoided because it may lead to wound enlargement.

9. **A** (S&F ch24)
This is pellagra, due to niacin deficiency. Deficiency of niacin is characterized by diarrhea, dementia, dermatitis, and death. Besides the workup listed above, urine should be analyzed for serotonin and 5-HIAA, and a 24-hour sample should be collected to test for carcinoid. Thiamine deficiency results in cardiomyopathy and neurologic disease. Riboflavin deficiency presents with angular stomatitis and seborrheic dermatitis. Pyridoxine deficiency results in cheilosis, peripheral neuropathy, and anemia. Folic acid deficiency results in megaloblastic anemia, glossitis, and diarrhea.

10. **D** (S&F ch25)
Suspicion for a Zenker diverticulum as the cause for this patient's oropharyngeal dysphagia and regurgitation of food should be examined by upper GI series with barium. Endoscopic evaluation can be difficult and potentially dangerous, in particular, due to his large diverticula originating from the Kilian triangle. Increasingly, endoscopic management of Zenker diverticula becomes the standard of care. Determining thyroid-stimulating hormone, referral to otolaryngology, or nonenhanced neck CT are not helpful during the initial workup.

11. **C** (S&F ch25)
The patient was diagnosed and treated for bacterial overgrowth with antibiotics. This is supported by a positive lactulose breath test and low vitamin B_{12} serum concentrations. However, the patient developed recurrent symptoms with findings that are consistent with malabsorption, as indicated by low albumin and microcytic anemia. These findings require further explanation. Following a repeat

course of antibiotics, it is worthwhile to examine the small bowel for underlying pathology with an imaging study. Either small bowel follow-through, or magnetic resonance enterography are of value in this scenario. However, given the increased radiation exposure with a small bowel follow-through in a woman of childbearing age, magnetic resonance enterography is the better choice to rule out strictures, fistulous tracts, or diverticuli.

12. A (S&F ch25)
Patients with small bowel diverticula are prone to develop severe dysmotility, which can lead to pseudoobstruction, characterized by abdominal distention and pneumoperitoneum. Conservative measures as outlined in option A are acceptable initial measures. Surgical consultation for exploratory laparotomy is indicated as a second-line intervention. Endoscopic decompression has no role in management of small bowel dysmotility and pseudoobstruction. Metoclopramide has no role in pseudoobstruction.

13. D (S&F ch25)
The estimated incidence of squamous cell carcinoma developing in a Zenker diverticulum is 1.5%. Carcinoma of the diverticulum usually presents with progressive dysphagia, regurgitation, and hematemesis. Radiographic studies usually reveal a filling defect within the diverticulum, which could be mimicked by entrapped food particles. One-step diverticulectomy is the treatment of choice for this condition. Conditions that have been associated with Zenker diverticulum include reflux disease, laryngocele, leiomyoma, cervical esophageal web, stenosis, hiatal hernia, and carotid body tumor. Infections, tonsillar carcinoma, adenocarcinoma, or squamous carcinoma of the esophagus has not been associated with Zenker diverticulum.

14. E (S&F ch25)
Enterolithiasis, single or multiple concretions, develop in the variety of GI diseases and modifications, including adhesions, strictures, diverticulosis, afferent loops, or intestinal tuberculosis. Intestinal concretions are present, ranging from 0.3% to 10%, depending on geographic location. Proximal enteroliths consist mostly of cholic acid salts, versus distal concretions that are predominantly calcium. Depending on the patient's infection with *Mycobacterium* tuberculosis and obstructive symptoms, surgery should be considered. Surgery remains the central line of therapy in definite intervention; however, this should be weighed against the patient's other comorbid conditions.

15. D (S&F ch26)
Development of incisional hernias is one of the most frequently occurring postoperative complications, particularly after a catastrophic event involving the abdomen, as in this patient with a gunshot injury. The incidence has been estimated ranging from 20% to 37% and has been reported as high as 50% in surgeries complicated by postoperative infection and dehiscence. Diagnosis can be a challenge, particularly in overweight patients. The two diagnostic modalities that have been shown to be of benefit are CT and abdominal ultrasound. In the event that CT does not identify the defect, it might be helpful to perform an abdominal ultrasound in an upright position, communicating your suspicion with the radiologist performing the procedure.

16. A (S&F ch26)
As suggested by history, physical exam, and imaging study, a gastric volvulus appears likely. Gastric volvulus has a 30% to 50% mortality without intervention. If the patient is hemodynamically stable, an attempt to temporarily correct the volvulus endoscopically could be made. Temporary correction with a standard upper endoscope is performed under fluoroscopic guidance, especially for patients who are surgical candidates. However, gastric volvulus has a high recurrence rate, and eventually surgery is required, fixating the stomach by gastropexy, hernia reduction, and Nissen fundoplication.

17. C (S&F ch26)
The patient has a large hiatal hernia and multiple erosions at the diaphragmatic pinch, consistent with Cameron erosions. These can lead to chronic blood loss and iron deficiency anemia. The other findings of nonerosive gastritis and duodenitis, small gastric polyps, and diverticulosis are not a cause of iron deficiency anemia.

18. C (S&F ch26)
Umbilical hernia incarceration following paracentesis is a surgical emergency that requires immediate attention and repair, regardless of coagulopathy, the presence of ascites, or thrombocytopenia. Mortality of incarcerated umbilical hernia has been estimated at 3.7%. Watchful waiting, the use of antibiotics, manual reduction, or replacing the paracentesis catheter do not address the underlying problem of entrapment and might make it even worse. Transjugular intrahepatic portosystemic shunt is a long-term solution.

19. C (S&F ch27)
Attempting to endoscopically remove the foreign bodies after endotracheal intubation is the correct management for this patient. Endotracheal intubation protects the airway and allows for a safe procedure. Other tools to use during the retrieval may include an overtube, Roth Net retriever, and an endoscopic protector hood. It is inappropriate to wait until after intoxication has resolved because this will miss the time window when endoscopic removal could be successful. Placing a NG tube and giving polyethylene glycol solution is inappropriate and potentially dangerous in this patient.

20. D (S&F ch27)
Current recommendations are to approach body packers conservatively, waiting for spontaneous evacuation without induction by laxatives. The use of paraffin oil has even been shown to lead to rupture of latex containers. Surgery should be reserved for cases in which the packets fail to pass spontaneously.

21. B (S&F ch27)
This is a case of accidental ingestion, leading to the immediate onset of chest pain, characteristic for acid exposure of the upper airways and GI tract. Acid exposure of the esophagus can lead to coagulation necrosis, as opposed to alkali exposure, which causes liquification necrosis. Endoscopically, esophageal injury is graded from I to IV. Grade I is characterized by mild erythema, grade IIA by bleeding and ulcerations, grade IIB by circumferential ulcerations, grade III by deep ulcerations with exudate, and grade IV by perforation. The patient's injury is consistent with grade III. Current recommendations are to admit the patient with a grade III esophageal injury due to caustic ingestion for close observation to the ICU. The patient should be kept from receiving anything by mouth, he should receive intravenous fluids, and a consultation should be in place

for an otolaryngology exam of the aerodigestive tract, especially in this case because the patient is complaining of hoarseness with increased salivation. NG tube placement, gastric lavage, regular diet, or placement of an esophageal stent are not indicated at this point, as manipulation of the esophagus should be minimized (see table at end of chapter).

22. **A** (S&F ch27)
Foreign bodies of less than 2.5 cm in diameter and less than 5 cm in length are more likely to pass through the pylorus, being expelled spontaneously. Larger objects, as described and options B through E, are less likely pass through physiologic narrowings of the intestinal tract, and the luminal diameter is decreased to less than 23 mm.

23. **C** (S&F ch27)
Ingestion of magnetic foreign bodies can lead to rapid pressure necrosis and possible perforation and peritonitis. Therefore, early intervention with the diagnostic and therapeutic endoscopy for magnetic foreign body retrieval is mandatory. If the magnet cannot be retrieved, surgery is indicated. Watchful waiting and conservative measures delay safe removal of the objects, leading to complications.

24. **B** (S&F ch27)
Food impactions that cannot be dislodged forward into the stomach should be attempted to be removed in a retrograde fashion using a snare, biopsy forceps, and a Roth Net retriever. The food bolus should be physically cut into smaller pieces for removal in a retrograde fashion. It is useful to use an overtube for airway protection to prevent dislodged fragments from passing through the vocal cords into the bronchi. Alternatively, clear plastic caps have been used to suction food boluses and their fragments into the overtube for safe removal. There is no role for glucagon, carbonated drinks, or a colonoscope in the management of this case.

25. **B** (S&F ch28)
A decrease in catheter output to 20 mL or less per 24 hours, in conjunction with improved imaging results, would allow for safe discontinuation of a percutaneous catheter.

26. **B** (S&F ch28)
Some patients with fistulizing Crohn's disease unresponsive to the combination of azathioprine and anti–tumor necrosis factor (TNF)-α might benefit from exchanging azathioprine with methotrexate. Methotrexate, dosed to 20 mg per week, leads to sustained closure of fistulas in 33% of cases. Alternatively, if dose adjustment of infliximab with the addition of methotrexate did not lead to a satisfactory response regarding fistula drainage, tacrolimus presents an alternative approach.

27. **D** (S&F ch28)
Fistulas originating from the small bowel can result in high output, ranging from 500 to 1000 mL per day, associated with electrolyte abnormalities and prerenal kidney failure. Besides correcting electrolyte abnormalities, imaging, and electrocardiogram, supplementation with intravenous fluids matching the fistulous tract output takes absolute priority. If, subsequently, difficulties are encountered correcting electrolytes, a stool sample should be analyzed for osmolite concentrations. This should be taken into account when managing and adjusting this patient's electrolytes.

28. **B** (S&F ch28)
Even with the advent of surgery and anti–TNF-α medications, postoperative recurrence rate for fistulae has been reported to range from 10% to 20%. A high rate of recurrence has been associated with complex fistulae, poor nutrition, disease activity, and high output fistulae. Aggressive management with medications proven to be effective in fistulizing Crohn's disease, including immunomodulators and anti–TNF-α medications, is mandatory to prevent future recurrence and complications.

29. **B** (S&F ch28)
Hounsfield units greater than 20 and the presence of extraluminal gas are highly predictive of an abscess. Differential diagnosis would include tumor necrosis, pseudocysts, and possibly hematomas. Given the size of the abscess being 7 cm x 3 cm, consideration has to be given to percutaneous drainage and culture and sensitivity.

30. **D** (S&F ch28)
Endoscopic drainage of sterile and infected intraabdominal fluid collections is possible for selected anatomic locations. Intraabdominal fluid collections amenable to ultrasound-guided endoscopic drainage include perihepatic, infradiaphragmatic, splenic, pancreatic, and rectal locations. For this approach, the lumen to abscess distance has to be equal to or less than 1 cm, without interposing vessels. Following EUS-supported guidance, the abscess is punctured with a needle, secured with a guidewire, balloon dilated, and patency maintained with a stent. Multiple stents can be placed in this fashion. Depending on location, success rates of 97% are reported.

31. **D** (S&F ch29)
Based on studies in adults with EoE, the frequencies of food triggers were as follows: wheat (60%), milk (50%), soy (10%), nuts (10%), eggs (5%) and seafood (<5%). The rationale for reintroducing foods is to start with the least likely trigger, seafood, and followed sequentially by eggs, nuts/soy, milk, and finally, wheat.

32. **E** (S&F ch29)
In general, EoE is a chronic, recurrent condition. Therefore, treatment is usually given indefinitely to maintain response. Short-term courses may temporally alleviate symptoms, but upon withdrawal, symptoms reappear and eventually strictures may develop. The dosing is aimed toward the least dose possible that suppresses signs and symptoms.

33. **D** (S&F ch29)
Prior to long-term immunosuppression for treatment of eosinophilic GI disorders (EGID), all patients should be evaluated for *Strongyloides stercoralis* infection. This infection can become life threatening in the setting of systemic immunosuppression. MRSA and *E. coli* may all be found in the stool without leading to clinical symptoms or requiring therapy. Testing for *G. lamblia* and *H. pylori* is not required prior to initiating steroid therapy.

34. **A** (S&F ch29)
The patient's symptoms are compatible with GERD or EoE. In a normal esophagus no eosinophils are found in the mucosa. In GERD <7 eos/HPF are seen, and in EoE, generally >15 eos/HPF are seen. This patient most likely has GERD, and a PPI trial should be given. All other therapies are used to treat EoE, which is not established in this patient.

35. B (S&F ch29)
In the pediatric population, the normal GI tract is populated with eosinophils in increasing density from oral to aboral (option B). The assumption is that this also holds true for the adult GI tract. The normal esophagus is devoid of eosinophils; 0 to 7 eos/HPF suggests GERD, and >15 eos/HPF is reported as EoE. Greater than 30 eosinophils/HPF is the hallmark of eosinophilic gastritis/gastroenteritis or colitis.

36. E (S&F ch29)
The clinical presentation and histologic findings are consistent with the diagnosis of eosinophilic gastroenteritis. IgA deficiency has been associated with this disorder. Deficiency of the other immunoglobulins is not associated with eosinophilic gastroenteritis.

37. C (S&F ch29)
The biopsy shows multiple eosinophils in addition to inflammation and fibrosis in the lamina propria, consistent with the diagnosis of eosinophilic esophagitis. The SFED (option C) has shown good success rates in inducing remission in EoE. Head-of-bed elevation and avoidance of fatty food and chocolate is recommended for patients with GERD. A FODMAP diet may be beneficial in patients with irritable bowel syndrome. Lactose intolerant/deficient patients benefit from a lactose free diet.

38. B (S&F ch29)
Endoscopic findings that can be found in patients with EoE include whitish exudates, longitudinal furrows, esophageal rings and furrows, narrow esophagus, strictures, and esophageal lacerations induced by passage of the scope ("crepe-paper" mucosa). On histology there are >15 eos/HPF. Esophageal webs are not a feature of EoE. EoE is more common in males and is treated with swallowed (rather than inhaled) Fluticasone.

39. C (S&F ch30)
The patient's clinical symptoms and laboratory studies are indicative of a protein-losing enteropathy. The small bowel biopsy shows two villi with dilated interstitial spaces and two normal villi pointing to a secondary intestinal lymphangiectasia as the underlying cause. Only constrictive pericarditis results in increased lymphatic pressures and subsequent lymphangiectasia. Eosinophilic gastroenteritis and celiac disease lead to increased mucosal permeability without erosions and subsequent intestinal protein loss. Sarcoidosis and amyloidosis show mucosal erosions, which result in intestinal protein loss.

40. B (S&F ch30)
The patient's clinical symptoms and laboratory studies are indicative of a protein-losing enteropathy, most likely secondary to the patient's SLE. The diagnostic test of choice is an α_1-AT plasma clearance. A 72-hour stool collection for fecal fat would diagnose steatorrhea, as seen in exocrine pancreatic insufficiency, but rarely leads to hypoproteinemia. A 24-hour urine protein collection is used to diagnose nephrotic syndrome but could not explain the diarrhea. An infectious diarrhea would have peripheral eosinophilia and could not explain the hypoproteinemia. Stool electrolytes are commonly abnormal in laxative abuse and rare villous adenomas.

41. D (S&F ch30)
This young patient's clinical symptoms are suggestive of primary intestinal lymphangiectasia. There is some association between the surgical correction of a congenital univentricular heart (Fontan's procedure) and protein-losing gastroenteropathy due to the high central venous pressures. The best treatment is a diet high in protein, low in fat, but enriched with MCT to minimize lymphatic flow. High dose diuretics are beneficial in protein-losing enteropathy due to some cardiac causes but less helpful in patients with a normal echocardiogram. Oral steroids may be of benefit in protein-losing enteropathies due to underlying inflammatory conditions (e.g., IBD, sarcoidosis, SLE). Gastrectomy may be the treatment of choice for Ménétrier's disease after conservative measures have been exhausted. A trial of metronidazole would be beneficial to treat bacterial overgrowth as the cause of the protein-losing enteropathy, but the patient does not report any underlying condition (e.g., previous intestinal surgery, scleroderma).

42. C (S&F ch30)
The patient's clinical symptoms are suggestive of a protein-losing enteropathy. In this condition, serum proteins are secreted into the intestinal lumen irrespective of their size, in contrast to the nephrotic syndrome. However, proteins with a short serum half-life (e.g., most clotting factors, prealbumin, insulin) are generally less affected due to the liver's capacity to rapidly synthesize them. The loss of proteins with longer half-lives (e.g., IgG, albumin, transferrin, fibrinogen) usually exceeds the liver's capacity to increase production, and leads to the subsequent decline in serum values.

43. E (S&F ch30)
The patient's clinical symptoms and endoscopic findings are compatible with Ménétrier's disease. In some instances, this is associated with *H. pylori* infection, and treatment of the infection has led to resolution of symptoms and protein-losing enteropathy. Therefore, this would be first-line therapy in this patient. Most patients with Ménétrier's disease are hypochlorhydric or achlorhydric, and PPI therapy would not be beneficial, although H2-blockers have shown symptomatic improvement. Octreotide is second line therapy, and gastrectomy is reserved for patients that have failed conservative measures. Antiemetics are used for symptomatic control of nausea but do not affect the underlying disease process.

44. C (S&F ch31)
The patient's lesion is most likely a GI lymphoma. Initial workup is directed at classifying the lymphoma. In order to differentiate B- and T-cell lymphomas, immunophenotypic analysis either by flow cytometry or immunohistochemistry is necessary. Once the diagnosis is verified, staging exams such as bone marrow biopsy and CT scanning are indicated. PCR for gene rearrangements is only indicated in T-cell lymphomas to provide prognostic information.

45. D (S&F ch31)
H. pylori eradication therapy is considered first line therapy for disease limited to the mucosa (stage I), and 75% of the patients respond. The patient could initially have an EUS for staging, but she would need definitive treatment. Lymphomas are generally not treated with local excision. Radiation and chemotherapy are generally second-line treatment after failure of *H. pylori* treatment or for advanced disease.

46. B (S&F ch31)
Current recommendations suggest semiannual EGDs for 2 years, then an annual EGD for follow-up of localized disease.

47. **D** (S&F ch31)
The patient's clinical symptoms and laboratory studies are indicative of a small bowel bleeding source. Patients with MALT lymphoma have an increased incidence of malignant transformation into DLBCLs. AVMs and NSAID enteropathy are common lesions of the small bowel but rarely present with brisk GI bleeding. GIST and carcinoid tumors are rare lesions that are not associated with lymphomas.

48. **E** (S&F ch31)
The patient most likely had a relapse of her MALT lymphoma, and this should be treated with a repeat course of *H. pylori* eradication therapy. Both chemotherapy and radiation therapy are reserved for patients who have failed repeated *H. pylori* therapy. Surgery has a very limited role in the treatment of MALT lymphoma. Gleevec is generally used in the treatment of GIST.

49. **C** (S&F ch31)
Although all mentioned lymphomas may occur in the small bowel or colon, the finding of multiple polyps ("lymphomatous polyposis") is characteristic of mantle cell lymphoma. Burkitt's lymphoma and DLBCL are aggressive lymphomas with rapid growth and a high malignant potential. MALT lymphoma and follicular lymphoma generally follow a more indolent course with slower growth but may transform into the above mentioned more aggressive lymphomas.

50. **A** (S&F ch31)
This young patient with symptoms of small bowel disease and infection with *G. lamblia* most likely has immunoproliferative small intestinal disease. This disease primarily affects young individuals from the Middle East and North Africa and has been nicknamed "Mediterranean lymphoma." Carcinoid tumors are focal lesions, although synchronous tumors may occur, and not a diffuse disease. Whipple's disease affects middle-aged white men, presents with arthralgias and neurologic manifestations in addition to GI symptoms, and generally does not show thickened folds on VCE. Enteropathy-associated T-cell lymphoma occurs in the setting of celiac disease and usually display ulcers in the small bowel. MALT lymphoma is generally more focal and does not affect the entire small bowel.

51. **C** (S&F ch31)
Large, pleomorphic, irregular T-lymphocytes are the most common finding in EATL (80%). Both monoclonal T-lymphocytes and T-cell receptor gene rearrangements can be seen in EATL; however, they are also prominent in refractory celiac disease and ulcerative jejunitis. These are the main alternative diagnoses in this patient with previously well controlled celiac disease and worsening symptoms. Villous atrophy is the hallmark of celiac disease and in this patient would indicate refractory celiac disease. Large irregular B-lymphocytes are seen in diffuse large B cell lymphoma, which is not commonly associated with celiac disease.

52. **B** (S&F ch31 and ch96)
Marginal zone lymphoma has been associated with hepatitis C and at times has regressed after successful hepatitis C treatment. Given the normal α-fetoprotein and lack of specific imaging characteristics, HCC is not the likely diagnosis. DLBCL is not associated with hepatitis C. Hemangioma and focal nodular hyperplasia are more common than lymphomas but have different imaging characteristics. Hemangiomas have a hypodense, avascular center and demonstrate peripheral "filling," whereas focal nodular hyperplasia show enhancement of the mass and the central stellate scar. Refer to chapter 96 for a detailed description of all hepatic lesions.

53. **B** (S&F ch31)
For DLBCL, an aggressive lymphoma, current data suggest chemotherapy plus rituximab as the best therapy. Some centers have added radiation therapy to this regimen. The number of cycles and duration are governed by the disease stage. Surgery is currently not recommended for DLBCL because chemotherapy appears to have superior success rates. *H. pylori* eradication therapy is primarily used in the treatment of localized MALT lymphoma but has been employed in a few cases of DLBCL limited to the mucosa. Deeper invasion (stage II or higher) generally requires more aggressive therapies. Radiation therapy alone and palliative care are generally not indicated for stage II disease.

54. **E** (S&F ch32)
The patient's lesion is most likely a GIST. About 80% of these lesions harbor c-KIT mutations. A smaller percentage (15%) contain platelet-derived growth factor receptor-A (PDGFR-A) mutations. Staining for SMA is the immunohistochemical hallmark of true leiomyosarcomas. CDH1 mutations are commonly found in hereditary diffuse gastric cancer, an autosomal-dominant disorder. Mutations of TP53 are the most common finding in sporadic gastric adenocarcinoma, which is a mucosal lesion.

55. **A** (S&F ch32)
The figure shows multiple spindle cells with elongated nuclei and eosinophilic cytoplasm, consistent with gastrointestinal stromal tumor (GIST). GISTs are an increasingly common incidental finding during endoscopic evaluations of the upper GI tract. Lesions less than 2 cm in size without worrisome EUS findings (e.g., cystic areas, inhomogeneous) have a low likelihood of progression and/or malignant transformation. Therefore, EUS evaluation and subsequent surveillance exams to monitor for growth are warranted in most patients. Surgical excision is generally recommended for larger lesions (>2 cm), symptomatic lesions or lesions that have displayed growth. Although the majority of small gastric GISTs do not change over time, a few lesions may show growth and would be referred for definitive therapy. Conventional systemic chemotherapy is not recommended for a gastric GIST. Endoscopic full thickness resection and subsequent closure has been reported in few patients but should be reserved for small lesions and performed in specialized centers as an investigational procedure.

56. **C** (S&F ch32)
The patient's GIST is large (>5 cm), and the primary treatment option of surgery carries significant morbidity. Therefore, trials have shown that prior therapy with imatinib can significantly reduce the tumor size and improve surgical outcomes. Palliative chemotherapy and radiation therapy have shown only limited clinical benefits in GIST and generally are not recommended unless the patient has failed all other treatment strategies (e.g., surgery, molecular therapy). Hospice care is reserved for patients not receiving any tumor-directed therapy.

57. **D** (S&F ch32)
The patient's clinical symptoms and laboratory studies are indicative of a small bowel bleeding source. Patients with neurofibromatosis type 1 *(NF-1)* have an increased incidence of GIST lesions as part of their disease manifestation. AVMs and NSAID enteropathy are common lesions of the small bowel but rarely present with brisk GI bleeding. Small bowel lymphomas and carcinoid tumors are rare small lesions that are not associated with *NF-1.*

58. **B** (S&F ch32)
The patient's clinical symptoms and laboratory studies are compatible with an advanced stage GIST. These tumors have been shown to frequently respond to molecular therapy with imatinib (Gleevec). Both palliative chemotherapy and radiation therapy are not efficacious in GIST. Surgery is generally not used in advanced disease, although debulking of large tumors has been used to treat obstructive symptoms. Hospice care is employed once tumor directed therapy options have been exhausted.

59. **E** (S&F ch32)
Although all the imaging options are able to visualize the gastric submucosal mass, PET-CT provides both anatomic and functional assessment of lesions >1 cm. Both EGD and EUS may give information about the gastric tumor size but generally are not able to adequately assess for disseminated disease (liver). Only half of gastric GIST have somatostatin receptors and hence would show on somatostatin receptor scintigraphy. MRI has limited utility in assessing gastric lesions due to wall motion artifacts.

60. **A** (S&F ch32)
The patient has the incidental finding of a small submucosal mass in the stomach. Most commonly, these lesions are GISTs. Both carcinoid tumors and MALT lymphomas are mucosally based lesions and diagnosed with simple biopsies. Duplication cysts are rare in the stomach. Pancreatic rests, albeit more common, are frequently diagnosed with simple mucosal biopsy.

61. **C** (S&F ch32)
With the increasing use of colonoscopy, a number of incidental findings in the colon and rectum are encountered. The differential diagnosis of submucosal rectal lesions is limited (GIST, carcinoid, cyst, lipoma). For small lesions (<2 cm) endorectal ultrasound has been shown to have the highest diagnostic yield. In addition to assessing the density of the mass, endorectal ultrasound can image the layers of the rectal wall and provide information on the depth or layer of origin (submucosa vs. muscularis propria). MRI and PET-CT are reserved for larger lesions and to assess for distant spread. A repeat colonoscopy is warranted for adenomatous polyps. Transanal resection should be reserved for lesions with malignant potential.

62. **B** (S&F ch32)
A National Institutes of Health consensus conference noted that the "rule-of-five" (size >5 cm, >5 mitoses/50 HPFs) portended a poor prognosis, and several studies have shown that adjuvant imatinib in this scenario is beneficial. CD117 immunostaining and c-KIT mutations are commonly found in gastric GISTs, but the presence or absence does not influence the decision to start imatinib therapy. PDGFR-A mutations are relatively rare (15%) and not prognostically significant. Likewise, the morphologic subtype (epitheloid vs. spindle cell) is not very useful in determining whether to give adjuvant therapy or not.

63. **B** (S&F ch32)
This patient with advanced GIST disease showed an initial response to molecular therapy but subsequently progressed. This is most likely due to an acquired mutation and loss of efficacy. Further continuation or dose escalation of imatinib beyond 800 mg per day would not regain clinical response and would add toxicity. Switching to a different molecular therapy (Sutent) has been shown to regain clinical control of disease in several studies. Palliative chemotherapy and radiation therapy have not shown clinical benefit in advanced GIST disease. Surgery is reserved for patients with curative intent.

64. **D** (S&F ch33)
The patient's abnormal fasting test is positive for insulinoma (plasma insulin to glucose ratio greater than 0.3). The vast majority of tumors are within the pancreas and, generally, small (less than 1 cm). EUS of the pancreas is the most sensitive test for these small lesions. CT and MRI are superior tests to detect distant metastatic disease; however, metastasis is present in less than 10% of the patients with insulinoma on presentation. Transabdominal ultrasound has a low sensitivity in detecting small pancreatic tumors. Somatostatin receptor scintigraphy is generally useful in the workup of neuroendocrine tumors; however, more than half the insulinomas do not contain somatostatin receptors 2 or 5, the receptors utilized in this test.

65. **C** (S&F ch33)
This young patient suffers from severe reflux esophagitis and is treated with high dose PPIs. The most common reason for elevated serum gastrin levels <1000 pg/mL is the PPI dosing. Even though this patient may have ZES, the incidence of ZES is so rare (1:1,000.000), that elevation due to PPI therapy via feedback inhibition is much more common. The second most common reason for elevated serum gastrin levels is atrophic gastritis. Serum gastrin levels may be elevated due to renal failure due to impaired clearance, but generally not more than 500 pg/mL. Serum gastrin levels may also be elevated due to *H. pylori* infection.

66. **B** (S&F ch33)
The hallmark of gastrinomas is secretion of gastrin by the tumor with loss of feedback inhibition and a tumor. The loss of feedback inhibition would be documented in the face of a low pH (high acid production), with an elevated serum gastrin level. Repeating the elevated gastrin level will not differentiate tumor-related elevation from physiologic increases in gastrin (atrophic gastritis). A serum PPI level may be helpful in monitoring patient adherence to PPIs. The parietal cell antibody is elevated in atrophic gastritis, a common differential diagnosis of elevated serum gastrin levels. SRS generally is indicated once the biochemical diagnosis of ZES has been made to localize a potential tumor.

67. **C** (S&F ch33)
The patient most likely has a small rectal carcinoid. Current recommendations favor an attempt at endoscopic removal for lesions less than 1 cm or pedunculated lesions. Larger lesions or those that invade the rectal muscle layer generally require surgery. Chemotherapy is

reserved for advanced-stage disease. The postresection surveillance guidelines have not been formally studied, but most authorities recommend initial close follow-up with subsequent interval increases following negative exams. Watchful waiting does remain an option, because most rectal carcinoids do not show growth. However, the small size and easy accessibility of rectal carcinoids make it a good target for endoscopic removal.

68. **B** (S&F ch33)
The patient's clinical symptoms and laboratory studies are compatible with an advanced-stage neuroendocrine tumor. These tumors have been shown to frequently respond to molecular therapy with somatostatin analogues. Both palliative chemotherapy and radiation therapy are not very successful in neuroendocrine tumors. Surgery is generally not used in advanced disease, although debulking of large tumors has been used to treat obstructive symptoms. Hospice care is employed once tumor-directed therapy options have been exhausted.

69. **A** (S&F ch33)
The patient most likely has a gastric carcinoid type 1 on the basis of atrophic gastritis. These are the most common small gastric neuroendocrine tumors with limited growth potential. They are usually superficial, and most can be resected endoscopically. PPI therapy in patients with atrophic gastritis is not useful. Somatostatin analog injections are effective in disseminated carcinoid or patients with carcinoid syndrome. They are not indicated in small gastric carcinoids. Surgery is usually not necessary in small gastric carcinoids. Watchful waiting may be indicated in the older, debilitated patient or when multiple small gastric carcinoids are present.

70. **D** (S&F ch33)
The patient has an ileal carcinoid. Chromogranin-A has been shown in several studies to have prognostic value, preoperatively as well as postresection. On the other hand, tumor size does not have the same predictive value as in adenocarcinomas (46% of tumors less than 1 cm are associated with liver metastases). Serotonin and histamine levels may be helpful in the evaluation of carcinoid syndrome. Smoking is not known to be a risk factor in neuroendocrine tumors of the ileum.

71. **C** (S&F ch33)
The patient has small gastric carcinoids. Since he has biochemical evidence of ZES, the previous history of parathyroidectomy points to underlying multiple endocrine neoplasia type 1 (MEN1). The most useful imaging exam at this time would be a somatostatin receptor scintigraphy to evaluate for pancreatic and liver lesions. EUS may be more helpful in evaluating pancreatic lesions; however, some liver lesions would be missed. Cross-sectional imaging with MRI or PET-CT can be helpful but may be less specific. Genetic testing is indicated for this patient, primarily for prognostic value (surgery vs. no surgery) and family consultation.

72. **C** (S&F ch33)
In this patient with ZES, multiple endocrine neoplasia type 1, and small gastric carcinoids, the chance of surgical cure is very limited (<10%). Most patients have several pancreatic tumors, which makes selective resection of the functionally active lesion near impossible. Most centers would opt for medical control with high-dose PPI therapy to suppress the excess acid expression and make the patient asymptomatic. Gastrectomy and pancreatectomy are not usually employed in the treatment of MEN1 patients. Chemotherapy has a limited role in ZES treatment. Endoscopic resection of the gastric carcinoid type 2 are technically possible but do not effect the natural history of the disease process.

73. **E** (S&F ch33)
This patient with an incidentally found appendiceal carcinoid shows all the features of a favorable prognosis (size <1 m, well differentiated, less than 3 mm invasion into mesoappendix, with clear surgical margins). These patients are sufficiently treated with the appendectomy and do not require further investigation or surgery. This patient would only benefit from a routine screening colonoscopy at this time.

74. **C** (S&F ch34)
Candida albicans is the most common esophageal infection in AIDS and is consistent with the clinical scenario above. CMV esophagitis is less common than *Candida* and typically presents with severe odynophagia or chest pain. Endoscopic findings of CMV often include large, deep ulcers. HSV esophagitis is uncommon in AIDS, and endoscopy typically reveals large shallow ulcerations. Idiopathic esophageal ulcerations can occur in late-stage AIDS and acute HIV seroconversion, and appear very similar to CMV ulcers. Although food allergies can be related to eosinophilic esophagitis, the endoscopic findings would differ from *Candida* and could include a feline esophagus with linear furrows, small whitish specks rather than diffuse white plaques and mucosal rings.

75. **A** (S&F ch34)
It is reasonable to empirically treat for esophageal candidiasis in AIDS patients presenting with oral thrush and typical symptoms. An EGD should be performed if the patient does not respond to treatment in 1 week. An upper GI would not likely be sufficient for establishing a diagnosis. Prednisone is used for the treatment of idiopathic ulcers. Intravenous ganciclovir would be used for CMV esophagitis.

76. **D** (S&F ch34)
The EGD findings of large, deep ulcerations in a patient with advanced AIDS is suspicious for CMV esophagitis. A biopsy of the base of an ulcer is the most useful for detecting viral cytopathic effect. Viral cultures are not sensitive, and brushings/cytology will not establish the diagnosis. Biopsies from the margins of esophageal ulcers are used to detect HSV esophagitis, as this is the site of viral replication. Midesophageal biopsies are used to detect eosinophilic esophagitis.

77. **A** (S&F ch34)
Cryptosporidium diarrhea presents with severe diarrhea and most commonly affects the small bowel, although it can be in all regions of the GI tract. An acid-fast stain of the stool is typically used to make the diagnosis, with stool antigen testing and PCR as helpful additional tools. The diagnosis can also be made with small bowel or rectal biopsies.

78. **C** (S&F ch34)
Improvement of the immune system has been found to be the most helpful in treating *Cryptosporidium*. Nitazoxamide, paramomycin, and azithromycin can be tried, but they have not been shown to be very helpful. Trimethoprim-sulfamethoxazole is used to

treat *Cyclospora* and *Isospora*. Metronidazole is used for microsporidia. Amphotericin B and fluconazole is used to treat fungi such as *Cryptococcus* infection and coccidiomycosis.

79. **B** (S&F ch34)
The clinical scenario describes that of disseminated *mycobacterium avium* complex (MAC) infection involving the GI tract, which can occur in AIDS. The duodenum is most commonly involved, although MAC can also infect the colon, rectum, ileum, jejunum, stomach, and esophagus. Granulomas are rarely present in AIDS patients with this diagnosis. Blood cultures are often positive. Unfortunately, eradication is difficult with antibiotic therapy, and starting HAART may prove to be the most helpful. Fecal acid-fast smears have low sensitivity. In contrast to *M. tuberculosis*, many patients with MAC in the GI tract are asymptomatic.

80. **B** (S&F ch34)
HPV types 16 and 18 are linked to most cases of anal squamous cell carcinomas in HIV patients, particularly as their disease progresses. HPV types 6 and 11 are commonly linked to anogenital warts. HHV-8 is correlated to Kaposi's sarcoma. EBV has been linked to lymphoma in HIV patients. HSV-2 causes genital or oral herpes infections.

81. **B** (S&F ch34)
The case describes AIDS cholangiopathy, which is characterized by findings resembling sclerosing cholangitis with papillary stenosis. The most common inciting infections include *Cryptosporidium*, CMV, microsporidia, and *Isospora*. The treatment is primarily biliary sphincterotomy, which is safe and not associated with increased complications. Jaundice is not common in this disease. Cholangiopathy usually occurs in advanced AIDS (CD4 count less than 100/μL), and the survival in this disease depends on the degree of immunodeficiency. Although infectious pathogens are usually the etiologic factor, antibiotic therapy is not effective treatment.

82. **D** (S&F ch34)
With the increasing number of antiretroviral medications available, drug-induced liver injury is quite common. Risk factors of drug-induced liver injury in HIV include concurrent HBV or HCV infection, preexisting liver fibrosis, elevation in liver enzymes prior to treatment, older age, history of alcohol abuse, and concurrent treatment with antituberculous therapies. MAC is a very frequent finding in advanced HIV disease. Fungal infections are not uncommon in advanced disease as well. CMV does not commonly cause hepatitis in HIV patients. Hepatic lymphoma may present in advanced AIDS and tends to be aggressive.

83. **E** (S&F ch34)
In HIV patients with no evidence of HBV or HAV, it is best to vaccinate when the immune function is preserved. A high prevalence of HBV and HCV is found in HIV populations, as risk factors such as intravenous drug use and sexual transmission are common for both. Unfortunately, coinfection with HIV confers a higher mortality risk and increased rate to progression to cirrhosis and the presence of HCC. However, HBV and HCV are not linked to progression of the HIV disease.

84. Answers C (S&F ch35)
The peak time period for CMV infection after organ transplant is 4 to 6 months, after antiviral prophylaxis is complete. The clinical features can vary from asymptomatic to fevers, malaise, bone marrow suppression, or invasive disease. HSV and VZV are the next most common pathogens, whereas EBV and HHV-6 infections are less common.

85. **A** (S&F ch35)
Nausea, vomiting, and diarrhea are common side effects of mycophenolate mofetil (Cellcept), whereas mycophenolic acid delayed release tablets (Myfortic) have fewer GI side effects and are better tolerated. One does need to be aware, however, that mycophenolate mofetil can cause histologic changes similar to that of GVHD. Gastroparesis in this scenario is unlikely with the presence of diarrhea, and although seen often in the case of lung transplant patients, is not common in kidney transplants. Intravenous ganciclovir would be indicated if invasive CMV disease was identified, but there is no evidence in this case. There is no evidence of *H. pylori* infection in this case, and the incidence is not increased in transplant patients. Although supportive care may be helpful, it is not the best answer in this scenario.

86. **D** (S&F ch35)
This case is consistent with posttransplant CMV infection. This most commonly occurs within 3 months of discontinuing CMV prophylaxis and is suggested in this clinical scenario by evidence of fever, bone marrow suppression, elevated aminotransferases, and GI involvement. GI CMV infection occurs in up to 40% of liver transplant recipients. *C. difficile* colitis can occur in the posttransplant setting and present as severe disease, but the endoscopic and histologic findings are not consistent in this case. Ulcerative colitis is less likely in this clinical setting, and the pathology description does not support this diagnosis. Eosinophilic colitis has been described with the use of tacrolimus, but biopsies usually show eosinophilic infiltrates, and peripheral eosinophilia are also noted. HSV colitis is extremely rare and would not show the histologic appearance mentioned in the case presentation.

87. **A** (S&F ch35)
Lymphoma is increased in the posttransplant setting. All of the other malignancies listed are not increased in the posttransplant setting. Additional tumors that have been found to be higher than the general population include posttransplant lymphoproliferative disorders, lung cancer, anal cancer, and other skins cancers.

88. **B** (S&F ch35)
The clinical findings are most consistent with the conditioning therapy required prior to bone marrow transplant. GVHD typically occurs after day 20. CMV infection typically occurs around day 50 to 150 after transplant, or sooner if CMV infection was present prior to transplant or the patient received a cord blood transplant. CMV infection is less common now due to prophylaxis. Fungal infections such as *Candida* are less likely due to antifungal prophylaxis, and the case scenario does not suggest this. Norovirus is possible but less likely.

89. **D** (S&F ch35)
This case is most consistent with acute GVHD, based on the timing (less than 20 days posttransplant), endoscopic, and clinical findings. Severe disease may present with diffuse mucosal sloughing and ulcerations. Treatment involves immunosuppressive therapy with steroids. Supportive care alone would not be effective in treating

GVHD and therefore is not the correct answer. Intravenous ganciclovir would be used for invasive CMV disease. Metronidazole would be indicated in the case of *C. difficile* colitis, which is not consistent in this case due to negative stool studies and concurrent upper GI involvement. Octreotide and oral loperamide may be helpful in cases of severe diarrhea due to conditioning therapy, which usually resolves by day 15 posttransplant.

90. **E** (S&F ch35)
The diagnostic yield for GVHD of the gut is highest when biopsies are obtained from the distal colon and stomach, or colon and ileum.

91. **C** (S&F ch35)
The case is consistent with an intramucosal esophageal hematoma, which can occur in posthematopoietic transplant patients due to repeated retching and severe thrombocytopenia. The care is supportive, with typical slow resolution over 1 to 2 weeks. EGD is typically not performed due to the risk of perforation. Esophageal adenocarcinoma is unlikely in this case scenario. Pill esophagitis can occur after ingestion of some medications, but the CT scan findings do not suggest this, nor GERD with erosive esophagitis. HSV esophagitis is rare due to antiviral prophylaxis and would not likely present like this on CT scan.

92. **B** (S&F ch35)
Biliary complications occur in about 25% of liver transplant patients and include bile leaks and strictures. Strictures usually occur at 2 to 6 months posttransplant. These can be treated with endoscopic therapy if a duct-to-duct anastomosis present. If a choledochojejunostomy is present, percutaneous or surgical therapy is indicated. GI CMV infection occurs in up to 40% of orthotopic liver transplant patients, and CMV hepatitis is actually the most common CMV manifestation. Currently, recurrence of hepatitis C occurs in most liver allografts and progresses to cirrhosis within 5 years. Invasive fungal infections occur more commonly in liver transplant patients compared to other solid organ transplants, particularly when antifungal prophylaxis is not given and the mortality is high.

93. **C** (S&F ch35)
If the donor and recipient are HBV DNA positive, the recipient should be given antiviral therapy before conditioning. HBV-naïve recipients require at least 1 year of antiviral therapy if the donor is HBsAg positive and HBV DNA negative. Active hepatitis B donors will transmit virus to the recipient. If there are two equally matched c donors available, the uninfected donor would be best. Donors who have prior exposure to hepatitis B as evidenced by anti–HBc-positive and HBsAg-negative serologies can be used if peripheral blood stem cells and serum are HBV DNA negative. Donors who are HBsAg positive and serum HBV DNA negative can donate to patients with no prior history of HBV; however, antiviral therapy is required after transplant. Treatment of chronic hepatitis B with entecavir or tenofovir in the donor is indicated to prevent passage of the virus. A recipient who is HBsAg positive or anti-HBc positive will benefit from an anti–HBc-positive donor, as adoptive transfer of immunity may assist in clearance of the virus.

94. **D** (S&F ch36)
This patient is taking NSAIDs, which are the most likely cause of upper GI symptoms in those with RA. Rheumatoid vasculitis, an inflammatory condition of the small- and medium-sized vessels, occurs typically in those with severe RA and is often associated with abnormalities of the skin and peripheral nervous system. Pancreatitis is less likely in the setting of a normal lipase. The patient does not complain of dysphagia, and therefore, an esophageal stricture is less likely. A bowel infarction can occur in patients with rheumatoid vasculitis, and the patient's presentation would likely be much more severe than the clinical scenario above.

95. **C** (S&F ch36)
The clinical scenario is consistent with a diagnosis of Behçet's disease, with the findings of oral ulcers, arthritis, uveitis, colonic ulcerations, erythema nodosum, and genital ulcerations. It primarily affects small veins and venules, leading to ulcer formation. GI involvement is common in Behçet's disease, particularly in Japan and the United Kingdom. Recurrences occur in 50% of patients after surgery, usually at the anastomotic site. Some of the findings may mimic Crohn's disease, but Behçet's disease rarely causes bowel strictures and perianal disease. The vasculitis primarily affects the ileocecal region.

96. **C** (S&F ch36)
Progressive systemic sclerosis mainly affects the smooth muscle in the lower two thirds of the esophagus. The upper esophagus, composed of striated muscle, is usually spared. These abnormalities may be seen in other diseases as well, such as amyloidosis, diabetes, chronic alcoholism, esophageal candidiasis, severe reflux, hypothyroidism, or other connective tissue diseases. Aperistalsis of the entire esophagus and incomplete LES relaxation is suggestive of achalasia. Hypertensive LES pressure is characterized by pressures greater than 40 mm Hg that relaxes normally, with normal peristalsis of the esophagus. Abnormally low pharyngeal contraction and upper esophageal sphincter pressure is suggestive of polymyositis. Simultaneous contractions throughout the esophagus are seen in diffuse esophageal spasm.

97. **C** (S&F ch36)
Cholelithiasis occurs in 70% of sickle cell patients and is due to pigmented stones from elevated bilirubin excretion due to chronic hemolysis. Elective cholecystectomy is indicated given symptomatic gallstones. ERCP or MRCP are not necessary as she has no signs of choledocholithiasis. The patient is symptomatic and therefore should not be observed only. Delayed gastric emptying is not likely in this patient, and therefore, a gastric emptying study is not indicated.

98. **A** (S&F ch36)
The biopsies are consistent with systemic mastocytosis. The treatment for this is aimed at reducing mast cell degranulation and controlling pathologic mast cell infiltration, by the use of H1 and/or H2 receptor antagonists, oral disodium cromoglycate, or glucocorticoids. Cytoreductive therapy is reserved for aggressive disease with organ dysfunction. There is no evidence of *H. pylori* in the biopsy specimens. Delayed gastric emptying is not characteristic of this disorder, and therefore, metoclopramide would not be helpful. Although there are eosinophils present in the biopsy specimens, the presence of mast cells are not typical for eosinophilic gastroenteritis.

99. **C** (S&F ch36)
This case is most consistent with hepatic dysfunction due to sepsis, which usually occurs within a few days after

the onset of bacteremia. Bilirubin levels are mostly direct and typically peak between 5 mg/dL and 10 mg/dL. The picture is not consistent with choledocholithiasis or acute cholecystitis, as neither are suggested by the ultrasound imaging. Gilbert syndrome is a common cause of indirect hyperbilirubinemia. There is no evidence of liver failure as evidenced by a normal prothrombin time. The serum aminotransferases are typically significantly elevated in ischemic hepatitis.

100. B (S&F ch36)
Constipation is very common in this patient population and may occur before the diagnosis of Parkinson's disease is made. The incidence of cholelithiasis, pancreatitis, diarrhea, and GI bleeding is not increased in Parkinson's disease. All stages of swallowing can be abnormal in these patients. Delayed gastric emptying is found in most Parkinson's disease patients, and metoclopramide is contraindicated as it aggravates Parkinson's disease.

101. E (S&F ch36)
The diagnosis of amyloidosis is suggested by the presence of macroglossia (pathognomonic), upper GI symptoms, and malabsorption. GI amyloid is most commonly present in the small bowel. Diagnosis is made by performing a serum protein electrophoresis (SPEP) and urine protein electrophoresis (UPEP), bone marrow biopsy, and biopsy of common sites, including the GI tract. Celiac disease, chronic pancreatitis, and small bowel bacterial overgrowth may present with diarrhea and signs of malabsorption, but the other clinical symptoms are not consistent with these diseases. Sarcoidosis may have some overlapping symptoms but overall is not consistent with the above scenario.

102. C (S&F ch36)
The clinical scenario suggests lupus vasculitis, which typically affects medium to small arteries, with the jejunum and ileum being the most commonly involved segments of the bowel. Glucocorticoids are usually effective, although cyclophosphamide may be used in more severe cases. Endoscopy may show ischemia and intermittent punched out ulcers. The presentation of lupus vasculitis can range from mild symptoms to an acute abdomen. Complications include ischemia, infarction, stricture formation, bleeding, and perforation.

103. C (S&F ch36)
This case is consistent with neutropenic enterocolitis or typhlitis, which is a necrotizing process involving the terminal ileum, cecum, and ascending colon. Given the clinical history, Crohn's disease or adenocarcinoma is less likely. Ischemic colitis is possible but less likely, given the location of the colon involvement. Acute appendicitis is also possible, but there is no comment on the appearance of the appendix in the imaging exam and, given the clinical history, neutropenic enterocolitis is more likely. When sepsis is present in this disease process, gram-negative bacteria are the most frequently identified pathogens. Management includes intravenous fluids, transfusion of blood and platelets, granulocyte colony-stimulating factors, and broad-spectrum antibiotics. Surgery is reserved for rare complications.

104. E (S&F ch37)
Observation is best in this case, as the patient is asymptomatic with very low risk of bleeding. Argon plasma coagulation (APC) could be performed in an actively bleeding angioectasia or in the case of iron deficiency anemia. Bipolar electrocoagulation can also be used to treat angioectasias but is less preferred than APC and is not indicated in this patient, who is asymptomatic. Biopsy of the lesion is not recommended as the pathology is usually nonspecific and there is a risk of bleeding. Hormonal therapy is typically reserved for multiple angioectasias throughout the GI tract.

105. B (S&F ch37)
The patient likely has a bleeding colonic angioectasia. Angiography is the next best step in localizing the source and treating the bleeding. Capsule endoscopy would be helpful if bleeding is suspected to be in the small bowel. A right hemicolectomy would be reserved for instances in which the angioectasia is identified and a colonoscopy and angiography are unsuccessful or cannot be performed. Thalidomide, which has antiangiogenic effects, may be helpful, but it is not the next best step in management.

106. A (S&F ch37)
Diagnosis of HHT requires thee out of the following four criteria:
- Recurrent spontaneous epistaxis
- Multiple telangiectasias on the skin, lips, face, nose, or mouth
- Visceral lesions in the internal organs (lungs, brain, liver, intestines, stomach, and spinal cord)
- A first degree relative with HHT

Symptoms typically arise in childhood; however, this is not part of the diagnostic criteria. Caput medusae (distended epigastric veins) and aphthous ulcers are not manifestations of this disease.

107. C (S&F ch37)
Therapy with a nonselective β-blocker, such as propranolol, confers a lower rebleeding rate at 12 months in patients with bleeding from portal hypertensive gastropathy. In refractory cases, TIPS is effective in most cases. Octreotide, which is a somatostatin analog, can also be effective for acute hemorrhage from portal hypertensive gastropathy (PHG) but is not the best answer. Observation would not be appropriate due to the severe IDA. There is no role for testing and treating *H. pylori* in PHG.

108. C (S&F ch37)
A Dieulafoy lesion is a vascular lesion that can be found anywhere in the GI tract but is most commonly found 6 cm distal to the cardioesophageal junction, where the arteries that supply the stomach are largest. It is two times more common in men than women. Massive hemorrhage can occur due to this lesion. If the lesion is identified, it should be marked with tattoo to easily identify it in the case that it rebleeds. Rebleeding rates are about 40%. Therapeutic techniques include injection therapy, heater probe, band ligation and hemoclip. Endoscopic bleeding can usually be achieved by use of multiple modalities; however, in a small subset of cases, surgery is required to control bleeding.

109. A (S&F ch37)
This patient's presentation is suspicious for an aortoenteric fistula, due to his history of abdominal aortic aneurysm repair 3 years ago and negative EGD. A high index of suspicion is required to make this diagnosis. Fistulas can occur when abdominal aortic aneurysm repairs are performed and usually occur in the third or fourth portions of the duodenum. The average time to development of an aortoenteric fistula is 44 months.

A CT angiography is most helpful in establishing the diagnosis. A capsule endoscopy would not be indicated to make this diagnosis. A colonoscopy would only be performed if an aortoenteric fistula was ruled out. A tagged red blood cell scan would not be as helpful in establishing the diagnosis and could delay it. Prompt surgical repair is needed to treat this life-threatening complication.

110. C (S&F ch37)
The clinical scenario describes that of superior mesenteric artery syndrome, which occurs with compression of the duodenum due to a narrowing of the wall of the aorta and the superior mesenteric artery to less than 25 degrees. This leads to gastric and intestinal obstruction. Superior mesenteric artery syndrome has been associated with marked rapid weight loss in adults, rapid growth in children, and full body casts with immobilization. Diagnosis is best made by CT angiography or MR angiography, and barium studies may also be helpful. The other listed studies are not helpful in the diagnosis.

111. B (S&F ch37)
Klippel-Trenaunay syndrome is composed of a vascular nevus of the lower limb, varicose veins only on the affected side, hypertrophy of the tissues of the affected limb, and a variety of vascular lesions. Lesions may occur in the GI tract (up to 20% of patients) liver, spleen, bladder, kidney, lung, and heart. When bleeding occurs from the GI tract, it is usually from the distal colon and rectum. Endoscopic therapy with thermal ablation can be helpful when lesions are localized. Otherwise, surgical intervention may be needed. Blue rubber bleb nevus consists of venous malformations that may involve the GI tract and other sites throughout the body, and orthopedic abnormalities may be present. Diffuse intestinal hemangiomatosis is defined by numerous cavernous type lesions, which affect the stomach, small bowel and colon, as well as skin and soft tissues of the head and neck. Osler-Weber-Rendu (hereditary hemorrhagic telangiectasia) is characterized by telangiectasias of the skin and mucous membranes and does not have orthopedic abnormalities present.

112. C (S&F ch37)
The clinical presentation combined with a pulsatile mass in the abdomen is consistent with a ruptured abdominal aortic aneurysm. Prompt surgical intervention is indicated in this scenario. Pancreatic edema and stranding suggests pancreatitis, which is not likely based on the normal lipase. The CT scan is unlikely to be normal given unstable vital signs and anemia, along with the clinical symptoms the patient has had. Colonic wall thickening at the splenic flexure is suggestive of ischemic colitis. Small bowel protruding through an abdominal wall defect is suggestive of an incarcerated abdominal wall hernia, which was not detected on physical exam in this patient.

113. D (S&F ch37)
This case is consistent with gastric antral vascular ectasia (GAVE), also known as watermelon stomach. GAVE is often seen in middle-aged and older woman with connective tissue diseases, achlorhydria, atrophic gastritis, and other diseases, as well as in patients with cirrhosis and portal hypertension. Initial treatment includes argon plasma coagulation, with antrectomy reserved for severe refractory cases. Epinephrine is not used to control bleeding in GAVE. A PPI is used for peptic ulcer disease, and octreotide is useful in bleeding from portal hypertensive gastropathy and variceal bleeding.

114. C (S&F ch38)
Pseudomyxoma peritonei is a clinical condition in which cancerous cells (mucinous adenocarcinoma) produce abundant mucin or gelatinous ascites. It is most common in women between 45 to 75 years of age. Ovaries and the appendix are the two most common sites of origin for this tumor. The tumor causes gelatinous implants of the peritoneum. Liver, kidney, uterus, and cervical cancer are not associated with pseudomyxoma peritonei.

115. C (S&F ch38)
Castleman's disease is a group of lymphoproliferative disorders that share common lymph node histologic features and may be localized to a single lymph node (unicentric) or occur systemically (multicentric). It is rare and caused by the HHV-8 virus. The unicentric form of the disease usually involves the central lymph node of the mediastinum or mesentery. All other viruses are not involved in the etiology of Castleman's disease.

116. A (S&F ch38)
Retroperitoneal fibrosis is more common in men and usually presents as a retroperitoneal mass. Open biopsy of the retroperitoneal mass shows inflammation and fibrosis. Use of immunosuppressives with glucocorticoids is the treatment of choice. Mesentric cysts are typically large and fluid filled and can be treated with excision of the cyst. Castleman's disease is a group of lymphoproliferative disorders that share common lymph node histologic features and may be localized to a single lymph node (unicentric) or occur systemically (multicentric). Surgical removal of the mass in unicentric form is recommended. Multifocal leiomyomas can be malignant and hormone sensitive. It can develop during pregnancy or estrogen therapy and regress by hormone withdrawal. The treatment of hemangiopericytomas is surgical resection.

117. A (S&F ch38)
Subphrenic abscess can be the etiology of postoperative hiccups, therefore, an abdominal CT scan is recommended. All other choices are reasonable for treatment of persistent and benign hiccups.

118. A (S&F ch38)
Staphylococcus epidermidis contamination of the indwelling catheter is the most common etiology for peritonitis in patients receiving peritoneal dialysis. Other choices, including *Pseudomonas*, fungal infection, *Mycobacterium tuberculosis*, and *E. coli* are less common organisms related to peritonitis secondary to peritoneal dialysis.

119. D (S&F ch38)
Chlamydia peritonitis can present with fever, abdominal pain, and abdominal distention with presence of ascites. History of pelvic inflammatory disease is a risk factor for this condition. Ascites fluid analysis usually demonstrates high WBC count with neutrophilic predominance and high protein levels. Laparoscopic evaluation is often needed to establish the diagnosis by specific findings of perihepatic adhesions, also called "violin slings" or "bridal veil" adhesions that extend from abdominal wall to liver. Spontaneous bacterial peritonitis occurs in patients with liver cirrhosis. This condition is usually associated with high serum ascites albumin gradient level and high WBC count in ascites fluid analysis. Ascites fluid in patients with secondary bacterial peritonitis has elevated WBC counts and is usually polymicrobial when cultured. Fungal peritonitis is

often associated with elevated ascites fluid WBC count with neutrophilic predominance. However, a history of pelvic inflammatory disease and characteristic findings during laparoscopy does not favor the diagnosis of this condition. Starch peritonitis has been described in the past and develops secondary to irritation from glove powder. This condition is unlikely to develop in a patient with no history of recent laparotomy. In addition, manufacturers have replaced cornstarch with more inert substances.

120. A (S&F ch38)
Risk factors for tuberculosis peritonitis include cirrhosis, HIV, underlying malignancy, and diabetes mellitus. Patients have elevated ascites WBC counts with lymphocytic predominance, along with high adenosine deaminase levels. This can differentiate between peritoneal carcinomatosis and tuberculosis peritonitis. Cytology will be positive in more than 90% of the cases of peritoneal carcinomatosis. Cirrhotic patients are at risk for spontaneous bacterial peritonitis. This condition is usually associated with high serum to ascites albumin gradient and high WBC counts in ascites fluid analysis. Secondary bacterial peritonitis usually is polymicrobial and is associated with high neutrophil counts in ascites fluid. Fungal peritonitis usually is associated with high WBC count and neutrophilic predominance in ascites fluid.

121. C (S&F ch39)
Choices A, B, D, and E are incorrect as pregnant patients must remain on medications to treat Wilson's disease because discontinuation of therapy may cause sudden copper release associated with hemolysis, acute liver failure, and death. Penicillamine is potentially teratogenic (FDA pregnancy class D), but appears to be safe during pregnancy at doses necessary for copper chelation. Zinc salt does not appear to be teratogenic, and some experts favor its use during pregnancy.

122. B (S&F ch39)
AFLP presents late in pregnancy, and patients frequently present with altered mental status, elevated INR, and leukocytosis on laboratory exams. Serum aminotransferase are moderately elevated, and jaundice is common. Acute viral hepatitis is the most common cause of acute hepatitis in pregnancy. It is usually associated with higher elevation of liver enzymes. Intrahepatic cholestasis of pregnancy usually presents with mild jaundice (bilirubin <5 mg/dL) and elevated serum bile acids. Sepsis is unlikely in this patient and would not cause such a presentation. Eclampsia presents with hypertension, edema, and proteinuria.

123. C (S&F ch39)
AFLP may develop if the fetus is deficient in LCHAD and carries at least one allele for LCHAD mutation. AFLP is usually seen late in pregnancy and is more common in women with multiple gestations and male fetuses. Patients with AFLP have a greater number of male fetuses compared to female fetuses (2.7:1 ratio). Liver biopsy shows microvesicular fatty infiltration of the liver that is most prominent in hepatocytes surrounding central veins. Periportal hemorrhage and intrasinusoidal fibrin deposition are characteristics of the HELLP syndrome and are not found in AFLP. Most affected women recover completely with supportive care and delivery, and they do not need liver transplantation.

124. E (S&F ch39)
Pregnancy is associated with an alteration in bile composition and increased size of the bile acid pool, which would lead to greater residual gallbladder volumes. Pregnant women have normal gastric secretion. Progesterone has a direct inhibitory effect on gut smooth muscles, leading to slow motility and prolonged intestinal transit time. Furthermore, the velocity of peristaltic waves is decreased in the distal esophagus, and resting LES tone progressively declines during gestation.

125. C (S&F ch39)
The pathogenesis of GERD in pregnant women is related to the effect of pregnancy-related hormones on esophageal motility, LES tone, increased intraabdominal pressure caused by enlarged uterus, and compression of the stomach. Risk factors for GERD during pregnancy include multiparity, older maternal age, and history of reflux during prior pregnancy. EGD is rarely required for the assessment of symptomatic GERD in pregnant women. Ranitidine remains treatment of choice for patients with persistent heartburn despite antacid therapy and PPIs should be reserved for refractory cases. Omeprazole is pregnancy FDA class C, whereas all other PPIs are class B.

126. A (S&F ch39)
The infants of mothers with a positive HBsAg should receive hepatitis B immune globulin at birth and hepatitis B vaccination during the first day of life and at ages 1 and 6 months. Breast-feeding by mothers with chronic hepatitis B does not impose any additional risk of viral transmission as long as the baby has had appropriate immunoprophylaxis. Treatment with tenofovir in the third trimester of pregnancy is safe and effective in preventing vertical hepatitis B viral transmission. Vertical transmission of HCV is rare, and the incidence of perinatal HCV does not seem to be related to the mode of delivery.

127. E (S&F ch39)
Hyperemesis gravidarum (HG) is a severe and persistent vomiting, which requires medical intervention that is associated with acid-base imbalance, nutritional deficiency, and weight loss. HG is associated with slight increases in serum aminotransferase and bilirubin levels in 25% to 40% of cases. Antiemetic and antireflux medications are first-line therapies. Phenothiazines and vitamin B_6 have been shown to reduce symptoms in those who failed initial pharmacotherapy. Patients are often advised to eat multiple small meals high in carbohydrates. The etiology of HG is likely multifactorial, including hormonal changes, GI dysmotility, *H. pylori* infection, and psychosocial factors.

128. D (S&F ch39)
Methotrexate is a class X medication and could be used with caution in patients during childbearing age. The optimum period to abstain from this medication before conception is unknown, but a minimum of 6 months is recommended. Evidence regarding human use of azathioprine and its metabolites has failed to show teratogenicity seen in animal studies. Experts recommend against their discontinuation before or during pregnancy. Glucocorticoid regimens have been used to treat pregnant patients with moderate to severe IBD, as the risk of fetal malformations with this class is very low. 5-Aminosalicylic acid is widely used during pregnancy for treating mild IBD.

129. C (S&F ch39)
The presentation is consistent with HELLP syndrome. Liver biopsy in HELLP syndrome demonstrates intrasinusoidal fibrin deposition, periportal hemorrhage, and irregular areas of liver cell necrosis. However, the diagnosis of HELLP syndrome is mainly established clinically on the basis of the features of the illness at the time of presentation. Laboratory blood work may show evidence of increased serum aminotransferase levels, fragmented red blood cells on blood smears, as well as decreased platelet counts. Abdominal imaging may be helpful in making the diagnosis by showing evidence of intrahepatic hemorrhage and infarction. HELLP syndrome is seen in 12% of women with severe preeclampsia and occurs in 0.2% to 0.8% of all pregnancies. Management of HELLP syndrome includes delivery of the baby in patients who are more than 34 weeks pregnant or have evidence of abnormal fetal testing, or severe maternal disease and disseminated intravascular coagulation.

130. A (S&F ch39)
Spontaneous rupture of the liver may complicate preeclampsia and HELLP syndrome, usually in the third trimester of pregnancy. This condition should be suspected in a pregnant patient who present with abdominal pain, distension, and cardiovascular collapse. Other options are not associated with spontaneous hepatic rupture during pregnancy.

131. C (S&F ch39)
Progesterone directly inhibits gut smooth muscles and results in slower motility. Therefore, gastric emptying and intestinal transit times will be prolonged, and resting LES tone progressively declines. Maternal alkaline phosphatase levels are normally elevated during the third trimester, largely due to placental production. Absorptive capacity of the small bowel will be increased during pregnancy.

132. C (S&F ch40)
Radiation enteritis could result in fibrosis and narrowing of the intestinal lumen due to stricture formation. Small intestinal bacterial overgrowth can be seen in patients who underwent radiation as a result of dilated loops and stasis proximal to stricture. A trial of antibiotics is recommended to treat small intestinal bacterial overgrowth and to control diarrhea. Hyperbaric oxygen therapy and subcutaneous octreotide therapy may reduce risk of acute and chronic radiation enteritis. Antidiarrheal agents and a low residue diet will help to control symptoms of diarrhea but will not help with treating the underlying etiology of diarrhea.

133. D (S&F ch40)
Combining chemotherapy with radiation increases the risk of radiation-induced injury. Toxicity is higher in women, and in IBD but appears to fare better in quiescent IBD than patients with active disease. Other risk factors include thin patients (possibly due to the larger amount of bowel in the pelvis); vasculopathy in patients with comorbid conditions, such as history of diabetes, peripheral vascular disease, hypertension, and cardiovascular disease; as well as a history of collagen vascular disease. Radiation treatment in the prone position with external compression is associated with less toxicity possibly due to exclusion of small bowel from the radiation field. Additionally, radiation dose and volume of the bowel exposed to radiation are important determinants of the severity of radiation-induced toxicity.

134. D (S&F ch40)
This patient has radiation colitis with telangiectasias noted on endoscopy. He is also anemic. Coagulation techniques, such as argon plasma coagulation, are useful for the treatment of bleeding secondary to radiation-induced colorectal ulcerations. This is the best initial treatment. Glucocorticoid suppositories can be helpful for radiation proctitis and can be considered for long-term management. Prostaglandins suppositories such as misoprostol have been investigated as potential radio protective agents. Similarly, short-chain fatty acids and amino acids, which nourish and protect the colonic mucosa, could also be potentially protective against radiation-induced injury. Sucralfate enemas, by forming protective complexes with rectal mucosae, may alleviate radiation proctitis.

135. D (S&F ch40)
The figure shows acute radiation induced esophageal injury with ulcerations and abundant fibroblasts. Amifostine is a free-radical scavenger and has been found to reduce radiation-induced esophageal injury. Glutamine deficiency can occur in the setting of hypercatabolic states like cancer, and its supplementation protects against oxidative injury to normal mucosa during radiation. Both amifostine and glutamine have been studies in trials to prevent radiation-induced injury. Acute radiation-induced esophagitis can be managed by topical anesthetics, gastric antisecretory agents, such as H2 blockers and PPIs, and dietary modifications. Combining of chemotherapy and radiation therapy increases the risk of esophageal toxicity.

136. A (S&F ch40)
Irradiation of the intestinal mucosa primarily affects the clonogenic intestinal stem cells within the crypts of Lieberkuhn. These are the cells that provide replacement cells to the intestinal villi. This leads to a decrease in cellular reserves for the villi and results in shortened villi and decrease absorptive area. In chronic radiation enteritis, the foam cells invade the intima of the arteriolar walls and contribute to obstructive vasculopathy. Although muscle cell, macrophages, and neuronal cells are affected with acute radiation injury, they are not the most critical cells damaged and leading to the pathophysiology of acute radiation enteritis.

137. C (S&F ch41)
Transgastric drainage of pancreatic pseudocysts requires prophylactic antibiotics to prevent cyst infection. Antibiotics are not indicated for a routine EGD in a patient with pancreatic pseudocyst. Prevention of infectious complications, such as spontaneous bacterial peritonitis, with antibiotics is needed before performing EGD in cirrhotic patients who present with acute GI bleeding, but not all patients with GI bleeding (or hepatitis C infection). Patients with prosthetic joints do not require prophylactic antibiotics. Prophylactic antibiotic treatment during FNA of lymph nodes or solid masses is not evidence-based and is not recommended.

138. A (S&F ch41)
Colon perforation occurs most commonly in the sigmoid colon, where it is most likely to encounter looping of the colonoscopy probe. Perforation can also be seen in other sites of colon, including the cecum, transverse colon, ascending colon, and descending colon, but it is not as frequent as the sigmoid colon.

139. C (S&F ch41)
Risk factors for post-ERCP pancreatitis include suspected sphincter of Oddi dysfunction, young age, history of post-ERCP pancreatitis, and normal bilirubin. Gender does not seem to increase risk of post-ERCP pancreatitis. Dilation of the biliary tract will not cause post-ERCP pancreatitis. Pancreatic duct manipulation, including injection, guidewire placement, sphincterotomy, and tissue sampling will increase risk of post-ERCP pancreatitis.

140. A (S&F ch41)
Prophylactic pancreatic stent placement and use of rectal indomethacin prevent post-ERCP pancreatitis in high risk patients. Manipulation of pancreatic duct but NOT bile duct will increase risk of post-ERCP pancreatitis. Other choices have not been shown to prevent post-ERCP pancreatitis.

141. E (S&F ch41)
High-level disinfection would kill most of the pathogens, including HBV, HCV, HIV and *C. difficile*, except prions. Prions are not found in saliva, blood, intestinal tissue, and feces, and therefore are not considered infectious for the purpose of infection control.

142. D (S&F ch41)
Intestinal obstruction, stricture, fistula or extensive Crohn's disease, swallowing disorders, ileus, and intestinal pseudo-obstruction are contraindications to capsule endoscopy. Relative contraindications include pregnancy, long-standing NSAID use, Zenker diverticulum, gastroparesis, previous abdominal pelvic surgery or radiation therapy, and presence of cardiac pacemaker or implantable cardioverter defibrillators.

143. B (S&F ch41)
Post polypectomy syndrome consists of a constellation of signs and symptoms, including fever, abdominal pain with rebound tenderness on exam, and leukocytosis. It typically occurs 1 to 5 days after a procedure and is best treated with hydration, bowel rest, and broad-spectrum antibiotics. Abdominal imaging should be performed to rule out localized perforation if worrisome findings are noted on serial abdominal exam. Mild cases can be treated with antibiotics in an outpatient setting; however, this does not apply to this patient given the presence of significant leukocytosis and rebound tenderness. Urgent laparotomy in the absence of any evidence of perforation is not necessary.

144. D (S&F ch41)
Medication-induced venodilation is usually the cause of hypotension during endoscopy, which is often responsive to administration of intravenous fluids. The oropharynx or cervical esophagus is the most common site of perforation during upper gastroesophageal endoscopy. Up to 78% of patients undergoing variceal sclerotherapy develop ulceration. Other complications of sclerotherapy include perforation, stricture formation, aspiration, as well as pericardial and pleural effusions. Methemoglobulinemia and severe anaphylactoid reaction can develop in those receiving topical lidocaine as a local anesthetic. Methemoglobinemia can be reversed with intravenous methylene blue. Whenever possible, endoscopic therapy should be considered, especially in small perforations that can be treated with clips. Stents and suturing devices are also used in the appropriate settings.

145. A (S&F ch41)
After percutaneous coronary interventions involving drug-eluting stent placement, elective GI procedures (e.g., screening colonoscopy) should be delayed, given the need for dual antiplatelet therapy and an increased risk for bleeding. The decision to continue antiplatelet agent will relate to the risk of thromboembolic event. Clopidogrel needs to be held before a procedure that involves polypectomy as it increases the risk of bleeding. Stopping aspirin and clopidogrel will put this patient at risk of stent thrombosis and is not recommended.

TABLE FOR ANSWER 21 Endoscopic Grades of Caustic Injury

Grade	Endoscopic findings
I	Edema and erythema
IIA	Hemorrhage, erosions, blisters, ulcers with exudate
IIB	Circumferential ulceration
III	Multiple deep ulcers with brown, black, or gray discoloration
IV	Perforation

CHAPTER

5

Esophagus

George M. Philips, Ravi Vora, and Field F. Willingham

QUESTIONS

1. A 55-year-old man has an upper endoscopy for a 15-year history of heartburn. On endoscopy, mild erythema with an irregular Z line is visualized at the gastroesophageal junction. What are biopsies at the gastroesophageal junction most likely to show?
A. Epithelial cells with neutrophilic infiltrate
B. Epithelial cells with eosinophilic infiltrate (>15/hpf)
C. Basal cell hyperplasia and protrusion of rete pegs
D. Epithelial cells with lymphocytic infiltrate
E. Columnar epithelium with goblet cells

2. A newborn is regurgitating saliva, and prenatal exams demonstrated polyhydramnios and an absent stomach bubble. Esophageal atresia is suspected. What diagnostic testing is indicated to confirm the diagnosis?
A. Ultrasound of the esophagus
B. Thoracic computed tomography (CT)
C. Abdominal x-ray
D. Barium swallow
E. Passage of a nasogastric (NG) tube and concurrent chest radiograph

3. A 7-year-old boy was doing well until he began having recurrent hospitalization with dyspnea, cough, and low-grade fevers. On each admission, he was found to have a right lower lobe infiltrate on chest x-ray, consistent with a pneumonia. Esophagography suggested no abnormalities. What is his most likely diagnosis?
A. Isolated esophageal atresia
B. Cystic fibrosis
C. H-type tracheosophageal fistula
D. Distal-type tracheoesophageal fistula
E. Esophageal stenosis

4. A newborn is diagnosed with esophageal atresia and undergoes surgical correction. Which of the following conditions or symptoms is he most likely to develop in later life?
A. Barrett's esophagus
B. Heartburn with esophagitis
C. Esophageal adenocarcinoma
D. Dysphagia
E. Candidal esophagitis

5. A 34-year-old man who is obese and a smoker reports a 5-year history of worsening dysphagia to solid foods. He undergoes an upper endoscopy, which is only notable for a submucosal lesion in the midesophagus. On subsequent endoscopic ultrasound, the lesion is described as an anechoic 15-mm lesion with no associated wall thickening or lymphadenopathy. What is the most likely diagnosis?
A. Esophageal squamous cell carcinoma
B. Esophageal adenocarcinoma
E. Esophageal lipoma
D. Duplication cyst
E. Gastrointestinal stromal tumor (GIST)

6. A 45-year-old man is found to have dysphagia to solids and liquids. On endoscopy he is found to have a symmetrical band of hypertrophied muscle that constricts the tubular esophagus in the lower third of the esophagus. What is the accepted optimal management to relieve the symptoms of dysphagia?
A. Passage of a 50-French mercury-weighted dilator
B. Balloon dilation
C. Heller myotomy
D. Peroral endoscopic myotomy
E. Pneumatic dilation

7. A 45-year-old man reports intermittent dysphagia to solids. An upper endoscopy is performed, and the patient is found to have a Schatzki ring. What is the most likely diameter of the esophageal lumen?
A. 12 mm
B. 14 mm
C. 16 mm
D. 18 mm
E. 15 mm

8. A 50-year-old woman with dysphagia has an upper endoscopy which confirms a Schatzki ring. The ring is bougie dilated. What should be recommended to prevent a recurrence of a Schatzki ring?
A. H2 receptor antagonists
B. Carafate
C. Proton pump inhibitor (PPI) therapy
D. Repeat endoscopy with dilation
E. Weight loss

9. A 43-year-old woman is found to have iron deficiency anemia. A colonoscopy is normal to the terminal ileum. An upper endoscopy is performed and she is found to have a thin horizontal membrane protruding from the anterior wall in the upper esophagus and midesophagus. What is a person with this condition at increased risk for?
A. Squamous cell carcinoma of the pharynx
B. Adenocarcinoma of the esophagus
C. Peptic stricture
D. Eosinophilic esophagitis
E. Achalasia

10. A 25-year-old man presents to your office with dysphagia. Earlier in childhood, he had recurrent upper respiratory tract infections. You obtain a barium esophagram prior to an endoscopic evaluation and it shows a pencil-like indentation at the level of the fourth thoracic vertebra. What are you most likely to find at endoscopy?
   A. Esophageal web
   B. Esophageal ring
   C. Peptic stricture
   D. A patent esophageal lumen
   E. Esophageal adenocarcinoma

11. A newborn is found to have esophageal atresia. In what other organ system is he most likely to have an associated anomaly?
   A. Pancreas
   B. Skin
   C. Eyes
   D. Heart
   E. Lymphatic

12. A 67-year-old man has a cerebrovascular accident (CVA). Subsequently, the patient is confirmed to have recurrent aspiration and difficulty transferring food bolus into the esophagus. Which portion of the esophagus has been compromised by the CVA?
   A. Skeletal muscle
   B. Smooth muscle
   C. Lower esophageal sphincter
   D. Myenteric plexus
   E. Meissner's plexus

13. A newborn is confirmed to have esophageal atresia and undergoes surgical correction. The overall outcome of the newborn is dependent on which of the following?
   A. Severity of cardiac abnormalities
   B. Nutritional status of the mother
   C. Severity of renal abnormalities
   D. Severity of limb abnormalities
   E. Type of esophageal atresia

14. A 65-year-old woman with a history of stroke complains of coughing and sputtering with wet swallows. What is the correct sequence of actions in the highly coordinated pharyngeal swallow response?
   A. Nasopharyngeal closure by elevation and retraction of the soft palate → upper esophageal sphincter (UES) opening → laryngeal closure → tongue loading and pulsion → pharyngeal clearance
   B. Tongue loading and pulsion → nasopharyngeal closure by elevation and retraction of the soft palate → UES opening → laryngeal closure → pharyngeal clearance
   C. Tongue loading and pulsion → laryngeal closure → nasopharyngeal closure by elevation and retraction of the soft palate → UES opening → pharyngeal clearance
   D. Nasopharyngeal closure by elevation and retraction of the soft palate → tongue loading and pulsion → pharyngeal clearance → UES opening → laryngeal closure
   E. Laryngeal closure → nasopharyngeal closure by elevation and retraction of the soft palate → UES opening → pharyngeal clearance → tongue loading and pulsion

15. A 34-year-old woman presents to your clinic complaining of dysphagia to both solids and liquids. She has undergone workup at another facility and brings her records from that evaluation. She was noted to have an integrated relaxation pressure greater than 10 mm Hg and aperistalsis on esophageal manometry. As you discuss her likely diagnosis and treatment options she asks what is the mechanism underlying her condition. What best explains the pathophysiology behind the most likely diagnosis?
   A. Degeneration of the vagus nerve
   B. Diffuse muscular hyperplasia in the distal esophagus
   C. Degeneration of the dorsal motor nucleus
   D. Excess of cholinergic drive
   E. Loss of ganglion cells within the myenteric plexus

16. A 63-year-old man presents to the emergency department for dysphagia. He reports dysphagia to solids and liquids, regurgitation, and chest pain for the past year. He is Spanish speaking only and reports that he also has an abnormal heart. He undergoes an EGD without evidence of a mechanical obstruction, and is awaiting esophageal manometry. Given his history and presentation, what additional testing might be diagnostic of the underlying etiology?
   A. Electrocardiogram
   B. Myocardial biopsy
   C. Esophageal biopsy
   D. Peripheral smear
   E. Polymerase chain reaction

17. A 72-year-old woman presents to your clinic with complaints of dysphagia to both solids and liquids occurring abruptly over the last 4 months. She reports weight loss due to an inability to tolerate peroral intake. She has a medical history significant for hypertension and acid reflux disease. She takes lisinopril and omeprazole daily. Given her symptoms you perform an upper endoscopy and find moderate resistance in passing the endoscope across the gastroesophageal junction (GEJ); however, no mass lesions, nodules, or strictures are seen. What is the next best step in the management for this patient?
   A. Biopsies at the GEJ and site of resistance
   B. Order a barium swallow study
   C. Dilation of the GEJ
   D. Increase PPI to twice daily
   E. Trial of amyl nitrite during manometry study

18. Which of the following statements regarding contrast imaging of swallow function (i.e., modified barium swallow) is correct?
   A. Peristalsis is best evaluated in the upright position
   B. Images are obtained in the anterior projection to best evaluate oropharyngeal function
   C. Primary peristaltic waves manifests as an inverted "V"
   D. Smooth tapering at the esophagogastric junction suggests normal relaxation
   E. Fluoroscopically, a corkscrew appearance can be normal

19. A 34-year-old woman is referred to your office for high-resolution esophageal pressure topography with symptoms of dysphagia and chest pain. As you review her test results, you notice that the integrated relaxation pressure (IRP) is 19 mm Hg. Which of the following statements regarding her study results thus far are false?
   A. IRP is the optimal measurement for quantifying deglutitive relaxation of the esophagogastric junction
   B. Normal IRP is 20 mm Hg or less
   C. IRP is both very sensitive and very specific in distinguishing between achalasia and other diagnoses
   D. IRP is the average pressure for the 4 seconds of greatest relaxation within the relaxation window
   E. IRP cannot be measured with conventional manometry

20. A 24-year-old man presents for follow-up after undergoing high-resolution esophageal manometry for dysphagia and regurgitation. Based on his results, he is diagnosed with achalasia subtype II. Which of the following manometric findings would you expect to find on his study?

A. Mean integrated relaxation pressure (IRP) 18 mm Hg, premature contractions in the distal esophagus
B. Mean IRP 10 mm Hg, absent peristalsis
C. Mean IRP 15 mm Hg, absent peristalsis
D. Mean IRP 21 mm Hg, weak peristalsis
E. Mean IRP 17 mm Hg, absent peristalsis with panesophageal pressurization

21. A 39-year-old woman with dysphagia undergoes high resolution manometry and is found to have normal to slightly weak peristalsis with an integrated relaxation pressure of 16 mm Hg. Which of the following would be the next best step in management?

A. Botox injection
B. Heller myotomy
C. Nonpneumatic dilation
D. CT scan of the chest
E. Impedance measurement

22. A 43-year-old woman presents for follow-up after being diagnosed with achalasia. She has continued to have symptoms and is inquiring about treatment options. Regarding treatment options for achalasia, which of the following statements is true?

A. Two thirds of patients who receive botulin toxin injections will have improvement in their symptoms for 6 months
B. Isosorbide dinitrate is effective in reducing lower esophageal sphincter (LES) pressure for approximately 30 minutes
C. Sildenafil reduces the LES pressure by stimulating phosphodiesterase type 5
D. Response to surgical myotomy is good, even with multiple failed attempts, with pneumatic dilation
E. Therapeutic dilation requires distension of the LES to 45 mm

23. A 34-year-old, Caucasian woman who is overweight is seen for noncardiac chest pain. She is asking about treatment options and has been consulting the internet for medical treatments. Of the following medications, which one is the best and first line therapy for treating esophageal hypersensitivity?

A. Imipramine
B. Trazodone
C. Theophylline
D. Citalopram
E. Ativan

24. A 63-year-old man presents to your clinic for high-resolution manometry. While reviewing his study results, you see that his integrated relaxation pressure (IRP) and distal contractile interval are both normal. Of the following statements, which is correct regarding the different measurements used in high-resolution esophageal manometry?

A. IRP of less than 10 mm Hg is considered abnormal
B. Distal contractile interval is used to measure the velocity of distal peristalsis
C. The contractile deceleration point landmark approximates the distal margin of the upper esophageal sphincter
D. Distal latency is the interval between the upper sphincter relaxation and the contractile deceleration point
E. Contractile force velocity and the IRP are used to define anomalies in propagation

25. A 41-year-old woman is evaluated after undergoing high-resolution manometry for chest pain and dysphagia. Her manometry indicates a normal integrated relaxation pressure of 9 mm Hg, a distal contractile interval of greater than 9000 mm Hg-s-cm, and a normal distal latency. Peristalsis was present. Given her symptoms and findings on manometry, what is her most likely diagnosis based on the Chicago Classification?

A. Distal esophageal spasm
B. Hypertensive peristalsis
C. Achalasia type II
D. Achalasia type III
E. Jackhammer esophagus

26. A 60-year-old woman is seen in clinic with a history of intermittent oropharyngeal dysphagia for the past year. A barium esophagogram was previously performed that showed a Zenker's diverticulum and a cricopharyngeal bar. Which of the following statements is true regarding these conditions?

A. Zenker's diverticula develop due to reduced compliance of the cricopharyngeus muscle.
B. Transcervical myotomy combined with diverticulopexy without diverticulectomy is associated with low success rates
C. Diverticulectomy alone is associated with good results in 80% to 100% of patients
D. Cricopharyngeal myotomy increases resistance to flow across the upper esophageal sphincter
E. Patients with dysphagia and cricopharyngeal bars without diverticula do not benefit from myotomy

27. A 34-year-old man has been deemed to be a failure to treatment for achalasia subtype II. He first presented 6 months ago after he was diagnosed with achalasia subtype II by high-resolution manometry. He was tried on calcium channel blockers and isosorbide dinitrate without relief. He then underwent botulinum toxin injections. Following injection, he felt well for a few days and then returned back to his baseline of dysphagia, chest pain, and regurgitation. Multiple pneumatic dilations were attempted; however, he did not improve. He presents with questions regarding further therapies. What would be the next best step in management?

A. Repeat high-resolution manometry
B. Trial of isosorbide dinitrate for 3 more months
C. Perform pneumatic dilation again
D. Refer for Heller myotomy
E. Trial of PPI twice daily

28. A 51-year-old Caucasian man is being seen in your office for dysphagia, regurgitation, severe heartburn, and chest pain. He undergoes upper endoscopy and high-resolution esophageal manometry and was found to have aperistalsis with a normal integrated relaxation pressure. Given his most likely diagnosis, which of the following interventions would be helpful in managing his disease state?

A. Lifestyle modifications, liquid intake while eating, postural maneuvers, and acid suppression
B. Low dose tricyclic antidepressant
C. Calcium channel blocker

D. Endoscopic ultrasound for further evaluation of the esophagogastric junction
E. Repeat EGD with pneumatic dilation

29. A 55-year-old man complains of chronic heartburn and has been on chronic PPI therapy. What is the most likely finding on upper endoscopy?
A. Pancreatic rest
B. Fundic gland polyp
C. Inflammatory gastric polyp
D. Hyperplastic polyp
E. Gastric inlet patch

30. A 60-year-old man with Barrett's esophagus has been taking omeprazole for the last 15 years. The patient is at greatest risk for which of the following?
A. Pneumonia
B. Gastric adenocarcinoma
C. Esophageal squamous cell carcinoma
D. Folic acid deficiency
E. Thiamine deficiency

31. A 45-year-old man reports daily symptomatic heartburn with odynophagia during his clinic visit. An upper endoscopy is performed. On upper endoscopy three mucosal tears greater than 5 mm involving 75% of the lower esophagus were discovered. What is the optimal medical management for this condition?
A. PPI therapy
B. H2 receptor antagonists
C. Carafate
D. Misoprostol
E. Antacid therapy

32. 55-year-old obese male with a long history of gastroesophageal reflux disease (GERD) with esophagitis that is currently on maximal PPI therapy presents with persistent symptoms of heartburn. He has optimized his lifestyle to minimize his GERD-related symptoms. What is the next step in the management?
A. Add H2 receptor antagonists
B. Add antacids
C. Additional PPI for breakthrough symptoms
D. Refer for surgery
E. Botulinum toxin injection at the gastroesophageal junction

33. A 38-year-old woman with a history of recurrent pulmonary embolism on warfarin returns to your office as follow-up for GERD. She has been taking maximal doses of lanzoprazole, but due to insurance coverage will need to switch to omeprazole. Her proton pump inhibitor therapy is switched to omeprazole. After the switch, she is at risk for which condition?
A. Pulmonary embolism
B. Hemorrhagic stroke
C. Esophageal adenocarcinoma
D. Acute tubular necrosis
E. Discoid lupus

34. A 40-year-old man with gastroesophageal reflux returns to clinic after being on a course of twice daily PPI therapy. On examination, he reports that he has been taking the PPI consistently with lunch and prior to bed. His symptoms have not improved despite the trial of medication. What is the best next step in management?
A. Switch to H2 receptor antagonists
B. Add baclofen
C. Add metoclopramide
D. Counsel to take the PPI 30 minutes before meals
E. Refer for antireflux surgery

35. A 36-year-old man presents to your office with daily heartburn and odynophagia. What is the best next step in management?
A. Prescribe PPI therapy for 4 weeks with a return clinic visit
B. Prescribe H2 receptor antagonist therapy for 4 weeks with a return clinic visit
C. Prescribe PPI therapy and schedule an upper endoscopy
D. Prescribe PPI therapy for 8 weeks with a return clinic visit
E. Check *Helicobacter pylori* stool antigen

36. A 50-year-old overweight woman returns to your office for GERD. She has had a normal upper endoscopy, and has taken twice-daily PPI therapy. What is the next best step in her further management?
A. Referral to surgery for antireflux surgery
B. Ambulatory reflux pH testing
C. Switch to H2 receptor antagonist therapy
D. Biofeedback
E. Referral to bariatric surgery

37. A 35-year-old man with multiple allergies presents for endoscopy with symptoms of heartburn and dysphagia to solid and liquids. Endoscopic exam is unremarkable. What is the next best step in management?
A. Empirically dilate the esophagus to 13 mm
B. Biopsy the distal esophagus to confirm reflux esophagitis
C. Biopsy the distal, mid, and proximal esophagus
D. Schedule the patient for pH/impedance testing
E. Prescribe PPIs and schedule office follow up

38. A 60-year-old otherwise healthy man has an upper endoscopy for new onset gastroesophageal reflux symptoms. On upper endoscopy, Los Angeles (LA) grade D erosive esophagitis is discovered. The patient is placed on twice daily PPI therapy and the upper endoscopy is repeated after 3 months. The erosive esophagitis is unchanged. What is the next best step in management?
A. Check anti-SCL 70
B. Check fasting serum gastrin
C. Check chromogranin A
D. Order an octreotide scan
E. Order a secretin stimulation test

39. What is the most dominant mechanism for gastroesophageal reflux episodes?
A. Increased transient lower esophageal sphincter relaxations
B. Swallow-induced lower esophageal sphincter relaxation
C. Absent basal lower esophageal sphincter pressure
D. Straining
E. Acid hypersecretion

40. A 53-year-old Caucasian man undergoes upper endoscopy for refractory GERD. Upon examination of the gastroesophageal junction it is noted that red, salmon colored mucosa extends proximally from the Z line. Biopsies are performed for histology. Which of the following is the most likely finding on biopsy?
A. Squamous epithelium
B. Intestinal-type epithelium with goblet cells
C. Intestinal-type epithelium without goblet cells

D. Eosinophils in the lamina propria layer
E. Gastric foveolar epithelium

41. A 57-year-old African-American man presents to clinic with concerns of developing Barrett's esophagus. His colleague was recently diagnosed with Barrett's esophagus and he would like to know if he has any risk factors of the disease. Which of the following is a risk factor for developing Barrett's esophagus?
A. Obesity
B. Nonsteroidal antiinflammatory drugs
C. Alcohol use
D. Gastric ulcer
E. Non-Caucasian race

42. Which of the following genetic alterations contributes to the neoplastic progression in patients with Barrett's esophagus?
A. Decreased expression of epithelial growth factor receptor
B. Inactivation of *p16*
C. Activation of *TP53*
D. Inactivation of telomerase
E. Increased cadherin-catenin formation

43. After performing an upper endoscopy with multiple biopsies for surveillance of Barrett's esophagus with high grade dysplasia, you are reviewing the pathology slides. Which of the following changes would you expect to see histologically?
A. Increase in cytoplasmic maturation
B. Atypical mitosis
C. Less crowding of tubules and villiform surfaces
D. Hypochromatism
E. Decreased size of the nuclei

44. A 63-year-old man presents to your office for a routine visit. He has a history of Barrett's esophagus first diagnosed 5 years ago with four quadrant biopsies on an upper endoscopy for refractory GERD. Subsequently he has had two EGDs for surveillance; the last one was performed 1 month ago by your colleague. Biopsy results revealed high grade dysplasia. You discuss therapeutic options to decrease risk of malignancy and he asks about the likelihood of progression to cancer. What is the yearly rate of progression to cancer in patients with high-grade dysplasia?
A. 0.25%
B. 6%
C. 12%
D. 20%
E. 50%

45. A 51-year-old man was recently diagnosed with Barrett's esophagus after a longstanding history of GERD. His symptoms were not controlled with PPI therapy. He reports today that he has been off of the PPI therapy and has been asymptomatic for 2 months, attributing this to lifestyle modifications. What would you advise him to do regarding GERD therapy?
A. Continue lifestyle modifications
B. Restart PPI daily
C. PPI as needed
D. H2 antagonist nightly
E. Refer for fundoplication

46. A 49-year-old Caucasian man is referred to your office for further management of his GERD. His symptoms have been controlled on daily PPI therapy. He is obese with a body mass index of 31 kg/m^2 and is an active smoker. What would you recommend for further management in addition to counseling regarding weight loss and smoking cessation?
A. Change PPI to dosing on an as needed basis
B. Change the PPI to a histamine receptor antagonist
C. Schedule an EGD for Barrett's esophagus screening
D. Increase PPI to twice daily given his risk factors
E. Continue the daily PPI

47. A 54-year-old woman has been referred to you after being diagnosed with short segment dysplastic Barrett's esophagus 1 month ago. A repeat EGD is performed with four-quadrant biopsies every 1 cm throughout the Barrett's epithelium. There are no nodules or mucosal irregularity. Biopsies confirm low-grade dysplasia. She suffers from chronic GERD for which she takes a PPI, but otherwise has no significant medical history. What would be the best management of her Barrett's esophagus?
A. Repeat EGD in 3 months
B. Repeat EGD in 3 to 5 years
C. Repeat EGD in 6 to 12 months
D. Endoscopic mucosal resection (EMR)
E. Cryoablation

48. A 63-year-old man presents to your office after an EGD for Barrett's esophagus surveillance. Mucosal irregularities were present on that examination. Biopsies revealed high-grade dysplasia and were confirmed by two pathologists. He has a history of chronic GERD, coronary artery disease, prior stroke, and low back pain. He takes a daily PPI and is on a full dose aspirin. He is anxious regarding his biopsy results and inquires about the next step. Which of the following recommendations would you make regarding his high-grade dysplastic Barrett's esophagus?
A. Endoscopic ultrasound
B. Endoscopic mucosal resection followed by radiofrequency ablation
C. Whole body PET-CT
D. Argon plasma coagulation
E. Discontinue aspirin due to an increased risk of bleeding and progression to cancer

49. Which of the following is *true* regarding ablative therapy for dysplastic Barrett's esophagus?
A. Photodynamic therapy (PDT) is a one-step process involving ultraviolet light
B. Thermal, cold, and photodynamic energy, along with endoscopic mucosal resection can be used to treat Barrett's epithelium, and have similar side effects
C. Radiofrequency ablation (RFA) delivers microwave energy via electrodes to ablate the mucosa in a uniform fashion.
D. Photodynamic therapy has no significant side effects
E. Radiofrequency ablation and photodynamic therapy are not equally as effective for ablating Barrett's esophagus

50. A 62-year-old man presents to your clinic following an EGD with biopsies for chronic GERD performed 1 week ago. Upon endoscopic evaluation he was noted to have LA class C esophagitis as well as distal esophageal mucosal irregularities. EMR of the nodular appearing mucosa was performed. Histologic exam revealed intestinal metaplasia with high grade dysplasia/intraepithelial neoplasia extending through the lamina propria and muscularis mucosa into the submucosa. Pathology of the other

esophageal biopsies taken is consistent with esophagitis. What is the next best step in management?
A. Increase PPI twice a day and repeat EGD with four-quadrant biopsies of the irregular appearing mucosa in 8 weeks
B. Plan for ablative therapy with radiofrequency ablation
C. Repeat EGD with multiple biopsies now
D. Schedule for endoscopic ultrasound (EUS)
E. Schedule for CT of the chest and abdomen

51. A 64-year-old woman presents to your clinic for follow-up after EMR of her known Barrett's epithelium revealed high grade dysplasia. All other mucosal biopsies revealed nondysplastic Barrett's esophagus. She is inquiring if there are any further steps that need to be taken to reduce risk of recurrence. What would you recommend?
A. Radiofrequency ablation
B. Repeat EGD in 3 months
C. Treat with PPI twice daily for 6 months and then perform ablation therapy
D. Schedule endoscopic ultrasound
E. Perform pH study to verify control of the esophageal acid exposure therapy

52. A 49-year-old man is being seen in your office for a second opinion. He underwent an EGD 1 month ago and has intestinal metaplasia of the distal esophagus. His medical history is significant for tobacco use, coronary artery disease, hypertension, and GERD, which is well controlled on a PPI. He is obese with a BMI of 35 kg/m^2. He is worried about his new diagnosis and wants to know what else to do for treatment. What is the next best step for management of his disease?
A. Perform chromoendoscopy
B. Repeat EGD in 3 years
C. Repeat EGD now with biopsies
D. Refer for ablation with radiofrequency ablation
E. Increase PPI twice daily

53. A 48-year-old man presents to your clinic with GERD refractory to PPI twice daily. You schedule him for an EGD, and upon inspection see salmon-colored mucosa extending 5 cm above the Z line in the distal esophagus. What is the next best step in regard to this irregular appearing mucosa?
A. Perform chromoendoscopy
B. Take four large capacity biopsies within the salmon colored mucosa for histology
C. Take one set of four-quadrant biopsies distal to the Z line and one set proximally
D. Take four-quadrant biopsies every 2 cm within the salmon colored mucosa
E. Take jumbo four-quadrant biopsies every 1 cm within the salmon colored mucosa

54. A 56-year-old woman presents to the hospital for abdominal pain. She undergoes a CT scan of the abdomen in the emergency department, which reports a possible gastric outlet obstruction. Given her findings and symptoms, an EGD is performed. She has no evidence of gastric outlet obstruction; however, on withdrawal she is noted to have a small hiatal hernia and 3 cm of salmon colored mucosa extending proximally from the Z line. Random biopsies are attempted of the pink appearing mucosa; however, due to her intolerance of the procedure only one biopsy can be obtained. The pathology report reveals intestinal epithelium with goblet cells and low grade dysplasia. Which of the following would be indicated at this time?
A. Repeat EGD with four-quadrant biopsies every 2 cm
B. Repeat EGD in 6 to 12 months
C. Refer for radio frequency ablation
D. Repeat EGD with four-quadrant biopsies every 1 cm
E. Refer for cryoablation

55. A 60-year-old woman with GERD is placed on alendronate for osteoporosis and a prior hip fracture. In reading online, she found out that alendronate can result in severe esophageal injury. She called your office for recommendations to prevent such injury. Which of the following should be recommended?
A. Take the alendronate with a PPI
B. Switch alendronate to pamidronate
C. Remain upright at least 30 minutes following ingestion
D. Take alendronate with sucralfate
E. Take alendronate with a meal

56. A 65-year-old woman with a prior hip fracture and known osteoporosis is placed on alendronate. Several months later she presents to your clinic with new symptoms of odynophagia and substernal chest pain. On endoscopy, a severe, circumferential, exudative, erosive esophagitis is visualized in the midesophagus, consistent with alendronate induced esophageal injury. What is the next best management step?
A. Twice daily PPI therapy for 3 months then endoscopic re-evaluation
B. Substitution of alendronate with risedronate
C. Concomitant use of sucralfate with alendronate
D. Substitution of alendronate with pamidronate
E. Suggest taking alendronate with a clear liquid

57. A 67-year-old man with an atrial arrhythmia underwent radiofrequency ablation. Approximately 2 weeks later, he became febrile and developed aphasia with hemiparesis. On MRI of the brain, he was found to have a cerebrovascular accident (CVA). Echocardiography showed air bubbles in the left atrium. What is the most likely source of these findings?
A. Acute hemorrhagic CVA
B. Intracranial abscess
C. Embolic CVA
D. Endocarditis
E. Myelitis

58. A 45-year-old woman presents to the local emergency department with retrosternal chest pain, dysphagia, and hematemesis for the past 24 hours. A chest CT demonstrates a diffusely thickened esophagus with obliteration of the esophageal lumen and a double-barrel appearance. Urgent endoscopy demonstrates obliteration of the esophageal lumen and a long, deep, friable blue submucosal mass. What is the most likely diagnosis?
A. Boerhaave syndrome
B. Candidal esophagitis
C. Mallory-Weiss tear
D. Esophageal hematoma
E. Esophageal cancer

59. A 55-year-old man from Ecuador presents to your clinic with dysphagia for the past 4 weeks. He has trouble swallowing breads and meat, which he overcomes by raising his hands above his head. On endoscopy, he has severe

white, exudative esophagitis with superficial ulcers. What are esophageal biopsies most likely to confirm?
A. Candidal esophagitis
B. Herpes simplex virus (HSV) esophagitis
C. Cytomegalovirus (CMV) esophagitis
D. Human immunodeficiency virus (HIV) esophagitis
E. Pill-induced esophagitis

60. A 35-year-old Asian-Indian man presents to the hospital with hemoptysis, chronic cough, fevers, and dysphagia for the past 3 months. A chest CT demonstrates focal esophageal thickening as well as paratracheal and paraesophageal lymphadenopathy. An upper endoscopy is performed and there is an esophageal mass with ulceration in the midesophagus. What is the most likely diagnosis?
A. Cytomegalovirus esophagitis
B. Post-transplant lymphoproliferative disease
C. Tuberculosis
D. Systemic lupus erythematosus
E. Churg-Strauss disease

61. A 23-year-old man presents to the emergency department with a gunshot wound to the chest. Chest radiography reveals pleural free air. A gastrograffin swallow study demonstrates extravasation of contrast in the distal esophagus. The emergency department team requests your opinion regarding emergent upper endoscopy and endoscopic closure. What is the next best step in the management of the patient?
A. Perform upper endoscopy to evaluate the lesion
B. Perform upper endoscopy and place an enteral stent
C. Recommend antibiotics and emergent surgical referral
D. Obtain a chest MRI to further evaluate the injury
E. Obtain a lateral chest x-ray to confirm distal esophageal injury

62. A 21-year-old man presents to the emergency department with hematemesis after a recent episode of binge drinking and active retching. On upper endoscopy you see a linear 5 mm tear in the lower esophagus oozing blood. What is the most likely diagnosis?
A. Mallory-Weiss tear
B. Boerhaave syndrome
C. LA grade B esophagitis
D. Cameron ulcer
E. NG tube trauma

63. A 30-year-old man visits your office for new onset symptoms of dysphagia, odynophagia and low-grade fevers. An upper endoscopy is performed to further characterize his symptoms. On upper endoscopy, rounded 1 to 3 mm vesicles in the mid and distal esophagus are visualized; some with ulcerated centers. Biopsies are obtained and the histologic description is multinucleated giant cells, ballooning degeneration, and Cowdry type A inclusion bodies. What is the optimal first-line treatment for this condition?
A. Fluconazole
B. Foscarnet
C. Prednisone
D. Valacyclovir
E. Nystatin

64. A 55-year-old healthy man is transferred to the trauma center after an accident at a construction site, when a heavy object fell over his chest and abdomen. He presents with hemodynamic shock after the sudden onset of chest pain, subcutaneous emphysema, and crepitus on exam with a left lower lobe effusion. The effusion has a mildly elevated amylase level. What is the most likely diagnosis?
A. Acute pancreatitis
B. Acute myocardial infarction
C. Esophageal trauma
D. Dissecting aortic aneurysm
E. Thoracic duct injury

65. There are four mechanisms for drug-induced esophageal injury. Tetracycline is known to cause esophageal injury by which mechanism?
A. Direct toxicity to esophageal mucosa
B. Production of caustic acidic solution
C. Production of caustic alkaline solution
D. Creation of a hyperosmolar solution
E. Inhibition of cellular regeneration

66. A 55-year-old woman presents to endoscopy for Barrett's esophagus surveillance. On endoscopy she has a 15 mm esophageal nodule at 33 cm from the incisors, within the Barrett's mucosa. What is the next best approach?
A. Referral to surgery
B. Band ligation and hot snare resection
C. Radiofrequency ablation
D. Cryotherapy
E. Shortened surveillance intervals

67. A 65-year-old man presented to endoscopy for Barrett's esophagus surveillance and was found to have a 4 mm nodule. Endoscopic mucosal resection was performed as well as four-quadrant biopsies from the other regions of salmon-colored Barrett's epithelium. The nodule was found to be an adenocarcinoma with extension to the lamina propria, no lymphovascular invasion, and negative deep and lateral margins. The biopsies reveal intestinal metaplasia with low-grade dysplasia. What is the next best step in management?
A. Referral to surgery
B. Cryotherapy
C. Aggressive monthly endoscopic surveillance
D. Radiofrequency ablation in 8 weeks
E. Endoscopic mucosal resection of the remaining Barrett's mucosa

68. A 55-year-old man presents for evaluation of long-segment Barrett's esophagus with a 18 mm nodule located within Barrett's mucosa. The nodule was biopsied by the referring provider and was found to be an adenocarcinoma. What is the next step in management?
A. Radiofrequency ablation
B. Monthly surveillance biopsies
C. Surgical referral
D. Cryoablation of the remaining Barrett's esophagus
E. Endoscopic ultrasound

69. A 70-year-old man with Barrett's esophagus and 18 mm nodule located within the Barrett's mucosa undergoes endoscopic mucosal resection. The histologic examination confirms the lesion as a T1b tumor. What is the deep extent of the tumor involvement?
A. Mucosal layer
B. Muscularis mucosa layer
C. Submucosal layer
D. Muscularis propria layer
E. Adventitia

70. A 28-year-old college student was noted to have fleshy tissue protrude from his mouth after an episode of vomiting. On endoscopy, the patient was noted to have a pedunculated polyp in the cervical esophagus. What is the most likely finding called?
A. Hamartoma
B. Hemangioma
C. Fibrovascular polyp
D. Lipoma
E. Granular cell tumor

71. A 60-year-old man presents to endoscopy with symptoms of chronic heartburn. On endoscopy, a 6 mm submucosal lesion is seen in the midesophagus. An endoscopic ultrasound reveals a smooth submucosal mass with a homogenous and hyperechoic echotexture. Which of the following is the most likely diagnosis?
A. Hamartoma
B. Gastrointestinal stromal tumor
C. Granular cell tumor
D. Leiomyoma
E. Lipoma

72. On diagnostic upper endoscopy performed for dyspepsia, an erythematous, 8 mm polyp is visualized in the midesophagus. On biopsy, concentric, perivascular fibroblast proliferation with increased eosinophils is seen. What is the next best step in management of this polyp?
A. Repeat endoscopy for resection
B. Referral to surgery
C. Watchful waiting
D. Treat with swallowed steroid and re-evaluate
E. Prescribe PPI therapy

73. A 55-year-old man presented to endoscopy for Barrett's esophagus surveillance and was found to have a nodule. Endoscopic mucosal resection was performed and the nodule was found to be adenocarcinoma. The lesion extends into the deep submucosal layer, is well differentiated, and there is limited lymphovascular invasion. Endoscopic ultrasound and PET-CT confirms no lymph node invasion or distant metastases. What is the next step in management?
A. Radiofrequency ablation
B. Cryotherapy
C. Repeat endoscopy with four-quadrant biopsies
D. Refer for neoadjuvant chemotherapy
E. Refer for surgical resection

74. A 58-year-old morbidly obese man with a BMI of 36 kg/m^2, a long history of GERD and known Barrett's esophagus with ongoing tobacco and alcohol use presents for surveillance endoscopy. What is his strongest risk factor for progression to esophageal adenocarcinoma?
A. GERD with Barrett's esophagus
B. Alcohol use
C. Tobacco use
D. Obesity
E. Male gender

75. A 34-year-old man returned to your office for follow-up of dysphagia. He has had a normal upper endoscopy, and esophageal manometry confirmed aperistalsis with failure of relaxation of the lower esophageal sphincter. What complication is this patient at risk for in the future?
A. Esophageal adenocarcinoma
B. Melanoma
C. Esophageal squamous cell carcinoma
D. Lymphoma
E. Granular cell tumor

76. A 42-year-old competitive eater reports progressive dysphagia over the past 2 months. An upper endoscopy is performed, and a large 22 mm submucosal lesion is visualized in the lower third of the esophagus with a negative pillow sign. An endoscopic ultrasound confirms a large, hypoechoic, heterogeneous structure arising from the fourth echoendoscopic layer. What would be the best next step in management?
A. Endoscopic submucosal dissection
B. Endoscopic mucosal resection
C. Watchful waiting
D. Surgical referral
E. Fine-needle aspiration

77. Which of the following are the most common benign esophageal tumors?
A. Granular cell tumors
B. Leiomyomas
C. Hamartomas
D. Hemangiomas
E. Fibrovascular polyps

78. A 62-year-old obese man presents for further management of nodular Barrett's esophagus. On endoscopy, two adjacent 20 mm nonulcerated nodules are found. Endoscopic mucosal resection is performed successfully; subsequently, the patient undergoes radiofrequency ablation with eradication of dysplasia. What is the most likely delayed complication that may occur in this patient?
A. Bleeding
B. Perforation
C. Stricture
D. Esophageal cancer
E. Fistulae

79. A 75-year-old woman presents with dysphagia, and an upper endoscopy confirms multiple midesophageal lesions with biopsies suspicious for metastatic disease. What is the most likely primary cancer?
A. Breast cancer
B. Renal cell carcinoma
C. Lung cancer
D. Pancreatic cancer
E. Endometrial cancer

80. A 60-year-old man undergoes an upper endoscopy for evaluation of dysphagia. He is found to have a soft, black nodular lesion in the midesophagus. Biopsies confirm melanoma. What is the next best step in management?
A. Endoscopic ultrasound
B. Surgical referral
C. PET-CT
D. MRI
E. Endoscopic resection

ANSWERS

1. **C** (S&F ch42)
The patient has a clinical history consistent with gastroesophageal reflux. Basal cell hyperplasia and protrusion of rete pegs (downward projections of the squamous epithelium) are associated with GERD on biopsies, and therefore choice C is the best option. Neutrophilic, eosinophilic, lymphocytic epithelial infiltrates are nonspecific changes that can occur with a variety of conditions.

2. **E** (S&F ch42)
Esophgeal atresia is the most common developmental anomaly of the esophagus. A scaphoid abdomen with salivary regurgitation occurs at birth. The diagnosis is confirmed with failure to pass an NG tube into the stomach combined with the presence of air contrast in the upper esophageal segment on a chest x-ray. Barium swallow, thoracic CT, and abdominal x-ray are not indicated. Prenatal esophageal ultrasound can suggest a blind ending and has a high specificity but low sensitivity for esophageal atresia.

3. **C** (S&F ch42)
H-type tracheoesophageal fistula typically have a delayed presentation of recurrent aspiration pneumonia and/or bronchiectasis in early childhood or adulthood, as in this question. Esophagography may not reveal any abnormalities due to the small size of the communication. Ingestion of methylene blue followed by bronchoscopy to search for the blue-stained fistula site aids in making the diagnosis. Isolated esophageal atresia presents in infancy and is not typically associated with recurrent pneumonia. Cystic fibrosis has recurrent multifocal pneumonia due to abnormal clearance but not fistula (multifocal penumoniae). Distal type tracheoesophageal fistulae typically present in infancy and do not have a delayed presentation. Esophageal stenosis presents with dysphagic symptoms, and not recurrent pneumonia. It should also have been present on the esophagography.

4. **D** (S&F ch42)
After surgical correction of esophageal atresia, the esophagus is prone to dysmotility as well as the possibility of anastomotic strictures. Dysphagia is reported in 85% of patients after surgical correction. Esophagitis is reported to be prevalent in 25% to 90% of patients. Barrett's esophagus and esophageal adenocarcinoma have been reported in a minority after surgical correction. The prevalence or incidence of candidal esophagitis is not known in this patient population.

5. **D** (S&F ch42)
A duplication cyst is a congenital anomaly characterized as a fluid-filled submucosal lesion, which may present with symptoms of dysphagia. The cystic component can be confirmed as an anechoic structure on endoscopic ultrasound. Esophageal squamous cell carcinoma and esophageal adenocarcinoma are mucosal processes that would be detected and appear as irregular mass lesions on examination. Lipoma and GIST are submucosal lesions that do not appear anechoic or cystic on EUS.

6. **A** (S&F ch42)
The description is of a type A esophageal ring. Symptomatic rings can be treated by passage of a dilator greater than 15 mm or botulinum toxin injection. Heller myotomy, peroral endoscopy myotomy, and pneumatic dilation are used to treat achalasia, which has not been described in this patient. Balloon dilation is possible; however, it has not been reported to be more effective than a mercury-weighted dilator with both radial and linear forces.

7. **A** (S&F ch42)
A Schatzki ring is typically symptomatic at 13 mm or less. The obstructing ring can be visualized radiographically by entrapment of a 13 mm marshmallow or barium tablet. However, the presence of Schatzki ring of any diameter in a patient with dysphagia warrants endoscopic dilation to disrupt the ring to try to improve the patient's symptoms.

8. **C** (S&F ch42)
Use of PPIs has been shown to decrease the recurrence of an obliterated Schatzki ring. There is no evidence to suggest that H2 receptor antagonists or carafate will prevent a ring. Repeat endoscopy is only indicated if dysphagia persists despite obliteration. There is no direct evidence to suggest that weight loss can prevent a recurrent Schatzki ring.

9. **A** (S&F ch42)
The syndrome characterized by iron deficiency anemia, dysphagia, and cervical esophageal webs is known as Plummer-Vinson syndrome. This syndrome identified a group of patients at increased risk for squamous cell cancer of the esophagus and pharynx.

10. **D** (S&F ch42)
The historical description and esophagogram findings are most consistent with dysphagia lusoria. This is a term given for symptoms associated with vascular compression of the esophagus by an aberrant right subclavian artery. It characteristically shows as a pencil-like indentation at the level of the third or fourth vertebra. On endoscopy, there will be no structural sources identified as indicated by choices A, B, C, and E.

11. **D** (S&F ch42)
Esophageal anomalies are often associated with anomalies in other organ systems, as defined by the acronym VACTERL, a mnemonic for the association of anomalies of the vertebral, anal, cardiac, tracheal, esophageal, renal, and limb systems. Only choice D involves one of the identified organ systems.

12. **A** (S&F ch42)
A CVA can affect skeletal muscle. This type of injury is suggested by the presentation with difficulty with bolus transfers from the oropharynx to the esophagus (transfer dysphagia). Skeletal muscle comprises about 5% to 33% of the upper esophagus and then intermixes with smooth muscle. The distal 50% of the esophagus is composed of smooth muscle.

13. **A** (S&F ch42)
Esophageal anomalies are often associated with anomalies in other organ systems, as defined by the acronym VACTERL, a mnemonic for the association of anomalies of the vertebral, anal, cardiac, tracheal, esophageal, renal, and limb systems. Low birth weight and severity of associated cardiac abnormalities are the main determinants of outcome after surgical correction of esophageal atresia.

14. **A** (S&F ch43)
The pharyngeal swallow rapidly configures pharyngeal structures from a respiratory to an alimentary pathway and then reverses this reconfiguration within 1 second. This is a highly coordinated response but can be dissected into separate actions. First there is nasopharyngeal closure

by elevations and retraction of the soft palate. This is followed by upper esophageal sphincter opening and laryngeal closure. Tongue loading or ramping occurs followed by pulsion of the food bolus. This entire process is completed with clearance of the pharynx, stripping the last residue from the pharyngeal walls.

15. E (S&F ch43)
The patient is presenting with achalasia, as observed by both her clinical symptoms of dysphagia to both liquids and solids, as well as her manometry findings of an increased relaxation pressure and absent peristalsis, per the Chicago Classification of Esophageal Motility Disorders. The proposed mechanisms for achalasia have included A, C, and E; however, only the loss of ganglion cells is well substantiated in the literature. Diffuse muscular hyperplasia in the distal third of the esophagus is seen in distal esophageal spasm, not achalasia. In a hypercontractile (jackhammer) esophagus, it is proposed that excess cholinergic drive or reactive compensation for increased esophagogastric junction outflow obstruction leading to myocyte hypertrophy are driving the hypercontractility.

16. E (S&F ch43)
The patient could have Chagas' disease given the symptoms suggestive of achalasia and the history of an abnormal heart. Chagas' disease is spread by a tick bite that transmits the parasitic infection, *Trypanosoma cruzi.* The diagnosis can be confirmed by serologic testing (PCR or complement fixation), if it is in the nonacute phase. An ECG can be useful if there is suspicion for Chagas' disease due to its multiorgan involvement, which can lead to chronic cardiomyopathy and arrhythmias; however, this would not be specific for the diagnosis. Biopsies of the esophagus would not be likely to yield any additional information. Myocardial biopsy is invasive and would not be the correct choice at this point. In the acute setting, a peripheral smear visualizing the parasite in the blood is diagnostic; however, it usually takes 20 years for the chronic phase of the disease to develop, with the destruction of the autonomic ganglion cells throughout the body. Therefore at this point, a peripheral smear is not likely to be helpful.

17. A (S&F ch43)
Her presentation is concerning for pseudoachalasia as opposed to idiopathic achalasia given her advanced age (greater than 50 years), abrupt and recent onset (less than 1 year), and weight loss. Though the presenting features make pseudoachalasia more common than idiopathic achalasia, they have a poor positive predictive value. Anatomical evaluation with endoscopy is indicated for every new case of achalasia as was done appropriately in this case. Resistance to passage of the endoscope across the EGJ should raise suspicion of pseudoachalasia. In idiopathic achalasia, the endoscope should pass through with gentle pressure. Given the high index of suspicion for pseudoachalasia in this case, the next best step would be to take endoscopic biopsies or obtain imaging (MRI or CT or endoscopic ultrasound) to further evaluate for infiltrative disease (including malignancy). A barium swallow would not be necessary at this stage given anatomical evaluation with endoscopy already completed. Empiric dilation would not be appropriate given the uncertainty of her diagnosis. There is no role to increase PPI daily given no complaints of uncontrolled GERD and no evidence on endoscopy of uncontrolled reflux disease. A trial of amyl nitrite (a smooth muscle relaxant) during esophageal manometry is used to observe if there is relaxation of the EGJ high-pressure zone, which is observed with a hypertensive sphincter (versus no effect with mechanical causes such as fundoplication). This would not be an incorrect choice; however, first it would be necessary to exclude an infiltrative process causing pseudoachalasia.

18. C (S&F ch43)
The primary peristaltic wave manifests as an inverted "V" representing the tail of the bolus. Abnormalities of peristalsis are inferred by a retrograde escape of the bolus through the wavefront ultimately resulting in incomplete esophageal emptying. Peristalsis is best evaluated in the prone position so that clearance is not aided by gravity. The lateral projection is better for evaluation of the esophagus because it will capture the oropharynx, palate, proximal esophagus, and the proximal airway. Normally the EGJ will become widely patent when approached by the bolus and impaired relaxation is suggested when there is either a smooth tapering at the EGJ or an impairment of bolus transit. Spastic contractions are demonstrated by a classic corkscrew appearing esophagus and are not normal.

19. B (S&F ch43)
The integrated relaxation pressure (IRP) is the optimal measurement for quantifying relaxation of the EGJ within the deglutitive relaxation window. Normal is 15 mm Hg or less, and greater than 15 mm Hg would be considered abnormal. IRP is both very sensitive and specific, 98% and 96% respectively, for distinguishing well-defined achalasia patients from control subjects and patients with other diagnoses. Conventional manometry does not have any standard measurements to define incomplete deglutitive EGJ relaxation.

20. E (S&F ch43)
The patient has been recently diagnosed with high-resolution manometry (HRM) with achalasia subtype II, which is defined, per the Chicago Classification, as an increased IRP greater than 10 mm Hg along with no esophageal contractions and panesophageal pressurization with equal to or greater than 20% of swallows. An increased IRP of 18 mm Hg and premature contractions in the distal esophagus is most consistent with achalasia subtype III. Absent peristalsis is defined as a normal IRP and 100% of swallows with failed peristalsis. Absent peristalsis with an increased IRP is the most obvious form of achalasia, or subtype I. An increased IRP with weak peristalsis is most consistent with an EGJ outflow obstruction, which can either be an early achalasia subtype or a mechanical obstruction.

21. D (S&F ch43)
With her manometry study results, she may have an EGJ outflow obstruction given the peristalsis with an increased IRP suggesting impaired relaxation. Such findings may be seen with a mechanical obstruction or either a variant or an earlier phenotype of achalasia. However, before diagnosing the disorder as a variant achalasia, it is important to exclude pseudoachalasia. The initial evaluation requires more testing than endoscopy alone, preferably including EUS or cross-sectional imaging (CT, MRI). Botulinum toxin injection, Heller myotomy, and nonpneumatic dilation may all be treatment options for variant achalasia; however, pseudoachalasia should be first excluded and the response to botulinum toxin and simple dilation is usually transient. Impedance measurement is not necessary or useful in differentiating between a mechanical obstruction or an early presentation of achalasia.

22. D (S&F ch43)
Subsequent response to surgical myotomy is *not* influenced by a history of previous dilations. Divided doses of botulin toxin are injected into the sphincter at 4 quadrants with a sclerotherapy catheter to decrease LES pressure by 33%; improvement in symptoms lasts up to 6 months in two thirds of patients. Isosorbide dinitrate has shown to be effective in reducing LES pressure; however, it has not been compared to placebo. Sildenafil (Viagra) inhibits phosphodiesterase type 5 and is another option for the treatment of achalasia; however, its use is limited due to cost and potential side effects. Pneumatic dilation for achalasia requires at least 3 cm diameter distension at the LES for a lasting reduction in LES pressure achieved presumably by disrupting the circular muscle of the sphincter.

23. A (S&F ch43)
Primarily, tricyclic antidepressants (e.g., imipramine), trazodone, and selective serotonin reuptake inhibitors are known to be effective in reducing hypersensitivity. Benzodiazepines are not used for noncardiac chest pain. Generally, low doses of tricyclic antidepressants and trazodone suffice and avoid the mood-altering effects. Evidence also suggest that the use of theophylline, presumably through adenosine receptor blockade, will increase the threshold for chest pain and relax the esophageal wall.

24. D (S&F ch43)
The distal latency is an interval measured in units of time between upper sphincter relaxation and the CDP. DL values less than 4.5 seconds define premature contractions. IRP is used to quantify deglutitive relaxation of the lower esophageal sphincter (LES) and a value greater than 15 mm Hg is considered abnormal. DCI measures the vigor of the distal esophageal contraction and is measured in mm Hg/s/cm. The CDP landmark approximates the proximal margin of the LES (not the UES) and is identified as the inflection point along the isobaric contour where deceleration of the contractile front occurs. CFV and DL are used to define anomalies in propagation (IRP measures the relaxation of the LES as described earlier).

25. E (S&F ch43)
The patient has a normal integrated relaxation pressure (IRP) and a very high distal contractile interval (DCI) which is seen in a hypercontractile esophagus or jackhammer esophagus. Distal esophageal spasm, formerly called diffuse esophageal spasm, is characterized by premature contractions and a decreased DL. Hypertensive peristalsis or nutcracker esophagus can be mistaken for jackhammer esophagus given the normal IRP and increased DCI; however, in this entity, the DCI is not as high as in jackhammer esophagus, usually greater than 5000 mm Hg-s-cm but less than 8000 mm Hg-s-cm. Both C and D are subtypes of achalasia, which by definition have an increased IRP.

26. A (S&F ch43)
Zenker's diverticula develop due to a restrictive process associated with diminished compliance of the cricopharyngeus muscle. This leads to increased hypopharyngeal intrabolus pressure which may lead to formation of hypopharyngeal diverticula. Transcervical myotomy combined with diverticulectomy or diverticulopexy is associated with good or excellent results in 80% to 100% of patients. Diverticulectomy or diverticulopexy alone without myotomy is not recommended as it does not treat the increased resistance at the upper esophageal sphincter. Cricopharyngeal myotomy decreases resistance to flow across the upper esophageal sphincter. Patients with oropharyngeal dysphagia and a cricopharyngeal bar should be considered bougie dilation or myotomy to decrease sphincter pressure and improve symptoms.

27. A (S&F ch43)
Repeat high-resolution esophageal manometry should be performed to evaluate if there has been any response to the integrated relaxation pressure as a measure of the lower esophageal sphincter pressure. Continuing the same failed pharmacotherapy is not recommended. The patient should be referred for a Heller myotomy, however after he is reevaluated to see if LES relaxation pressures are normal. Repeating pneumatic dilation after multiple failed attempts might be considered but may have diminishing returns and should follow repeat manometry. Increasing the PPI to twice daily is unlikely to be beneficial.

28. A (S&F ch43)
The patient is presenting with absent peristalsis. Absent peristalsis is defined as no evidence of contractions and a normal IRP. If the patient had an elevated IRP along with absent peristalsis, these manometric findings would be consistent with achalasia type I. Choices B through E could be acceptable interventions for achalasia type 1. In absent peristalsis, no medications have been shown to significantly improve peristalsis, and treatment is aimed at minimizing complications. These patients may require PPI at higher than FDA approved dosing.

29. B (S&F ch44)
Fundic gland polyps are benign growths that are associated with chronic PPI therapy. They carry a negligible malignant potential, and are considered incidental findings on routine upper endoscopy.

30. A (S&F ch44)
Long-term PPI therapy has been associated with a few conditions, including pneumonia and enteric infections such as *Clostridium difficile*. Chronic PPI therapy has been associated with increased fracture risk and vitamin B_{12} and iron deficiency. PPI therapy is also associated with benign fundic gland polyposis but not gastric adenocarcinoma or esophageal squamous cell carcinoma.

31. A (S&F ch44)
This patient has GERD with erosive esophagitis, LA grade D. On large series and meta-analyses, PPI therapy was found to be more effective than H2 receptor antagonists at 4 to 8 weeks of treatment. The number needed to treat (NNT) with PPI in order to prevent one episode of erosive esophagitis was 3. Misoprostol has been used for gastric ulcers and NSAID-induced ulcer prevention; however, its use is limited by diarrhea. Antacid therapy is useful for immediate heartburn relief but not for erosive esophagitis healing. Carafate has been useful as adjunctive therapy, but does not treat the underlying source of esophageal injury, namely acid reflux.

32. D (S&F ch44)
The patient in the case has had maximal medical therapy with objective evidence of acid reflux injury and minimal symptom improvement. Therefore, antireflux surgery should be considered in this patient. The addition of a supplemental medication may be considered, but would not be the optimal choice in the setting of refractory GERD despite maximal PPI therapy. There is no role for endoscopic botulinum toxin injection at the lower esophageal sphincter in treatment of GERD.

33. B (S&F ch44)
Omeprazole decreases the clearance of warfarin by inhibiting the cytochrome P450 enzyme 2C19. Therefore, patients on warfarin have an increased risk of life-threatening hemorrhage, and possibly hemorrhagic stroke. Omeprazole alone can cause idiosyncratic interstitial nephritis in 1% of patients; however, this has not been associated with concomitant warfarin use, and acute tubular necrosis is rare. According to indirect evidence, esophageal adenocarcinoma may be prevented with use of PPI therapy. Discoid lupus is a condition associated with various drugs; however, neither omeprazole nor warfarin has been strongly associated with this condition.

34. D (S&F ch44)
Prior to making any medication changes or referral for surgery, the PPI compliance for optimal effectiveness needs to be assessed. In this case, the PPI was not used to optimize effectiveness. The patient should be counseled to take the PPI at least 30 minutes before a meal; typically at breakfast and if needed before dinner. PPI have consistently been shown to be more effective at acid suppression than H2RA. Baclofen has been shown to decrease transient lower esophageal sphincter relaxations; however, clinical effectiveness in patients has been limited. Antireflux surgery can be considered only when GERD has been refractory to optimal medical management.

35. C (S&F ch44)
Typically GERD does not warrant early endoscopic evaluation unless there are alarm features elicited in the clinical history. Clinical alarm features include age greater than 55, weight loss, persistent vomiting, gastrointestinal bleeding, dysphagia, or odynophagia. In this question, the patient has exhibited dysphagia, which warrants early endoscopic therapy. A trial of PPIs is recommended in this otherwise young man if there are no other alarm features.

36. B (S&F ch44)
Ambulatory reflux pH testing is the only test that reliably records episodes of reflux and correlates with patient symptoms. It has indicated uses in four scenarios: (1) prior to antireflux surgery, (2) GERD-like symptoms resistant to treatment with equivocal endoscopic findings, and (3) to verify that extraesophageal symptoms of GERD are occurring. The patient in this case scenario has equivocal endoscopy results and persistent symptoms despite maximal PPI therapy. Therefore, ambulatory pH testing is the best next test to identify if the patient symptomatology is gastroesophageal reflux-related.

37. C (S&F ch44)
The current indication for esophageal biopsies in the evaluation of GERD is to exclude eosinophilic esophagitis, especially in those patients who complain of dysphagia. The most accepted protocol is to take at least two biopsies from the distal, mid, and proximal esophagus to optimize the sensitivity to detect eosinophilic esophagitis. A trial of PPI therapy and scheduling a patient for ambulatory pH/impendence testing may be considered if the biopsies for eosinophilic esophagitis are negative. Empiric dilation is not considered a standard management strategy in GERD without any mucosal abnormalities, and may increase the risk of perforation in a patient with untreated eosinophilic esophagitis.

38. B (S&F ch44)
GERD with erosive esophagitis can be associated with several conditions, including Zollinger-Ellison syndrome, scleroderma, prolonged nasogastric intubation, and post-Heller myotomy. In this clinical scenario, the patient has severe, refractory erosive esophagitis; therefore, evaluation for a gastrinoma should be initiated with a fasting serum gastrin. Evaluation for scleroderma may be considered; however, the patient has no other systemic findings that would make this condition possible. Chromogranin A is unlikely to have any utility in this clinical situation, and may be falsely elevated due to PPI therapy. Secretin stimulation and octreotide scan testing could be considered after testing with fasting serum gastrin.

39. A (S&F ch44)
Increased frequency of transient lower esophageal sphincter relaxations are the most dominant mechanism for GERD. These relaxations have four characteristic features: (1) occur independently of swallowing, (2) are not associated with peristalsis, (3) persist longer (greater than 10 seconds), (4) are accompanied by inhibition of the crural diaphragm.

40. B (S&F ch45)
This patient has salmon colored mucosa in the distal esophagus starting at the Z line, which is suspicious for Barrett's esophagus. Finding intestinal-type epithelium with goblet cells is clear evidence of metaplasia in the esophagus and confirms the clinical suspicion of Barrett's esophagus. The normal esophagus is lined with squamous epithelium. Multiple eosinophils would be found with eosinophilic esophagitis and would not be consistent with Barrett's esophagus. Though both intestinal type epithelium without goblet cells and gastric type epithelium have been considered to carry an increased risk of malignancy, intestinal type epithelium with goblet cells is the most consistent with a diagnosis of Barrett's esophagus.

41. A (S&F ch45)
Obesity, tobacco use, and GERD are known risk factors for Barrett's esophagus. Alcohol consumption is a strong risk factor for squamous cell carcinoma of the esophagus, but is not considered to be a risk factor for the development of Barrett's esophagus or esophageal adenocarcinoma. Gastric ulcer is not a risk factor for Barrett's esophagus. Barrett's esophagus typically affects white middle-aged men. It is less common in African Americans and Asians.

42. B (S&F ch45)
During carcinogenesis, the Barrett's epithelial cells accumulate multiple genetic and epigenetic alterations that endow the cells with the core physiologic attributes of malignancy. Reactivation of telomerase allows cells to replace the telomeres needed for cell division and thus allowing limitless replicative properties. Expression of oncogenes, growth factors, and growth factor receptors, such as epithelial growth factor receptor, enable Barrett's cells to acquire self-sufficiency in growth signals. Inactivation of tumor suppressor genes (e.g., *TP53* and *p16*) allows the cell to evade apoptosis and antigrowth signals. To allow tumor invasion and metastasis, the cells must dissociate themselves from surrounding cells by disrupting cell adhesion proteins, such as cadherins and catenins.

43. B (S&F ch45)
Dysplasia is recognized by cytologic and architectural abnormalities, which include nuclear changes such as enlargement (as opposed to decreased size), hyperchromatism, pleomorphism, stratification, and atypical mitosis. Loss of cytoplasmic maturation and crowding of tubules and villiform surfaces may also be found.

44. B (S&F ch45)
For patients with high-grade dysplasia the risk of progression to cancer is approximately 6% per year. The overall incidence of cancer development in patients with Barrett's esophagus is approximately 0.25% per year.

45. B (S&F ch45)
Generally the approach for treatment of GERD is the same for patients with or without Barrett's esophagus. One important difference, however, is that patients with Barrett's esophagus should be maintained on PPI therapy irrespective of symptoms or signs of esophagitis. There is indirect evidence suggesting that acid reflux promotes carcinogenesis in Barrett's disease and thus control of acid reflux may interfere with carcinogenesis. Fundoplication is not more effective than antisecretory therapy in preventing cancer in Barrett's esophagus, and thus should not be solely performed for cancer prevention.

46. C (S&F ch45)
Multiple medical societies, including the American Gastroenterological Association (AGA), the American Society of Gastrointestinal Endoscopy (ASGE), and the American College of Physicians (ACP), have published guidelines that recommend endoscopic screening for Barrett's esophagus in patients with multiple risk factors for esophageal adenocarcinoma. Risk factors include chronic GERD, age of 50 years or older, white race, male gender, hiatal hernia, elevated BMI, increased intraabdominal body fat, nocturnal reflux symptoms, and tobacco use. Changing to a PPI on an as-needed basis could be considered; however, his symptoms are controlled on his current regimen, and given his risk factors, he should first undergo EGD for screening. If he did not have evidence of Barrett's esophagus this could be considered. If he has Barrett's esophagus, he should be continued on the PPI irrespective of his symptoms. Lifestyle modifications should always be discussed—in addition to their other adverse consequences, obesity and tobacco use are risk factors for developing Barrett's esophagus and esophageal adenocarcinoma. Twice daily PPI therapy is not indicated for Barrett's esophagus alone and, given his controlled symptoms, this would not be a correct choice.

47. C (S&F ch45)
The patient has low-grade dysplasia confirmed on repeat EGD. Current guidelines recommend individualization of therapy for patients with Barrett's esophagus with low-grade dysplasia. Patients may be followed with serial surveillance endoscopy or the Barrett's esophagus may be treated with radiofrequency ablation. Cryotherapy has been incompletely studied in this setting and guidelines would not recommend cryotherapy for this patient. There was no nodularity or mucosal irregularity and EMR would not be performed in this setting. She should undergo a repeat EGD in 6 to 12 months with four-quadrant biopsies every 1 cm. The extent of Barrett's esophagus (short segment versus long segment) does not alter the frequency of screening or the need for 1 cm biopsy intervals.

48. B (S&F ch45)
The correct next step in management of high-grade dysplasia with mucosal irregularity would be to perform EMR followed by ablation therapy, preferably radiofrequency ablation, given the side effect profile associated with photodynamic therapy. Dual therapy is now preferred, first removing foci of neoplastic cells via EMR followed by eradication of all of the Barrett's mucosa. Given mucosal irregularities, EMR would be best to stage his disease and confirm that the involvement is limited to the mucosa. If there is invasion, the next steps could include further staging, chemotherapy, and/or esophagectomy. There is a small risk of lymph node involvement even in patients with high-grade dysplasia or intramucosal carcinoma. Aspirin and NSAIDs have been shown to have a protective effect against esophageal adenocarcinoma, progression to cancer in Barrett's esophagus, and even development of Barrett's metaplasia. Currently there is no recommendation to routinely prescribe aspirin or NSAID therapy for chemoprevention in patients with Barrett's esophagus, but patients with the disease should be screened and started on aspirin if there are other indications.

49. C (S&F ch45)
Radiofrequency ablation (RFA) delivers a circumferential thermal injury and uniform mucosal ablation. Photodynamic therapy (PDT) uses a systemic dose of a light-activated chemical, which is taken up by esophageal cells. Irradiation by a low-power laser activates the chemical and transfers that energy to form a singlet oxygen, a toxic molecule that destroys the abnormal cells and their vasculature. PDT has significant side effects including photosensitivity and esophageal stricture formation, which can be difficult to treat. RFA can cause esophageal strictures; however, this is considerably less common, the strictures are easier to manage, and the procedure does not result in systemic photosensitivity. Though PDT and RFA have not been tested in head-to-head trials, they appear to be equally effective in ablating Barrett's esophagus. Thermal, cold, and photodynamic energy, along with endoscopic mucosal resection can be used to treat Barrett's epithelium; however, there are more side effects with PDT versus RFA.

50. D (S&F ch45)
The patient was incidentally found to have high-grade dysplasia and early adenocarcinoma in the setting of longstanding GERD and increased acid exposure in the distal esophagus. Following EMR of the mucosal irregularity there is histologic evidence of submucosal involvement, increasing the likelihood of lymph node involvement or metastases. The best answer choice is to schedule the patient for an EUS to evaluate for lymph node spread. A CT scan would be more useful for distant metastasis but is not the next best choice for staging. Though the patient has esophagitis both histologically and endoscopically, it would be incorrect to wait 8 weeks given the presence of esophageal adenocarcinoma on biopsies. Prior to staging, ablative therapies should not be performed.

51. A (S&F ch45)
The patient has evidence of high-grade dysplasia within the Barrett's epithelium. Complete resection by EMR was achieved and the next step in management would be to survey her disease as well as prevent recurrence of metachronous lesions. Ablative therapy (primarily RFA) of non-neoplastic Barrett's epithelium following EMR reduces the risk of metachronous lesions compared to EMR of neoplastic foci alone. Repeat EGD is indicated after complete eradication; however, this follows the ablative therapy. EUS is not necessary for staging given the absence of deeper involvement on her histology. pH studies are not routinely recommended to document normalization of acid exposure after PPI therapy.

52. C (S&F ch45)
The correct answer is to repeat EGD now with biopsies. If nondysplastic Barrett's esophagus is confirmed,

surveillance EGD can be performed after 3 years. Non-neoplastic Barrett's esophagus does not require endoscopic eradicative therapy. Because his GERD is controlled, there is no need to increase his PPI to twice daily.

53. D (S&F ch45)
The patient has irregular appearing mucosa suspicious for Barrett's epithelium; thus, biopsies need to be taken to confirm the presence of intestinal metaplasia. The best answer is D. Four-quadrant biopsies every 2 cm should be taken to sample this irregular appearing mucosa. Chromoendoscopy could be performed; however, it is not required and would not preclude sampling the mucosa. There is no need to take biopsies of regular appearing mucosa such as that found distal to the Z line. Any mucosal irregularities or nodularity should be targeted and sampled separately. Four-quadrant biopsies should still be taken in addition to targeted biopsies. Biopsies at 1 cm intervals are performed for Barrett's esophagus with dysplasia.

54. D (S&F ch45)
The patient has Barrett's esophagus with low grade dysplasia. The next best step would be to repeat EGD with four-quadrant biopsies every 1 cm. Any mucosal irregularities or nodularity should be sampled separately. This exam may need to be performed with anesthesia to improve the procedural tolerance. The goal is to confirm that she does not have high-grade dysplasia or esophageal adenocarcinoma. Two centimeter intervals are used to sample nondysplastic Barrett's esophagus. It would also be incorrect to repeat in 6 months since a thorough sampling could not be completed at diagnosis. Ablation or endoscopic eradication therapy is not always performed for low-grade dysplasia. Ablation procedures would not be considered prior to complete sampling and assessment.

55. C (S&F ch46)
No treatment has been proven to be effective in preventing pill-induced esophagitis; however, proper administration may decrease the likelihood of an esophageal injury. Therefore, it is recommended that medications such as alendronate, which have been associated with pill-induced esophagitis, be taken with at least 8 ounces of a clear liquid, and that the patient should remain upright for at least 30 minutes after ingestion of the medication.

56. B (S&F ch46)
Given the patient history, bisphosphonate therapy is indicated. Risedronate is the one bisphosphonate that has not been associated with esophageal injury. Therefore, the best recommendation would be a substitution of alendronate with risedronate. PPI and sucralfate therapy may assist with the esophagitis but will not treat the underlying causative mechanism of injury. Use of alendronate with clear liquid may partially mitigate the injury; however, the patient will also need to be advised to remain upright. Also, given the endoscopic description, there is a high risk of stricture formation without cessation of the alendronate therapy.

57. C (S&F ch46)
Cardiac radiofrequency ablation procedures have been associated with atrial-esophageal fistulas. This can present with subsequent air emboli or massive gastrointestinal hemorrhage. The initial presentation can include fever and neurologic abnormalities and can be fatal. Air in the atrium is a clue to the presence of a fistula and makes the other answer choices less apt explanations.

58. D (S&F ch46)
Spontaneous esophageal hematoma typically presents with a classic triad of retrosternal chest pain, dysphagia, and hematemesis in middle-aged women. CT radiography of the chest may demonstrate a diffusely thickened esophagus with a double barrel appearance and obliteration of the esophageal lumen as seen in this patient. Endoscopy shows a long, blue submucosal mass with esophageal obliteration, consistent with a compressive intramural esophageal hematoma. Therefore, spontaneous esophageal hematoma is the most likely diagnosis. Boerhaave syndrome does not present with a submucosal mass. Candidal esophagitis, Mallory-Weiss tears, and esophageal cancer are mucosal, not submucosal processes.

59. A (S&F ch46)
The patient has clinical features suggestive of achalasia, which is associated with esophageal stasis and candidal superinfection. The endoscopic description of white exudates is most consistent with candidal esophagitis. CMV and HIV present endoscopically as broad-based ulcers, and HIV esophagitis typically presents as an isolated, nonhealing ulcer. HSV esophagitis typically has a "volcano-like" ulcer with heaped borders. Pill-induced esophagitis is more commonly acute than chronic, and there is no history of medication ingestion in the stem.

60. C (S&F ch46)
The patient is from a region with endemic tuberculosis and has typical clinical, radiographic, and endoscopic findings. On sampling, the tissue should be sent for acid-fast staining, mycobacterial culture, and polymerase chain reaction. CMV esophagitis usually presents with ulceration and not typically with a mass-like lesion. There is no history of transplantation. An esophageal mass lesion would not be consistent with systemic lupus erythematosis or Churg-Strauss disease.

61. C (S&F ch46)
Endoscopic visualization is not contraindicated for distal esophageal injuries; however, the utility of an endoscopic examination is reduced when the injury has been localized by other radiographic means. A surgical team should evaluate the patient and help guide the decision-making process. Enteral stents have been utilized for esophageal injuries; however, with penetrating trauma to the esophagus, there may be other injuries which need to be addressed. A CT scan might demonstrate other findings and show the location of the foreign body; however, MRI would be relatively contraindicated with a metallic foreign body, such as a bullet in the chest. Decompression with an NG tube, antibiotics, and emergent surgery are more likely to optimize the outcome for the patient.

62. A (S&F ch46)
Mallory-Weiss tears typically occur after a sudden increase in intraabdominal pressure with forceful gastric herniation. As in this case, the classic history is an episode of vomiting and/or retching followed by hematemesis. Boerhaave syndrome is a complete transmural tear, which has a more severe clinical presentation. Although LA grade B esophagitis is possible, the clinical history of forceful vomiting and hematemesis makes this less likely. There is no documentation of NG tube placement. Cameron erosions or ulcers occur due to diaphragmatic "pinch" on the gastric mucosa in patients with large hiatal hernias. The erosions do not affect the esophagus.

63. D (S&F ch46)
The endoscopic and pathologic description is most consistent with herpes simplex virus esophagitis in an immunocompetent host. The optimal first-line treatment for this condition is acyclovir or valacyclovir. Fluconazole and nystatin are used for candidal esophagitis. Prednisone may be used for an HIV-induced esophageal ulcer. Foscarnet is second line therapy for cytomegalovirus esophagitis.

64. C (S&F ch46)
This patient presents with signs of esophageal injury after blunt trauma. This presents with shock, severe chest pain, and pneumomediastinum. The diagnosis can be confirmed by a gastrograffin swallow study. The clinical presentation can mimic an acute cardiac event or aortic dissection; however, crepitus and an amylase-rich left lobe pleural effusion is not consistent with these etiologies. Acute pancreatitis and thoracic duct injury may result in a left sided, amylase-rich pleural effusion; however, they typically do not progress to hemodynamic shock as rapidly. In addition, subcutaneous emphysema and crepitus would not be typical of these etiologies.

65. A (S&F ch46)
Medications can damage the esophageal mucosa through four basic mechanisms. Direct drug toxicity is the mechanism by which tetracycline, doxycycline, and doxycycline derivatives cause mucosal injury. Production of a caustic acidic solution, as generated by vitamin C (ascorbic acid) or ferrous sulfate, is a second mechanism. Alternatively, some medications like alendronate and the bisphosphonates produce a caustic alkaline solution. Finally, medications like potassium chloride create a local hyperosmolar state that causes local injury.

66. B (S&F ch47)
Endoscopic mucosal resection (either band-assisted or cap-assisted resection) is the best method for evaluating esophageal nodules within Barrett's metaplasia. Surgical referral is premature prior to evaluation. RFA ablation has become standard of care for flat dysplastic Barrett's esophagus; however, RFA must follow resection of nodularity and mucosal irregularity. Shortened surveillance intervals may be recommended as one option, depending on the final results from the EMR and biopsies, but would not be the most appropriate management strategy at this time.

67. D (S&F ch47)
The patient has an intramucosal adenocarcinoma, which has been completely removed by endoscopic mucosal resection. There is an increased likelihood of metachronous cancer and high-grade dysplasia in the remaining Barrett's esophagus. Radiofrequency ablation is indicated for the remaining Barrett's esophagus whether dysplasia is present or not. Surgery, cryotherapy, and increased surveillance would not be indicated at this point in the management. Concentric EMR is associated with a high rate of stricture formation, and is not the recommended treatment for flat Barrett's mucosa once all nodularity and mucosal irregularity has been addressed.

68. E (S&F ch47)
The patient has been found to have an adenocarcinoma in a nodule in Barrett's esophagus. The next step in the management requires proper evaluation and staging. Cross sectional imaging and endoscopic ultrasound should be performed as well as possible endoscopic mucosal resection in this setting. Radiofrequency ablation is not indicated for nodularity in Barrett's esophagus and should not precede the proper staging. Endoscopic treatment modalities would not be indicated if EUS demonstrated lymph node metastases or metastatic disease. Surgical referral may be indicated, but would follow staging. Cryoablation should not be performed prior to evaluation and staging.

69. C (S&F ch47)
T1b lesions are defined by their penetration into but not through the submucosal layer. The distinction between T1a lesions and T1b lesions in addition to nodal status is critical in determining the proper management. T1a lesions do not penetrate to the submucosa, and in the absence of nodal involvement, may be amenable to endoscopic treatment. Nodal involvement is directly related to the depth of tumor invasion. T2 tumors penetrate into but not through the muscularis propria layer. T3 tumors penetrate through the muscularis propria layer.

70. C (S&F ch47)
The clinical and endoscopic description is most consistent with a fibrovascular polyp. This is a benign pedunculated polyp that arises from the cervical esophagus and may present incidentally as a fleshy mass that protrudes through the mouth during episodes of vomiting or coughing. It has been rarely associated with asphyxiation; therefore, endoscopic or surgical removal is recommended.

71. E (S&F ch47)
This incidental submucosal lesion has echoendosonographic features consistent with a lipoma (smooth, hyperechoic, and homogenous). The other tumors are not hyperechoic by EUS. Leiomyoma is the most common submucosal esophageal mass but presents as a hypoechoic mass arising most commonly from the muscularis propria layer.

72. C (S&F ch47)
The incidental polyp has endoscopic and histologic features of an inflammatory polyp. There is no role for endoscopic or surgical resection for this benign, asymptomatic lesion. The inflammatory polyp is not associated with eosinophilic esophagitis or gastroesophageal reflux with erosive esophagitis, and therefore medical management is not recommended with fluticasone or PPIs, respectively.

73. E (S&F ch47)
The endoscopic mucosal resection has confirmed that the esophageal adenocarcinoma has extended into the submucosal layer, confirming a T stage of at least T1b. In addition, there is lymphovascular invasion. For patients with deeper T1b tumors (sm2 and sm3) as well as tumors with lymphovascular invasion, endoscopic management is not indicated if the patient is an operative candidate. Without evidence of lymph node involvement, the standard of care is esophagectomy. Neoadjuvant therapy may be considered with lymph node involvement, which was not the case in this clinical scenario. There is no role for surveillance in this clinical scenario.

74. A (S&F ch47)
GERD with Barrett's esophagus is accepted as the strongest risk factor for progression to esophageal adenocarcinoma. Obesity and tobacco use are risk factors for progression of Barrett's esophagus to esophageal adenocarcinoma. Male gender is a risk factor for Barrett's esophagus. Alcohol

use has not been associated with Barrett's esophagus nor progression to esophageal adenocarcinoma.

75. C (S&F ch47)
The clinical symptoms and manometric findings are consistent with achalasia. Achalasia, Plummer-Vinson syndrome, and tylosis are associated with esophageal squamous cell carcinoma.

76. D (S&F ch47)
On endoscopy there is a 2 cm hypoechoic lesion, with a negative pillow sign (no indentation with palpation using a closed biopsy forceps) arising from the muscularis propria. This is most consistent with a leiomyoma or gastrointestinal stromal tumor (GIST). Based on size criteria, a GIST may be malignant or the lesion could represent a leiomyosarcoma. Most important, the lesion is progressively symptomatic. Thus he needs surgical evaluation and likely resection. Endoscopic resection methods are not well suited for submucosal lesions arising from the muscularis propria due to the risks of perforation and the likelihood of a positive deep margin with endoscopic resection. Fine needle aspiration with endoscopic ultrasound can be performed and may be diagnostic for lesions of this size; however, given the features and symptoms, a negative biopsy or leiomyoma on the biopsy would not change the indications for resection.

77. B (S&F ch47)
The most common benign esophageal tumor is a leiomyoma. Leiomyomas are fat deposits made up of adipocytes that may appear in different portions of the gastrointestinal tract. They typically present at endoscopy as a submucosal lesion, occasionally with a yellow hue. On probing with biopsy, the lesion is soft and readily indents, which is referred as the "pillow sign." On echoendosonographic exam, the submucosal lesion appears hyperechoic, well-circumscribed, and arises from the submucosa. These lesions do not warrant surveillance or excision unless symptomatic.

78. C (S&F ch47)
Endoscopic mucosal resection has been shown to be a safe endoscopic technique; however, it is associated with certain complications. Bleeding occurs in up to 10% of patients, generally around the time of the ablation. Perforation may occur in up to 3% of patients. Strictures are a late complication of endoscopic mucosal resection and depend on the length and circumference of mucosectomy. Strictures were seen in 7% of patients with Barrett's esophagus being managed with radiofrequency ablation. Given the clinical description in the context of an extensive endoscopic mucosal resection, a stricture is the most likely late or delayed complication.

79. A (S&F ch47)
The two most likely cancers to metastasize to the esophagus are breast cancer and malignant melanoma.

80. C (S&F ch47)
Approximately 4% of melanoma occurs in the esophagus as the primary source. The PET-CT helps to evaluate for metastatic melanoma. Endoscopic ultrasound and endoscopic resection are not recommended in the management of melanoma. Surgical referral is premature without adequate staging. MRI is considered inferior to PET-CT for the staging of melanoma.

CHAPTER

6

Stomach and Duodenum

Stephen Hans Berger, Parit Mekaroonkamol, Behtash Ghazi Nezami, and Shanthi Srinivasan

QUESTIONS

1. A 66-year-old man with past medical history of hypertension, chronic kidney disease stage III, chronic obstructive pulmonary disease (COPD) and chronic back pain with heavy nonsteroidal antiinflammatory drug (NSAID) use presented to the emergency department with abdominal pain and black tarry stools for the past 2 days. His blood pressure on arrival was 90/60 mm Hg with a heart rate of 120 bpm. He was admitted the medical intensive care unit and underwent an esophagogastroduodenoscopy (EGD) which showed a 2 cm gastric ulcer located at the fundus of the stomach with a visible bleeding vessel. Despite multiple attempts at hemostasis endoscopically, the procedure had to be aborted secondary to hypoxia and incomplete visualization. The patient was emergently rushed to interventional radiology for embolization. Given the patient's chronic kidney disease and need for minimal contrast use, which arterial distribution would give the highest yield in finding the culprit vessel for embolization?
   A. Short gastric arteries, supplied from splenic artery
   B. Right gastric artery, supplied by the common hepatic artery
   C. Left gastric artery, supplied by the celiac artery
   D. Right gastroepiploic artery, supplied by the gastroduodenal artery
   E. Left gastroepiploic artery, supplied by the splenic artery

2. A 56-year-old man complains of dyspepsia symptoms over the last 3 months. An EGD shows normal mucosa in the body and antrum of the stomach. Random biopsies were taken from the antrum, incisura, and body of the stomach to rule out *H. pylori*. What type of cells would one expect to find in the antrum of the stomach on pathologic exam?
   A. Basophilic staining cells responsible for synthesis of pepsinogen
   B. ATPase-dependent acid secreting cells
   C. Gastrin secreting cells
   D. Intrinsic factor secreting cells
   E. Neuroendocrine cells

3. A 54-year-old man with a history of chronic tension headaches thought to be exacerbated by his stressful corporate lifestyle has been taking naproxen twice daily for the last 2 weeks and is seen in the emergency department for abdominal pain. Initial vital signs show the patient to be afebrile with a heart rate of 110 bpm and blood pressure 100/50 mm Hg. His physical exam is notable for exquisite tenderness diffusely with rebound and guarding. CT is ordered immediately, which shows an area in the proximal duodenum that is inflamed and notable for air under the diaphragm, concerning for a perforated duodenal ulcer. He is taken to the operating emergently for an exploratory laparotomy. Which statement is correct in regards to anatomy of the duodenum?
   A. The gastroduodenal artery, bile duct, and portal vein lie posterior to the first portion
   B. The superior mesenteric artery (SMA) courses posterior to the third part of the duodenum
   C. The fourth portion of the duodenum is separated from the jejunum by falciform ligament
   D. The duodenum in its entirety is retroperitoneal
   E. The minor papilla is located in the third portion of the duodenum

4. A 65-year-old man presented to the hospital with severe periumbilical abdominal pain acutely over the last hour. He has never had anything like this before. His physical exam reveals an irregular rhythm and abdominal pain out of proportion to palpation. Laboratory studies show a lactic acidosis. A CT abdomen with intravenous contrast shows occlusions in branches of the superior mesenteric artery. An echocardiogram done bedside shows a large left ventricular thrombus. Which of the following portions of the GI tract would most likely be affected by ischemic changes on imaging?
   A. Esophagus
   B. Body and fundus of the stomach
   C. Antrum of the stomach
   D. Proximal Duodenum
   E. Distal duodenum

5. A 39-year-old gravid woman comes to the emergency department in her third trimester with complaints consistent with uterine contractions of labor. The pregnancy was not medically monitored. Bedside ultrasound appears within normal limits other than an excess amount of amniotic fluid. She has an uncomplicated vaginal birth. During the first feeding, the newborn begins having forceful, bilious emesis. On physical exam, there are notable features such as slanted palpebral fissures, a protruding tongue and palmar creases. What congenital anomaly does this child likely suffer from?
   A. Duodenal duplication cyst
   B. Duodenal atresia
   C. Infantile hypertrophic pyloric stenosis
   D. Gastric atresia
   E. Annular pancreas

6. A 25-year-old man undergoes a CT of the abdomen with oral contrast for right lower quadrant abdominal pain and was found to have appendicitis. He undergoes an appendectomy, recovers well, and is ready for discharge. Upon chart review, the CT scan notes a well-rounded, well-delineated pouch with air fluid level located adjacent to

the esophagogastric junction. The patient states he has no symptoms of dysphagia, dyspepsia, vomiting, or epigastric pain. Which of the following is the most appropriate next step in management?

A. Barium upper GI study
B. Check *H. pylori*
C. Endoscopic ultrasound
D. Repeat imaging in 1 year
E. Reassurance

7. A 3-month-old male infant presents to his pediatrician for vomiting and continued discomfort with feedings per the mother. His past medical history is notable for premature and difficult delivery. Abdominal ultrasound demonstrates a solid and cystic extragastric area along the greater curvature of the stomach. A noncontrast CT shows calcifications within the mass but no regional infiltration. What is the likely origin of this mass, and what further workup is needed?

A. Hypertrophic circular muscles, a pyloromyotomy should be performed
B. All three germ cell layers, tumor excision
C. Gastrointestinal stroma, endoscopic ultrasound, and possible excision
D. All three germ cell layers, endoscopic ultrasound, and possible excision
E. Gastrointestinal stroma, tumor excision

8. A 40-year-old man presents to the hospital with abdominal pain, nausea, postprandial fullness, and vomiting. Physical exam is unremarkable other than some mild epigastric tenderness. EGD was performed and notable for a 4 cm x 4.5 cm bulge of mucosa just beyond the ampulla. Endoscopic ultrasound is performed and shows an anechoic lesion consistent with a cyst. The diagnosis of duodenal duplication cyst is suspected. Which of the following is true about this diagnosis?

A. Histological criteria include gastrointestinal mucosa, a smooth muscle layer in the wall of the cyst, and an association with the duodenal wall
B. Pancreatitis has not been described in association with duodenal duplication cysts
C. Duodenal cysts in adults have low malignant potential
D. Duodenal cysts generally do not communicate with the duodenal lumen
E. Most common type of mucosa in the cyst is gastric type mucosa

9. A 3-month-old infant presents with postprandial vomiting and evidence of malnutrition. The child appears volume depleted and on further questioning, the mother notes diarrhea shortly after feedings. An Upper GI contrast study is performed and is notable for an enlarged esophagus and a tubular appearing stomach. What is the most likely cause?

A. Microgastria
B. Gastric duplication
C. Gastric atresia
D. Pyloric Stenosis
E. Gastric diverticulum

10. A 44-year-old woman with past medical history of type 1 diabetes mellitus presents to your clinic with complaints of abdominal bloating, nausea, and postprandial vomiting of 6 months duration. She had an EGD performed last week, which was normal. Her gastric emptying study shows delayed gastric emptying. Her vital signs show normal temperature, heart rate of 70 bpm, and blood pressure of 124/77 mm Hg. Physical exam is non-revealing. Which of the following is true in regards to interstitial cells of cajal (ICC) and diabetic gastroparesis?

A. Etiology of gastroparesis is thought to be from depletion ICC in the fundus
B. The greater the depletion of ICC, the higher likelihood of response to gastric electrical stimulation
C. ICCs are only located in submuscular and intramuscular layers
D. ICCs in the fundus are the most active areas of depolarization and are the pacemakers for slow waves
E. Myenteric ICCs establish the dominant pacemaker frequency

11. A 60-year-old man presents to your clinic with complaints of bloating, early satiety, and cramps with periods with diarrhea alternating with constipation. He previously had undergone extensive workup including an EGD, gastric emptying study, and abdominal imaging, all of which were non-revealing. The patient is new to your clinic and is presenting with his EGD report. He is inquiring about the images and how the food he eats ends up moving into his intestines. Which of the following is true in regards to normal gastric neuromuscular function?

A. Gastric slow waves normally occur at 8 cycles per minute
B. The pacemaker region is located in the greater curvature of the stomach
C. The pylorus is not an electrical barrier between slow waves of the antrum and duodenum
D. Higher plateau potentials do not correlate with stronger gastric contractions
E. Fundic smooth muscle resting membrane potential lies below the threshold for contraction

12. An otherwise healthy 36-year-old woman is admitted to the hospital for a fractured fibula suffered during a competitive sporting event. She is to undergo surgery the next morning and recieves nothing by mouth after midnight. Her surgery is scheduled for 9:00 AM and her last meal was at 9:00 PM. What is true in regards to 12 hours of fasting and the enteric neuromuscular activity of the migrating myoelectical (motor) complex (MMC)?

A. There are four phases of the MMC complex
B. Approximately 15 of these complexes can be expected during a 12-hour fast
C. Phase two consists of irregular random contractions
D. Phase three always originates in the stomach and migrates down to the ileum
E. Postvagotomy patients will lose the MMCs

13. A 38-year-old woman presents with 15-pound weight loss over the last 2 months. She has stated that during this time she has been feeling full more quickly while eating regular meals. She denies vomiting, but has some nausea when eating liquids or solids. She denies any melena or blood in her stools. Her vital signs show normal temperature, a heart rate of 60 bpm, and blood pressure 109/50 mm Hg. She states that prior to these last few months, she had been eating and drinking normally. During consumption of a meal, fundic tone relaxes to accommodate food and prevent early satiety. Which of the following causes an increase muscle tone of the gastric fundus?

A. Ingestion of solid foods
B. Acetylcholine and substance P
C. Duodenal and antral distension
D. Colonic distension
E. Intraluminal perfusion of the duodenum with lipid or protein

14. A 56-year-old man with history of gastroparesis on medical management is coming into clinic today shortly after the thanksgiving holiday. He said he has been doing well but definitely felt symptoms of his gastroparesis after all of the holiday feasts he had partaken in. He recalls eating turkey with gravy, mashed potatoes with extra butter, and fruit salad. He asks you about specific types of food that he should try to stay away from that may cause more symptoms than others. Which meal-related factors are more likely to delay the rate of gastric emptying?

A. Decreased acidity
B. Foods low in tryptophan
C. Foods higher in fat
D. Decrease in meal volume
E. Decrease in osmolarity

15. A 58-year-old man presents to your clinic with intermittent nausea. His past medical history is significant for type 2 diabetes mellitus, hypertension, and asthma as a child. He states that he cannot pinpoint the exact association with his nausea, but says that he believes it is sometimes associated with eating. He has been checking his blood glucose regularly and has had no recent change to his medications. His vital signs reveal a temperature of 37° C, heart rate of 80 bpm, and blood pressure 128/78 mm Hg. Which of the following scenarios is associated with a reduction in gastric emptying?

A. Blood glucose of 150 mg/dL
B. Ileum exposure to diet-derived proteins
C. Reduction in cholecystokinin (CCK)
D. Increase in corticotropin-releasing factor
E. Diarrhea

16. A 55-year-old-man with a past medical history of stroke is being consulted for percutaneous gastrostomy tube placement due to severe dysphagia and risk for aspiration. The patient and his family inquire into his nutritional status following gastrostomy tube placement and about his overall feelings of hunger. Which of the following should suppress hunger the greatest in normal individuals?

A. 600 mL volume, low calorie meal ingested by mouth
B. 300 mL volume, high calorie meal ingested by mouth
C. 600 mL volume, low calorie meal ingested directly via PEG tube
D. 300 mL volume, low calorie meal ingested by mouth
E. 600 mL volume, low calorie meal ingested via nasogastric tube placed post-pyloric

17. A 32-year-old man with morbid obesity is presenting to your clinic for routine follow-up. He has tried multiple lifestyle modifications for weight loss, including portion control, diet changes, and exercise programs without success. He has also attempted multiple medical weight loss medications without success. He is requesting surgical consultation regarding gastric bypass. He has read online about the alteration of anatomy, but also the change in hormones that aid in the weight loss and wants to know more about how these hormones affect his appetite and fullness. Which of these hormones is decreased after ingestion of meals and plays important roles in the sensation of fullness?

A. cholecystokinin
B. Leptin
C. Ghrelin
D. Glucagon-like peptide-1 (GLP-1)
E. Apolipoprotein A-IV

18. A 44-year-old man has a past medical history of coronary artery disease, peripheral vascular disease, and previous multiple strokes. He is currently on aspirin and clopidogrel. He is admitted to the hospital for persistent nausea and vomiting for the last week. His vital signs show normal temperature, heart rate of 110 bpm, and blood pressure of 108/60 mm Hg. His physical exam is notable for an obese male, mild epigastric tenderness, but no rebound or guarding. An abdominal bruit is appreciated. Which of the following diagnostic modalities would be consistent with a diagnosis of gastroparesis?

A. Wireless motility capsule takes approximately 5 hours to reach the duodenum
B. Scintigraphy showing 20% retained gastric contents after 120 minutes
C. Ingestion of 800 mL of Ensure over 30 minutes in 5 minute intervals evokes nausea and gastric dysrhythmia
D. Scintigraphy showing 5% retained gastric contents after 4 hours
E. Full thickness biopsies of gastric tissue shows depletion of interstitial cells of Cajal (ICC)

19. A 28-year-old woman with a past medical history of diabetes type 1 since age 12 is presenting to your clinic for routine follow-up of her gastroparesis. Overall her symptoms are very difficult to manage but she has been maintaining her nutritional intake and her weight has been stable while on medications. She mentions how her uncle is also a diabetic diagnosed in his 40s around the same time as her and was also given the diagnosis of gastroparesis just a few years ago. What is typically true in regards to type 1 and type 2 diabetic gastroparesis?

A. Type 2 diabetic gastroparesis tends to be more severe
B. Early satiety is more severe in type 2 diabetics
C. Incidence of gastroparesis is higher in patients with type 2 than in type 1 diabetes
D. Type 1 diabetics tend to have fewer hospitalizations for gastroparesis compared to type 2 diabetics
E. Prior to diagnosis of gastroparesis, hyperglycemia is usually present for a longer duration in type 1 diabetics as compared to type 2 diabetics.

20. A 56-year-old man presents to the hospital with a 6-month history of early satiety, bloating, and postprandial fullness. His past medical history is significant for nonobstructive coronary artery disease for which he takes a baby aspirin daily. He also has diabetes mellitus type 2 diagnosed 3 years ago managed on metformin. His surgical history is notable for vagotomy 2 years ago in the setting of peptic ulcer disease. His vital signs reveal a temperature of 37° C, a heart rate of 90 bpm, and blood pressure of 134/77 mm Hg. He otherwise is compliant with annual visits to his general practitioner. An EGD is performed showing a 5 mm sessile polyp in the body of the stomach with a smooth surface contour. Biopsies were taken showing pathologic features consistent with a fundic gland polyp. Which of the following is the most likely etiology of the patient's symptoms?

A. Diabetic gastroparesis
B. Postsurgical gastroparesis
C. Fundic gland polyp
D. Ischemic gastroparesis
E. Pylorospasms

21. A 37-year-old woman with no past medical history presents with nausea and vomiting. She states that she had just come back from a week-long cruise approximately 2 to 3 weeks ago. At that time she and multiple other passengers developed a flu-like illness with fevers, nausea, and vomiting. This acute episode resolved, but now over the last week abdominal pains developed, and nausea and

vomiting returned. She is unable to keep anything down, including solids and liquids. Which of the following is true in regards to this cause of gastroparesis?
A. Patients have been shown to have smooth muscle dysfunction with a thickened basal lamina on pathology
B. It is not related to the recent illness
C. Symptoms can resolve completely over the next 1 to 2 years
D. It can sometimes be associated with multiple courses of antibiotics
E. Compared to patients with diabetes, this type of gastroparesis tends to have more severe depletion of interstitial cells of Cajal

22. A 44-year-old man with a past medical history of diabetes diagnosed 12 years ago, history of gastroesophageal reflux disease and alcohol abuse is presenting abdominal pain. He states pain is located on the right side. He has never had this pain before and otherwise is taking all his medications as prescribed, including metformin and omeprazole. He denies any association with eating. Pain is worsened with anterior abdominal muscle contraction and there is noticeable tenderness on a previously healed incision. What is the most likely origin of the patient's pain?
A. Pancreatitis
B. Gastroparesis
C. Gastroesophageal reflux disease (GERD)
D. Abdominal wall syndrome
E. Functional dyspepsia

23. A 28-year-old woman with diabetes type 1 underwent a scintigraphy for gastric emptying 2 months ago and showed approximately 15% of radiolabeled food at 4 hours post ingestion. She was started on metoclopramide and ondansetron with good results and is presenting now with 2 days of protruding tongue movements, bulging of the cheeks, and repetitive chewing. She describes main symptoms of gastroparesis to be nausea and vomiting, which were improved with metoclopramide but have restarted since she stopped her medication when these side effects began. Her vital signs show a temperature of 37° C, a heart rate of 100 bpm, and blood pressure of 150/80 mm Hg. Abdominal exam reveals a soft, nontender abdomen. What is the most appropriate next step in management?
A. Discontinue metoclopramide, consider cisapride
B. Discontinue metoclopramide, consider domperidone
C. Restart metoclopramide but give a dose of intramuscular diphenhydramine first
D. Discontinue metoclopramide, add erythromycin
E. Refer for gastric electrical stimulator

24. A 55-year-old man is presenting with chronic abdominal complaints. His history is significant for chronic back pain, hypertension, and history of abdominal surgeries. He previously had been on high-dose nonsteroidal antiinflammatory medications for his back pain; however, he developed a large ulcer in the gastric antrum requiring surgical resection and Billroth II procedure. He states that for the last few months, he has been noticing abdominal bloating, nausea, and sometimes vomiting. This occurs shortly after eating and is followed by diarrhea. Two to 4 hours afterwards, he will start feeling sweaty and lightheaded. An EGD is performed, showing findings of prior surgery, consistent with Billroth II anatomy. There are no strictures or ulcerations around the surgical anastomosis. What is the most likely underlying cause for his sweats and lightheadedness?
A. Gastroparesis
B. Distension of the small bowel from dumping
C. Osmotic diarrhea causing dehydration
D. Rapid carbohydrate absorption
E. Functional dyspepsia

25. A 65-year-old Caucasian man with a history of gastrinoma who underwent a distal pancreatectomy presents to his gastroenterologist's office for a follow-up visit at 6 months after his surgery. He complains of intermittent epigastric pain, for which he is taking omeprazole with some relief. His chromogranin A (CgA) level, even though decreased from his baseline prior to surgery of 680 ng/mL, remains elevated at 115 ng/mL. (Normal range is less than 36.4 ng/mL.) A somatostatin receptor scintigraphy using ^{111}In-DPTA-D-phe1-octreotide showed no uptake activity. Which of the following is the most appropriate next step in management?
A. MRI of the abdomen
B. Endoscopic ultrasound (EUS)
C. Check pancreatic polypeptide level
D. Repeat CgA level in 3 months
E. Stop omeprazole and repeat CgA level

26. A 50-year-old Asian woman presents with a 1-year history of epigastric abdominal pain. She has empirically tried esomeprazole twice a day for the past 6 months but stopped taking it for the past 4 weeks as it provided her with only minimal relief. A subsequent EGD found three small clean base duodenal ulcers. Random gastric biopsy was positive for *H. pylori*. Which of the following best describes the effect of *H. pylori* infection in pathogenesis of this patient's ulcer disease?
A. Antral gastritis causing decreased somatostatin secretion
B. Interference with transcription of H^+/K^+ ATPase inhibiting acid secretion
C. Secretion of IL-1β and TNF-α that inhibit parietal cell secretion
D. Direct inhibition of the parietal cell by a constituent of the bacterium
E. Rebound acid hypersecretion after stopping proton pump inhibitor (PPI) therapy

27. Which of the following inhibits gastrin release from antral G cells?
A. Cholecystokinin
B. Glucagon
C. Somatostatin
D. Secretin
E. Leptin

28. Proton pump inhibitor (PPI) is the drug of choice in reducing gastric acid secretion. Which of the following statement is true regarding this class of medications?
A. PPI has best efficacy if taken in a fasting state because it requires an acidic environment for the conversion to its active form
B. Stopping PPI after chronic acid suppression can cause enterochromaffin-like (ECL) cell hyperplasia
C. Because PPI can directly inhibit H^+/K^+ ATPase, it does not get affected by gastric pH
D. PPI should be taken at breakfast time because this is when most H^+/K^+ ATPase pumps are inserted
E. PPI can be taken with meal because it normally reaches the peak plasma concentration within 30 minutes

29. Which of the following is found in gastric body?
A. Parietal cell
B. Pyloric gland
C. G cell

D. D cell
E. Squamous epithelial cells

30. Which of the following stimulates gastric acid secretion by the parietal cells?
A. Calcitonin gene–related peptide (CGRP)
B. Norepinephrine
C. Somatostatin
D. Acetylcholine
E. Amylin

31. A 39-year-old woman presents to her primary care physician's office with a 1-month history of nausea and vague epigastric pain that is worse after meals. She denies weight loss, vomiting, dysphagia, hematemesis, or rectal bleeding. She takes estrogen-based oral contraceptives and occasionally ibuprofen for headaches. Physical exam reveals mild tenderness to deep palpation in the epigastric area. Laboratory values are as follows:

Hemoglobin	13.5 g/dL
WBC	6000/µL
Platelet count	300,000/µL

She is advised to stop ibuprofen and is started on pantoprazole 40 mg per day. She returns to the office after 8 weeks and her symptoms are not changed. What is the next best therapeutic test?
A. EGD with random biopsy
B. *H. pylori* serology and treatment if positive
C. *H. pylori* stool antigen testing and treatment if positive
D. Empirically treat *H. pylori*
E. Add H2 blocker to pantoprazole therapy

32. A 52-year-old man is admitted to the hospital with abdominal distension and intractable vomiting. CT with contrast reveals thickening of the antrum with gastric outlet obstruction, as well as preaortic lymphadenopathy. An EGD is performed, revealing a 1 cm, superficial white-based ulcer within the antrum. Biopsy of the ulcer reveals sheets of mature lymphoid cells expressing CD19, CD20, and CD79a, but is CD5-negative. *H. pylori* organisms were present. *H. pylori* organisms were present. What is the best course of treatment?
A. External beam radiation therapy
B. Rituximab
C. Antrectomy
D. Combination chemotherapy
E. Antibiotics and proton pump inhibitor therapy

33. A 40-year-old man is seen in clinic for follow-up of dyspepsia. He was seen in clinic 3 months ago for symptoms of postprandial pain and burning in the epigastric area. He tested positive for *H. pylori* using urea breath test. He was treated with standard triple therapy for *H. pylori* (amoxicillin, clarithromycin, proton pump inhibitor [PPI]). He had resolution of his symptoms initially, but now he has developed recurrence of dyspepsia. An EGD is performed, showing a small shallow ulcer in the gastric fundus. Rapid urease test is positive for *H. pylori* organisms. Which of the following is the best next step in management?
A. Repeat initial therapy, extended to a 21-day duration
B. PPI + levofloxacin + amoxicillin for 14 days
C. PPI + doxycycline + metronidazole + bismuth for 14 days
D. PPI + amoxicillin + rifabutin for 14 days
E. Repeat EGD and biopsy for *H. pylori* culture and sensitivity

34. A 61-year-old man undergoes an upper endoscopy for abdominal pain. A 4 cm gastric ulcer in noted on the lesser curvature of the stomach. Biopsies from the antrum are positive for *H. pylori* infection. The patient is seen back in your office after taking the prescribed therapy for *H. pylori* eradication. His symptoms have resolved. which of the following is the best next step in management?
A. Discharge from clinic
B. Continue proton pump inhibitor (PPI) indefinitely and observe
C. Repeat endoscopy
D. Repeat noninvasive *H. pylori* testing
E. Stop PPI and test for *H. pylori* in 2 weeks

35. A 50-year-old man is seen in your office for persistent gastric ulcers. He has persistent *H. pylori* infection after being treated with a standard course of a proton pump inhibitor (PPI) + clarithromycin + amoxicillin and a second regimen of PPI + clarithromycin + metronidazole. He does not use any medications other than recent *H. pylori* regimens. He drinks one to two beers daily and smokes one packet of cigarettes daily. On his most recent endoscopy performed a few days before his visit, he continues to have two clean-based duodenal ulcers and *H. pylori* organisms are seen on biopsy. His stomach mucosa appeared normal. What is the next course of treatment?
A. PPI + bismuth + metronidazole
B. PPI + clarithromycin + nitroimidazole + amoxicillin
C. Ask the patient to stop smoking and retreat with PPI + clarithromycin + amoxicillin
D. PPI + clarithromycin + amoxicillin for 6 weeks
E. Rifabutin + PPI + metronidazole twice daily for 14 days

36. Which factor is essential for colonization of *H. pylori* in the stomach?
A. Absence of toll-like receptor 4
B. Intestinal metaplasia
C. *H. pylori* motility
D. Lewis antigens expressed on the bacteria
E. Minimum amount of *H. pylori* infection

37. Patients with antral-predominant *H. pylori* infection have increased predisposition to which of the following conditions?
A. Gastric peptic ulcer disease
B. Barrett esophagus
C. Duodenal peptic ulcer disease
D. Pangastritis
E. Gastric adenocarcinoma

38. A 35-year-old woman with new onset abdominal epigastric burning and nausea has a positive stool *H. pylori* antigen. She is treated with conventional triple therapy for 2 weeks, but her symptoms do not improve. She has no alarming symptoms such as weight loss, black stool, or hematemesis. On physical exam there is mild epigastric tenderness. The rest of the exams are within normal limits. Laboratory results are as follows:

Hemoglobin	13 g/dL
WBC	7200/µL
Platelet count	380,000/µL

A repeat stool *H. pylori* antigen is negative. What is the next best course of action?
A. Computed tomography (CT) of the abdomen
B. Upper endoscopy
C. Quadruple therapy
D. Reassurance and follow-up in 3 months
E. Tricyclic antidepressants

39. A 41-year-old morbidly obese woman is seen in your clinic for retrosternal burning pain for 3 months. The pain seems to be exacerbated by eating, and is also worse at night. She currently smokes one half pack per day of cigarettes, and drinks two glasses of wine every week. Her daughter has noticed frequent belching and malodorous breath. She denies recent weight loss, dysphagia, or vomiting blood. A recent cardiac stress test was negative. Which of the following is the most appropriate next step in management?
   A. Upper endoscopy
   B. *H. pylori* stool antigen testing
   C. C-14 urea breath test
   D. *H. pylori* serology
   E. Proton pump inhibitor (PPI) therapy

40. Which of the following processes is involved in the host response to *H. pylori* infection?
   A. Natural killer cell activation
   B. NF-κB–mediated gene expression
   C. $CD8^+$ T cell recruitment
   D. Altered cholecystokinin signaling
   E. Increased mucous production

41. Which of the following statements regarding *H. pylori* epidemiology is true?
   A. Most infected individuals are symptomatic carriers
   B. Over 75% of the world population is seropositive
   C. Infection is commonly acquired in adulthood in developing countries
   D. Spontaneous clearance of bacteria is common
   E. In the United States, *H. pylori* infection is more common in Hispanics than in African Americans

42. Which of the following processes is a step in gastric oncogenesis with *H. pylori* infection?
   A. Reduced angiogenesis
   B. Gastric hypertrophy
   C. Intestinal metaplasia
   D. Superficial *H. pylori* gastritis
   E. Loss of KRAS tumor suppressor

43. Which of the following statements about the risk of peptic ulcer disease (PUD) is true?
   A. *H. pylori* infection alone increases the risk of PUD by fourfold
   B. Nonsteroidal antiinflammatory drug (NSAID) use alone increases the risk of PUD by threefold
   C. Long term NSAID use and *H. pylori* infection increase the risk of PUD by sixfold
   D. *H. pylori* infection does not increase the risk of PUD in patients taking low-dose aspirin
   E. Smoking, excessive alcohol intake, and Type A personality are all strong risk factors for PUD

44. Which statement about diagnostic testing for *H. pylori* is correct?
   A. Proton pump inhibitors (PPIs) should be discontinued 2 weeks prior to fecal antigen or serology testing
   B. Serological testing has better positive predictive value for detecting *H. pylori* infection in the Mexican population than in the American population
   C. The specificity of urea breath testing will decrease if performed earlier than 4 weeks after completion of antibiotic therapy
   D. The sensitivity and specificity of urea breath testing and fecal antigen testing is less than 70% to 80% in untreated patients who are not taking PPIs, bismuth, or antibiotics
   E. *H. pylori* serology can be used to confirm eradication

45. A 37-year-old Chinese immigrant presents with postprandial epigastric fullness and occasional nausea for the past 2 months. She denies heartburn, weight loss, or dark stool. Her review of systems is otherwise normal. She has been taking omeprazole, with partial improvement. She does not use tobacco, alcohol, or illicit drugs. Her vital signs are normal. On physical exam, she has mild epigastric tenderness on deep palpation. What is the best next step in management of this patient?
   A. EGD with biopsies for *H. pylori*
   B. EGD with rapid urease test
   C. Stop PPI for 4 weeks and test with urea breath test
   D. Serology testing for *H. pylori*
   E. Start empiric conventional triple therapy for *H. pylori*

46. A 55-year-old Hispanic man is admitted to the hospital for abdominal distension and epigastric pain for 3 days. He received an allogenic bone marrow transplantation 2 months ago for acute lymphocytic leukemia and takes mycophenlylate and prednisone. Upper endoscopy reveals a narrowed gastric antrum with edema of the antral mucosa and multiple deep linear ulcerations. What is the most likely diagnosis?
   A. Infiltrating antral adenocarcinoma
   B. Leukemic recurrence
   C. *Candida* infection
   D. Cytomegalovirus (CMV) gastritis
   E. Crohn's disease

47. What are the classic histopathologic findings in a patient with cytomegalovirus gastritis?
   A. Signet ring cells with disorganized mucus cells
   B. Lymphocytic infiltration of the muscularis propria
   C. Polymorphonuclear infiltrate with enlarged epithelial cells containing nuclear inclusion bodies
   D. Numerous histiocytes
   E. lymphocytic-predominant infiltrate with cytoplasmic inclusion bodies

48. A 60-year-old man is admitted to the intensive care unit for respiratory failure due to severe pneumonia. He is intubated and placed on low tidal volume ventilation. Nasogastric tube aspirate shows small amount of coffee ground material. An upper endoscopy reveals edema, erythema, and multiple shallow erosions throughout the gastric body and antrum. What is the most likely cause of his gastritis?
   A. *H. pylori* infection
   B. Nasogastric tube–related injury
   C. Stress gastritis
   D. Drug-induced gastritis
   E. Autoimmune gastritis

49. A 65-year-old Caucasian man is seen in the emergency department due to 1 month of severe fatigue, loss of balance, and mouth pain. He has a history of essential hypertension and rheumatoid arthritis. Physical exam reveals tender glossitis, scleral pallor, tachycardia with a systolic flow murmur, and decreased joint proprioception bilaterally. Which of the following laboratory findings would be most likely in this patient?
   A. Vitamin B_{12} <200 pg/mL
   B. Megaloblastic anemia on peripheral blood smear
   C. Antiparietal cell antibodies
   D. Intrinsic factor antibodies
   E. Elevated methylmalonic acid (MMA) level

50. A 55-year-old Caucasian man is evaluated is referred to gastroenterology for endoscopic evaluation of occult blood loss

anemia. An EGD is performed, which shows erythema and edema in the gastric mucosa just below the esophagogastric junction. Biopsy reveals atrophic gastritis and Warthin silver stain reveals *H. pylori* organisms. The patient is at higher risk for which of the following conditions?
A. Junctional squamous cell carcinoma
B. Adenocarcinoma
C. Duodenal ulcer
D. Gastrointestinal stromal tumor
E. Achalasia

51. A 38-year-old man is evaluated for gnawing epigastric pain, which has been worsening since a laparoscopic cholecystectomy 2 months ago for uncomplicated biliary colic. He has not been able to maintain his weight due to severe postprandial pain. He is referred for urgent endoscopy, which shows red streaky erosions in the antrum and bile-stained mucosa. What is the best initial treatment for this condition?
A. Pyloroplasty
B. Roux-en-Y diversion
C. Cholestyramine
D. Proton pump inhibitor and antacid therapy
E. Appetite stimulant

52. A 26-year-old man with type 1 diabetes mellitus is admitted to intensive care unit with altered mental status. Initial evaluation reveals severe diabetes ketoacidosis (DKA) and protease positive urinary tract infection. He is comatose and intubated for airway protection. During intubation the patient has 100 mL of coffee ground emesis and some visible blot clots. Oral gastric tube is inserted and lavage reveals coffee ground material and dark red blood streaks in gastric content. He has not had hematochezia or melena since admission. Abdomen is soft and nondistended with hypoactive bowel sound. Vital signs include a blood pressure of 140/90 mm Hg and heart rate of 72 bpm. Laboratory results are as follows:

Hemoglobin	15.8 g/dL
Creatinine	2.9 mg/dL
Urea nitrogen	65 mg/dL
WBC	26,000/µL
pH	6.9
INR	1.3
Platelet count	470,000/µL

What is next best step in management?
A. Gastric lavage
B. Proton pump inhibitor (PPI) infusion followed by EGD
C. Octreotide infusion
D. Urgent upper endoscopy
E. Intravenous PPI once daily and observation

53. What hormone is expected to increase in a patient with diffuse corporal atrophic gastritis?
A. Cholecystokinin
B. Glucagon
C. Gastrin
D. Secretin
E. Vasoactive intestinal peptide

54. A 42-year-old man with history of duodenal ulcers and conventional triple antibiotic therapy for *H. pylori* infection 3 months ago, undergoes routine follow up EGD. He complains about epigastric fullness and pain in the past 5 days. He takes ibuprofen for his knee pain. EGD shows extensive erosive gastritis and a single, 1 cm ulcer in the duodenum close to ampulla of Vater. Which of the following processes is involved in the pathogenesis of this condition?
A. COX-2 Inhibition
B. Mast cell infiltration
C. Hypergastrinemia
D. Increased prostaglandin E2 synthesis
E. Increased neutrophil infiltration

55. A 48-year-old woman is evaluated for abdominal pain and nausea for the past 3 months. She has lost 5 pounds in the past month. She is afraid to eat as it results in the abdominal pain. An upper endoscopy reveals erythema and inflammation in the gastric body and antrum. Biopsies are taken and shown below (see figure). What is the diagnosis of this patient?
A. Lymphocytic gastritis
B. Autoimmune gastritis
C. Adenocarcinoma
D. Eosinophilic gastritis
E. Ménétrier disease

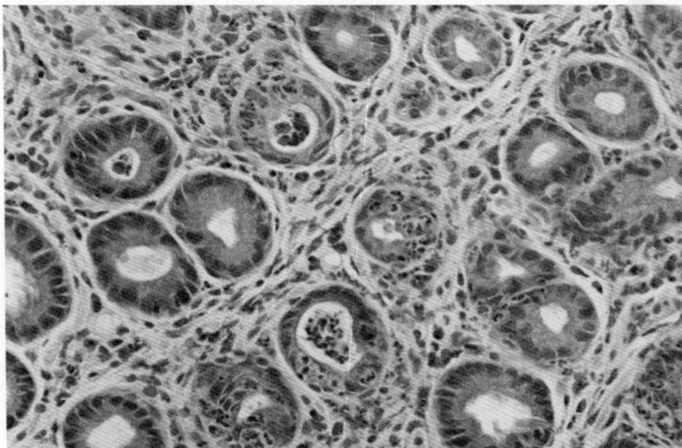

Figure for question 55.

56. A 42-year-old man comes to the physician complaining of epigastric discomfort for 4 months. He was treated with proton pump inhibitor therapy, but had no relief in his symptoms. He has recently developed diarrhea and has lost 10 pounds unintentionally. EGD is performed, which shows diffusely thickened rugae with antral sparing. Gastric biopsy shows exuberant foveolar hyperplasia with cystic dilation, minimal gastritis, and increased mucus glands (see figure). What is the most likely diagnosis?
A. Acute gastritis
B. Eosinophillic gastritis
C. Ménétrier disease
D. Gastric adenocarcinoma
E. Chronic gastritis

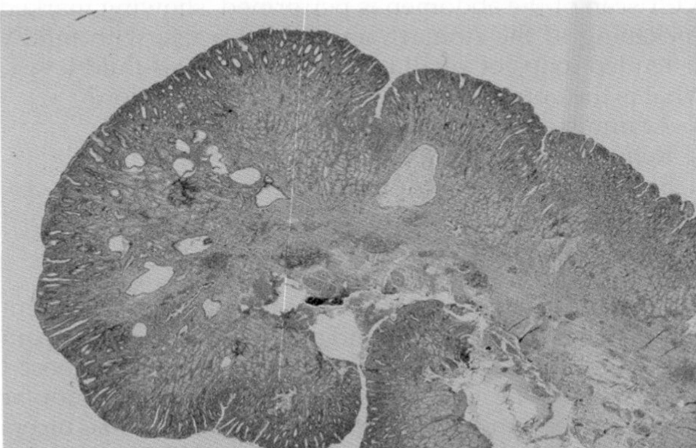

Figure for question 56.

57. A 48-year-old man patient is referred to you by his primary care physician for chronic osmotic diarrhea, anemia, and a sore tongue. Laboratory evaluation reveals macrocytic anemia. Atrophic gastritis is suspected. What findings are necessary to confirm the diagnosis?
A. Three random biopsies from the gastric fundus, cardia, and antrum
B. Single random biopsy from the gastric body
C. Anti–intrinsic factor antibody titer
D. Hypersegmented neutrophils on peripheral blood smear
E. A set of five biopsies taken from the gastric body, incisura, and antrum

58. A 24-year-old patient with advanced HIV/AIDS is admitted to the intensive care unit for *Pneumocystis* pneumonia, complicated by septic shock. On the third day of mechanical ventilation, he develops melena and hypotension. An EGD is performed urgently and shows a single large clean-based ulcer in the antrum. Biopsy shows copious yeast with pseudohyphae. What is the likely diagnosis?
A. Gastric candidiasis
B. Angioinvasive aspergillosis
C. Disseminated cryptococcal infection
D. Stress ulcer
E. Histoplasmosis

59. A 31-year-old woman is brought into the emergency department by paramedics after she develops sudden intractable bilious emesis and excruciating abdominal pain during an argument with her husband. She reports developing an upper respiratory infection the week prior. She is adopted, and her medical history is remarkable only for asthma and childhood eczema. Laboratory evaluation reveals peripheral blood eosinophilia of 8%. CT scan shows severe edema of the gastric mucosa and small bowel wall. What is the most likely diagnosis?
A. Acute mesenteric ischemia
B. Angioedema
C. Viral gastroenteritis
D. Gastrointestinal anaphylaxis
E. Eosinophilic gastritis

60. A 22-year-old male college student is evaluated in the emergency department for 2 days of fever, nausea, abdominal pain, nonbilious vomiting, and watery diarrhea. His dormitory roommate developed similar symptoms concurrently. On exam, his abdomen is scaphoid, soft, and mildly tender diffusely, with hyperactive bowel sounds. A CT scan of the abdomen is performed, showing marked thickening of the stomach and bowel walls, with mildly distended loops of small bowel and three air-fluid levels. What is the appropriate therapy for this condition?
A. Administer corticosteroids
B. Rehydration and reassurance
C. Surgical consultation for exploratory laparotomy
D. A course of ciprofloxacin
E. Diagnostic endoscopy

61. A 35-year-old man undergoes endoscopy for iron deficiency anemia, weight loss, and progressive epigastric pain for 2 weeks. He has a history of anterior uveitis diagnosed 3 years ago. The endoscopist notes patches of nodular gastric mucosa and several serpiginous fissure-like ulcers in the antrum and proximal duodenum. No fistulae are appreciated. Biopsy shows transmural granulomatous inflammation with submucosal fibrosis. A recent colonoscopy done for weight loss was normal. What is the first line of therapy?
A. Biologic therapy
B. Truncal vagotomy
C. Sucralfate
D. Proton pump inhibitor therapy
E. Corticosteroids

62. A 71-year-old woman is admitted to the hospital for symptomatic iron deficiency anemia and periodic epigastric pain for the last 4 months. Her medical history includes ischemic stroke 2 years ago and peripheral artery disease with moderate claudication. Endoscopy demonstrates red streaky gastric mucosa with several subepithelial hemorrhages. Biopsy demonstrates foveolar hyperplasia and erosions of the lamina propria. What is the most likely diagnosis?
A. Cholesterol embolization
B. Environmental metaplastic atrophic gastritis
C. Chronic ischemic gastritis
D. Portal hypertensive gastropathy
E. Drug-induced gastropathy

63. Which food item is most strongly associated with allergic gastritis?
A. Shellfish
B. Goat's milk
C. Egg
D. Honey
E. Cow's milk

64. A 57-year-old man undergoing chemoradiation for locally advanced non–small cell lung carcinoma develops severe nausea and vomiting several weeks after treatment is completed. Restaging positron emission tomography (PET) is performed, demonstrating reduced size of the primary tumor and new areas of bright PET-avidity in the gastric fundus and body. An endoscopy is performed to evaluate this. What is the most likely histopathologic finding?
A. Metastatic carcinoma
B. Small vessel vasculitis
C. Focal collagen deposition
D. Epithelial erosion and foveolar hyperplasia
E. Adenocarcinoma

65. A 37-year-old Japanese woman is seen in your clinic for chronic dyspepsia and iron deficiency anemia. She has a history of dysfunctional uterine bleeding and menorrhagia. It is decided to proceed with endoscopy, which reveals diffuse rugal thickening. Biopsy reveals a dense mononuclear infiltrate consisting of $CD56^+$ cells. A specimen is also sent for *H. pylori* culture. What is the best next course of therapy?
A. Interferon
B. Reassurance
C. Triple therapy
D. External beam radiation
E. Repeat endoscopy in 8 weeks

66. A 60-year-old obese African-American man with a history of hypertension, diabetes, and hypercholesterolemia presented to the emergency department for epigastric pain and symptomatic anemia. Two months ago, he suffered from a traumatic knee pain for 4 weeks and took ibuprofen 600 mg 2-3 times/day. He also takes aspirin 81 mg daily. He was found to have melena on digital rectal exam and hemoglobin of 6 g/dL. Subsequent EGD found a 1-cm ulcer with visible vessel in gastric body. Epinephrine injection and endoclips placement were performed successfully. His serum *H. pylori* antibody was positive. A 14-day course of antibiotics, along with omeprazole twice daily was started. He was advised to avoid further NSAIDs. He came back for a follow-up 10 weeks after his hospital discharge. A repeat EGD showed a healed ulcer. *H. pylori* eradication was confirmed. Which of the following is the most appropriate recommendation regarding his aspirin and proton pump inhibitor use?

A. Continue current aspirin and omeprazole dose
B. Switch omeprazole to daily dose and continue aspirin
C. Stop omeprazole; he can continue taking aspirin
D. Start misoprostol along with aspirin use
E. He should no longer take aspirin

67. Which of the following is associated with increased risk of peptic ulcer disease due to mucosal ischemia?

A. Smoking
B. Cocaine use
C. Corticosteroid intake
D. Bisphosphonate therapy
E. Type A personality

68. A 40-year-old woman presents to his gastroenterologist's office for chronically persistent epigastric pain for the past 3 months. The pain is dull, associated with bloating, often occurs at night, and is relieved by food. She takes oxycodone daily for pain with good relief. She reports constipation in the past 2 months. The pain also improves with bowel movement. She has no nausea, vomiting, or weight loss. She denies any NSAID use. She is not aware of any family history of stomach cancer or colon cancer. Her stool *H. pylori* antigen test was negative. Which of the following is the most appropriate next step in management?

A. EGD
B. Colonoscopy
C. Check CT of the abdomen
D. Trial of proton pump inhibitor therapy for 6 weeks
C. Trial of stimulant laxative, avoid opioid use

69. A 65-year-old Asian man with no significant past medical history presents to his gastroenterologist's clinic for a 2-month history of epigastric pain. The pain is intermittent, pressure-like, worsens with food, and relieved with antacid. He started taking ranitidine 150 mg twice daily 2 weeks ago with good symptomatic improvement but has not yet completely resolved. He has normal bowel movement and denies nausea, vomiting, dysphagia, NSAID use, weight loss, or family history of gastrointestinal cancer. Which of the following is the most appropriate next step in management?

A. Continue ranitidine for another 4 weeks and reevaluate
B. Switch ranitidine to a proton pump inhibitor (PPI); continue PPI for 6 weeks and reevaluate
C. Check CT of the abdomen
D. EGD
E. Check stool *H. pylori* antigen

70. A 60-year-old woman presents to her gastroenterologist's clinic after a recent EGD 8 weeks ago. She initially complained of a 6-month history of epigastric pain with 10 pounds unintentional weight loss, which prompted an EGD that revealed a white base 6-mm ulcer at the gastric antrum. Biopsy at the edge of the ulcer was benign. Random gastric biopsy, however, was positive for *H. pylori* infection. She completed her 14-day course of antibiotics 6 weeks ago with resolution of all her symptoms. Her weight is back to baseline. She ran out of pantoprazole 2 weeks ago and has been taking ranitidine instead. She came into clinic today for a refill of her medication. Stool *H. pylori* antigen today is negative. Which of the following is the most appropriate next step in management?

A. Refill her pantoprazole and continue for another 4 weeks, then reevaluate
B. Repeat EGD now
C. Stop ranitidine and recheck stool *H. pylori* antigen
D. Stop ranitidine, then reevaluate in 4 weeks
E. No further management is needed

71. Which of the following medications are is not metabolized by the liver and can be given at bed time?

A. Famotidine
B. Cimetidine
C. Ranitidine
D. Nizatidine
E. Rabeprazole

72. Which of the following statement is true regarding histamine-2 receptor antagonists?

A. Dose reductions are recommended when the creatinine clearance is below 50 mL/min
B. Dose adjustments are necessary in dialysis patients
C. Dose reductions are necessary in patients with hepatic dysfunction
D. Tolerance to the antisecretory effect is rare
E. When used with warfarin, ranitidine is preferred over famotidine because it does not bind to hepatic CYP-450 system

73. A 60-year-old man with history of gout, hypertension, hypercholesterolemia, and diabetes comes to see you in the clinic and asked for advice regarding ulcer prevention treatment. He denies any history of peptic ulcer disease. He requires pain medication intermittently for his knee pain from gouty arthritis. He tried multiple doses of acetaminophen without any relief. He takes 81 mg of aspirin at home for primary cardiovascular prevention. He was prescribed tramadol for pain, but he cannot tolerate drowsiness and constipation. He states that the ibuprofen has worked in the past but he was told not to take it because of risk of developing gastric ulcer. His stool *H. pylori* antigen is negative. What is the most appropriate drug regimen to control his pain and minimize his risk of gastric ulcer?

A. Naproxen and omeprazole
B. Ibuprofen and misoprostol
C. Naproxen and misoprostol
D. Naproxen and stop aspirin
E. Celecoxib at the lowest effective dose

74. A 55-year-old woman with history of asthma, polysubstance abuse, epigastric pain, and postprandial nausea whose recent EGD revealed a 1-cm clean base ulcer at gastric body and *H. pylori* infection comes in to her gastroenterologist's office for a follow-up visit. She took clarithromycin 500 mg twice daily and amoxicillin 1 g twice daily for 14 days, and has been taking esomeprazole 40 mg daily for the past 8 weeks with only minimal relief of her symptom. Stool *H. pylori* antigen today was negative. A repeat EGD revealed a 6-mm clean base ulcer at the same location with only slight improvement. Which of the following factors can contribute to her refractory ulcer?

A. Size of the ulcer
B. Caffeine intake

C. *H. pylori* infection
D. Ulcerative colitis
E. Inadequate duration of treatment

75. A 65-year-old man with multiple medical problems which include epilepsy, hypertension, atrial fibrillation, and congestive heart failure presents to his gastroenterologist's office for a 3-month history of epigastric pain. The pain was cramping in nature and associated with hunger. Food seems to alleviate the pain. A subsequent EGD reveals a clean base duodenal ulcer. Random gastric biopsy was negative for *H. pylori.* A proton pump inhibitor was prescribed for his ulcer disease. His other medications are warfarin, amlodipine, phenytoin, and furosemide. Which of the following medications has the highest likelihood of drug interaction?
A. Omeprazole
B. Esomeprazole
C. Lansoprazole
D. Pantoprazole
E. Rabeprazole

76. A 75-year-old woman with history of NSAID-induced duodenal and gastric ulcers comes to her gastroenterologist's office for a follow-up. She states that despite her greatest effort, she cannot discontinue NSAID use entirely due to her rheumatoid arthritis. She still uses NSAID three to four times per week when her joint pain "flares up." However, she has not used any NSAID in the past 2 weeks. She also reports epigastric pain that is worsened with food. Her other medical problems include uncontrolled diabetes, hypertension, and mild diastolic heart failure. Her physical exam today is unremarkable. Laboratory results show worsening kidney function with creatinine clearance decrease from 55 mL/min 6 months ago to 35 mL/min. Besides, stopping all NSAID, which of the following medications can be continued without any dose adjustment?
A. Ranitidine
B. Bismuth subsalicylate (Pepto-Bismol)
C. Misoprostol
D. Aluminium hydroxide
E. Sucralfate

77. Which of the following ulcers is most likely to have the best outcome and lowest risk of re-bleeding?
A. A 2.5-cm clean base ulcer at the antrum
B. A 1-cm ulcer in the cardia with a flat pigmented spot
C. A 1.5-cm clean base ulcer at the fundus
D. A 0.5-cm ulcer with pigmented spot at the posterior duodenal bulb
E. A 1-cm ulcer at the gastric body with adherent clot

78. A 70-year-old woman with a past medical history of hypertension, hypercholesterolemia, and osteoarthritis presents with a 2-week history of progressively diffuse abdominal pain that is worsened with food intake. The pain is associated with nausea and vomiting. The emesis is described as large amount of yellow fluid that comes 1 to 2 hours after a meal. She has had three to four non-bloody emesis per day during the last week. Yesterday the pain got worse with 10 vomiting episodes. She felt some pain relief after vomiting but noticed a small amount of blood in her vomit yesterday. This morning after she woke up, she vomited "a full cup of bright red blood," hence the emergency department visit. She admits taking naproxen twice daily for the past 2 months to help relieve her hip pain. Physical exam revealed a heart rate of 125 bpm, blood pressure of 100/60 mm Hg, severely tender epigastric area with marked distension but soft, no guarding or rebound tenderness; no chronic liver stigmata was seen. Laboratory results showed hemoglobin of 8.5 g/dL, decreased from her baseline of 12 g/dL, hypokalemia of 3.1 mEq/L, hypernatremia of 152 mEq/L, HCO_3 of 32 mEq/L, platelet count of 215/μL, and INR of 0.9. Which of the following is the next best step in management?
A. A stat abdominal x-ray and nasogastric tube insertion
B. An urgent upper endoscopy
C. Esomeprazole 80 mg intravenous bolus, then 8 mg/hr continuous drip
D. Type and cross for blood transfusion
E. Normal saline bolus

79. A 70-year-old woman with a past medical history of hypertension, hypercholesterolemia, and osteoarthritis who presents with a 2-week history of progressively diffuse abdominal pain that is worsened with food intake. The pain is associated with nausea and vomiting. The emesis is described as large amount of yellow fluid that comes 1 to 2 hours after meal. She has had three to four non-bloody emesis per day within the last week. Yesterday the pain got worse with 10 vomiting episodes. She felt some pain relief after vomiting but noticed a small amount of blood in her vomit yesterday. This morning after she woke up, she vomited a "a full cup of bright red blood", hence the emergency department visit. She admits taking naproxen twice daily for the past 2 months to help relieve her hip pain. Physical exam revealed a heart rate of 125 bpm, blood pressure of 100/60 mm Hg, severely tender epigastric area with marked distension but is soft, no guarding or rebound tenderness, no chronic liver stigmata was seen. Laboratory results showed a hemoglobin of 8.5 g/dL, decreased from her baseline of 12 g/dL, otherwise normal results. An urgent endoscopy was performed and showed a linear mucosal tear at the distal esophagus, consistent with a Mallory-Weiss tear. There was no bleeding stigmata that warranted an endoscopic intervention. A large amount of fluid was seen in the stomach. After aggressive suctioning, a large, clean base 3-cm pyloric channel ulcer, obstructing the pylorus was seen. An ultrathin gastroscope was used to traverse the pylorus and revealed normal duodenum. Which of the following is the next best step in management?
A. Consult surgery for antrectomy
B. Check serum *H. pylori* antibody and treat if positive
C. Continuous esomeprazole infusion and start total parenteral nutrition
D. Biopsy the ulcer edge and check carcinoembryonic (CEA) level
E. Endoscopic balloon dilation

80. Which of the following patients should receive proton pump inhibitor for peptic ulcer disease prophylaxis?
A. A 35-year-old woman with lupus flare who has been started on a 6-week course of high dose prednisone
B. A 55-year-old man with decompensated alcoholic cirrhosis and an INR of 2.5 who is admitted for hepatic encephalopathy
C. A 75-year-old woman who is admitted for hip fracture and has had nothing to eat or drink (NPO) for the past 3 days due to delayed surgery schedule
D. A 40-year-old woman who is admitted for chronic obstructive pulmonary disease exacerbation and has required mechanical ventilation for the past 2 days
E. A 20-year-old man who is admitted to the intensive care unit (ICU) due to severe metabolic acidosis from diabetic ketoacidocis

81. Which of the following is a risk factor for gastric adenocarcinoma?
   A. Acute gastritis
   B. History of duodenal surgery
   C. Peutz-Jeghers syndrome
   D. Caucasian ethnicity
   E. Multiple fundic gland polyps

82. Which of the following statement is true regarding the association of *H. pylori* infection to gastric adenocarcinoma?
   A. *H. pylori* infection is associated with intestinal-type gastric adenocarcinoma, not diffuse-type
   B. With the declining prevalence of *H. pylori* infection, the incidence of adenocarcinoma at the gastric cardia has decreased
   C. Patients with untreated *H. pylori*-induced duodenal ulcers have increased risk of gastric adenocarcinoma
   D. The development of dysplasia or invasive cancer usually occurs when *H. pylori* is fully colonized and actively replicating
   E. The most important cofactor in the induction of *H. pylori*-related adenocarcinoma is host immune response, particularly CD4 T cell reaction

83. Which of the following genes is the most commonly mutated gene in gastric cancer?
   A. Adenomatous polyposis coli gene *(APC)*
   B. Fragile histidine triad gene *(FHIT)*
   C. MutL homologs 1 *(MLH1)*
   D. *RAS* gene
   E. *TP53* gene

84. A 55-year-old man with a past medical history of gastroesophageal reflux disease who has been taking pantoprazole once daily for the past 5 years presents to the emergency department because of a 5-day history of black tarry stool and progressive dyspnea on exertion. He was found to have hemoglobin of 6.5 g/dL, decreased from his previous baseline hemoglobin of 11 g/dL 1 year ago. A subsequent EGD revealed a 1-cm duodenal ulcer with visible vessel in the bulb. An endoclip, together with epinephrine injection, yielded a successful hemostasis. Incidentally, three polyps were found in the fundus, size 0.5 cm to 1 cm. He denies any nausea or vomiting, dysphagia, nonsteroidal antiinflammatory drug (NSAID) use, weight loss, or family history of gastrointestinal cancer. Which of the following statement is true regarding the management of his gastric polyps?
   A. They are most likely hyperplastic polyps
   B. The risk of malignant transformation is low and no further management is needed
   C. They often regress after *H. pylori* eradication
   D. Repeat EGD is warranted for biopsy of the polyps
   E. Increasing his proton pump inhibitor (PPI) to twice daily may help polyp regression

85. A 40-year-old woman presented to her gastroenterologist's office for a 6-month history of epigastric pain. Her stool *H. pylori* antigen was positive, prompting a 14-day course of clarithromycin, amoxicillin, and omeprazole. She came back to clinic 6 weeks after completion of her antibiotics with ongoing abdominal pain. She felt no relief with omeprazole 20 mg daily. A subsequent EGD revealed cobblestone-appearing gastric mucosa with a 2.5 cm pedunculated polyp at the fundus. Random gastric biopsy and biopsy of the polyp were performed. Pathology showed chronic atrophic gastritis without evidence of *H. pylori* infection. The polyp biopsy showed hyperplastic fragment without dysplasia. Which of the following is the most appropriate next step in management?
   A. Reassurance
   B. Repeat EGD in 6 to 12 months for surveillance biopsy
   C. Increase omeprazole to 20 mg twice daily
   D. Repeat EGD and polypectomy
   E. Endoscopic ultrasound

86. A 70-year-old man presented to the emergency department after a motor vehicle accident. CT of the abdomen incidentally found thickening of gastric antrum. He denies any chronic abdominal pain, nausea, or family history of gastrointestinal cancer. However, his review of systems was positive for early satiety and 20 lbs unintentional weight loss over the past year. He adamantly refused an upper endoscopic workup because his father passed away from a procedural complication of a colonoscopy. He asked if there is any blood test that can help make the diagnosis of cancer. Which of the following statement is true regarding serum markers of gastric cancer?
   A. Low serum pepsinogen (PG) and hypergastrinemia are associated with intestinal metaplasia
   B. Only a few gastric cancers detected by serum pepsinogen level are early adenocarcinoma
   C. High ratio of PG-I to PG-II is suggestive of high risk pre-neoplastic lesions
   D. Serum carcinoembryonic antigen (CEA) cannot be used for surveillance of gastric cancer recurrence
   E. Serum CEA has a high sensitivity for early cancer detection

87. A 65-year-old Asian man presented to his gastroenterologist's office for a 6 months history of early satiety, 15 lbs weight loss, and epigastric pain. Physical exam and laboratory results were non-revealing. A subsequent EGD showed a 2 cm sessile mass in the antrum. Biopsy showed adenomatous polyp with high grade dysplasia and fragments of moderately differentiated adenocarcinoma. Which of the following is the most appropriate next step in management?
   A. Subtotal gastrectomy
   B. Endoscopic submucosal dissection
   C. Endoscopic ultrasound
   D. Diagnostic laparoscopy with peritoneal lavage
   E. PET scan

88. A 65-year-old African American woman presents with a 1-year history of progressive epigastric pain, nausea, vomiting, and unintentional weight loss. An EGD found a mass at the gastric body measuring 3.5 cm. Biopsy showed moderately differentiated adenocarcinoma. CT of the abdomen showed five to six enlarged perigastric lymph nodes, ranging from 1.0 to 1.5 cm in size. There is no evidence of distant metastasis seen on CT. Her carcinoembryonic antigen (CEA) level 18 ng/dL (normal is <2.5 ng/dL). Which of the following is the most important factor to determine her prognosis?
   A. Size of the tumor
   B. Depth of invasion
   C. Location of the tumor in relation to the gastroesophageal (GE) junction
   D. Presence of lymph node metastasis
   E. Her CEA level

89. A 60-year-old man with diabetes, gout, and hypercholesterolemia presents with a 3-day history of melena. He underwent an EGD and was found to have a 3.5 cm ulcerated mass at the antrum. Biopsy confirmed gastric adenocarcinoma. A CT of chest, abdomen, and pelvis showed multiple perigastric enlarged lymph nodes, but no distant

metastasis. An endoscopic ultrasound revealed infiltration in subserosal layer. Which of the following is the most appropriate next step of management?

A. Total gastrectomy
B. Partial gastrectomy with extended lymphadenectomy
C. Endoscopic submucosal dissection
D. Diagnostic laparoscopy
E. Neoadjuvant chemotherapy

90. A 65-year-old woman who was previously healthy was found to have hemoglobin of 10.5 g/dL on routine annual laboratory test. Subsequent colonoscopy showed only small hyperplastic polyps. An EGD found a 1-cm ulcer with a heaped-up margin at the greater curvature of the gastric body. The biopsy at the edge of the ulcer is shown in the figure. An endoscopic ultrasound showed tumor invasion to subserosal space. Which of the following is the most appropriate next step in management?

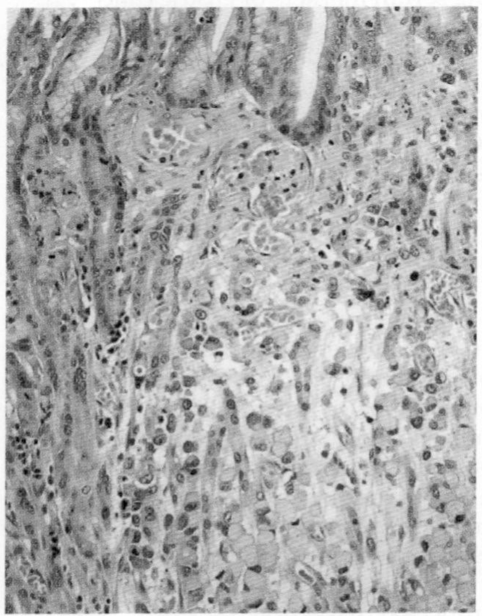

Figure for question 90.

A. Total gastrectomy
B. Partial gastrectomy
C. Endoscopic submucosal dissection
D. Endoscopic mucosal resection
E. Neoadjuvant chemotherapy

91. Which of the following factors is important in determining the resectability of early gastric cancer?

A. Histology type
B. location in the cardia
C. location in the lesser curvature
D. location in the fundus
E. location in the antrum

92. A 60-year-old woman with a past medical history of hypertension, hypercholesterolemia, and osteoarthritis presentes with a 2-week history of progressive dysphagia. She had difficulty swallowing both solid and liquid diet. She also complained of postprandial nausea and vomiting. An EGD showed a 1.5 cm mass at the cardia, 3 cm below gastroesophageal junction. An endoscopic ultrasound showed tumor invasion to subserosal space. Which of the following is the next best step in management?

A. Neoadjuvant chemotherapy and total gastrectomy
B. Total gastrectomy and perioperative chemotherapy
C. Total gastrectomy and adjuvant chemotherapy
D. Neoadjuvant chemotherapy and partial gastrectomy
E. Partial gastrectomy and adjuvant chemotherapy

93. A 65-year-old woman presents to the emergency department for five episodes of melena. Her hemoglobin upon arrival is 6.3 g/dL. An urgent EGD is performed and three ulcerated mass-like lesions were found in the gastric body and antrum, ranging from 1 cm to 3 cm. Biopsy showed malignant histologic features that are not consistent with gastric adenocarcinoma. What is the most common primary site of metastatic disease to the stomach?

A. Ovary
B. Lung
C. Colon
D. Liver
E. Breast

94. A 60-year-old man with known gastric adenocarcinoma presents to his gastroenterologist's office for postoperative follow-up. He was diagnosed 2 months ago after a traumatic CT protocol done for a fall incidentally found a gastric mass with multiple intraabdominal lymphadenopathy. An EGD confirmed a 4 cm mass at the lesser curvature of the gastric body, 5 cm below the gastroesophageal junction. Biopsy revealed gastric adenocarcinoma. He underwent a total gastrectomy with extended lymphadenectomy 3 weeks ago. Final pathology results revealed a large, poorly differentiated intestinal-type adenocarcinoma invading to the serosal layer of the stomach wall. The margins of the resected specimen were negative. Ten out of 18 lymph nodes were positive for cancer. Intraoperative peritoneal washing was positive for malignant cells. Whole body PET scan obtained last week showed no flurodeoxyglucose (FDG) uptake. Which of the following is the most appropriate next step in management?

A. Surveillance endoscopy and repeat whole body CT in 3 months
B. Repeat diagnostic laparoscopy for restaging
C. Empiric whole abdominal radiation
D. Intraperitoneal chemotherapy
E. Consult palliative care

95. A 40-year-old woman presents with chronic progressive epigastric pain and unintentional weight loss. Her brother and maternal aunt passed away from gastric cancer. An EGD revealed a 4 cm necrotic ulcer with a heaped-up edge in the gastric body. Biopsy confirmed adenocarcinoma. She subsequently underwent a total gastrectomy. Pathology revealed diffuse type gastric adenocarcinoma with ERBB2 (formerly HER2) overexpression and 12/15 positive lymph node involvement. CT abdomen showed more than ten small rim-enhanced hepatic lesions. Which of the following is the most appropriate next step in management?

A. Check bilateral mammogram
B. EOX regimen (Epirubicin, Oxaliplatin, and Capecitabine)
C. Cisplatin and 5-FU
D. Irinotecan and trastuzumab
E. Consult palliative care for pain control

96. A 40-year-old man visits his primary care physician's clinic for an annual physical exam. He has no significant medical history and is not taking any medication. He does not drink alcohol or smoke. His brother was just diagnosed with gastric cancer 1 month ago. He also had a paternal uncle who passed away from gastric cancer when he was 60 years old. He asks if there is any medication that can prevent him from getting gastric cancer. Which of the following agents has the most promising potential to be a chemoprotective agent to development of gastric cancer?

A. Rabeprazole
B. Aspirin
C. Atorvastatin
D. Carotenoids
E. Green tea extract

97. Which of the following is the most common site of metastasis of primary gastric adenocarcinoma?

A. Left supraclavicular lymph node
B. Periumbilical lymph node
C. Liver
D. Ovary
E. Lung

ANSWERS

1. A (S&F ch48)
This patient has an active bleeding vessel in the setting of a gastric ulcer. He also has chronic kidney disease (CKD) stage III, and it is important to minimize contrast to find the culprit vessel. Given the location of the ulcer in the fundus of the stomach, the most likely vascular supply would be via the short gastric arteries that arise from the splenic artery. The right and left gastric arteries are supplied from common hepatic and celiac arteries respectively; they supply the lesser curvature of the stomach. The right and left gastroepiploic arteries are supplied by gastroduodenal and splenic arteries, but they supply the greater curvature.

2. C (S&F ch48)
The correct answer is gastrin secreting cells or G cells. Answer A is referring to chief cells, which are found in the oxyntic glands of the fundus and body of the stomach. These cells are responsible for synthesis and secretion of pepsinogens I and II. B and D are referring to parietal cells also found in the oxyntic glands of the fundus and stomach and are responsible for production of hydrochloric acid and secretion of intrinsic factor, which is vital in uptake of vitamin B_{12}.

3. A (S&F ch48)
The gastroduodenal artery, bile duct, and portal vein lie posterior to the first portion of the duodenum. The superior mesenteric artery (SMA) courses anterior (not posterior) to the third portion. This anatomic location is clinically significant, as the SMA can lead to compression of the third portion of the duodenum when there is loss of the mesenteric fat pad. This is generally referred to as "superior mesenteric artery syndrome." The stomach is completely invested by peritoneum, except for a small bare area at the esophagogastric junction. The first few centimeters of the duodenum are covered by anterior and posterior elements of the peritoneum, but the remainder of the duodenum lies posterior to the peritoneum (retroperitoneal). The fourth portion of the duodenum is separated from the jejunum by the ligament of Treitz. The minor papilla is located in the second portion of the duodenum.

4. E (S&F ch48)
The distal duodenum is supplied by branches of the superior mesenteric artery. The arterial supply to the duodenum is rich and based on its embryonic origin. Branches of the celiac trunk supply the proximal duodenum. While the antrum of the stomach is derived from the distal foregut, its arterial blood supply is also derived from branches of the celiac artery. Imaging therefore may show focal or segmental bowel wall thickening, intestinal pneumatosis, bowel dilation, or solid organ infarction.

5. B (S&F ch48)
This child most likely has Trisomy 21 (Down syndrome). Duodenal atresia is a congenital defect characterized by complete obstruction of the duodenum. Trisomy 21 is strongly associated with duodenal atresia. Atresias occur most commonly by a complete membrane obstructing the lumen. Most lesions are near the ampulla of Vater. Etiology may be secondary to failure to recanalize the duodenal lumen. Radiographs may show the classic "double-bubble" sign representing air in the stomach and first portion of the duodenum. Duodenal duplication cysts are located posterior to the first and second portion of the duodenum, but they do not generally communicate with the duodenal lumen and are not known to be associated with Trisomy 21. Hypertrophic pyloric stenosis and gastric atresia should not give bilious vomiting.

6. E (S&F ch48)
The lesion described is most consistent with a gastric diverticulum incidentally found on imaging. While imaging cannot distinguish between acquired and congenital, most congenital diverticula are located on the posterior wall of the cardia of the stomach. These contain all layers of the gastric tissue. If patients are asymptomatic, no treatment is necessary.

7. B (S&F ch48)
Gastric teratomas are benign neoplasms of the stomach. They contain all three layers of embryonic germ cells and are generally not associated with other tumors. If the teratoma does not have intramural extension, then excision is adequate and no further workup is needed. Answer A is referring to infantile hypertrophic pyloric stenosis. This is not associated with calcifications and generally presents as forceful, rarely bilious vomiting at 3 to 4 weeks of age. Gastrointestinal stromal tumors (GISTS) are usually intraluminal, rare in infancy, and generally require endoscopic ultrasound.

8. E (S&F ch48)
Duodenal duplication cysts are rare and most commonly located posterior to the first or second portion of the duodenum. They generally do not communicate with the duodenal lumen but do share its blood supply. Histologic criteria for a duodenal duplication cyst include GI mucosa, a smooth muscle layer in the wall, and an association with the duodenal wall. Most often the mucosa is duodenal, though gastric mucosa is described in 15% of cases. Pancreatitis and small bowel obstructions have been described in association with duodenal duplication cysts. Treatment in adults should include consideration for surgical excision given the potential for invasive carcinoma.

9. A (S&F ch48)
This clinical scenario is most consistent with microgastria. It is an extremely rare congenital anomaly of the caudal part

of the foregut. Treatment is typically frequent small-volume feedings. Surgical creation of a double-lumen Roux-en-Y pouch has been described. Gastric duplication generally presents as an abdominal mass and failure to gain weight. Contrast radiography may demonstrate the duplication via a mass effect on the stomach. Gastric atresia shows complete obstruction of the stomach on imaging. Gastric diverticula are typically asymptomatic and found incidentally.

10. **E** (S&F ch49)
Myenteric interstitial cells of Cajal (ICCs) are located between circular and longitudinal muscle layers and are responsible for the generation of the slow waves. ICCs are located in submuscular, intramuscular, myenteric, and subserosal layers of the gastric wall. The most active area of depolarization and repolarization of the ICCs is located in the pacemaker region between fundus and proximal corpus. The fundus itself lacks slow waves. Depletion of ICCs from the corpus-antrum is associated with gastroparesis.

11. **B** (S&F ch49)
The pacemaker region is located on the greater curvature of the stomach, between the fundus and the proximal corpus. This gives rise to 3 cycles per minute of slow waves. The pylorus serves as an electrical barrier and higher plateau potentials correlate with stronger gastric contractions. The fundic smooth muscle resting membrane potential lies at or above the threshold for contraction to promote sustained smooth muscle contraction and ongoing fundic tone.

12. **C** (S&F ch49)
There are three phases to the MMC complex. Phase one is a period of quiescence wherein little or no contractile activity is recorded. Phase two consists of random, irregular contractions. Phase three, however, consists of regular high-amplitude contractions that last from 5 to 10 minutes. They occur every 1.5 to 2 hours with about 6 to 8 cycles in a 12-hour period. Phase three originates either from the stomach or the duodenum and migrates slowly throughout the small intestines down to the ileum. Patients will still develop MMCs after vagotomy, indicating that nonvagal mechanisms initiate and sustain MMC activity.

13. **B** (S&F ch49)
Acetylcholine and substance P are excitatory neurotransmitters that stimulate smooth muscle contractions. Solid food that is delivered from the esophagus into the fundus is associated with receptive relaxation of the fundus. Relaxation of the fundus is a vagal nerve–mediated event that requires nitric oxide and vasoactive intestinal peptide (VIP). Antral distention, duodenal distention, duodenal acidification, intraluminal perfusion of the duodenum with lipid or protein, and colonic distension all decrease fundic tone.

14. **C** (S&F ch49)
Delay in gastric emptying can be affected largely by the type of food we eat. Foods high in acidity and tryptophan are associated with a delay in emptying. The more volume and osmolarity is ingested, the longer the delay in gastric emptying. Carbohydrates and protein tend to accelerate the rate of gastric emptying when compared to foods that are higher in fat content. The patient's thanksgiving meal, which was likely high in tryptophan from the turkey, as well as foods high in fat content most likely contributed to his delay in gastric emptying thus producing his symptoms.

15. **D** (S&F ch49)
Corticotropin-releasing factor works to decrease gastric emptying thus an increase in this factor should decrease gastric emptying. Hyperglycemia has been shown to increase fundic compliance and decrease sensations related to fundic distension. Typically, blood glucose levels greater than 220 mg/dL result in decreased antral contractions, decreased gastric emptying, and induced gastric dysrhythmias. Ileum exposure to carbohydrates and fatty acids is the so-called "ileal break" and delays gastric emptying. Usually colorectal distention with constipation slows gastric emptying.

16. **A** (S&F ch49)
Volume of food ingested suppresses hunger and stimulates the sense of fullness more than calorie content of the meal. Typically, the average volume of water ingested to achieve fullness is 600 mL. Also it has been showing that nutrients taken by mouth suppress hunger greater than infusion of nutrients into the stomach or duodenum. Postprandial fullness is not completely understood physiologically but is believed to be due, in large part, to stretch on the stomach walls and secretion of gastric juices.

17. **C** (S&F ch49)
Ghrelin is decreased during the fed state and increased during fasting and stimulates food intake. It is also called the hunger hormone. Cholecystokinin (CCK) is released from duodenal mucosa and receptors to CCK participate in fullness and nausea sensations. Leptin is synthesized in the stomach and works via the central nervous system regulation to reduce food intake. GLP-1 enhances fullness after a meal. Apolipoprotein A-IV is released during absorption of triglycerides. It decreases food intake and gastric motility partly via CCK and vagal pathways.

18. **E** (S&F ch49)
The underlying pathophysiology of gastroparesis is largely thought to be representative of pathologic loss of interstitial cells of Cajal as is described in answer E. This scenario likely represents ischemic gastroparesis. An abnormal scintigraphic study showing retention of greater than 60% of food at 2 hours and greater than 9% retention of food at 4 hours would be consistent with gastroparesis. Four-hour testing has been shown superior to 2-hour testing. Both answers B and D are normal scintigraphic tests. In healthy subjects, wireless motility capsule takes approximately 5 hours to empty into the duodenum and thus answer A represents a normal finding. Answer C is a normal sensation in healthy subjects.

19. **B** (S&F ch49)
Early satiety is more severe in patients with type 2 diabetic gastroparesis. Typically, type 1 diabetic gastroparesis tends to be more severe, have a higher incidence, and have more hospitalizations compared to type 2 diabetics. Hyperglycemia is typically present for a longer duration prior to the diagnosis in type 2 diabetics as compared to type 1 diabetics.

20. **B** (S&F ch49)
This patient most likely has postsurgical gastroparesis resulting from his vagotomy. After vagotomy, the fundus fails to relax normally after meals, resulting in rapid filling of the antrum. Vagotomy is also associated with gastric dysrhythmias, decreased antral contractions, and poor antropyloroduodenal coordination. While diabetic gastroparesis is possible, this seems less likely given his recent diagnosis and routine follow-up. A small fundic gland polyp does not

cause any symptoms. Ischemic gastroparesis also appears less likely given his nonobstructive coronary artery disease. Pylorospasms typically give right upper quadrant pain and would be less likely in this clinical scenario.

21. **C** (S&F ch49)
The history and symptoms are consistent with idiopathic gastroparesis. Occasionally, patients may describe flu-like illness prior with fever, nausea, and vomiting. Postviral gastroparesis resolves completely over 1 to 2 years in the majority of patients. Similar to the presented case, Norwalk virus can be implicated as a potential cause. Smooth muscle dysfunction can be seen, but typically only seen in diabetic gastroparesis.

22. **D** (S&F ch49)
The patient is likely describing pain originating from the anterior abdominal rectus muscles. On physical exam he is positive for Carnett sign. There is no association with eating and symptoms and physical exam appear more consistent with abdominal wall syndrome. Nothing in the patient's history is consistent with worsening GERD, and functional dyspepsia is a diagnosis of exclusion after other potential diseases are ruled out.

23. **B** (S&F ch49)
This patient is manifesting symptoms of tardive dyskinesia, and metoclopramide should be discontinued. Intramuscular diphenhydramine is the treatment for acute dystonia and not for tardive dyskinesia. Domperidone is a dopamine antagonist that decreases nausea, corrects gastric dysrhythmias, and increases gastric emptying rates. It could be obtained through a new drug application process with the FDA. Adding erythromycin is unlikely to be helpful in this patient who has predominant symptoms of nausea and vomiting. Also, erythromycin is not a good long-term agent given its potential for tachyphylaxis. Cisapride and tegaserod were withdrawn from the market. They are 5HT4 antagonists and were not approved for gastroparesis. A gastric electrical stimulator should not be the next step until all medical options are exhausted.

24. **D** (S&F ch49)
The most likely diagnosis in this patient is Dumping syndrome. This occurs in the setting of patients who have had vagotomy and pyloroplasty or Billroth I or II gastrojejunostomy. Etiology of the sweats and lightheadedness that develop afterwards are most likely due to rapid carbohydrate absorption and mismatch of hyperglycemia with insulin, causing hypoglycemia. Distension of the small bowel will correspond to the initial abdominal bloating and nausea, which can sometimes be mistaken for gastroparesis. Osmotic diarrhea can develop but usually does not cause sweats or lightheadedness.

25. **E** (S&F ch50)
Chromogranin A (CgA), which is a glycoprotein within neuroendocrine cells, can be used as a marker for the diagnosis of neuroendocrine tumors (e.g., carcinoid and gastrinoma). Serum CgA is normally derived from gastric enterochromaffin-like (ECL) cells. Therefore, elevated circulating CgA concentrations can be seen in patients with ECL hyperplasia caused by hypergastrinemia as a result of atrophic gastritis or treatment with proton pump inhibitors (PPIs). Thus, CgA level can be falsely elevated in patients who are taking PPIs. The correct answer is to stop the PPI and repeat the level again. After discontinuation of PPI therapy, serum CgA gradually declines with a half-life of 4 to 5 days. Almost all gastrinomas contain somatostatin receptors, therefore somatostatin receptor scintigraphy (SRS) using ^{111}In-DPTA-D-phe1-octreotide is the diagnostic test of choice to localize the tumor. Further imaging study such as MRI or EUS is not necessary at this time. Pancreatic polypeptide is a less specific biomarker than CgA for neuroendocrine tumor and has no role in this case.

26. **A** (S&F ch50)
Patients chronically infected with *H. pylori* mainly develop pangastritis with reduced acid secretion. This is because of functional inhibition of parietal cells by either products of *H. pylori* itself or products of the inflammatory process. Small amount of patients (10% to 15%) manifests increased acid secretion, as in this patient. They tend to have antral-predominant inflammation and are predisposed to duodenal ulcer. Pathophysiology is believed to be a result of reduced antral somatostatin (SST) content with elevated basal and stimulated gastrin secretion (see figure). Acute infection also results in decreased acid secretion and pangastritis via multiple pathways, as described in choice B, C, and D. These mechanisms include direct inhibition of the parietal cell and enterochromaffin-like cell by a constituent of the bacterium (e.g., vacuolating cytotoxin, lipopolysaccharide, acid-inhibitory factor) and indirect inhibition through changes in cytokines such as IL-1β and TNF-α. *H. pylori* itself interferes with the transcription, translation, and insertion of human H^+/K^+ ATPase. Rebound acid hypersecretion after discontinuing long-term PPI therapy, which is a result of hypergastrinemia-induced increases in parietal and enterochromaffin-like cell masses, does not occur in *H. pylori*-infected individuals because *H. pylori* and cytokines produced by the inflammatory infiltrate can inhibit acid secretion and mask the rebound.

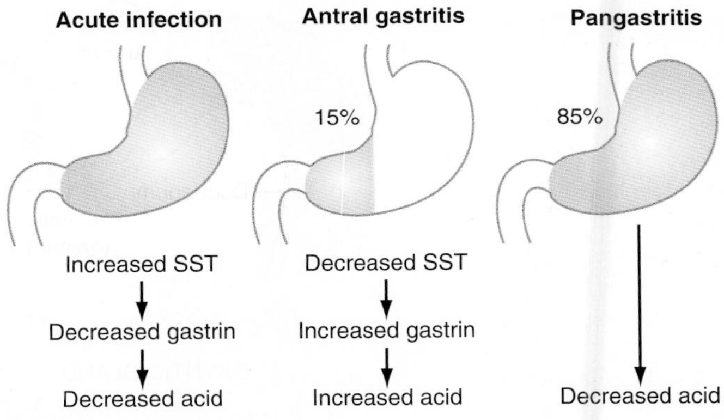

Figure for answer 26.

27. **C** (S&F ch50)
Somatostatin inhibits acid secretion by directly acting on parietal cells and by inhibiting gastrin release from antral G cells. The other hormones mentioned in the answer choices do not affect gastrin secretion.

28. **D** (S&F ch50)
It is recommended that PPIs be taken 30 minutes to 1 hour before the first meal since most pumps are inserted during breakfast. If greater inhibition is needed, an additional dose should be taken before dinner. PPIs are weak bases that concentrate in acidic environment within the body especially where pH is less than 4. They are membrane permeable when it is unprotonated. In blood, PPIs are predominantly unprotonated and thus pass readily into cells.

They later become protonated and trapped intracytoplasmically. Since only the apical-membrane inserted H+,K+ ATPase is blocked by PPIs, and an acid environment is necessary for trapping and converting the PPI to its active form, the potency of PPIs is decreased when administered during the fasting state (between meals), when acid secretion is inhibited. Acid suppression by a PPI causes hypergastrinemia. Gastrin promotes growth factors in normal and neoplastic tissues, therefore hypergastrinemia results in parietal and ECL cell hyperplasia. Stopping PPI will reverse ECL-cell hyperplasia after 2 to 3 months.

29. A (S&F ch50)
The stomach consists of three anatomic (fundus, corpus or body, and antrum) and two functional (oxyntic and pyloric gland) areas (see *top portion* of figure). The gastric body and fundus constitute the oxyntic gland area, which carries oxyntic or parietal cells. The pyloric gland area is found in the antrum, which contains G cells. Oxyntic gland also contains D cells (somatostatin and amylin), enterochromaffn-like cells (histamine and parathyroid hormone–like hormone), enterochromaffn cells (atrial natriuretic peptide [ANP], serotonin, and adrenomedullin), and A-like or Gr cells (ghrelin and obestatin), while the pyloric gland contains G cells (gastrin) and D cells (somatostatin and amylin) (see *bottom portion* of figure).

30. D (S&F ch50)
Acid secretion by the parietal cell is controlled by neurohormonal mechanisms (see figure). Somatostatin is synthesized by the D cells in the antrum. It inhibits acid secretion through its action on the receptors of the parietal cells, G cells, and enterochromaffin cells. Stimulation of the vagus nerve through the cephalic, gastric, and intestinal phase results in the release of acetylcholine, which acts on the muscarinic cholinergic receptors of the parietal cells to increase acid secretion. Gastrin is synthesized by the G cells and stimulates the enterochromaffin cells to release histamine and cause increased acid secretion. Histamine increases acid secretion by stimulating H2 receptors on the parietal cells.

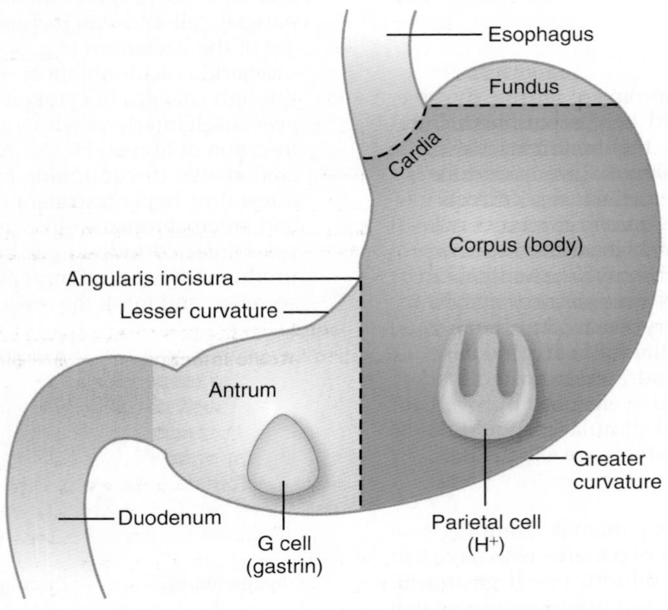

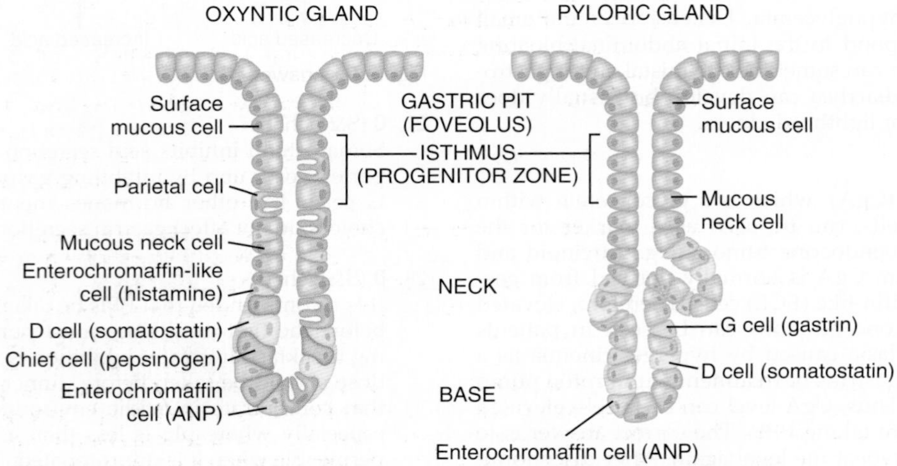

Figure for answer 29.

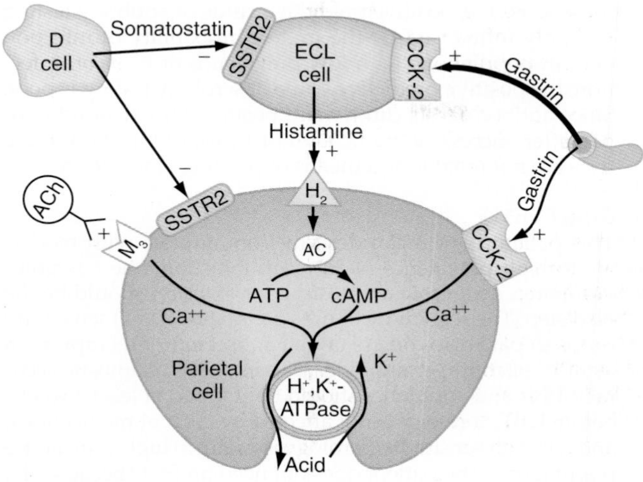

Figure for answer 30.

31. **C** (S&F ch51)
The method for detecting *H. pylori* depends on the clinical situation, population prevalence and pretest probability of infection, test availability, and cost. *H. pylori* serology testing is not useful in distinguishing a current active infection from past infections, and it has lower sensitivity and specificity compared to stool antigen. Given that she had an inadequate response to proton pump inhibitor therapy, the next step would be to test and treat for *H. pylori*. EGD should not be performed only to obtain biopsies for the diagnosis of *H. pylori* infection. In this patient, symptoms did not improve with pantoprazole, and the addition of a H2 blocker has no role in the management of this patient (see figure).

32. **E** (S&F ch51)
In this patient CD markers and histopathology characteristics are consistent with mucosa-associated lymphoid tissue (MALT) lymphoma. MALT lymphoma is the only malignancy that can be cured with antibiotics and is closely associated with *H. pylori* infection (95% of the time). All the other choices include treatments that are not indicated as a first-line therapy for MALT lymphoma.

33. **C** (S&F ch51)
Initial treatment with *H. pylori* triple therapy can fail in up to 25% of patients, which is partially attributed to clarithromycin resistance. Treatment of a first relapse involves switching to alternate first-line therapy, preferably containing metronidazole. The patient should not be treated with the previously used combination. Therapy with levofloxacin (B) or rifabutin (D) are considered as salvage therapy and are given if both triple and quadruple therapies fail, in patients who have failed therapy at least two times. Culture-based selection therapy should be considered for patients who do not respond to multiple treatment courses, but is not routinely performed after failure of first line regimens.

34. **C** (S&F ch51)
H. pylori-associated gastric ulcer requires confirmatory endoscopy after a course of eradicative treatment to document ulcer healing. Since this is a large gastric ulcer that was not biopsied on previous exam, it is important to confirm healing by endoscopy and in addition biopsies can be obtained for *H. pylori* testing to confirm eradication. Although noninvasive testing can help confirm *H. pylori*

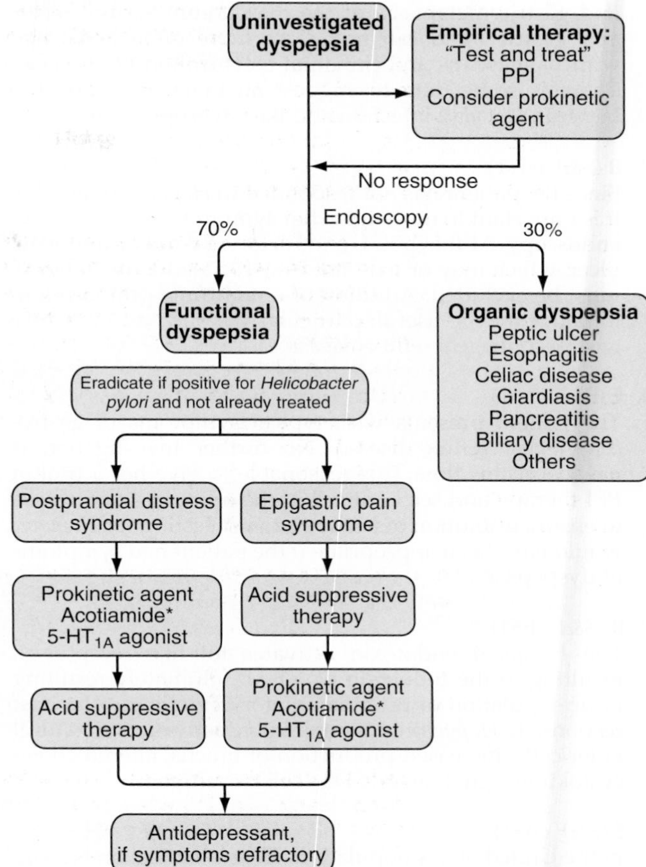

Figure for answer 31.

eradication, it is important to document the gastric ulcer healing.

35. **B** (S&F ch51)
Treatment of second recurrence is called rescue therapy and usually involves concomitant therapy with a penicillin and metronidazole as seen in choice B. Longer duration of the same regimen has not been proven useful for rescue therapy of *H. pylori*. Other rescue regimens include rifabutin + PPI + amoxicillin twice daily for 14 days. Although smoking can increase the chance of treatment failure, it is not recommended to use the same regimen again that has failed previously. PPI + bismuth + metronidazole + tetracycline is one of the first line therapy that is inexpensive but is a complex regimen for the patient to take.

36. **C** (S&F ch51)
One of the main factors for colonization of *H. pylori* is its ability to be motile. *H. pylori* will not colonize mucosa with intestinal metaplasia. The other factors important for colonization of *H. pylori* are the presence of gastric mucosa, expression of Lewis (Le) antigen by host cells that serve as a receptor for *H. pylori* binding, the presence of toll-like receptors (TLRs) on gastric epithelial cells and the secretion of urease that helps *H. pylori* adapt to the gastric acidic milieu.

37. **C** (S&F ch51)
The location of *H. pylori* in the stomach can determine its disease manifestations. Antral *H. pylori* infection leads to hyperacidity and dramatically increases the risk of duodenal ulceration due to increased antral proton production

and gastric metaplasia of the duodenum. Gastric ulcers and gastric adenocarcinoma are more often associated with pangastritis and proximal colonization of *H. pylori.* There is some data to suggest an inverse relationship between *H. pylori* infection and Barrett esophagus.

38. B (S&F ch51)
Since the patient has not responded to *H. pylori* treatment, it is important to investigate her symptoms with an upper endoscopy. At this point, a refractory gastric or duodenal ulcer, which may or may not be associated with *H. pylori,* must be excluded. Addition of a nighttime proton pump inhibitor maybe useful; particularly if she had refractory gastroesophageal reflux disease.

39. E (S&F ch51)
The patient presents with typical symptoms of gastroesophageal reflux disease. No further investigation is needed at this time; it is reasonable to give her a trial of PPI therapy and see her back in the office in 4 to 6 weeks to ensure resolution of her symptoms. Testing for *H. pylori* would have been appropriate if the patient had symptoms of dyspepsia.

40. B (S&F ch51)
The *H. pylori* endotoxin activates toll-like receptor 4, resulting in the induction of NF-κB, ultimately resulting in up-regulation of proinflammatory cytokines. The host response to *H. pylori* does not involve activation of natural killer cells, increased production of mucus, altered cholecystokinin signaling, or CD8+ cell recruitment.

41. E (S&F ch51)
In the United States population, *H. pylori* infection is more common in Hispanics (58%) than African Americans (51%) and Caucasions (27%). Most carriers are asymptomatic and approximately 50% of the world population is seropositive. Infection in the developing countries is usually acquired at an early age. Spontaneous clearance of infection is not common and *H. pylori* infection usually persists until it is treated with antibiotics.

42. C (S&F ch51)
Intestinal metaplasia is associated with the pathogenesis of gastric oncogenesis with *H. pylori* infection. In addition, increased angiogenesis, gastric hypotrophy, and *H. pylori* gastritis can all participate in the pathogenesis of gastric cancer. KRAS tumor suppressor mutation is not involved in *H. pylori* oncogenesis.

43. C (S&F ch51 and ch53)
The most common predisposing factors for peptic ulcer disease are NSAID use and *H. pylori* infection. Smoking and alcohol are not associated with PUD, but may delay healing of ulcers. *H. pylori* infection alone increases the risk of PUD by 1.79-fold, NSAID use alone increases the risk by 4.85-fold and *H. pylori* infection in long term NSAID users increased the risk by sixfold. Although associated with PUD, smoking, excessive alcohol intake, and Type A personality have not be proven to be strong risk factors. *H. pylori* infection does increase the risk of PUD in patients taking low dose aspirin.

44. B (S&F ch51)
Urea breath testing (UBT) and fecal antigen testing are highly accurate means of primary *H. pylori* testing. However, recent use of PPIs, bismuth, or antibiotics can reduce the sensitivity of the UBT and fecal antigen test. For this reason, PPIs should be withheld for at least 4 weeks prior to performing these tests. The positive predictive value of antibody testing is highly influenced by the pretest probability of infection and, in populations with low prevalence of *H. pylori* infection, the positive predictive value of serology testing is poor. Since antibody tests can remain positive for extended periods after successful eradication of *H. pylori* infection, these tests are not reliable as a means of proving eradication.

45. C (S&F ch51)
This patient is of Asian descent from an area with moderate to high prevalence of *H. pylori* infection. She has uninvestigated dyspepsia and testing for *H. pylori* should be the next step. The sensitivity of urea breath test (UBT) sensitivity drops in patients who are taking antisecretory therapy such as PPIs, bismuth, or antibiotics. To improve diagnostic accuracy, PPIs and antibiotics should be stopped at least 4 weeks before UBT. Serology is not affected by current medications, and has high sensitivity. Serology is useful in high-prevalence populations. The patient does not need an EGD because she is greater than 55 years old without alarm symptoms.

46. D (S&F ch52)
CMV gastric disease occurs in severely immunosuppressed patients and presents with multiple deep linear ulcerations. This presentation is not consistent with adenocarcinoma or *Candida* infection. The patient just underwent bone marrow transplantation and therefore leukemic recurrence is unlikely. Crohn's disease only rarely involves the gastric mucosa and is unlikely in this patient on multiple immunosuppressants.

47. C (S&F ch52)
CMV gastritis is characterized by a neutrophil-predominant infiltration with nuclear inclusions ("owl-eye appearance") (see figure). Signet ring cells are seen in gastric adenocarcinoma. Lymphocytic infiltration is seen in *H. pylori* infection.

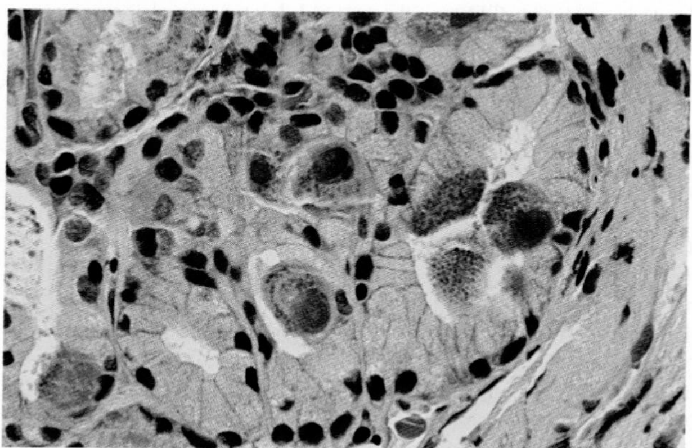

Figure for answer 47.

48. C (S&F ch52)
Several factors predispose this patient to stress gastritis. These include sepsis, shock, mechanical ventilation, and possible coagulopathy. Although *H. pylori* infection may be a cause for chronic gastritis, it is unlikely the cause of acute gastritis. Nasogastric tube trauma tends to be patchy and linear but would not affect the whole body and antrum. All the other choices do not fit with the current presentation of the patient, however, these are all known causes of gastritis.

49. C (S&F ch52)
Antiparietal cell antibodies are found in 90% of patients with pernicious anemia. Vitamin B_{12} level is neither sensitive nor specific, as numerous conditions may result in

altered B_{12} absorption (e.g., inflammatory bowel disease, celiac sprue), and patients with pernicious anemia may have normal levels due to anti-IF antibody interference with the assay. Megaloblasic anemia is a late finding of severe B_{12} or folate deficiency, occurring after the development of simple macrocytosis.

50. **B** (S&F ch52)
Atrophic carditis is considered a precursor lesion of adenocarcinoma at the gastroesophageal junction. Proximal *H. pylori* infection is also associated with gastric adenocarcinoma. Atrophic carditis does not predispose to junctional squamous cell carcinoma, duodenal ulcer, GIST, or achalasia.

51. **D** (S&F ch52)
First-line therapy for acute bile reflux gastritis includes the combination of PPI and antacid therapy. Bile acid sequestrants and sucralfate can be used in addition to the above if symptoms are not improving, but have not been shown to produce consistent benefit. In severe cases failing medical therapy, surgery may be indicated. An appetite stimulant is not indicated in this patient.

52. **E** (S&F ch52)
This patient is hemodynamically stable and has not had a significant drop in his hemoglobin. A self-limited hemorrhagic gastritis occurs in 25% of patients with DKA. It does not require specific endoscopic intervention. Therefore, it is appropriate to give intravenous PPI and watch this patient, and to perform endoscopy urgently only if there is evidence of active ongoing bleeding.

53. **C** (S&F ch52)
In diffuse corporal atrophic gastritis, patients exhibit achlorhydria or hypochlorhydria, and secondary hypergastrinemia due to low or absent gastric acid. The destruction of parietal cells, which secretes hydrochloric acid (HCl), leads to decreased acid secretion. G cells secrete Gastrin, which stimulate parietal cells to secrete HCl. If acid levels decrease in the stomach, the G cells secrete more gastrin to normalize its acid levels.

54. **A** (S&F ch52)
The most common cause for peptic ulcer disease is *H. pylori* infection and NSAID use. This patient was recently treated for *H. pylori* and continues to use NSAIDS. NSAIDs have COX-2 inhibitory effect that results in *decreased* mucosal prostaglandin synthesis, which leads to ulcer formation. NSAIDS do not cause hypergastrinemia or infiltration of mast cells and/or neutrophils.

55. **D** (S&F ch52)
This patient has symptoms, endoscopic features, and histopathology consistent with eosinophilic gastritis. The characteristic features as seen in the figure are abnormal eosinophilic infiltrate (>20 eosinophils/high power field), necrosis with neutrophil infiltration, and epithelial regeneration. The histologic features are not consistent with the other choices presented.

56. **C** (S&F ch52)
The presented histopathologic findings are consistent with Ménétrier disease. Ménétrier disease has been associated with infections such as *H. pylori* and human immunodeficiency virus and with cytomegalovirus gastritis. Ménétrier disease can be associated with protein-losing enteropathy. The histological features presented are not consistent with gastric adenocarcinoma, nor with acute, chronic, or eosinophilic gastritis.

57. **E** (S&F ch52)
The patient clinically presents with signs of pernicious anemia, which is consistent with autoimmune atrophic gastritis. Diagnosis is made endoscopically with five biopsies from the gastric body, incisura, and antrum (see figure).

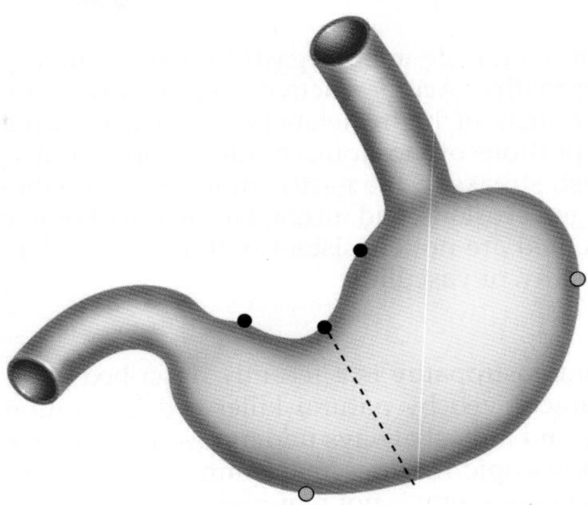

Figure for answer 57.

58. **D** (S&F ch52)
Candida colonization of ulcer surfaces is a nearly universal finding in critically ill immunosuppressed patients who have been exposed to antibacterial therapy. True *Candida* gastritis is rare, and would present with multiple widespread aphthous erosions and linear ulcers. In this patient, the most likely cause of ulceration is stress ulcers with the predisposing factors being shock, sepsis, hypotension, critical illness, and mechanical ventilation.

59. **B** (S&F ch52)
Hereditary angioneurotic edema is characterized by hyper acute episodes of bowel edema, which can mimic anaphylactoid states. This is most consistent with the patient's current acute presentation. Eosinophilic gastritis presents with enlarged folds and mucosal ulceration, and tends to present with a more indolent/chronic course. The presence of eosinophilia is a nonspecific finding, and may be due to her asthma.

60. **B** (S&F ch52)
The patient has acute viral gastroenteritis; therefore, rehydration and reassurance is best in this scenario. CT imaging may demonstrate diffuse gastric and bowel edema. At this time there is no need for a surgical consultation or starting antibiotics and/or steroids.

61. **D** (S&F ch52)
This patient has gastric-limited Crohn's disease. This is uniquely responsive to PPI therapy alone. In this patient, corticosteroids or immunosuppressive therapy would not be the first line of treatment. Truncal vagotomy is not indicated for gastric-limited Crohn's disease.

62. **C** (S&F ch52)
Chronic gastric ischemia due to atherosclerotic disease results in histologic changes of reactive erosive gastropathy. This patient has other evidence of vascular disease and therefore is predisposed to chronic gastric ischemia. The patient's history and pathological findings are not consistent with atrophic gastritis or portal hypertensive/drug-induced gastropathy.

63. **E** (S&F ch52)
Children with food allergy have no higher incidence of allergic gastritis than those without food allergy. The only

exception is in infants who are allergic to cow's milk, in whom hematemesis and endoscopic signs of gastritis (erythema, erosion, and friability of the gastric mucosa) can occur. Symptoms resolve when cow's milk formula is changed to other formulas.

64. D (S&F ch52)
This patient has an acute erosive gastritis also known as reactive gastropathy. Acute reactive gastropathy often presents with areas of high metabolic activity, favoring the proximal portions of the stomach. Endoscopic finding include reddish streaks in the gastric mucosa, subepithelial hemorrhages, erosions, and ulcers. The histopathologic features presented are not consistent with cancer, collagenous gastropathy, or vasculitis.

65. B (S&F ch52)
Lymphomatoid gastropathy is a recently described clinical entity characterized by natural killer cell infiltration (CD56+ cells), and almost always undergoes spontaneous remission. Endoscopic findings may mimic gastric lymphoma. Repeat endoscopy is not required.

66. C (S&F ch53)
H. pylori infection increases the risk of peptic ulcer disease (PUD) in patients receiving low-dose aspirin. Among patients with *H. pylori*-related ulcer bleeding who continued to take low-dose aspirin, successful eradication of *H. pylori* infection resulted in a very low risk of recurrent ulcer bleeding similar to that seen with aspirin/omeprazole co-therapy. In contrast, aspirin users with bleeding ulcers but without *H. pylori* infection were at high risk of recurrent ulcer bleeding with continued enteric-coated aspirin treatment. In this case, as *H. pylori* eradication was confirmed, there is no need to continue along with aspirin. Misoprosol is a protective agent for NSAID-induced ulcer; however, for reasons stated above, his risk of re-bleeding after resuming low dose aspirin is low and a protective medication is not needed.

67. B (S&F ch50)
The principal risk factors of PUD are *H. pylori* infection and NSAID use (see figure). Other risk factors of peptic ulcer disease include cocaine and methamphetamine use (presumably due to mucosal ischemia), bisphosphonate therapy, selective serotonin reuptake inhibitors (SSRI), smoking, stress, type A personality, and excessive alcohol intake. There is little if any risk for PUD in patients taking only glucocorticoids. In combination with NSAIDs, however, glucocorticoids increase the risk of PUD above the risk with NSAIDs alone.

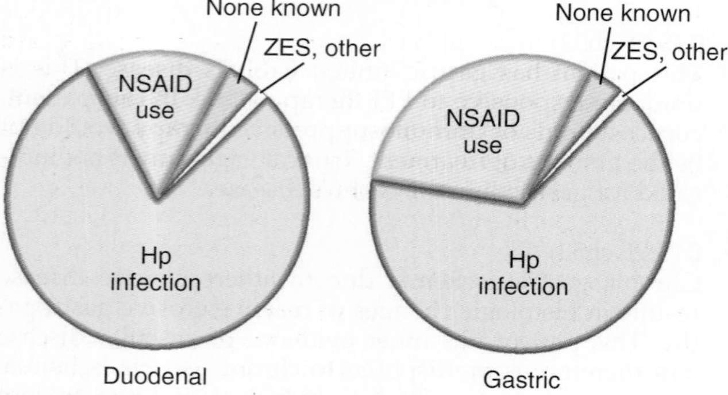

Figure for answer 67.

68. D (S&F ch53)
This patient has classic symptoms of peptic ulcer disease. It is associated with hunger, occurs at night, and is often relieved by food and antacids. Often patients complain of dyspeptic symptoms such as a bloating and fullness, with no alarming features (see box at end of chapter). Based on American Gastroenterological Association guideline, the "test and treat" approach is preferred over prompt EGD (see figure). A trial of a PPI should be started first before endoscopic evaluation. Her constipation and bloating is most likely associated with narcotics use. Her clinical course is sub-acute and is not suggestive of irritable bowel syndrome (<6 months). Her pain preceded the constipation, thus treating constipation alone will not help. She does not have risk factors for colon cancer or pancreatic cancer; colonoscopy or abdominal CT scan is not indicated at this point.

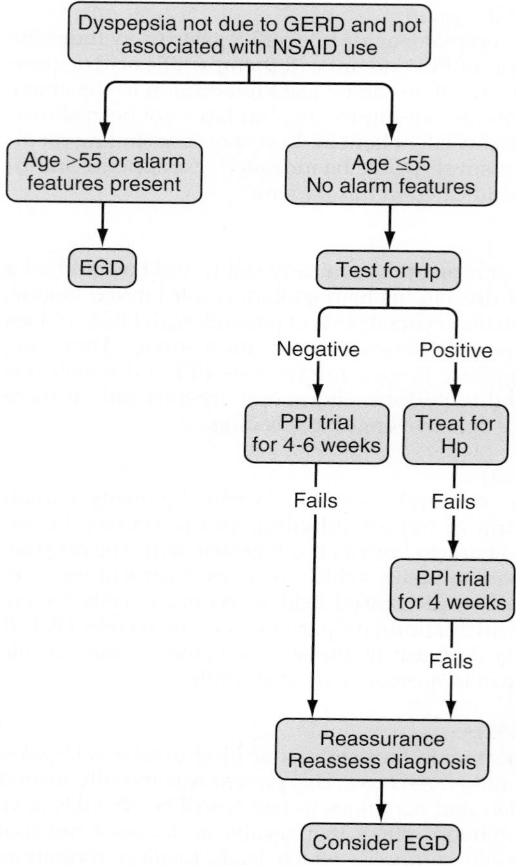

Figure for answers 68 and 69.

69. D (S&F ch53)
This patient has symptoms suggestive of peptic ulcer disease (diet-related epigastric pain that is relieved by antacids). Even though his symptoms are improving with ranitidine, a new onset dyspepsia at his age (>55 years old) is an alarming feature (see box at end of chapter). Based on American Gastroenterological Association guidelines, a prompt EGD is warranted (see figure). A "test and treat" strategy with a trial of antisecretory agents (answers A, B, and E) can be considered in patients younger than 55 years old with no alarming symptoms, but not in this case. If the EGD is non-revealing and pain persists, CT of the abdomen may be considered to evaluate for other causes of abdominal pain, such as a pancreatobiliary lesion; however, it is not the initial test of choice.

70. B (S&F ch53)
Because up to 4% of apparently benign gastric ulcers (GUs) at initial endoscopy are subsequently found to be

malignant, it is recommended that EGD should be repeated 8 weeks later to confirm healing of the gastric ulcer even if the initial biopsies are benign. Since eradication of *H. pylori* is confirmed after she stopped the PPI for 2 weeks (*H. pylori* antigen can be falsely negative if tested while taking a PPI) and all of her symptoms have resolved, if EGD confirmed a healed ulcer, no further management is needed.

71. D (S&F ch53)
Histamine-2 receptor antagonists (H2RAs) are competitive inhibitors of histamine-stimulated acid secretion. They markedly suppress both basal and meal-stimulated acid secretion. H2RAs administered in the evening are effective in suppressing nocturnal acid output. H2RAs are well absorbed after oral dosing, and their absorption is not affected by food. H2RAs cross the blood-brain barrier and the placenta. All H2RAs (cimetidine, ranitidine, and famotidine) undergo first-pass hepatic metabolism, which reduces their bioavailability by 35% to 60%, except for nizatidine which is the only H2RA that does not undergo first-pass metabolism. Its bioavailability approaches 100% with oral dosing. Rabeprazole is a proton pump inhibitor (PPI) that requires acidic environment for activation; therefore, it binds predominantly to those proton pumps that are actively secreting acid. Most of the proton pumps actively secrete acid after being stimulated by diet. Thus, PPIs are most effective if they are administered immediately before meals. Its potency will significantly decrease if administered during fasting state before bed time. It is also metabolized in the liver.

72. A (S&F ch53)
Both cimetidine and ranitidine bind to the hepatic cytochrome P-450 (CYP). This binding can inhibit the elimination of other drugs that are metabolized through the same system, including warfarin, theophylline, phenytoin, lidocaine, and quinidine. In contrast, famotidine and nizatidine have no significant avidity for the CYP system. H2RAs are eliminated by a combination of renal excretion and hepatic metabolism. Dose reductions are recommended when the creatinine clearance is below 50 mL/min, but are not necessary when the patient is on dialysis or has hepatic failure. Despite unclear mechanism, tolerance to the H2RAs can develop quickly and frequently.

73. A (S&F ch53)
Due to the previously reported cardiovascular adverse effects, patients with high cardiovascular risk should avoid using COX-2 inhibitors and most nonselective NSAIDs. If an NSAID is needed in patients at high cardiovascular risk, naproxen is a preferred drug because it will not increase the cardiothrombotic risk. This patient has one risk factor for NSAID ulcer (concomitant use with aspirin) and is considered as having a moderate gastrointestinal risk. He has multiple cardiovascular risk factors requiring low dose aspirin for primary prevention, making him a high cardiovascular risk patient (see table at end of chapter). Since his knee pain requires ongoing NSAID treatment, concomitant use of NSAIDs and low-dose aspirin will markedly increase the risk of ulcer complications over that incurred with NSAIDs alone. Thus, co-therapy with a PPI or misoprostol is necessary even if patients do not have other GI risk factors (see other table at end of chapter). Patients known to have high cardiovascular risk should receive low-dose aspirin irrespective of NSAID use. Since glucocorticoids alone (without NSAID) do not increase the risk of ulcer, it can be considered if short-term antiinflammatory therapy is required for acute, self-limiting arthritis (e.g., gout).

74. C (S&F ch53)
Refractory ulcer is an ulcer lesion that does not heal within 8 weeks of initiation of antisecretory therapy or beyond 12 weeks for a large ulcer (>2 cm). Possible causes for nonhealing ulcer include noncompliance; penetrating ulcer to the pancreas, liver, or other organ; *H. pylori* infection; nonsteroidal antiinflammatory drugs (NSAIDs); cigarette smoking; inadequate duration of treatment; Zollinger-Ellison syndrome; primary or metastatic neoplasms; infections (e.g., cytomegalovirus); cocaine use; eosinophilic gastroenteritis; and Crohn's disease. Her ulcer was small and treatment duration of 8 weeks is considered adequate. Her stool *H. pylori* antigen test was performed while she is taking PPI, which can cause a false negative result.

75. A (S&F ch53)
PPIs are metabolized via the hepatic cytochrome (CYP) P450 system and therefore they have the potential to alter the metabolism of other drugs that are eliminated by CYP enzymes, such as warfarin, phenytoin, theophylline, diazepam, and clopidogrel. Among available PPIs, omeprazole has the highest avidity to CYP450 system and thus the greatest potential for such drug interactions, whereas lansoprazole, pantoprazole, and rabeprazole do not appear to interact significantly with drugs metabolized by the CYP system.

76. C (S&F ch53)
This patient has chronic kidney disease with worsening kidney function to the point that her creatinine clearance is less than 50 mL/min. Many pharmaceutical agents for peptic ulcer disease require dose adjustment or discontinuation in this population. However, proton pump inhibitors (PPIs) and misoprostol do not require dose adjustment and are considered safe in patients with renal insufficiency. All antacids must be used with caution in patients who have chronic kidney disease, due to risk of hypermagnesemia, hypercalcemia, and neurotoxicity (when aluminum-containing antacids is used). As H2RAs are eliminated by a combination of renal excretion and hepatic metabolism, dose reductions are recommended when the creatinine clearance is below 50 mL/min, but dose adjustments are not necessary for dialysis patients. Sucralfate is a complex aluminum salt of sulfated sucrose that can cause aluminum accumulation and possible neurotoxicity, similar to aluminum containing antacid. Short-term, standard-dose therapy with bismuth is acceptable with minor risk of toxicity. However, when administered in high dose or long duration especially in patients with chronic kidney disease, there is the potential for bismuth encephalopathy with neuropsychiatric symptoms. Misoprostol has no effect on hepatic CYP450. Dose reductions of misoprostol are unnecessary in patients with chronic kidney disease.

77. C (S&F ch53)
Size, location, and bleeding stigmata are most important prognostic factors of the ulcer. According to Forrest classification, ulcers with flat pigmentation and clean base do not require endoscopic interventions given low risk of rebleeding (see table at end of chapter). Ulcer size (>2 cm) and location (either high on the lesser curvature of the stomach or in the superior or posterior duodenal bulb) are important prognostic factors associated with poorer outcomes. These are locations where ulcers can erode into major

arteries, such as the left gastric artery and the gastroduodenal artery, respectively. These ulcers occur mostly in older adult patients, often with significant comorbidities, who often present with hemodynamic instability. Among all options, choice C is the only one with no high-risk features.

78. **E** (S&F ch53)
This patient presented with hematemesis and severe dehydration. Hypochloremic, hypokalemic metabolic alkalosis is a common finding in patients with severe vomiting. Peptic ulcer disease (PUD) remains the leading cause of acute upper gastrointestinal (UGI) bleeding, especially in patients who have no history of chronic liver disease with a normal platelet count and INR, as in this case. Patients with acute UGI bleeding should be assessed promptly on presentation. Volume resuscitation should take priority and precede endoscopy. An urgent endoscopy, together with antisecretory agent (e.g., proton pump inhibitor infusion) should promptly follow an adequate fluid resuscitation and initial clinical stabilization. The rationale for antisecretory therapy in bleeding PUD is based on the fact that increased intragastric pH facilitates pepsin activity and platelet aggregation. A gastric pH of 6 or greater is critical for clot stability and hemostasis. However, medical treatment should not take priority over volume resuscitation. Blood transfusion may be required, but over-transfusion should be avoided and goal hemoglobin should be around 7 to 8 g/dL. Her clinical presentation is concerning for gastric outlet obstruction, however, there was no signs of luminal perforation. An abdominal x-ray and nasogastric decompression may be required before the endoscopic intervention but should not precede volume resuscitation in patients with upper gastrointestinal bleeding.

79. **C** (S&F ch53)
This patient has severe peptic ulcer disease (PUD) with gastric outlet obstruction. Gastric outlet obstruction has become a much less frequent complication of PUD due to improved medical therapy. Its clinical manifestations include nausea and postprandial vomiting, abdominal fullness, pain, and early satiety. Patients with obstructing peptic ulcers are often volume depleted. The loss of fluid, hydrogen ions, and chloride ions in the vomitus leads to hypochloremic, hypokalemic metabolic alkalosis. The patient should be volume resuscitated with potassium replacement once urine output is adequate. Nasogastric tube placement for gastric decompression helps relieve vomiting, monitors fluid loss, and allows the stomach to regain its tone. Proton pump inhibitors facilitate ulcer healing, ameliorates inflammatory edema, and assists in resolving obstruction. If conservative management fails, endoscopic dilation should be attempted before surgery. In severely malnourished patients, parenteral nutrition may be required. Searching for the etiology of the ulcer is always essential. Stool *H. pylori* antigen is more specific than serum *H. pylori* antibody, and should be checked and treated if positive. If the ulcer fails to heal, biopsy to rule out malignancy should be performed, however, these tests are of no urgency at this point. Moreover, the etiology of the ulcer in her case is likely from nonsteroidal antiinflammatory drugs.

80. **D** (S&F ch53)
Stress-related gastric and duodenal mucosal injury (stress ulcers) is an illness of the critically ill. A small proportion of patients with stress-related mucosal lesions will have clinically overt GI bleeding. Routine use of stress ulcer prophylaxis in the ICU is not recommended unless the patient has a coagulopathy or is receiving mechanical ventilation. Significant bleeding occurred in 3.7% of the patients who had one or both of these risk factors and in only 0.1% of patients without these risk factors. There is negligible risk for PUD in patients taking glucocorticoids alone. However, glucocorticoids, when taken with NSAIDs, increase the risk of PUD above the risk with NSAIDs alone and require PPI prophylaxis. Even though the patient in option B has coagulopathy, he is not cared for in the ICU, hence the low risk for a stress ulcer. Being NPO or being in the ICU alone without coagulopathy, history of bleeding ulcers, or respiratory failure does not require PPI prophylaxis.

81. **C** (S&F ch54)
There are multiple definite and probable risk factors for gastric adenocarcinoma (see box at end of chapter). Major risk factors include *H. pylori* infection, chronic atrophic gastritis, intestinal metaplasia or dysplasia, cigarette smoking, history of gastric surgery, familial adenomatous polyposis, or Peutz-Jeghers syndrome. Obesity increases the risk of adenocarcinoma of the cardia. Fundic gland polyps do not predispose to gastric adenocarcinoma. Incidence of gastric adenocarcinoma is highest in black, Asian, and Pacific Islander population and is lowest in white population (see table at end of chapter)

82. **E** (S&F ch54)
The only statement that is true is E: the most important cofactor in the induction of *H. pylori*-related adenocarcinoma is host immune response, particularly CD4 T cell lymphocyte response. Development of gastric adenocarcinoma due to *H. pylori* infection is multifactorial and is dependent on many risk factors, including host genetic factors, the strain of bacteria, the duration of infection, and the presence or absence of other environmental risk factors (e.g., poor diet, smoking). A combination of a virulent bacterial strain, a genetically permissive host, and a favorable gastric environment are necessary for cancer to occur. Proposed carcinogenetic pathways include increased oxidative stress and the formation of oxygen free radicals, leading to DNA damage, increased $CD4^+$ T cells and myeloid cells, and elevated proinflammatory cytokine production, which will lead to accelerated cell turnover, reduced apoptosis, and the potential for faulty or incomplete DNA repair. Pangastritis with high intragastric pH is associated with higher risk of gastric cancer. *H. pylori*-induced duodenal ulcer disease is associated with a high gastric acid output as well as a reduced risk for developing gastric cancer. Patients who are genetically predisposed to developing atrophic gastritis in response to *H. pylori* infection (reduced acid output) are therefore predisposed to gastric cancer. *H. pylori* infection is associated with both diffuse-type and intestinal-type adenocarcinomas. In Western countries, *H. pylori*-associated gastric cancer is usually confined to non-cardia tumors. The development of dysplasia and invasive cancer tends to occur when *H. pylori* colonization has either declined or disappeared from the stomach and occurs in the setting of gastric atrophy.

83. **E** (S&F ch54)
TP53 is the most commonly mutated gene in gastric cancer, while mutations in *RAS*, *APC*, and *MYC* are much less frequent. Loss of heterozygosity at the *APC* locus and the deletion of the fragile histidine triad gene *(FHIT)* occur more commonly. Microsatellite instability (MSI) in dinucleotide repeats from defects DNA mismatch repair genes, such as *MLH1* and *MLH2* (mutL homologs 1 and 2) are

known as primary pathogenesis of colorectal cancer and hereditary nonpolyposis colorectoral cancer (HNPCC) syndrome. MSI may also play a role in the development of gastric cancer as suggested by high incidence of gastric cancer in HNPCC patients.

84. D (S&F ch54)
The British and American Societies of Gastrointestinal Endoscopy guidelines recommend that all gastric polyps should be biopsied, and all gastric adenomas, symptomatic polyps, and polyps with dysplasia should be removed. Further management plan for this patient's polyps should be based on the biopsy results and the type of polyps. Therefore, the risk of malignant transformation is unclear at this time. *H. pylori*, if present, should be eradicated in patients with hyperplastic or adenomatous polyps. Gastric polyps consist predominantly of fundic gland polyps (~50%), hyperplastic polyps (~40%), and adenomatous polyps (~10%). This patient has been taking chronic PPI suggesting that the polyps are most likely fundic gland polyps, rather than hyperplastic or adenomatous polyps. The clinical course of fundic gland polyps is generally benign with very low risk of malignant transformation (~1%) and confined to polyps larger than 1 cm. Hyperplastic polyps are generally benign, often multiple, and are typically found in the background of chronic inflammatory conditions (e.g., chronic atrophic gastritis), pernicious anemia, and at sites of gastroenterostomies. *H. pylori* eradication often helps regression of the polyps. Hyperplastic polyps rarely undergo malignant transformation and are usually predisposed by dysplastic areas or intestinal metaplasia first. They typically form a well-differentiated intestinal-type cancer. In contrast to other polyps of the stomach, gastric adenomas have a high rate of malignant transformation (11% within 4 years).

85. D (S&F ch54)
Hyperplastic polyps larger than 1 cm should be removed due to the risk of malignancy. Reassurance or surveillance EGD without polyp removal is not appropriate. As she did not respond initially to PPI, increasing the dose is unlikely to resolve her symptoms. Endoscopic ultrasound is not required to examine the polyp because it does not add useful information for this pedunculated polyp.

86. A (S&F ch54)
Low ratio of pepsinogen (PG)-I to PG-II is suggestive of high risk pre-neoplastic lesions. To date, there is no reliable serum marker with high enough sensitivity and specificity to help make the diagnosis of gastric cancer. Low serum PGI levels, low ratios of PGI to PGII, and hypergastrinemia can also be seen in patients with atrophic gastritis and intestinal metaplasia with mixed results on the gastric cancer detection. In chronic atrophic gastritis, production of PGI is reduced, whereas PGII levels remain relatively constant. Therefore, both low serum PGI levels (<70 mg/L) and a low PGI/II ratio (<3.0) are useful for the identification of patients with pre-neoplastic lesions. A positive PG test in combination with upper GI series may have some utility in identifying early gastric cancer. Serum CEA and carbohydrate antigen (CA) 19-9 have low sensitivity and specificity for early gastric cancer detection. These tumor markers can be used to monitor recurrence of gastric cancer, especially in patients who had elevated levels prior to surgical resection.

87. C (S&F ch54)
Accurate staging in gastric cancer is essential for treatment decisions before considering subtotal gastrectomy or endoscopic submucosal dissection. Currently, endoscopic ultrasound (EUS) is the diagnostic test of choice for the staging of gastric cancer, particularly in assessing tumor depth and nodal involvement. With improvements in imaging quality for CT and MRI, they are considered as alternatives to EUS. PET scanning alone is not recommended as a sole imaging test for gastric cancer staging, largely because most gastric adenocarcinomas have low FDG uptake and there are false positives as well. Approximately 50% of gastric cancer have metastatic disease involving the peritoneum, thus laparoscopy with peritoneal lavage for patients with seemingly resectable disease is recommended by National Comprehensive Cancer Network guidelines, especially for whom neoadjuvant chemotherapy is being considered. However, it is not the initial test of choice in this patient.

88. B (S&F ch54)
Overall, the 5-year survival rate in the United States from gastric cancer is 27%. The TNM classification is used to stratify gastric cancer into four clinical stages to help predict prognosis in patients treated with gastrectomy (see table at end of chapter). "T" indicates the depth of the invasion, not size. Large tumor size (>5 cm) is a independent risk factor associated with worse survival, independent of nodal status or overall tumor stage. Her tumor is only 3.5 cm. The best prognosis is when early gastric cancer is diagnosed. Early gastric cancer is defined as a cancer that does not invade beyond the submucosa, regardless of lymph node involvement. Location of the tumor helps determine the extent of the surgery. In general, total gastrectomy is performed for proximal gastric tumors and for diffuse gastric cancer, while partial gastrectomy is reserved for tumors in the distal stomach. According to AJCC staging system, cancer at cardia (tumors within 5 cm of and crossing the GE junction) is now classified together with esophageal and GE junction tumors. CEA level has low sensitivities. It is frequently used in recurrent disease but not for prognostic purpose.

89. D (S&F ch54)
This patient has a large mass invading through subserosa (T3) with CT revealing lymphadenopathy (at least N2), therefore his staging is at least stage III (see table at end of chapter). This puts him at high risk for peritoneal metastasis despite a normal CT. Approximately half of gastric cancer patients with metastatic disease have cancer involving the peritoneum. Current imaging techniques such as EUS and CT have limited sensitivity in detecting peritoneal seeding. As approximately 50% of gastric cancer has metastatic disease involving the peritoneum. Laparoscopy with peritoneal lavage for patients with seemingly resectable disease is recommended by National Comprehensive Cancer Network guidelines, especially patients for whom neoadjuvant chemotherapy is being considered. Total gastrectomy is performed for proximal gastric tumors and for diffuse gastric cancer, while partial gastrectomy is reserved for tumors in the distal stomach. His tumor is localized in the antrum, therefore partial gastrectomy is preferred. Extended lymph node resection is mainly performed in Japanese centers, not in the Western population. To prevent "understaging," the current recommendation is a minimum D1 lymphadenectomy with removal of at least 15 nodes. This patient's tumor is too large and invasive for endoscopic submucosal dissection (ESD). According

to Japanese expanded criteria, ESD can be considered when: (1) mucosal intestinal-type cancer of any size without ulceration, (2) mucosal intestinal-type cancer less than 3 cm with ulceration, and (3) submucosal intestinal-type cancer less than 3 cm and with submucosal invasion less than 500 μm.

90. A (S&F ch54)
This patient has diffuse-type adenocarcinoma as demonstrated by mucin-containing singly invasive tumor cells that lack any glandular structure (as compared to gland-like formation of tubular structure in the intestinal-type). Surgical treatment for diffuse-type gastric cancer is total gastrectomy. Partial gastrectomy is reserved for tumors in the distal stomach. As the tumor has invaded beyond submucosa, she has an advanced gastric cancer. EMR and ESD are not appropriate in this case.

91. A (S&F ch54)
Histologic subtype of gastric cancer is an important factor when considering endoscopic resectability of the tumor. Intestinal type is considered resectable, while diffuse type is not. The location of the lesion does not affect the appropriateness of endoscopic resection. Other factors to consider are tumor size, presence of ulceration, and venous and lymphatic invasion.

92. B (S&F ch54)
This patient presented with pseudoachalasia due to involvement of the lower esophageal sphincter of the inferior cardia cancer. According to AJCC staging system, cardia cancer (tumors within 5 cm of and crossing the gastroesophageal [GE] junction) is now classified together with esophageal and GE junction tumors. Preoperative chemoradiation was recommended for adenocarcinoma of the esophagogastric junction (AEG) type I (distal esophagus) and II tumors. For AEG type III (cardia) tumors, perioperative chemotherapy is preferred. Total gastrectomy is performed for proximal gastric tumors such as in this case and for diffuse gastric cancer, while partial gastrectomy is reserved for tumors in the distal stomach.

93. E (S&F ch54)
Metastatic disease to the stomach can occur with primary tumors of the breast, melanoma, lung, ovary, liver, colon, and testicular cancers, with breast cancer being the most common. Other rare malignant tumors that can involve the stomach are Kaposi sarcoma, myenteric schwannoma, glomus tumor, small cell carcinoma, and parietal cell carcinoma. Miscellaneous benign tumors of the stomach include lipomas, pancreatic rests, xanthelasma, and fundic gland cysts.

94. D (S&F ch54)
This patient has gastric cancer T4aN3M0 stage IIIc (tumor invading to serosa with more than 7 positive lymph nodes) (see table at end of chapter). The surgery was performed with curative intent. However, peritoneal washing was positive, suggesting peritoneal metastasis. Approximately 50% of gastric cancer patients have metastatic disease involving the peritoneum and may require diagnostic laparoscopy. Because systemic chemotherapy is ineffective for peritoneal dissemination, intraperitoneal (IP) chemotherapy should be considered in patients whose tumors are resected for cure but have a high likelihood of microscopic residual disease, especially in patients with stage III and IV disease, serosal invasion, and lymph node metastases. Hyperthermic IP chemotherapy is mainly used in clinical trials. In addition, adjuvant chemoradiation is the standard of care and is also warranted in this case, although the optimal chemotherapy regimen is not yet clear. Consulting palliative, surveillance CT or endoscopy, repeat laparoscopy, and radiation alone are not appropriate management in this case. Of note, PET scanning alone is not recommended as a sole imaging test for gastric cancer staging, largely because most gastric adenocarcinomas have low FDG uptake and there are false positives as well.

95. D (S&F ch54)
This patient has stage IV gastric adenocarcinoma and palliative chemotherapy is warranted. Adjuvant chemotherapy can improve survival and quality of life, and is currently the standard of care postoperatively or even in unresectable case. She has a ERBB2+ (formerly HER2+) gastric cancer. ERBB2 is a key driver of tumorigenesis in up to 34% of gastric cancers. Trastuzumab, a monoclonal antibody that interferes with the ERBB2 receptor is therefore warranted. Further manipulation of this pathway using the novel anti-ERBB2–directed agents, pertuzumab and T-DM1, together with dual EGFR/ERBB2 blockade with lapatinib can potentially have additional benefit. As a consequence, tumor assessment for ERBB2 overexpression should be performed, and trastuzumab should be added to palliative chemotherapy regimen for every patient with ERBB2+ gastric adenocarcinoma. Cisplatin-based chemotherapy and EOX regimen are first line chemotherapy for gastric cancer, however, starting them without trastuzumab is not an appropriate option. Monotherapy with docetaxel or irinotecan is a second-line chemotherapy. It has been shown to be superior to best supportive care and can be used for a palliative regimen.

96. B (S&F ch54)
H. pylori eradication is believed to be the cornerstone of chemoprevention of gastric cancers. Other potential protective factors include supplementation with antioxidants and the use of NSAIDs, COX-2 inhibitors, and statin. Out of these, aspirin and NSAID have most promising data. A meta-analysis reported a significant association between any NSAID use and reduced risk of gastric cancer. Given the lack of convincing evidence, the use of green tea and antioxidants such as carotenoids, vitamin C, and vitamin E cannot be recommended.

97. C (S&F ch54)
Gastric cancer is metastatic at the time of diagnosis in up to one third of cases. The most common sites of metastasis are the liver (40%) and peritoneum. Other sites of spread include periumbilical lymph nodes (Sister Joseph nodule), left supraclavicular sentinel nodes (Virchow node), the pouch of Douglass (rectal shelf of Blumer, palpated on digital rectal exam), and the ovaries (Krukenberg tumor). Gastric cancer has also been reported to metastasize to the kidney, bladder, brain, bone, heart, thyroid, adrenal glands, and skin. There are reports of unusual presentations of metastatic disease, such as shoulder-hand syndrome from bone metastasis, diplopia and blindness from orbital and retinal metastases, and virilization due to Krukenberg tumors.

TABLE FOR ANSWER FOR 73 Risk Factors for NSAID Ulcers*

Risk Factor	Risk Ratio
History of complicated ulcer	13.5
Use of multiple NSAIDs (including aspirin, COX-2 inhibitors)	9
Use of high doses of NSAIDs	7
Use of an anticoagulant	6.4
History of an uncomplicated ulcer	6.1
Age >70 years	5.6
H. pylori infection	3.5
Use of a glucocorticoid	2.2

*Not all NSAIDs pose the same risk.
NSAID, Nonsteroidal antiinflammatory drug.

TABLE FOR ANSWER FOR 73 Recommendations for Reducing the Risk of NSAID Ulcers as a Function of GI and Cardiovascular Risk

	GI risk*		
	Low	**Moderate**	**High**
Low CV risk	NSAID at the lowest effective dose	NSAID plus either a PPI or misoprostol	COX-2 inhibitor plus either a PPI or misoprostol
High CV risk†	Naproxen plus either a PPI or misoprostol	Naproxen plus either a PPI or misoprostol	Avoid NSAIDs or COX-2 inhibitors; use alternative therapy

**Low GI risk* denotes no risk factors (see other table for answer 73); *moderate GI risk* denotes 1 or 2 risk factors; *high GI risk* denotes ≥3 risk factors, prior complicated ulcer, or concomitant use of low-dose aspirin or anticoagulants. All patients with a history of ulcer who require NSAIDs should be tested for *H. pylori*, and if infection is present, eradication therapy should be given.
†*High CV risk* denotes the requirement for prophylactic low-dose aspirin for primary or secondary prevention of serious CV events.
CV, Cardiovascular; **PPI**, proton pump inhibitor.

TABLE FOR ANSWER 77 Frequency and Prognosis of Various Endoscopic Stigmata of Hemorrhage in Patients with a Bleeding Peptic Ulcer*

Endoscopic Characteristic†	Frequency (Range) (%)	Further Bleeding (%)	Surgery (%)	Mortality (%)
Active bleeding (type I)	18 (4-26)	55	35	11
Non-bleeding visible vessel (type IIa)	17 (4-35)	43	34	11
Adherent clot (type IIb)	17 (0-49)	22	10	7
Flat pigmentation (type IIc)	20 (0-42)	10	6	3
Clean base (type III)	42 (19-52)	5	0.5	2

†Classification by Forrest et al. is shown in parentheses.

TABLE FOR ANSWER 81 Gastric Cancer Incidence and Mortality Rates per 100,000 Cases (Age Adjusted) in the United States, 2005-2009

	Incidence		Mortality	
	Male	**Female**	**Male**	**Female**
All races	10.5	5.3	5.0	2.6
White	9.3	4.4	4.3	2.2
Black	17.0	8.7	10.3	4.8
Asian/Pacific Islander	16.4	9.9	9.0	5.3
American Indian/Alaska Native	13.6	7.3	8.3	3.8
Hispanic	14.4	8.5	7.3	4.3

TABLE FOR ANSWERS 88, 89, AND 94 Clinical Staging of Gastric Cancer Based on the TNM Classification

	N0	N1	N2	N3	M1 (Any N)
Tis	0	—	—	—	—
T1	IA	IB	IIA	IIB	IV
T2	IB	IIA	IIB	IIIA	IV
T3	IIA	IIB	IIIA	IIIB	IV
T4a	IIB	IIIA	IIIB	IIIC	IV
T4b	IIIB	IIIB	IIIC	IIIC	IV

is, In situ; **M**, metastases; **N**, node involvement; **T**, tumor.

BOX FOR ANSWERS 68 AND 69 Alarm Features in Patients with Upper GI Symptoms*

Age older than 55 years with new-onset dyspepsia
Family history of upper GI cancer
GI bleeding, acute or chronic, including unexplained iron deficiency
Jaundice
Left supraclavicular lymphadenopathy (Virchow node)
Palpable abdominal mass
Persistent vomiting
Progressive dysphagia
Unintended weight loss

*These features should prompt EGD and often other testing to establish a definitive diagnosis.

BOX FOR ANSWER 81 Risk Factors for Gastric Adenocarcinoma

Definite
H. pylori infection
Chronic atrophic gastritis
Intestinal metaplasia
Dysplasia*
Adenomatous gastric polyps*
Cigarette smoking
History of gastric surgery (especially Billroth II)*
Genetic factors:
- Family history of gastric cancer (first-degree relative)*
- Familial adenomatous polyposis (with fundic gland polyps)*
- Hereditary nonpolyposis colorectal cancer*
- Peutz-Jeghers syndrome*
- Juvenile polyposis*

Probable
High salt intake
Obesity (adenocarcinoma of the cardia only)
Snuff tobacco use
History of gastric ulcer
Pernicious anemia*
Regular aspirin or other NSAID use (protective)

Possible
Statin use (protective)
Heavy alcohol use
Low socioeconomic status
Ménétrier disease
High intake of fresh fruits and vegetables (protective)
High ascorbate intake (protective)

Questionable
Hyperplastic and fundic gland polyps
Diet high in nitrates
High green tea consumption (protective)

*Surveillance for cancer is recommended in patients with this risk factor.

CHAPTER

7

Pancreas

Hazem Hammad, Fazia Mir, Saurabh Chawla, and Emad Qayed

QUESTIONS

1. A 45-year-old man presents to the emergency department 2 days after being involved in a motor vehicle accident. He tells you that he was the restrained driver in the vehicle during a front-on collision at 50 miles/hour. He presented to another emergency department at that time but was discharged home as he had no complaints and no external signs of trauma. Today he complains of abdominal epigastric pain that started 12 hours ago. This is associated with nausea and nonbloody emesis. Medical history is significant for hypertension. His laboratory workup reveals a hemoglobin of 11.6 g/dL, WBC count of 18,000/μL and lipase level of 1750 IU/L. A computed tomography (CT) scan of the abdomen reveals pancreatic interstitial edema consistent with acute pancreatitis. Which part of the pancreas is most vulnerable to injury in the setting of restrained motor vehicle crash?
   A. Head of the pancreas
   B. Uncinate process
   C. Body of the pancreas
   D. Tail of the pancreas
   E. Pancreatico-duodenal arteries

2. Which of the following pancreatic cell type is responsible for the bulk of pancreatic secretion?
   A. Acinar cell
   B. Duct cells
   C. Stellate cell
   D. Beta cells
   E. Pancreatic polypeptide (PP) cells

3. A 67-year-old Caucasian man presents to the emergency department with large amount of hematemesis. He has a newly diagnosed mass in the body of the pancreas, suspicious for adenocarcinoma. He has no history of liver disease. On physical exam, his blood pressure is 90/50 mm Hg, pulse 110 bpm, and respiratory rate 14 breaths/min. Physical examination shows icteric sclera. He has abdominal epigastric tenderness to palpation. Laboratory values are as follows: hemoglobin 8 g/dL, platelet count 150,000/μL, WBC 11,000/μL. He is admitted to the intensive care unit for management. After resuscitation, upper endoscopy is performed, which reveals large amount of fresh blood in the stomach and fundal gastric varices. Proximity of the mass to which of the following structures is most likely responsible for this patient's presentation?
   A. Spleen
   B. Superior mesenteric artery (SMA)
   C. Inferior vena cava
   D. Splenic vein
   E. Pancreatico-duodenal artery

4. A 50-year-old woman with a history of hepatitis C cirrhosis is seen in clinic for follow-up. She has mild ascites controlled on furosemide 40 mg daily and aldactone 100 mg daily. She has a history of encephalopathy for which she takes lactulose. Abdominal exam reveals mild abdominal distension and fullness in the flanks. There is no tenderness. Laboratory values are as follows:

Hemoglobin	12 g/dL
Platelet count	190,000/μL
Total bilirubin	1.8 mg/dL
Creatinine	1.1 mg/dL
INR	1.3

An upper endoscopy is performed to screen for varices, and reveals a lesion in the antrum (see figure). What is the most likely diagnosis?

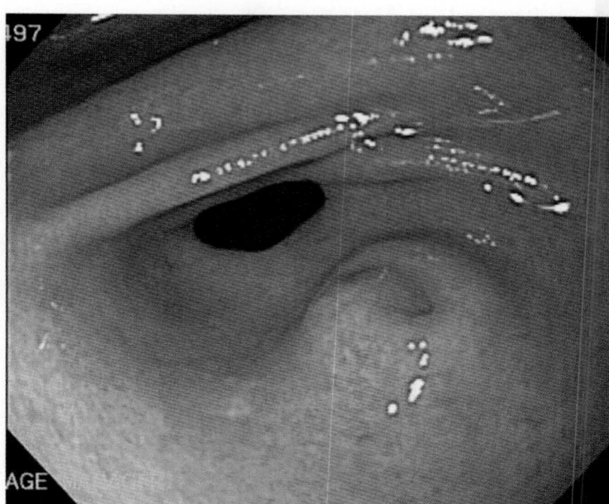

Figure for question 4.

   A. Gastrointestinal stromal tumor (GIST)
   B. Lipoma
   C. Carcinoid tumor
   D. Ectopic varix
   E. Ectopic pancreatic tissue

5. A 68-year-old man is seen in clinic with intermittent right upper quadrant abdominal pain of 2-month duration. He also reports pruritus, jaundice, and 10-pound weight loss. Magnetic resonance imaging (MRI)/magnetic resonance cholangiopancreatography (MRCP) shows a gallbladder mass with invasion into the surrounding liver, a hilar stricture, and dilated intrahepatic ducts. The pancreatic duct is normal in size. There is a common channel between the

pancreatic and bile duct that measures 22 mm. Which of the following correctly describes this biliary and pancreatic ductal anatomy?

A. Pancreaticobiliary malunion
B. Normal anatomy
C. Annular pancreas
D. Pancreas divisum
E. Pancreatic agenesis

6. A 40-year-old man presents with abdominal pain, nausea, and vomiting for the last 24 hours. He is otherwise healthy. Laboratory values are as follows:

Hemoglobin	13 g/dL
WBC	16,000/μL
Bilirubin	3.0 g/dL
Alkaline phosphatase	178 U/L
ALT	88 U/L
AST	125 U/L
Lipase	1700 IU/L

CT scan shows pancreatic interstitial edema and peripancreatic fat stranding. There is dilation of the proximal duodenum. Upper gastrointestinal (GI) series with contrast was performed for further evaluation (see figure). Which of the following is the most likely diagnosis?

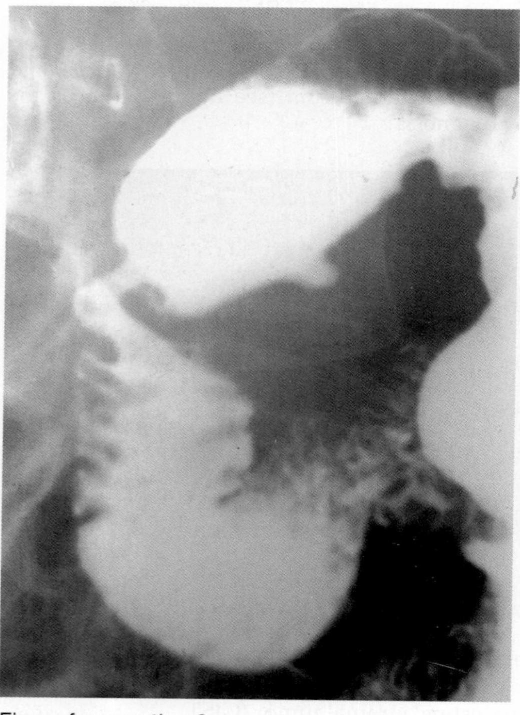

Figure for question 6.

A. Superior mesenteric artery syndrome
B. Gastric adenocarcinoma
C. Annular pancreas
D. Pancreas divisum
E. Choledochal cyst

7. Which of the following cells in the pancreas is responsible for fibrosis in chronic pancreatitis?

A. Acinar cells
B. Duct cells
C. Pancreatic stellate cells
D. Alpha cells
E. F cells

8. A 26-year-old woman is seen in the emergency department with acute onset epigastric pain, nausea, and vomiting. She has had similar episodes of pain over the past 2 years. She denies alcohol, tobacco, or drug use. On physical exam she has a temperature of 98° F, blood pressure of 100/50 mm Hg, and heart rate of 110 bpm. Abdominal exam reveals tenderness in the epigastrium. Laboratory values are as follows:

WBC	15,000/μL
ALT	20 U/L
AST	19 U/L
Alkaline phosphatase	120 U/L
Total bilirubin	2.2 mg/dL
Lipase	2000 IU/L

She is started on intravenous fluids and intravenous analgesia. A right upper quadrant ultrasound reveals no gallstones. An MRCP is performed (see figure). Which of the following is the most appropriate next step in management?

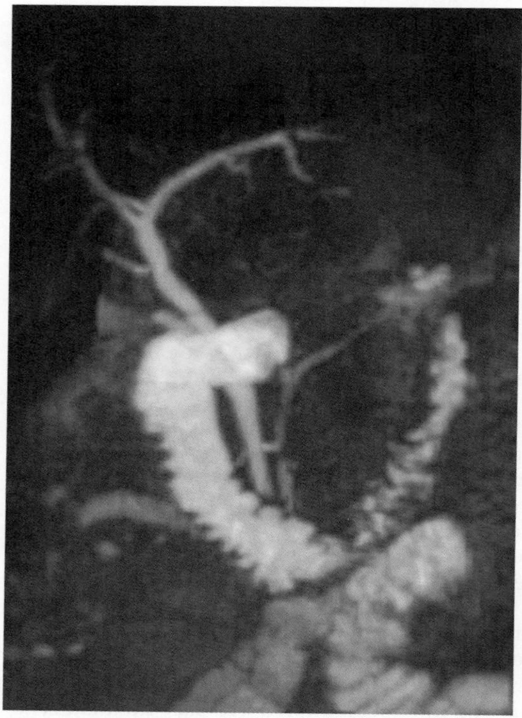

Figure for question 8.

A. Continue supportive care
B. Minor papilla sphincterotomy and stent placement
C. Major papilla sphincterotomy and stent placement
D. Whipple's procedure
E. Cholecystectomy

9. Which of the following is true regarding the acinar cell of the pancreas?

A. It is part of the endocrine pancreas
B. It is a cell that lines the pancreatic duct
C. It is responsible for secreting exocrine pancreatic digestive enzymes
D. The basolateral surface of the cell stores zymogen granules
E. It is responsible for secreting neurotransmitters

10. Which of the following anomalies results from failure of the ventral pancreas to rotate around the duodenum?
   A. Annular pancreas
   B. Pancreas divisum
   C. Anomalous pancreaticobiliary junction
   D. Bifid pancreatic duct
   E. Ansa pancreatica

11. Secretin is released from the neuroendocrine S cells in the duodenal mucosa. Which of the following is the molecular target of secretin?
   A. G protein–coupled receptor
   B. G protein–gated ion channel
   C. Cl^-/HCO^{3-} antiport pump
   D. Na^+/K^+ adenosine triphosphatase (ATPase)
   E. Cyclic adenosine monophosphate (cAMP)-dependent Cl channel

12. Which of the following is a true function of secretory trypsin inhibitor?
   A. Catalyzes the activation of proenzymes
   B. Forms a stable complex with trypsin
   C. Controls secretion of pancreatic enzymes
   D. Inhibits vagal stimulation of the pancreas
   E. Acts by enzymatic degradation of trypsin

13. The pancreas secretes many proenzymes that are activated when they reach the duodenum. Which of the following enzymes is secreted in its active from?
   A. Carboxypeptidase
   B. Phospholipase A2
   C. Lipase
   D. Trypsin
   E. Elastase

14. Exocrine pancreatic secretion has a cephalic, gastric, and intestinal phase. Which of the following neurotransmitters is the most important mediator of the cephalic phase of pancreatic secretion?
   A. Vasoactive intestinal peptide (VIP)
   B. Gastrin releasing peptide (GRP)
   C. Acetylcholine
   D. Secretin
   E. Cholecystokinin (CCK)

15. Which of the following is true regarding the intestinal phase of pancreas secretion?
   A. Secretin is the major mediator for meal stimulated enzyme secretion
   B. CCK is secreted when the pH in the duodenum drops to less 4.5
   C. CCK stimulates pancreatic bicarbonate and fluid secretion
   D. Vagovagal reflexes regulate enzyme and bicarbonate secretion
   E. Secretin is secreted from the duodenal mucosa in response to digested fat and protein in the duodenum.

16. You are called to evaluate a 3-day-old neonate who has been getting irritable and not taking feeds over the last 24 hours. On examination, he has abdominal distention and has not passed stool since birth; however, the abdomen is otherwise soft. A diagnostic enema was performed (see figure). What is the most likely diagnosis?
   A. Intestinal atresia
   B. Hirschsprung's disease
   C. Meconium ileus
   D. Annular pancreas
   E. Sigmoid volvulus

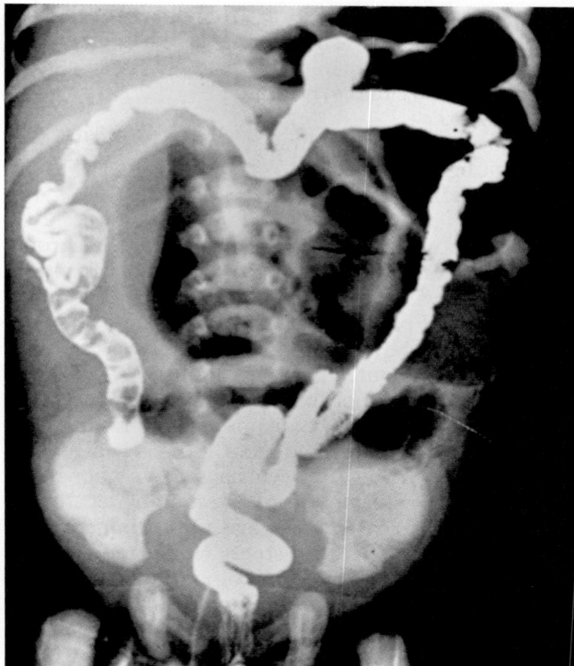

Figure for question 16.

17. A 4-year-old boy with pancreatic insufficiency due to cystic fibrosis is seen in clinic for evaluation. He is on chronic pancreatic enzyme replacement therapy for the last 2 years. His pediatrician has continued to modify his regimen as he has grown older. He is currently on 2500 lipase units/kg/meal and 1000 lipase units/kg for snacks. He is currently getting the enzyme supplements as enteric coated mini-microspheres. His mother reports that he still is having voluminous foul smelling stools with abdominal distention and discomfort and has been lagging on his growth chart. Which of the following is the most appropriate next step in management?
   A. Switch the pancreatic enzyme supplements from enteric coated mini-microspheres to uncoated enzyme supplements and add aluminum hydroxide.
   B. Increase the dosing of the supplements and titrate to symptoms up to a maximum of 7500 lipase units/kg/meal
   C. Continue enzyme replacement as such but modify diet to low fat, high protein and add a multivitamin preparation
   D. Continue enzyme replacement as such and add a histamine receptor-2 antagonist
   E. Continue enzyme replacement as such and cholestyramine

18. A 3-year-old boy is admitted to the hospital with failure to thrive. He has had recurrent episodes of infections, abdominal bloating, and foul smelling voluminous stools. On physical examination, he appears undernourished. X-rays of the pelvis show disorganization and calcification of the upper femoral and metaphysis. Chest x-ray shows short, flared ribs. He is below the 5% percentile for both height and weight. Laboratory values are as follows:

Hemoglobin	7 g/dL,
Platelet count	40,000/μL
WBC	2300/μL

Serum glucose and sweat chloride levels are reported as normal. Which of the following is the most likely diagnosis?

A. Shwachman-Diamond syndrome
B. Cystic fibrosis
C. Diamond-Blackfan syndrome
D. Pancreatic agenesis
E. Johanson-Blizzard syndrome

19. A 15-year-old boy presents to the hospital with chronic intermittent abdominal pain, which has been worsening over the last 2 days. The patient says that he has had intermittent abdominal pain for as long as he remembers. The pain has previously always resolved in a day or two with his grandmother's home remedies, though occasionally he has had to miss school for a day. This time, he has a similar dull, gnawing pain, which is not improving. The child and his parents migrated from India when he was 5 years of age and frequently travel back on vacations. The boy has recently spent 2 months of his summer vacation in India and returned back 3 months ago. On examination, he appears lean and in moderate distress. He has mild tenderness in epigastrium. Laboratory evaluation is significant for a fasting blood glucose of 180 mg/dL. An abdominal x-ray done in the clinic shows multiple rounded calcifications in the middle abdomen. Which of the following is the most likely diagnosis?

A. Pancreatitis secondary to *CFTR* mutations
B. Autoimmune pancreatitis
C. Hereditary pancreatitis
D. Tropical pancreatitis
E. Gallstone pancreatitis

20. A 10-year-old Caucasian boy is admitted to the hospital with acute pancreatitis. His mother reports that this is his fourth such admission over the last 2 years and wants to know why he is having these attacks of pancreatitis. The mother recalls that the boy's father also was diagnosed with pancreatitis, which was attributed to excessive alcohol use. The patient takes no medications. Previous ultrasound imaging is negative for gallstones. Lipid panel is normal. The patient does not have any other medical problems and otherwise seems to be doing well. His pediatrician suspects a genetic cause for his pancreatitis. Which of the following is the most appropriate recommendation?

A. Screening for *SPINK1* mutation
B. Perform a sweat chloride test and if negative evaluate for *CFTR* gene mutations
C. Perform a pedigree analysis and test for *PRSS1* mutations
D. Obtain a careful nutritional assessment and test for chymotrypsinogen-C *(CTRC)* gene mutation
E. Test for mutations in ubiquitin-ligase E3 *(UBR1)* gene.

21. A 10-year-old girl has just been diagnosed with hereditary pancreatitis and found to have a *PRSS1* gene mutation. Her mother has been researching the diagnosis on the internet and is very concerned about her risk for pancreatic cancer. Which of the following is true about the risk of pancreatic cancer in this hereditary pancreatitis?

A. Hereditary pancreatitis is associated with a minimally increased risk of pancreatic cancer
B. Screening is not recommended in patients with hereditary pancreatitis
C. 50% of patients with hereditary pancreatitis develop pancreatic cancer by age 50
D. Annual screening starting at age 18 is recommended
E. Tobacco smoking doubles the pancreatic cancer risk

22. An 18-year-old Indian exchange student presents with severe abdominal pain, nausea, and vomiting of 1-day duration. On examination he is mildly tachycardic and diaphoretic. Abdominal exam is significant for epigastric tenderness and mild hepatomegaly. Xanthomas are noted over the extensor surfaces of the arms, legs, and buttocks. He reports similar episodes of epigastric pain in the past, which resolve spontaneously. He denies any other significant medical history. He admits to occasional alcohol and marijuana use but denies tobacco smoking, other illicit drugs, or any prior exposure to needles. Laboratory values are as follows:

WBC	9000/μL
ALT	50 U/L
AST	60 U/L
Alkaline phosphatase	180 U/L
Total bilirubin	1.8 mg/dL
Lipase	2000 IU/L

The laboratory calls you to report that the patient's serum appears to be milky. Which of the following is the most likely etiology of pancreatitis in this patient?

A. *PRSS1* mutation
B. Gallstone disease
C. Familial hyperlipidemia
D. Marijuana use
E. Tropical pancreatitis

23. A 13-year-old boy who is visiting from India is admitted to the hospital due to inability to maintain oral intake. He has chronic recurrent abdominal pain, which has worsened over the past 2 days. The pain is associated with vomiting. He has lost more than 10 pounds over the last 6 months. The patient's father, mother, and sibling have no history of similar complaints. On physical exam the boy is thin and pale. The abdomen is soft but tender to palpation in the epigastric area. X-ray of the abdomen shows calcifications in the upper middle abdomen in the region of the pancreas. Ultrasound shows multiple pancreatic stones and a dilated pancreatic duct. Which of the following is the most likely diagnosis?

A. Hereditary pancreatitis
B. Tropical pancreatitis
C. Familial pancreatitis
D. Shwachman-Diamond syndrome
E. Johanson-Blizzard syndrome

24. Which of the following enhances trypsinogen activation?

A. Cystic fibrosis transmembrane conductance regulator *(CFTR)* activation
B. Serine protease inhibitor, Kazal type 1 *(SPINK1)*
C. Chymotrypsin-C *(CTRC)*
D. Protein Serine 1 *(PRSS1)*
E. Presence inside zymogen granule

25. Which of the following is correct about *SPINK1*?

A. It is considered a susceptibility gene in the development of chronic pancreatitis
B. It inhibits trypsin autoactivation
C. It inhibits *CFTR*
D. It enhances trypsin degradation
E. It enhances trypsin flushing into the duodenum

26. A 52-year-old woman presents to the emergency department with worsening epigastric pain for the last 2 days. The pain is sharp, severe, and radiates to the back. She reports a history of excessive alcohol drinking. Physical exam shows the following:

Temperature	100° F
Heart rate	95 bpm
Respiration	14 breaths/min
Blood pressure	95/65 mm Hg

Her abdomen is tender to palpation in the epigastrium. Laboratory values are as follows:

WBC	13,000/μL
Hematocrit	46%
Lipase	1150 IU/L
Amylase	1500 IU/L
Creatinine	1.1 mg/dL
BUN	25 mg/dL

The patient is admitted to the floor, started on IV fluids, IV analgesia, and nothing orally (NPO). Abdominal CT scan was obtained (see figure). Which of the following is the most appropriate next step in management?

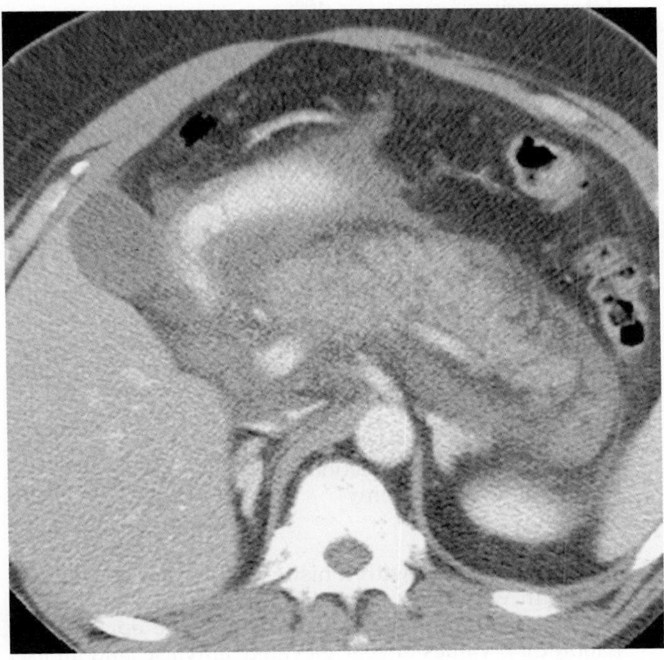

Figure for question 26.

A. Start IV antibiotics with piperacillin-tazobactam
B. CT-guided aspiration
C. Obtain blood cultures and start the patient on IV antibiotics
D. Consult surgery
E. Continue supportive care

27. A 55-year-old man with a history of alcohol abuse presents with worsening epigastric pain for the last 2 days. His abdomen is tender to palpation in the epigastrium. Laboratory studies reveal elevated amylase and lipase. Abdominal CT scan reveals interstitial pancreatitis with peripancreatic inflammatory changes without necrosis. The patient is admitted to the floor, started on IV fluids, IV analgesia, and kept NPO. He improves over the next 48 hours and is discharged uneventfully. He is seen in clinic 2 months later with mild epigastric discomfort. He denies nausea, vomiting, or weight loss. A repeat CT scan reveals a new low attenuation cystic lesion with a thin wall adjacent to the body of the pancreas measuring 7 cm. Which of the following is the most appropriate next step in management?
A. Conservative management
B. CT-guided aspiration of the cyst
C. Start ciprofloxacin and metronidazole
D. Obtain a surgical consult
E. Endoscopic cystgastrostomy

28. A 65-year-old obese man presents to the emergency department with altered mental status. He is unable to provide a detailed history. Physical exam reveals the following:

Temperature	100° F
Heart rate	115 bpm
Respiration rate	20 breaths/min
Blood pressure	95/65 mm Hg

He is lethargic and grimaces upon abdominal palpation. Laboratory values are as follows:

WBC	17,000/μL
Hemoglobin	15.5 g/dL
Lipase	3000 IU/L
Creatinine	3 mg/dL
BUN	60 mg/dL

An emergent CT scan reveals bilateral diffuse alveolar infiltrates, extensive pancreatic necrosis, and multiple peripancreatic fluid collections. Which of the following is true about the patient's condition?
A. This phase of acute pancreatitis lasts for about 1 week
B. Mortality is very high in the first 24 to 48 hours
C. The severity of this patient's pancreatitis has no relation to his extrapancreatic organ failure
D. Mortality in the first week is mostly due to infections
E. The condition can be largely reversed by surgical debridement of necrotic pancreatic tissue

29. A 22-year-old obese female presents with severe diffuse abdominal pain, nausea, and vomiting for the last 12 hours. Physical exam reveals diffuse marked tenderness to palpation in the abdomen. Her vital signs are as follows:

Temperature	103° F
Blood pressure	80/38 mm Hg
Heart rate	115 bpm

Laboratory values are as follows:

WBC	19,000/μL
AST	100 U/L
ALT	120 U/L
Alkaline phosphatase	100 U/L
Bilirubin	1.7 mg/dL
Serum amylase	290 IU/L (normal 28-100 IU/L)
Lipase	53 IU/L (normal 13-60 IU/L)

An ultrasound examination reveals intraperitoneal fluid. Which of the following is the most likely diagnosis?
A. Gallstone pancreatitis
B. Ruptured ectopic pregnancy
C. Acute cholecystitis
D. Infected pancreatic necrosis
E. Pancreatic pseudocyst from previous attack of pancreatitis

30. A 45-year-old Caucasian woman with suspected sphincter of Oddi dysfunction underwent an endoscopic retrograde cholangiopancreatography (ERCP) for evaluation of abdominal pain and mildly elevated liver enzymes. Cannulation was difficult and required precut sphincterotomy. Postprocedure, the patient developed severe abdominal pain. Laboratory work revealed that lipase was 2000 IU/L;

other laboratory parameters were in normal limits. Which of the following prophylactic measures could have been employed to prevent this complication?
A. Biliary stenting
B. Injection of botulinum toxin
C. Transdermal glyceryl trinitrate
D. Rectal indomethacin
E. Pancreatic sphincterotomy

31. A 40-year-old Caucasian woman with a history of Crohn's disease presents with abdominal pain, nausea, and vomiting. She reports passing loose stool two times per day with occasional rectal bleeding. Medication history reveals that the patient takes amlodipine 10 mg orally daily and was started on azathioprine (150 mg) and infliximab (5 mg/kg) 6 weeks ago. She denies drinking alcohol or smoking. Physical exam shows the following:

Temperature	99° F
Heart rate	95 bpm
Respiratory rate	16 breaths/min
Blood pressure	105/65 mm Hg

Her abdomen is tender to palpation in the epigastrium. Laboratory values are as follows:

AST	40 U/L
ALT	35 U/L
Bilirubin	1.0 mg/dL
Triglycerides level	320 mg/dL
Lipase	1000 U/L

Ultrasound of the right upper quadrant reveals no gallstones. Which of the following is the most likely cause of the patient's symptoms?
A. Crohn's colitis flare
B. Amlodipine
C. Azathioprine
D. Infliximab
E. Alcohol

32. A 35-year-old woman presents to the emergency department with nausea, vomiting, and epigastric pain of 6-hour duration. Significant past medical history includes hypertension for which she takes lisinopril. Physical exam shows the following:

Temperature	97° F
Heart rate	105 bpm
Respiratory rate	15 breaths/min
Blood pressure	120/65 mm Hg

Her abdomen is distended and is tympanic to percussion. There is tenderness to deep palpation in the epigastrium. Abdominal ultrasound reveals cholelithiasis. CBD was 6 mm in diameter. Laboratory values are as follows

WBC	11,000/μL
Hematocrit	40%
Hemoglobin	14 g/dL
Calcium	7.2 mg/dL
ALT	75 U/L
AST	83 U/L
Alkaline phosphatase	180 U/L
Bilirubin	2.5 mg/dL
Amylase	1200 IU/L
BUN	20 mg/dL

Which of the following is the most appropriate next step in management?
A. Abdominal CT scan
B. Fluid resuscitation
C. Wide-spectrum IV antibiotics
D. ERCP
E. Insert nasogastric (NG) tube

33. Based on the revised Atlanta classification of acute pancreatitis, which of the following best describe severe acute pancreatitis?
A. Persistent organ failure
B. Transient organ failure
C. Multiple fluid collections in and around the pancreas
D. Necrosis of >50% of the gland
E. Hematocrit >44%

34. A 67-year-old man is seen in clinic for evaluation of abdominal pain of 2-year duration. The pain occurs intermittently in the right upper quadrant, lasts for 2 hours, and then subsides slowly over the next 3 hours. He had a cholecystectomy 12 months ago for this type of pain, with minimal improvement. He denies a history of pancreatitis. Laboratory values are as follows:

WBC	8000/μL
Hematocrit	40%
Lipase	50 IU/L
Creatinine	0.7 mg/dL
AST	40 U/L
ALT	35 U/L
Total bilirubin	1.2 mg/dL

A right upper quadrant ultrasound showed a common bile duct of 6 mm. He had an upper endoscopy that was normal. The patient is referred for ERCP. An initial cholangiogram reveals a bile duct dilation to 8 mm. A large biliary sphincterotomy is performed. Pancreatogram shows normal pancreatic duct. A pancreatic sphincterotomy is performed. Which of the following is considered a risk factor for post-ERCP pancreatitis in this patient?
A. Male gender
B. Clinical presentation
C. Bile duct contrast injection
D. Biliary sphincterotomy
E. Age

35. A 70-year-old man with a history of alcohol abuse presents with worsening epigastric pain for the last 2 days. His abdomen is tender to palpation in the epigastrium. Laboratory values reveal elevated amylase and lipase. The patient is admitted to the floor, started on IV fluids, IV analgesia, and kept NPO. Over the next 2 days, he becomes increasingly short of breath and his mental status declines. Chest x-ray showed bilateral multilobar infiltrates consistent with acute respiratory distress syndrome (ARDS). He is intubated and placed on mechanical ventilation. CT scan of abdomen revealed nonenhancement of around 60% of the pancreas with multiple peripancreatic fluid collections and extensive fat stranding. Vital signs are as follows:

Temperature	100° F
Heart rate	93 bpm
Blood pressure	95/65 mm Hg

Laboratory values are as follows:

WBC	14,500/μL
Hematocrit	36%
Platelet count	350,000/μL
Lipase	1150 IU/L
Amylase	1500 IU/L
Creatinine	1.5 mg/dL

Which of the following is most appropriate next step in management?
- **A.** Start total parenteral nutrition
- **B.** Intravenous meropenem
- **C.** CT-guided aspiration of the peri-pancreatic fluid collections
- **D.** Place a nasoenteric feeding tube and start feeding as soon as possible
- **E.** Endoscopic drainage of the peri-pancreatic fluid collections

36. Which of the following statements is true regarding gallstone pancreatitis?
- **A.** Patients with elevated AST/ALT should undergo ERCP to clear the bile duct
- **B.** 15% of individuals with gallstones develops gallstone pancreatitis
- **C.** It occurs more commonly in men
- **D.** Most cases are due to stones <5 mm in size
- **E.** Recurrence is common after cholecystectomy and bile duct clearance.

37. A 48-year-old Caucasian woman is admitted to the general medical floor for treatment of acute gallstone pancreatitis. During her admission, she develops shortness of breath, and her oxygen saturation drops to 85% on room air. A chest x-ray is performed (see figure). Which of the following is true about this complication?

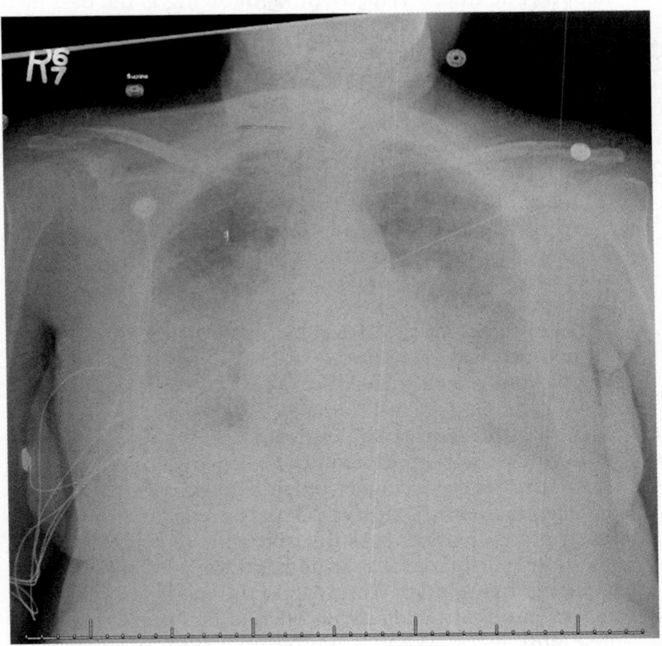

Figure for question 37.

- **A.** It usually occurs during the first 48 hours of admission
- **B.** Treatment consists of endotracheal intubation with high tidal volumes
- **C.** It usually results in pulmonary scarring and chronic impairment of lung function
- **D.** Administration of broad-spectrum antibiotics is required
- **E.** Phospholipase A2 plays a major role in pathogenesis

38. A 35-year-old woman who is 3 months postpartum presents with epigastric pain, nausea, and vomiting of 6-hour duration. She denies smoking but admits to drinking few beers on the weekends. Physical exam shows the following:

Temperature	101° F
Heart rate	110 bpm
Respiratory rate	14 breaths/min
Blood pressure	100/55 mm Hg

Her abdomen is distended and is tympanic to percussion. There is tenderness to deep palpation in the epigastrium. Laboratory values are as follows:

WBC	14,000/μL
Hemoglobin	15.0 g/dL
Lipase	500 IU/L
AST	40 U/L
ALT	35 U/L
Total bilirubin	2 mg/dL
Direct bilirubin	0.8 mg/dL
Creatinine	0.8 mg/dL

In addition to keeping her NPO and starting aggressive IV fluid hydration, which of the following is the most appropriate imaging study?
- **A.** CT scan of abdomen with IV contrast
- **B.** MRI with MRCP
- **C.** Right upper quadrant ultrasound
- **D.** Hepatobiliary (HIDA) scan
- **E.** Endoscopic ultrasound

39. A 60-year-old woman with a history of alcohol abuse presents with worsening epigastric pain for the last 2 days. Her abdomen is tender to palpation in the epigastrium. Laboratory values reveal elevated amylase and lipase, and a diagnosis of acute pancreatitis is made. The patient is admitted to the floor, started on IV fluids, IV analgesia, and kept NPO. Which of the scoring systems can be used within the first 12 hours of admission for early identification of patients at increased risk of in-hospital mortality?
- **A.** Ranson's score
- **B.** Bedside Index for Severity in Acute Pancreatitis (BISAP) score
- **C.** Acute Physiology and Chronic Health Evaluation (APACHE) II score
- **D.** Blatchford's score
- **E.** Rockall's score

40. A 51-year-old woman is seen in clinic for consultation regarding screening for pancreatic cancer. She has history of chronic alcoholic pancreatitis for the last 5 years. Which of the following is true regarding pancreatic cancer and chronic pancreatitis?
- **A.** Pancreatic cancer risk is increased in all forms of chronic pancreatitis
- **B.** Lifetime risk for developing pancreatic cancer in chronic pancreatitis is around 20%
- **C.** Chronic alcoholic pancreatitis carries the highest risk for developing pancreatic cancer
- **D.** CT scan with contrast is superior to endoscopic ultrasound (EUS) with fine-needle aspiration (FNA) for evaluation of malignancy
- **E.** Annual cancer antigen 19-9 is indicated in this patient for screening of pancreatic malignancy

41. A 52-year-old Caucasian man with a history of chronic alcoholic pancreatitis presents to your clinic with increased frequency of bowel movements for the past 8 months. He passes greasy, foul smelling stool up to 5 times per day. He reports a weight loss of 10 pounds. You suspect that he has developed pancreatic exocrine insufficiency. How much

reduction of the pancreatic enzyme secretion is needed before steatorrhea develops?
A. 25%
B. 40%
C. 60%
D. 75%
E. 90%

42. A 45-year-old Caucasian woman with a history of chronic pancreatitis presents to your clinic with increased frequency of bowel movements for the past 10 months. She passes greasy, foul smelling stool multiple times per day for the past 6 months. Deficiency of which of the following micronutrients is more likely to develop in this patient?
A. Vitamin A
B. Vitamin B_{12}
C. Vitamin C
D. Folate
E. Biotin

43. A 55-year-old Caucasian man is referred to your clinic for evaluation of chronic abdominal pain. He denies any diarrhea or weight loss. He had long history of alcohol use and tobacco smoking in the past but quit a few years ago. Chronic pancreatitis is suspected. Which of the following is the most sensitive diagnostic test for chronic pancreatitis?
A. Measurement of duodenal bicarbonate concentration after secretin stimulation
B. Serum trypsinogen
C. Fecal elastase
D. ERCP
E. 72-hour quantitative fecal fat excretion

44. A 48-year-old African-American man was referred for management of chronic abdominal pain. He has a diagnosis of chronic alcoholic pancreatitis for the last 5 years. He has been experiencing worsening abdominal pain over the past several months. He is requiring higher doses of tramadol. An ERCP is performed and the pancreatogram is shown (see figure). Which of the following is the most appropriate next step in management?

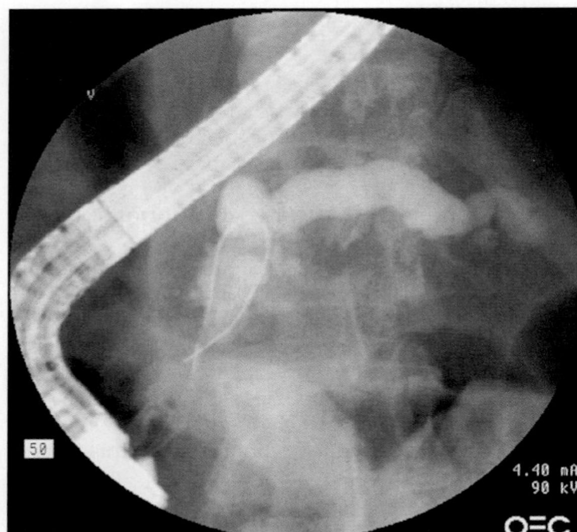

Figure for question 44.

A. EUS-guided celiac plexus block
B. Minor papilla sphincterotomy
C. Pancreatic duct stent placement
D. Whipple's procedure
E. Pancreas enzymes

45. A 70-year-old Caucasian man is referred for evaluation of jaundice. He reports having intermittent abdominal discomfort for the last 3 months and has lost 10 pounds. He denies fever or chills. Physical exam shows the following:

Temperature	100° F
Heart rate	95 bpm
Respiratory rate	14 breaths/min
Blood pressure	105/65 mm Hg

He has scleral icterus. His abdomen is tender to palpation in the epigastrium. Laboratory values are as follows:

WBC	6000/μL
Hemoglobin	11.5 g/dL
Creatinine	1 mg/dL
Bilirubin	3.5 mg/dL
Alkaline phosphatase	198 IU/L
ALT	65 IU/L
AST	72 IU/L
Amylase	190 IU/L
Lipase	286 IU/L

Abdominal CT reveals a diffusely enlarged sausage-shaped pancreas with delayed enhancement. EUS shows a diffusely enlarged and hypoechoic pancreas without focal lesions, along with mildly dilated extrahepatic and intrahepatic bile ducts. Which of the following is the best next step in management?
A. Whipple's procedure
B. Celiac plexus neurolysis
C. Lateral pancreaticojejunostomy
D. Prednisone
E. ERCP

46. Which of the following is true regarding autoimmune pancreatitis type 1?
A. Associated with ulcerative colitis
B. More common in females
C. High serum IgG4 levels
D. Histology is characterized by presence of neutrophils in medium and small ducts
E. Commonly present with cachexia and abdominal pain

47. A 45-year-old man with long-standing history of chronic pancreatitis is seen in clinic for follow-up of steatorrhea. You have previously prescribed pancreatic enzyme replacement therapy during his last appointment 3 months ago. He reports that he still complains of persistent foul smelling diarrhea and that he is taking the enzyme supplements twice a day. You review the medication list and inform him that the enzymes need to be taken with every meal and snack. What is the optimal dose of lipase that needs to be delivered to the intestine with each meal to eliminate steatorrhea?
A. 1000 IU
B. 4000 IU
C. 30,000 IU
D. 60,000 IU
E. 90,000 IU

48. A 67-year-old African-American man is brought to the emergency department after a syncopal episode. He complains of epigastric pain that started 12 hours ago. He has a history of chronic alcoholic pancreatitis and pseudocyst. Physical exam shows a blood pressure of 85/40 mm Hg and pulse of 115 bpm. He is alert and oriented. The abdomen is tender to palpation in the epigastrium. Digital rectal exam shows brown stool, fecal occult positive. Laboratory values are as follows:

WBC	7000/μL
Hemoglobin	7 g/dL
Creatinine	1 mg/dL
Bilirubin	2 mg/dL
Alkaline phosphatase	150 IU/L
ALT	35 IU/L
AST	42 IU/L
Amylase	120 IU/L
Lipase	90 IU/L

His laboratory results 2 months ago were as follows:

WBC	6000/μL
Hemoglobin	11 g/dL
Creatinine	0.6 mg/dL

Resuscitation with IV fluids was started. An upper endoscopy is unremarkable. Which of the following is the most appropriate next step in management?

A. Technetium-99m–labeled red blood cell scan
B. ERCP
C. Abdominal CT scan
D. Capsule small bowel study
E. Angiography

49. Which of the following is true regarding alcohol consumption and chronic pancreatitis?

A. Among heavy alcohol users, around 20% end up developing chronic pancreatitis
B. Pancreas ductal cells are key players in the pathogenesis of alcoholic chronic pancreatitis
C. 80% of the chronic pancreatitis cases are due to alcohol
D. Men are more likely to develop alcoholic chronic pancreatitis
E. In patients with established chronic pancreatitis, abstinence from alcohol drinking halts the progression of the disease

50. A 58-year-old Caucasian male with history of alcoholic chronic pancreatitis presents for evaluation of worsening intermittent abdominal pain, nausea, and vomiting. On physical exam, a bulge in the epigastrium is felt. Laboratory values are as follows:

Bilirubin	2.0 mg/dL
Alkaline phosphatase	175 U/L
ALT	40 U/L
AST	85 U/L
Lipase	350 U/L

CT scan showed a large 10 cm encapsulated pseudocyst anterior to the body of the pancreas. Which of the following is the best next step in management?

A. Watchful waiting, as most of these pseudocysts will resolve over the course of few months
B. Wait 4 to 6 weeks to allow the pseudocyst's capsule to mature
C. Percutaneous drainage of the pseudocyst
D. EUS-guided pseudocyst drainage
E. Surgical cystgastrostomy

51. Which of the following is consistent with the diagnosis of type 2 autoimmune pancreatitis?

A. Neutrophilic infiltration with microabscesses
B. Lymphoplasmacytic sclerosing pancreatitis
C. Storiform fibrosis
D. Presence of >10 IgG4-positive plasma cells per high-power field
E. Obliterative phlebitis

52. A 63-year-old Caucasian man with history of heavy alcohol use is being evaluated for chronic epigastric pain of 1 year duration. An upper endoscopy is performed, and it reveals normal findings. Due to reports of foul smelling stools, fecal elastase is ordered and found to be low (150 μg/g of stool). An upper endoscopic ultrasound (EUS) is performed to examine for chronic pancreatitis. Which of the following EUS features is suggestive of chronic pancreatitis?

A. Hypoechoic foci
B. Anechoic pancreatic duct margins
C. Pancreatic duct diameter of 2.3 mm in the body of the pancreas
D. Lobularity of pancreatic contour
E. Homogenous, granular pancreatic parenchyma

53. A 58-year-old Caucasian man with a history of chronic alcoholic pancreatitis and pseudocyst presents to the emergency department with worsening shortness of breath for the past 2 days. Four days prior to presentation, he was discharged from another hospital with a discharge diagnosis of community-acquired pneumonia with a parapneumonic pleural effusion. A chest tube was inserted for treatment, and removed 1 day prior to discharge. A chest x-ray performed at discharge is shown (see figure, part A). Upon arrival to the emergency department, he was noted to be in severe respiratory distress, with vital signs as follows:

Respiratory rate	30 breaths/min
Oxygen saturation	75% on room air
Heart rate	120 bpm
Blood pressure	110/70 mm Hg

A chest x-ray performed in the emergency department is shown (see figure, part B). He is subsequently intubated and sent to the medical intensive care unit. Which of the following will confirm the most likely etiology of his respiratory compromise?

A. Pleural fluid cytology
B. Pleural fluid amylase
C. Pleural fluid cell count and culture
D. Bronchoscopy and lavage
E. Chest CT scan

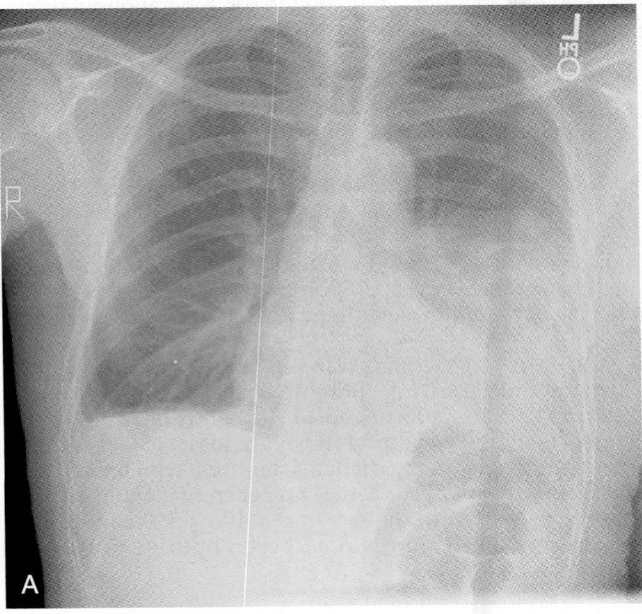

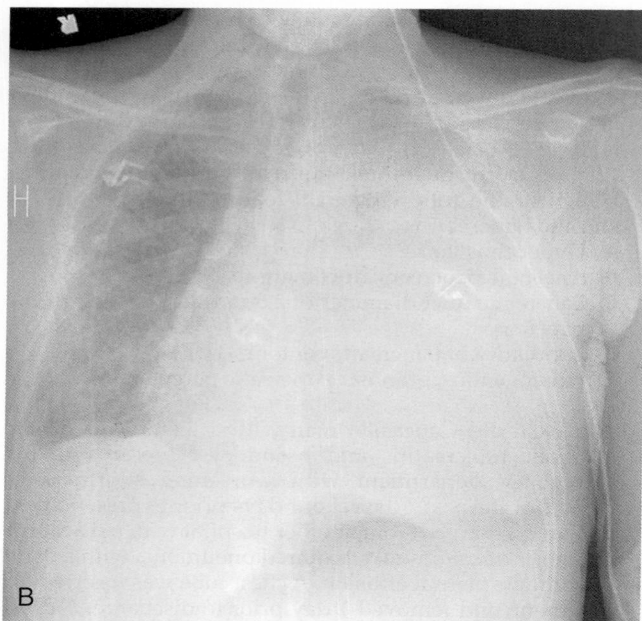

Figure for question 53.

54. Which of the following conditions carries the highest individual risk for development of pancreatic cancer by age 70?
  A. Hereditary breast/ovarian cancer syndrome
  B. Familial atypical multiple mole melanoma (FAMMM) syndrome
  C. Peutz-Jeghers syndrome
  D. Lynch syndrome
  E. Familial pancreatic cancer

55. A 35-year-old Caucasian man presents to your clinic to discuss screening for pancreatic cancer. The patient is a healthy nonsmoker who exercises regularly and does not have any significant past medical history. He is concerned because his father, who is 70 years old, was recently diagnosed with pancreatic cancer. Which of the following is true?
  A. The patient has a tenfold increased risk for pancreatic adenocarcinoma compared to the general population
  B. Screening is recommended for first degree relatives in a kindred with at least two affected first degree relatives, or those with specific gene mutations
  C. The patient should be scheduled for an MRI of the abdomen, which, if negative, needs to be repeated biannually
  D. You will suggest that starting at age 50 years, it is recommended that he undergoes annual noninvasive screening using salivary biomarkers
  E. The patient should be scheduled for EUS evaluation of his pancreas every 6 months for the first year and, if negative, follow an annual EUS surveillance protocol

56. A 65-year-old Vietnam War veteran presents for evaluation of dull, gnawing abdominal pain of 6 months duration. His pain is localized to the central abdomen and associated with a 30-pound weight loss. He feels that his weight loss is due to diabetes mellitus, which was diagnosed 1 year ago. He denies any current alcohol or illicit drug use but admits to being a 40-pack/year smoker. On exam, he is thin and cachectic but otherwise does not have any icterus, pallor, or lymphadenopathy. There is no organomegaly on abdominal exam but tenderness to deep palpation is appreciated in the epigastrium. Which of the following diagnoses should be strongly suspected?
  A. Pancreatic adenocarcinoma
  B. Autoimmune pancreatitis
  C. Pancreatic neuroendocrine tumors
  D. Chronic pancreatitis
  E. Solid pseudopapillary tumor

57. A 65-year-old woman presents to the emergency department with abdominal pain of 12 hours duration. Her pain is localized to the left lower quadrant and is associated with low-grade fevers. On exam, she appears comfortable, with mild left lower quadrant tenderness on abdominal exam. No rebound tenderness is noted. A contrast-enhanced CT of the abdomen and pelvis done in the emergency department shows localized diverticulitis in the sigmoid colon. Note is also made of an incidental 25 mm cystic lesion in the body of the pancreas with multiple microcysts with thin septations. What is the most likely etiology of the pancreatic mass?
  A. Mucinous cystic neoplasm
  B. Solid pseudopapillary neoplasm
  C. Serous cystadenoma
  D. Pancreatic adenocarcinoma
  E. Intraductal papillary mucinous neoplasm

58. A 61-year-old Hispanic woman was brought to the hospital by her daughter for right upper quadrant pain and worsening yellowness of the eyes. In addition, she has significant itching. Her daughter reports that she has had chronic right upper quadrant pain for the last several years, which has been worsening over the last 2 weeks. She has been taking 6 to 9 tablets of acetaminophen 500 mg daily for the pain. She denies any alcohol or illicit drug use. Past medical history is significant for cholecystectomy 15 years ago. In the hospital she undergoes a good quality contrast enhanced CT scan of the abdomen, which is reported as moderate intrahepatic and extrahepatic biliary ductal dilation, with cutoff in the distal common bile duct (CBD) near the duodenum. The spleen, pancreas, and adrenal glands are within normal limits. A coronal section shows the dilated CBD (see figure). What is the most appropriate next step in management?

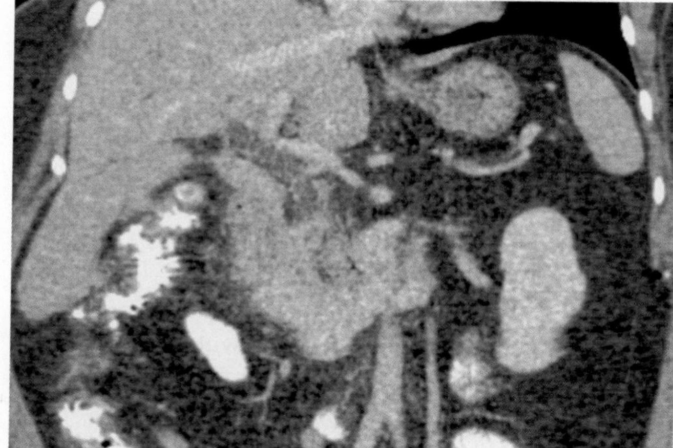

Figure for question 58.

A. MRI abdomen
B. Refer to surgery for a Whipple procedure
C. Bile duct excision
D. Liver biopsy
E. ERCP

59. A 70-year-old, previously healthy man presents with painless jaundice and itching over the last 2 months. He reports a 20-pound weight loss but denies any fevers, chills, or abdominal pain. Physical examination reveals a thin patient in no distress. Abdomen is soft but tender to deep palpation in the epigastric area. Laboratory values are as follows:

WBC	6300/μL
ALT	80 U/L
AST	68 U/L
Alkaline phosphatase	220 U/L
Total bilirubin	5.2 mg/dL
Direct bilirubin is	4.1 mg/dL

MRI of the abdomen shows a 3 cm solid mass lesion localized within the pancreatic head causing obstruction of the distal common bile duct (CBD). The mass does not abut the portal and the superior mesenteric veins and is well away from the celiac axis and the superior mesenteric artery. Which of the following is the most appropriate next step in management?
A. Schedule an ERCP
B. Schedule an EUS with FNA
C. Refer for pancreaticoduodenectomy
D. Refer him to medical oncology for neoadjuvant chemotherapy
E. Discuss palliative options, including internal or external biliary drainage

60. A 60-year-old woman who presented with obstructive jaundice and abdominal pain was found to have a 4 cm pancreatic head mass in the pancreas on MRI. The mass was abutting the superior mesenteric vein (SMV) and the portal vein confluence for more than 180 degrees but not involving the celiac axis or the superior mesenteric artery (SMA). Two small lymph nodes measuring 6 mm and 8 mm were noted in the periportal region. No celiac, periaortic, or retroperitoneal lymph nodes or distant metastases were visualized. Laboratory values are as follows:

Hemoglobin	11 g/dL
WBC	7000/μL
Total bilirubin	7.5 g/dL
Direct bilirubin	5.2 g/dL
Alkaline phosphatase of	378 U/L
ALT	188 U/L
AST	155 U/L

Which of the following is the most appropriate next step in management?
A. ERCP with endoscopic ultrasound
B. ERCP and uncovered metal stent placement
C. Whipple procedure
D. Chemoradiation
E. Hospice referral

61. A 67-year-old business executive has just been diagnosed with metastatic pancreatic cancer. His only symptoms are pruritus and icterus from obstructive jaundice. He is losing weight but continues to have a good appetite and denies any nausea or vomiting. He has done research before coming to you and says he understands that his survival is dismal and does not want unnecessary interventions or treatments that will not help him. Which of the following is the most appropriate recommendation for this patient?
A. Refer to home hospice
B. ERCP with metal stent placement
C. Biliary and duodenal bypass surgery
D. ERCP with metal stent placement plus combination chemotherapy
E. Neoadjuvant chemoradiation followed by tumor resection

62. A 57-year-old Caucasian man was admitted to your service for abdominal pain and weight loss. The patient has a history of abdominal pain radiating to the back for 6 days. His medical history did not show any other relevant diseases. The physical examination was significant for slight tenderness on palpation in the upper abdomen and tender circumscribed subcutaneous nodules over the legs. Laboratory examination shows the following:

Lipase	7143 U
Amylase	45 U/L
γ-Glutamyl transferase	440 U/L
Alkaline phosphatase	317 U/L

CT scan revealed a 5 cm exophytic, heterogenous, hypoenhancing mass with cystic components in the body and tail region of the pancreas. The common bile duct and pancreatic duct were not dilated. Multiple disseminated hypervascularized lesions of the liver were also detected. Which of the following is the most likely diagnosis?
A. Pancreatic adenocarcinoma with liver metastasis
B. Acute pancreatic fluid collection with multiple hepatic abscesses
C. Metastatic acinar cell carcinoma
D. Side-branch intraductal pancreatic mucinous neoplasm
E. Solid pseudo-papillary tumor

63. A 70-year-old man presents with abdominal pain and weight loss. During his workup, a CT scan of the abdomen is done that shows a 5 cm mass in the head of the pancreas. The mass is hypodense and homeogenous and infiltrating into peripancreatic tissue but not involving the vasculature. The pancreatic duct is not dilated. A few small round hypoechoic peripancreatic lymph nodes are also visualized. Laboratory values are as follows:

Hemoglobin	13 g/dL
WBC	16,000/μL
Total bilirubin	3.0 g/dL
Alkaline phosphatase	178 U/L
ALT	88 U/L
AST	115 U/L

The patient undergoes FNA of this mass, which shows abnormal lymphocytes with large nuclei with single to multiple prominent nucleoli in a background of abundant necrosis. Further testing shows these cells have CD20 expression. Which of the following is the most appropriate next step in management?
A. Staging laparoscopy followed by resection of tumor if no peritoneal seeding
B. Neoadjuvant chemotherapy followed by surgery

C. Nutritional support and serial imaging to evaluate spontaneous resolution of necrosis
D. Chemotherapy and radiation with curative intent
E. Supportive and palliative therapy

64. A 38-year-old woman presented to the emergency department after being involved in a low-impact motor vehicle accident, which involved her hitting a parked van while parking her car. She complained of some abdominal pain, which she said had been going on for several months. Her physical exam was significant for mild abdominal tenderness and fullness in the upper abdomen. A CT of the abdomen showed a large 8 cm well-encapsulated mass in the body of the pancreas. The mass was heterogeneous with solid and cystic components. Which of the following is the most likely diagnosis?
A. Serous cystadenoma
B. Pancreatic pseudocyst
C. Acinar cell carcinoma
D. Mucinous cystic neoplasm
E. Solid pseudopapillary tumor

65. A 62-year-woman is referred to you for an endoscopic ultrasound (EUS) for pancreatic cystic lesion in the body of the pancreas, found incidentally. She has no abdominal pain or other symptoms. On EUS, you notice a 5 cm well-circumscribed multicystic lesion, which shows honeycombing and central calcification. Which of the following is the most appropriate next step in management?
A. Follow-up imaging in 1 year
B. Surgical resection
C. Check serum chromogranin levels
D. ERCP
E. PET scan

66. A patient with abdominal pain and a dilated pancreatic duct is referred for ERCP for further evaluation. Upon introducing the side-viewing duodenoscope, the following finding is encountered as seen in the image (see figure). What is the most likely diagnosis?

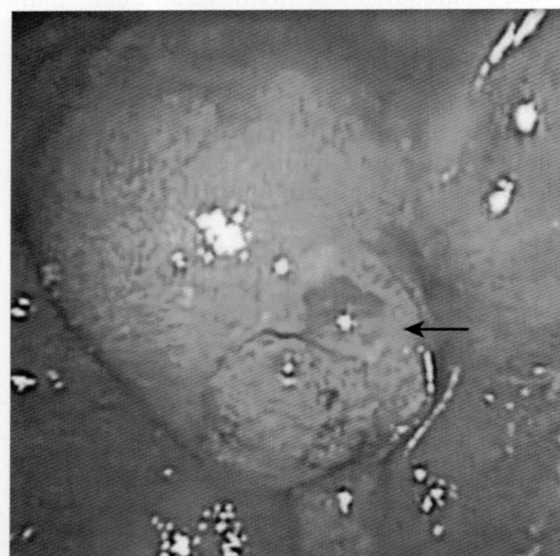

Figure for question 66.

A. Ampullary adenocarcinoma
B. Ampullary adenoma
C. Side-branch intraductal papillary mucinous neoplasm
D. Main-duct intraductal papillary mucinous neoplasm
E. Chronic pancreatitis

67. Which of the following is true regarding mucinous cystic neoplasms (MCN) of the pancreas?
A. MCNs are benign cystic lesions of the pancreas predominantly found in middle-aged men
B. MCNs are precursors to main-duct intraductal papillary mucinous neoplasms, which in turn are precursors to ductal adenocarcinoma of the pancreas
C. MCNs should be ablated by aspiration of cyst contents and injection of absolute alcohol
D. They are characterized by numerous tiny cysts separated by delicate fibrous septa
E. MCNs can be diagnosed histologically by the presence of ovarian type stroma within the tumor

68. A 56-year old woman with a history of congestive heart failure and hepatitis C cirrhosis undergoes MRI of the abdomen for hepatocellular cancer surveillance. There is no suspicious liver lesion, but a 5 cm thick-walled cystic lesion is found in the body of the pancreas with few septations. The common bile duct and the pancreatic duct are not dilated. She has no abdominal pain, nausea, or vomiting. Her exposure to hepatitis C was from a contaminated blood transfusion in 1978 when she had a complicated fracture of her femur. What would you recommend for the incidentally found pancreatic lesion?
A. No further treatment
B. Endoscopic cystogastrostomy
C. EUS with FNA
D. Repeat MRI in 6 months
E. Surgical referral for resection of pancreatic adenocarcinoma

69. A 63-year-old man undergoes a distal laparoscopic pancreatectomy for an intraductal papillary mucinous neoplasm localized to the tail of the pancreas. Histology of the resected specimen reveals high-grade ductal dysplasia but no invasion. The resected margins are not involved. What is the most appropriate follow-up for this patient?
A. Indefinite postoperative surveillance with MRI every 2 years
B. No postoperative surveillance
C. Total pancreatectomy
D. Annual surveillance with follow-up MRI for the first 3 years; if no recurrence is noted, no further follow-up is required
E. Repeat EUS and FNA of the remnant pancreas in 1 year

70. A 56-year-old woman is referred for an EUS to further evaluate a pancreatic cystic lesion, found incidentally. On EUS, a smooth-walled 2 cm, predominantly anechoic lesion is found in the neck of the pancreas. No honeycombing or central calcification is noted. FNA with fluid aspiration is performed. Cytology is nondiagnostic as only a few normal appearing columnar cells are present on the smears. Cyst fluid analysis is significant for an amylase level of 40 IU/mL and a carcinoembryonal antigen (CEA) level of 88 IU/mL. Which of the following is the most appropriate advice for the patient?
A. Reassure her that she has serous cystadenoma with an extremely low risk of malignant transformation, therefore no further follow-up is required

B. Discuss with her that she has mucinous cystadenoma; however, because the CEA levels are low, she does not have malignant transformation and therefore does not need further follow-up
C. Reassure her that she has a side-branch IPMN and does not need follow-up
D. Discuss with her that the results are not conclusive but not concerning for malignancy; she should follow up with serial imaging to monitor the cystic lesion
E. Discuss with her that the results are not conclusive, and malignancy cannot be ruled out; therefore, she should consider surgery for the cystic lesion in her pancreas

71. A 56-year-old woman presents to the emergency department with acute onset of abdominal pain of 24-hour duration. The pain started in the right upper quadrant and then localized to the midabdomen. The pain also radiates to the back. She complains of nausea and has had two episodes of emesis. She denies alcohol use and is not taking any medications. On examination, she has a body mass index of 30 kg/m^2 and is mildly diaphoretic. Vital signs are as follows:

Heart rate	100 bpm
Blood pressure	100/70 mm Hg
Temperature	37.4° C

Laboratory values are as follows:

Hemoglobin	14 gm/dL
WBC	12,000/µL
Total bilirubin	2.6 gm/dL
AST	50 IU/L
ALT	50 IU/L
Lipase	600 IU/mL

A bedside ultrasound reveals cholelithiasis. There is no intrahepatic biliary ductal dilation, and the common bile duct measures 5 mm. You are consulted for evaluation for an ERCP for gallstone pancreatitis. In addition to maintaining NPO, IV analgesia, and fluid resuscitation, which of the following is the most appropriate management?
A. ERCP within 24 to 48 hours
B. Intravenous antibiotics
C. MRI/MRCP
D. Emergency cholecystectomy
E. Abdominal CT scan with contrast

72. A 62-year-old man presents to the gastroenterology clinic for follow-up after a recent admission with alcohol-induced pancreatitis 4 weeks ago. That was his first presentation with pancreatitis. He had no complications during that hospital stay. He is recovering well, has regained his appetite, stayed abstinent, and is presently asymptomatic. A CT of the abdomen performed 2 days ago reported a new peripancreatic fluid collection measuring 6 cm. No pancreatic necrosis is reported. Laboratory values are as follows:

Hemoglobin	13 g/dL
WBC	8000/µL
Total bilirubin	1.5 g/dL
Alkaline phosphatase	128 U/L
ALT	28 U/L
AST	35 U/L
Lipase	120 IU/L

He was asked by his family doctor to discuss with you treatment options for this fluid collection. Which of the following is the best management approach?
A. Endoscopic drainage
B. Repeat abdominal imaging in 3 to 6 months
C. Transabdominal drainage
D. Surgical drainage
E. MRI/MRCP

73. A 45-year-old man presents for follow-up 3 months after undergoing a successful endoscopic cystogastrostomy for a symptomatic pseudocyst following an attack of acute alcoholic pancreatitis. A CT scan performed 6 weeks postprocedure showed almost complete resolution of the pseudocyst. The transgastric stents were subsequently removed from the cyst cavity. At this visit, the patient reports symptoms of gastric fullness and pain after eating, similar to the symptoms he had prior to endoscopic drainage. A repeat CT scan reveals recurrence of the pseudocyst (measuring 8 cm) without any evidence of necrosis. The patient would like to avoid a surgical procedure, if possible. Which of the following is the most appropriate next step in management?
A. Surgical pseudocyst drainage
B. Percutaneous drainage
C. Repeat cystogastrostomy
D. Conservative management with oral analgesia
E. Endoscopic retrograde pancreatography (ERP)

74. A 49-year-old woman is hospitalized with severe acute gallstone pancreatitis. After 5 days of hospitalization, she continuous to have severe abdominal pain and abdominal distention. Physical exam shows the following vital signs:

Temperature	100° F
Heart rate	95 bpm
Respiratory rate	18 breaths/min
Blood pressure	100/65 mm Hg

Her abdomen is tender to palpation in the epigastrium Laboratory values are as follows:

WBC	9000/µL
ALT	40 U/L
AST	100 U/L
Alkaline phosphatase	110 U/L
Total bilirubin	1.5 mg/dL
Lipase	350 IU/L

A CT of the abdomen is performed and shows pancreatic necrosis involving more than 50% of the pancreatic parenchyma. The next step in management would be:
A. Continue supportive care and provide enteral nutrition
B. Broad-spectrum antibiotics
C. Surgical pancreatic necrosectomy
D. Endoscopic pancreatic necrosectomy
E. Percutaneous drainage of necrosis

75. A 55-year-old woman is hospitalized with severe acute gallstone pancreatitis. On day 4, she continues to have abdominal pain, nausea, and inability to tolerate anything orally. A CT scan is performed that shows pancreatic necrosis involving more than 30% of the pancreatic parenchyma. A nasojejunal tube is placed for nutrition, and supportive care with IV fluids and IV analgesia is continued. On day 10, she continues to have abdominal pain. She has nausea and frequent vomiting. She is passing formed stool with no blood. Physical exam shows the following:

Temperature	103° F
Heart rate	110 bpm
Respiratory rate	18 breaths/min
Blood pressure	90/55 mm Hg

Her abdomen is tender to palpation in the epigastrium. Laboratory values are as follows:

WBC	14,000/μL
ALT	60 U/L
AST	120 U/L
Alkaline phosphatase	180 U/L
Total bilirubin	1.8 mg/dL
Lipase	450 IU/L

Chest x-ray shows bilateral small pleural effusions, with clear lungs otherwise. Abdominal x-ray reveals a normal bowel gas pattern. Urinalysis shows 3 RBC/HPF and 8 WBC/HPF. Blood cultures are pending. Which of the following is the most appropriate next step in management?

A. Start broad-spectrum antibiotics and antifungals
B. Surgical pancreatic necrosectomy
C. Endoscopic pancreatic necrosectomy
D. FNA of pancreatic necrosis
E. Stool *Clostridium difficile* testing

76. A 27-year-old Hispanic woman is seen in clinic for evaluation of abdominal pain of 2 years duration. The patient reports intermittent epigastric pain that radiates to the back. Each episode lasts from a few hours to a few days, and she frequently has to go to the emergency department during these episodes. Blood tests in the last two emergency department visits were significant for amylase levels of more than 500 IU/mL (range 25-100 IU/mL); other labs from the most recent visit are as follows:

WBC	6500/μL
ALT	20 U/L
AST	19 U/L
Alkaline phosphatase	120 U/L
Total bilirubin	1.2 mg/dL

MRI/MRCP performed during the last episode showed a common bile duct measuring 6 mm with no filling defects. There was no intrahepatic biliary ductal dilation. The pancreatic parenchyma appeared normal with no evidence of pancreatitis. The pancreatic duct was mildly dilated to 5 mm in the body of the pancreas. She recalls that she underwent a cholecystectomy 18 months ago at another hospital because she was then diagnosed with "gallbladder-related complications" for similar symptoms. Which of the following is the most appropriate next step in management?

A. Tramadol as needed
B. Ursodiol
C. Refer for pancreatic manometry
D. EUS of the pancreas
E. ERCP and cholangiogram

77. A 55-year-old Caucasian woman is seen in clinic for evaluation of intermittent lower abdominal pain of 2 years duration. The abdominal pain starts in the hypogastric region and radiates to both flanks. Each episode lasts for a few hours, but she has continuous dull pain in between episodes. The pain often gets worse postprandially and is only partially improved by defecation. She has intermittent diarrhea with urgency, with passage of a small volume of loose stools. Physical exam shows the following:

Temperature	99° F
Heart rate	75 bpm
Respiratory rate	12 breaths/min
Blood pressure	110/65 mm Hg

Her abdomen is mildly tender to palpation in the hypogastrium. Laboratory values are as follows:

WBC	15,000/μL
Hemoglobin	13 g/dL
ALT	22 U/L
AST	134 U/L
Alkaline phosphatase	128 U/L
Total bilirubin	1.2 mg/dL
Lipase	56 IU/L
Amylase	71 IU/L

A right upper quadrant ultrasound reveals cholelithiasis. The common bile duct measures 4 mm. CT abdomen performed during the emergency department visit was significant for complete pancreas divisum but was otherwise normal. Which of the following is the most appropriate next step in management?

A. ERCP with minor papilla cannulation
B. ERCP and cholangiogram
C. HIDA scan
D. Laparoscopic cholecystectomy
E. Colonoscopy

78. A 19-year-old Caucasian man was brought to the hospital after being involved in a motor vehicle accident. He underwent emergent abdominal laparotomy for hemoperitoneum and was found to have hepatic lacerations, splenic rupture, and pancreatic contusion. He underwent a splenectomy and repair of the liver lacerations. The pancreas was explored but no pancreatic laceration was noted; therefore, a drain was placed in the pancreatic bed. The patient had a prolonged postoperative hospitalization. Four weeks after the surgery, he continues to have significant output from the peripancreatic drain. A fluid analysis from the drain output was significant for an amylase level of 5000 IU/mL. A recent CT scan showed no peripancreatic fluid collection, and the pancreatic duct measured 4 mm in the body of the pancreas. Which of the following is the most appropriate next step in management?

A. Place on NPO status, start total parenteral nutrition (TPN), and continue to follow the drain output
B. Abdominal MRI/MRCP
C. Endoscopic retrograde pancreatography
D. Distal pancreatectomy for a distal pancreatic duct leak
E. Lateral pancreaticojejunostomy

79. A 60-year-old Caucasian man with chronic alcoholic pancreatitis presents to the emergency department with abdominal pain of 3 months duration. His pain is described as sharp, in the central abdomen, and made worse after eating. He has been abstinent for the last 6 months. At present, he is on opioid analgesics, which he usually takes after eating food when his pain is the worst. A recent MRI shows pancreatic parenchymal changes consistent with chronic pancreatitis. The pancreatic duct is dilated in the body and tail to 8 mm, with a 4 mm stone is visualized in the neck region of the pancreatic duct. Which of the following is most likely to result in pain improvement?

A. Convert the opioid analgesics to short acting formulations given with food, with nonsteroidal antiinflammatory drugs (NSAIDs) taken for baseline pain control
B. Celiac plexus block for pain control with weaning of opioid analgesics
C. ERCP with pancreatic duct dilation and stone removal
D. Distal pancreatectomy
E. Start him on uncoated pancreatic enzyme supplements combined with acid suppression

80. A 55-year-old man with chronic calcific pancreatitis is referred to you for possible endoscopic management of his pain. He describes his pain as dull, gnawing, continuous, and not related to food. It is localized in the central abdomen and does not improve with analgesics. He is presently on high doses of opioids and pancreatic enzyme supplements with no improvement. A recent abdominal MRI demonstrates atrophic pancreatic parenchyma with heavy parenchymal calcifications in the body and tail. There are multiple strictures and calculi in the pancreatic duct in the body and tail, and the downstream pancreatic duct in the head of the pancreas is not dilated. Which if the following is the most appropriate next step in management?
   A. Refer him to a pancreatic surgeon
   B. Refer him for external shock wave lithotripsy (ESWL)
   C. Perform an EUS-guided celiac plexus block
   D. Refer him for ESWL followed by ERCP for pancreatic duct stricture dilation
   E. Refer him for percutaneous pancreatic drainage and reassess in 6 months

ANSWERS

1. **C** (S&F ch55)
   The midline part of the body of the pancreas overlies the lumbar spine and makes this area susceptible to abdominal trauma. The head and neck of the pancreas are covered anteriorly by the duodenum. The tail is relatively mobile, and its tip rests at the hilum of the spleen.

2. **B** (S&F ch55)
   The pancreas duct cells secrete water and bicarbonate, which constitute the bulk of the pancreatic secretion. Acinar cells secrete small amounts of sodium chloride–rich fluid. Pancreatic stellate cell secretes extracellular matrix components to help maintain the pancreatic microstructure. *Beta* cells secrete insulin and amylin. *PP* cells secrete pancreatic polypeptide and adrenomodullin.

3. **D** (S&F ch55)
   The splenic vein runs posterior to the body of the pancreas. Due to this anatomic proximity, inflammatory or neoplastic diseases of the body and tail of the pancreas can lead to splenic vein thrombosis. This can lead to retrograde flow toward the splenic hilum and engorgement of the short gastric and left gastroepiploic veins, resulting in gastric varices.

4. **E** (S&F ch55)
   The endoscopic appearance is consistent with ectopic pancreatic tissue. This gastric submucosal lesion is usually found incidentally during an esophagogastroduodenoscopy. There is a characteristic central umbilication. The other lesions (GIST, lipoma, carcinoid tumor, and ectopic varices) can present as a submucosal gastric mass, but they do not have the characteristic central umbilication. EUS can be performed to confirm the diagnosis.

5. **A** (S&F ch55)
   Up to 75% of the general population has a common channel between the common bile duct and pancreatic ducts that ranges in length between 1 and 12 mm (average 4.5 mm). Other less common variants include completely separate openings or an interposed septum. Pancreaticobiliary malunion is a congenital malformation in which junction of the bile and pancreatic ducts occurs outside the duodenal wall, resulting in a long common channel (>15 mm) that leads to the duodenal lumen. This malunion allows reflux of bile into the pancreatic duct and pancreatic secretions into the bile duct, which leads to increased risk of pancreatitis, choledochal cysts, and biliary malignancies later in adulthood. Malunion is seen in up to 60% of adults with gallbladder cancer. Annular pancreas is a congenital anomaly that occurs when part of the pancreas forms a thin band around the duodenum. Pancreas agenesis is complete or partial absence of pancreas. Pancreas divisum results from failure of fusion between the dorsal and ventral pancreatic ducts. The majority of pancreatic secretions drain through the minor papilla.

6. **C** (S&F ch55)
   This patient has acute pancreatitis. The upper GI series shows a stricture in the second portion of the duodenum with proximal dilation, compatible with the diagnosis annular pancreas. This congenital condition can present in the pediatric age group or in adulthood. Adult patients usually present in the fourth through the seventh decades of life. Bypassing the narrowed duodenal segment with a duodenoduodenostomy is the preferred surgical treatment, rather than pancreatic resection or division. SMA syndrome refers to compression of the third portion of the duodenum by the SMA and the aorta, and presents with intermittent obstruction unrelated to pancreatitis. Pancreas divisum and choledochal cyst do not present with bowel obstruction and this characteristic finding on upper GI series.

7. **C** (S&F ch55)
   The pancreatic stellate cells secrete collagen and other extracellular proteins to preserve the pancreatic microarchitecture and facilitate acinar sell secretions. These cells get activated during pancreatic injury and provide the necessary matrix for healing. However, with persistent injury, they can induce significant fibrosis and result in chronic pancreatitis. The primary role for acinar cells is secretion of digestive enzymes. Duct cells primarily secrete bicarbonate and water. *Alpha* cells secrete glucagon. *F* cells (also called *PP* cells) secrete pancreatic polypeptide and adrenomedullin.

8. **B** (S&F ch55)
   The MRCP image shows the dorsal pancreatic duct opening into the minor papilla. This is seen above the major papilla, which is the opening of the common bile duct. There is no communication between the dorsal and ventral duct, consistent with a diagnosis of complete pancreas divisum. Although many patients with this condition are asymptomatic, some develop recurrent episodes of acute pancreatitis. This patient appears to have recurrent acute idiopathic pancreatitis. In a randomized control trial, 90% of patients with pancreatic divisum and acute pancreatitis noted symptomatic improvement with pancreatic duct stent placement. Other studies have shown response with minor papilla sphincterotomy and/or stent placement. Genetic mutations such as *SPINK1* and *CFTR* may need to be ruled out in symptomatic patients with pancreas divisum. Cholecystectomy is unlikely to be helpful in this case. Whipple's surgery is not indicated. ERCP with major papilla sphincterotomy and stent placement is not appropriate for pancreas divisum.

9. **C** (S&F ch55)
The functional unit of the exocrine pancreas is composed of the acinar cell and the ductule. The acinar cells synthesize and secrete digestive enzymes. The apical zone of the cell contains zymogen granules that store pancreatic enzymes. The cuboidal cells that line the pancreatic duct generate ATP for ion transport and contain carbonic anhydrase that produces bicarbonate.

10. **A** (S&F ch55)
Failure of the ventral pancreas to rotate around the duodenum leads to annular pancreas. Pancreas divisum occurs when the ventral and dorsal pancreatic buds fails to fuse. Anomalous pancreaticobiliary ductal junction occurs when the junction between the bile duct and pancreatic duct is located outside of the duodenal wall, with a long common channel (>15 mm) Bifid pancreatic duct and ansa pancreatic are abnormalities in the course and shape of the pancreatic ducts and not related to the rotation of the ventral pancreas.

11. **A** (S&F ch56)
Secretin binds to its receptors on the basolateral membrane of the pancreatic duct cell, increasing cAMP levels. This activates the chloride channels, leading to chloride secretion into the lumen. Chloride is exchanged, for bicarbonate in the lumen by the action of the Cl^-/HCO^{3-} antiport. The secretin receptor is not a G protein–gated ion channel, and it does not work on the Na^+/K^+ ATPase.

12. **B** (S&F ch56)
The pancreatic secretory trypsin inhibitor is a 56–amino acid peptide that inactivates trypsin by binding it near its catalytic site, forming a stable complex. The main function of the inhibitor is to inactivate and promote degradation of trypsin that is prematurely formed in the pancreas, thus preventing autodigestion and pancreatitis. It does not enzymatically degrade trypsin. The other functions listed in the answer choices are incorrect.

13. **C** (S&F ch56)
Amylase and lipase are stored and secreted in their active forms. Trypsinogen, chymotrypsinogen, proelastase, procarboxypeptidase, and prophospholipase A2 are stored in the pancreas and secreted into the duodenum as inactive proenzymes.

14. **C** (S&F ch56)
The vagal nerves mediate the cephalic phase of pancreatic secretion, which consists of stimulation of acinar cell enzyme secretion and ductal bicarbonate secretion. This is mediated mainly by acetylcholine. Cholinergic antagonists can significantly diminish pancreatic secretion in the cephalic phase. Other less important mediators include VIP and GRP. The gastric phase of stimulation of pancreatic secretion in response to a meal reaching the stomach and intestinal phase is when chyme first enters the duodenum. Secretin and CCK are important players in the intestinal phase of secretion.

15. **D** (S&F ch56)
Pancreatic enzyme and bicarbonate secretion is regulated by both hormonal and neural pathways. Vagovagal reflexes play a prominent role in this process. CCK, not secretin, is the major mediator for meal stimulated enzyme secretion, and it is secreted from the duodenal mucosa in response to digested fat and protein in the duodenum. Secretin, not CCK, is secreted when the pH in the duodenum drops to less 4.5, and it increases pancreatic bicarbonate and fluid secretion.

16. **C** (S&F ch57)
The clinical presentation and radiographic picture are consistent with meconium ileus. Contrast enema shows meconium in the distal ileum seen as filling defects, in addition to dilated upstream small bowel loops. Distal to the obstruction in the distal ileum, there is an empty and narrow "microcolon." Hirschsprung's disease can present with failure to pass meconium in the neonate; however, contrast enema usually shows a transition between the aganglionic bowel and the normal colon. Contrast enema in intestinal atresia does not show filling defects in the distal ileum. Sigmoid volvulus presents with intestinal obstruction in adults, and barium enema shows a distended loop of sigmoid colon. Annular pancreas may lead to duodenal obstruction, and upper GI series can show the "double-bubble" sign.

17. **D** (S&F ch57)
Treatment of maldigestion from pancreatic exocrine failure in cystic fibrosis requires delivery of active digestive enzymes to proximal small intestine with meals. The enzyme supplements may be inactivated by the low pH in the stomach or in the duodenum, and therefore enteric coated preparations are preferred to protect the enzymes from gastric acidity. This patient has symptoms despite maximal dosing. In these cases, it is recommended to try acid suppression with an H2 receptor antagonists or proton inhibitors to further decrease gastric acid secretions, which may be decreasing the duodenal pH due to impaired duodenal bicarbonate secretions. Switching to uncoated supplements and adding aluminum hydroxide will make the symptoms worse by further inactivating the enzymes. Higher doses of enzymes are no longer recommended due to concern of fibrosing colonopathy. Although multivitamin preparations are recommended, as these patients have malabsorption of vitamins, the underlying symptoms will persist. Most centers do not recommend dietary modification for concern of growth retardation.

18. **A** (S&F ch57)
The patient presents with symptoms of pancreatic insufficiency (steatorrhea), recurrent infections, skeletal malformations, and pancytopenia. This presentation is characteristic of Shwachman-Diamond syndrome (SDS). SDS is the second most common cause of pancreatic insufficiency in infancy and can be differentiated from cystic fibrosis by normal sweat chloride levels. Diamond-Blackfan syndrome is a rare congenital hypoplastic anemia that usually presents early in infancy. Pancreatic agenesis is extremely rare and, along with pancreatic exocrine insufficiency, presents with profound endocrine insufficiency, which this patient does not have. Johanson-Blizzard syndrome is a rare autosomal-recessive syndrome that leads to pancreatic exocrine insufficiency. Unlike SDS, patients with this syndrome have no hematologic abnormalities.

19. **D** (S&F ch57)
Tropical pancreatitis is a form of early onset idiopathic chronic pancreatitis with unique epidemiologic and clinical features. It is characterized by recurrent abdominal pain, pancreatic calculi (which may manifest as calcifications on abdominal x-ray), and diabetes mellitus. It occurs most commonly among children and young adults. Pancreatitis due to atypical *CFTR* mutations, hereditary pancreatitis, and autoimmune pancreatitis may also be diagnosed in adolescents but usually do not present as calcific pancreatitis associated with diabetes. Gallstone pancreatitis is a cause of acute pancreatitis in adolescents and adults, but does not lead to chronic pancreatitis.

20. C (S&F ch57)
The patient likely has hereditary pancreatitis, which is a syndrome of recurrent acute pancreatitis often leading to chronic pancreatitis. It is inherited in an autosomal-dominant pattern and most commonly caused by a gain-of-function mutation in the cationic trypsinogen gene *(PRSS1)*. Cystic fibrosis is more commonly associated with pancreatic insufficiency than recurrent acute pancreatitis. Pancreatitis develops in about 10% of cystic fibrosis patients. These patients usually present during late adolescence or early adulthood. The *SPINK1* mutation is a modifier gene mutation associated with tropical pancreatitis and may make patients with other gene mutations (e.g., *CFTR*) or environmental insults more susceptible to pancreatitis. *CTRC* gene mutations are uncommon gene mutations also associated with tropical pancreatitis. Mutations in the *UBR1* gene are associated with Johanson-Blizzard syndrome, which is a rare inherited disorder that leads to lipomatous transformation of the pancreas and exocrine insufficiency

21. E (S&F ch57)
The incidence of pancreatic cancer in patients with hereditary pancreatitis is significantly increased. Cancer develops about 30 to 40 years after the onset of pancreatitis. Pancreatic cancer can develop in both men and women, and the cumulative risk is 8% to 11% by age 50 and 40% to 55% by age 75. There are no strict guidelines for screening, but some experts recommend screening at age 40 or 45. Tobacco smoking doubles the pancreatic risk, and median age of diagnosis in smokers is 20 years sooner than nonsmokers; therefore, absolute lifetime abstinence from smoking should be strongly recommended and reinforced at each visit.

22. C (S&F ch57)
The patient presents with acute pancreatitis, which is most likely due to hypertriglyceridemia. This is suggested by the presence of xanthomas and also the lactescent serum, which occurs when the serum appears milky at very high triglyceride levels. The most likely cause of hypertriglyceridemic pancreatitis in a young male would be familial hypertriglyceridemia (usually type I, IV, and V) although it can also be seen in secondary hypertriglyceridemia in patients with other conditions such as diabetes, hypothyroidism, and pregnancy. The other choices may result in pancreatitis but are not typically associated with xanthomas and lactescent serum.

23. B (S&F ch57)
The patient's clinical presentation of chronic abdominal pain, pancreatic calcifications, and pancreatic duct stones is consistent with tropical pancreatitis. Familial pancreatitis refers to any type of pancreatitis that runs in families. It may or may not be caused by a specific genetic mutation. Hereditary pancreatitis is a subset of chronic pancreatitis that follows an autosomal-dominant pattern of inheritance. Shwachman-Diamond syndrome and Johanson-Blizzard syndrome lead to pancreatic exocrine insufficiency in childhood.

24. D (S&F ch57)
PRSS1 leads to trypsinogen activation. This is enhanced by the presence of calcium. Activation of *CFTR* "flushes" trypsin to the duodenum and protects from injury. *SPINK1* inhibits trypsin's effects on autoactivation and further damage. *CTRC* facilitates trypsin degradation. Trypsinogen is protected from activation inside the zymogen granule (see figure).

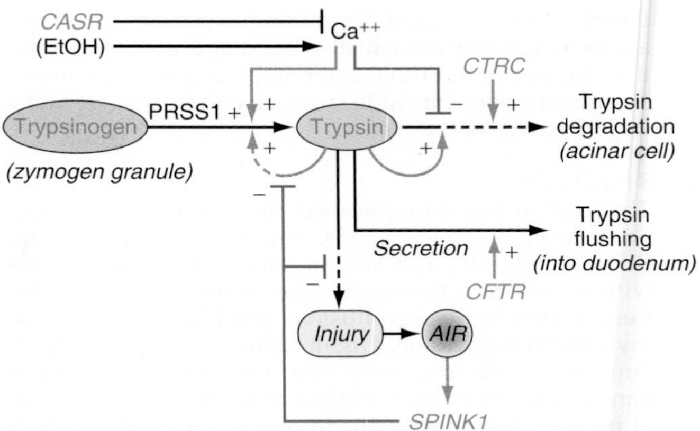

Figure for answers 24 and 25. Diagram of trypsin control mechanisms in the pancreas (*green arrows* are positive, and *red lines* are negative influences). Trypsinogen *(far left)* is protected from activation within the zymogen granules. Trypsinogen activation (*arrow* to trypsin) is supported by elevated calcium (Ca^{++}) and trypsin autoactivation (*green dashed arrow* from trypsin *to the left*). Trypsin degradation is inhibited by calcium, but facilitated by trypsin (*solid green arrow* from trypsin *to the right*) and chymotrypsin-C *(CTRC)*. Mutations in the calcium-sensing receptor gene *(CASR)* or in *CTRC* lead to excess trypsin and eventually pancreatic injury *(yellow)*. After pancreatic injury and an acute inflammatory response (AIR), there is a dramatic up-regulation of *SPINK1*, an acute-phase reactant that inhibits trypsin's effects on autoactivation and further damage. If trypsinogen (and trypsin) can be secreted into the duodenum by a *CFTR*-dependent mechanism, then the pancreas is protected by removal of trypsin from the gland. Blue letters indicate that mutations in the corresponding genes are associated with an increased risk of pancreatitis. Dashed lines indicate a pathway contingent on the absence of inhibition. *CFTR*, cystic fibrosis transmembrane conductance regulator; *PRSS1*, protease serine 1; *SPINK1*, serine protease inhibitor, Kazal type 1.

25. B (S&F ch57)
SPINK1 acts as the first line of defense against prematurely activated trypsinogen in the acinar cell and inhibits trypsin autoactivation. It is considered a modifier gene, rather than a susceptibility gene. A mutation affecting *SPINK1* does not by itself increase the risk of pancreatic disease. However, in someone with a *PRSS1* mutation, the presence of an additional *SPINK1* mutation strongly drives the pancreatic injury and resultant fibrosis. *CFTR l*, not *SPINK1*, leads to trypsin flushing into the duodenum. *CTRC* leads to trypsin degradation (see figure).

26. E (S&F ch58)
The abdominal CT scan shows interstitial pancreatitis without necrosis. There is diffuse swelling of the pancreas with peripancreatic inflammatory changes. Therefore, continuing current supportive care with IV fluids, analgesia, and NPO is appropriate. There is no indication for antibiotics, blood cultures, or surgical consult.

27. A (S&F ch58)
This patient has developed a pancreatic pseudocyst following an episode of acute interstitial pancreatitis. Regardless of their size, most pseudocysts are sterile and can be managed conservatively with clinical follow-up and interval monitoring. Intervention is indicated only if the cysts are symptomatic. This patient has mild abdominal pain but is able to maintain oral intake and not lose weight, and

therefore, he is a good candidate for conservative management. Pseudocysts can also be complicated with infection, rupture or bleeding, and require urgent intervention. Treatment options include surgical, endoscopic, or radiologic drainage of the cyst.

28. **B** (S&F ch58)
This patient has multiple risks for severe acute pancreatitis including age >55, WBC count >12,000/μL, obesity, BUN >20 mg/dL, and multiorgan failure. Some patients with severe pancreatitis develop acute respiratory distress syndrome, pleural effusions, renal failure, shock, and myocardial depression. Organ failure is the most important factor affecting morbidity and mortality in acute pancreatitis. Mortality is highest in the first 24 to 48 hours of presentation, mostly due to organ failure. Mortality in the second week is mostly due to infection and multiorgan failure. Patients who are older and have comorbid illnesses have a substantially higher mortality. Around 20% of patients develop a protracted course that lasts weeks to months. Surgical debridement of sterile pancreatic necrosis is not beneficial. When indicated, debridement is typically delayed for 5 or 6 weeks to allow for a less invasive approach (i.e., laparoscopic, percutaneous, or endoscopic).

29. **B** (S&F ch58)
This patient is presenting with a ruptured ectopic pregnancy mimicking acute pancreatitis. The serum amylase is elevated. Elevated serum amylase is not specific to pancreatitis and can be seen in many conditions such as disease of the ovaries and fallopian tubes (e.g., ectopic pregnancy), parotitis, intestinal infarction, and perforated viscus. Serum lipase is considered more specific to pancreatic disease and is normal in this patient, excluding the possibility of significant pancreatic disease.

30. **D** (S&F ch58)
Acute pancreatitis is the most common complication of ERCP. Pathogenesis of post-ERCP pancreatitis is incompletely understood. Factors predisposing to post-ERCP pancreatitis include young age, female gender, suspected sphincter of Oddi dysfunction, recurrent pancreatitis, difficult cannulation, and pancreatic sphincterotomy. NSAIDs, such as rectal diclofenac or indomethacin, have shown promise in decreasing the rate of post-ERCP pancreatitis. Pancreatic (not biliary) stent placement was also shown to be effective. Injections of botulinum toxin and nitroglycerin have not been shown to be effective in preventing post-ERCP pancreatitis.

31. **C** (S&F ch58)
Drug-induced pancreatitis accounts for <1% of pancreatitis cases and tends to occur 4 to 8 weeks after commencing a medication. The pathophysiology is likely a hypersensitivity reaction. Azathioprine is known to be associated with pancreatitis. Drug-induced pancreatitis is typically mild and self-limited once the offending medication is discontinued. Pancreatitis can recur upon reexposure to the medication. The diagnosis should only be considered after ruling out other more common etiologies, such as alcohol, gallstones, hypertriglyceridemia, and hypercalcemia. Although triglyceride level was high in this patient, levels associated with pancreatitis are typically >1000 IU/L. Amlodipine and infliximab are not known to be associated with pancreatitis.

32. **B** (S&F ch58)
Early aggressive IV fluid replacement in acute pancreatitis is extremely important to prevent progression and complications in acute pancreatitis. The goal is to decrease BUN and hematocrit and increase pancreatic perfusion. Adequate resuscitation should result in adequate urine output, which decreases the risk of renal failure. Fluid resuscitation is most beneficial in the first 12 hours of admission. Generally 250 mL to 400 mL/hour of lactated Ringer's solution or normal saline is adequate for the first 24 to 48 hours. Antibiotics are not recommended for the management of mild acute pancreatitis without evidence of infection. ERCP could be indicated in this patient if the bilirubin increases or if an MRCP shows a common bile duct stone. However, there is no evidence of cholangitis at this time, and fluid resuscitation remains the most important treatment. Inserting an NG tube is appropriate because the patient has nausea and abdominal distension, but it is not a priority. Abdominal CT scan is not really needed at this time because the diagnosis of pancreatitis is established. It should not delay aggressive IV fluid resuscitation.

33. **A** (S&F ch58)
Based on the 2012 revised Atlanta classification of acute pancreatitis, severe acute pancreatitis is defined as pancreatitis associated with persistent (>48 hours) single or multiorgan system failure. Other accepted definitions of severe pancreatitis include three or more of Ranson's 11 criteria for non-gallstone pancreatitis and APACHE II score >8 (see box at end of chapter).

34. **B** (S&F ch58)
The patient presents with suspected sphincter of Oddi dysfunction, which increases the risk of post-ERCP pancreatitis (PEP). Female, rather than male, gender is associated with PEP. Pancreatic sphincterotomy and injection, rather than biliary sphincterotomy or injection, are risk factors for PEP. Younger age is associated with PEP. Other risk factors for PEP in this patient include his normal bilirubin level (see box at end of chapter).

35. **D** (S&F ch58)
In severe acute pancreatitis, enteral feeding was shown to be safer than parenteral nutrition and is associated with less septic complications. Therefore, total parenteral nutrition (TPN) should be avoided as much as possible. There is no indication for prophylactic antibiotics or CT-guided aspiration unless there are signs of infection. Infections usually occur after the first week. Interventions to treat pancreatic fluids collections and necrosis, if needed, are better delayed for 4 to 5 weeks. This allows the formation of a fibrous wall around the fluid or necrotic materials, and a less invasive drainage or debridement procedure can be performed.

36. **D** (S&F ch58)
Small stones are more likely to pass through the cystic duct and cause obstruction at the ampulla. Therefore, pancreatitis is more likely to occur when the gallstones are small (<5 mm). ERCP is not indicated in all cases of elevated liver enzymes. It is performed in patients with suspected cholangitis or when other predictors of persistent choledocholithiasis are present (dilated CBD, elevated bilirubin, or abnormal imaging). Only 3% to 7% of individuals with gallstones develop pancreatitis. The disease is more common in women. Recurrence is extremely rare after cholecystectomy and bile duct clearance.

37. **E** (S&F ch58)
The chest x-ray shows multilobar alveolar infiltrates and interstitial thickening, which is consistent with acute

respiratory distress syndrome (ARDS). This is a serious pulmonary complication of acute pancreatitis and can lead to significant hypoxia and increased mortality. Pancreatic phospholipase A2 plays a major role in pathogenesis. It digests lecithin, a major component of surfactant in the pulmonary alveoli, and results in interstitial edema. Symptoms and signs usually commence between the second and seventh day. It results in bilateral pulmonary interstitial edema secondary to increased alveolar capillary permeability. Patients usually need endotracheal intubation with positive end-expiratory pressure ventilation. Low tidal volumes are preferred to prevent pulmonary volutrauma. Unless infection is suspected, there is no need for antibiotics. With supportive treatment, lung function and structure is expected to return to normal after recovery from the acute injury.

38. **C** (S&F ch58)
Abdominal ultrasound is indicated in acute pancreatitis to check for gallstones. CT scan is mainly indicated to exclude other intraabdominal etiologies of abdominal pain if the diagnosis of acute pancreatitis is not clear. It is also indicated if patients do not improve within 48 to 72 hours to check for complications. MRI/MRCP is excellent modality to check for choledocholithiasis when suspected based on the laboratory tests and ultrasound. HIDA scan is indicated to check for acute cholecystitis if ultrasound is inconclusive. EUS is not indicated for evaluation of the pancreas in acute pancreatitis. EUS is very sensitive (as good as MRCP and ERCP) for the detection of choledocholithiasis and could be helpful in certain patients suspected to have bile duct stones.

39. **B** (S&F ch58)
Unlike the Ranson and APACHE-II scores, the BISAP score is a simple scoring system for acute pancreatitis that can be used within the first 12 hours to predict severity and identify patients at risk for complications and mortality. This score gives one point for each of the following: BUN >25 mg/dL, impaired mental status, systemic inflammatory response syndrome, age >60, and pleural effusion. A score of 4 or 5 indicates a sevenfold to twelvefold increased risk of organ failure. The Rockall and Blatchford scores are used to assess severity in acute upper GI bleeding, not in acute pancreatitis.

40. **A** (S&F ch59)
Pancreas cancer risk is increased in all forms of chronic pancreatitis (lifetime risk is round 4%), but the highest risk is seen in hereditary pancreatitis, particularly in smokers, with a cumulative risk up to 40%. EUS (despite being challenging in the settings of chronic pancreatitis) is superior to CT scan for the detection of pancreatic adenocarcinoma, especially small lesions. Serum level of cancer antigen 19-9 is increased in up to 80% of patients with pancreas adenocarcinoma. The use of this marker and other screening strategies for pancreas cancer is not considered cost-effective (and is not recommended) for patients with chronic pancreatitis, although patients with hereditary pancreatitis may benefit from screening.

41. **E** (S&F ch59)
Steatorrhea and azotorrhea (protein maldigestion) do not usually occur until pancreatic enzyme secretion is reduced to <10% of the maximum output. Affected patients may present with diarrhea and weight loss. Some patients present with bulky foul smelling stools or even frank oil droplets in the stool. Steatorrhea is a late manifestation of chronic pancreatitis, with a median time of onset of 13 years in patients with alcoholic chronic pancreatitis.

42. **A** (S&F ch59)
Malabsorption and deficiency of fat-soluble enzymes (A, D, E, and K) could develop in patients with steatorrhea. The other micronutrients (folate, vitamin B_{12}, biotin, and vitamin C) are not particularly affected in cases of steatorrhea.

43. **A** (S&F ch59)
Direct hormonal stimulation is the most sensitive test for chronic pancreatitis. This is usually done by measurement of bicarbonate or enzyme output after administration of a secretagogue (secretin, CCK, or both). These tests are only available in specialty referral centers. Very low blood level of trypsinogen and low fecal elastase can be seen in advanced chronic pancreatitis, but the sensitivity is generally low in early disease. Abnormal fecal fat excretion can be seen in substantial steatorrhea but is not sensitive in early disease. ERCP is sensitive for chronic pancreatitis, especially in the advanced stages (up to 90%); however, hormonal stimulation is more sensitive and specific than ERCP. Subtle abnormalities of the pancreatic duct seen during ERCP can be age related and nonspecific.

44. **C** (S&F ch59)
Endoscopic therapy for chronic pancreatitis is appropriate in patients with dilated pancreatic duct with a single dominant stricture or stone in the head of the pancreas. Surgical drainage procedures (e.g., lateral pancreaticojejunostomy) are an alternative in patients who are fit for surgery. Given the short-term effect, celiac plexus block is not routinely used in patients with chronic pancreatitis. There is no evidence of pancreas divisum on the pancreatogram, and minor papilla sphincterotomy is not indicated. Pancreas enzymes replacement may be helpful in female patients with idiopathic chronic pancreatitis (small duct disease). Whipple's procedure is usually reserved for patients in whom malignancy cannot be ruled out or there is associated biliary or duodenal obstruction.

45. **D** (S&F ch59)
This patient presents with classic presentation of autoimmune pancreatitis type 1. Given no evidence of malignancy on CT and EUS, it is reasonable to proceed with a trial of glucocorticoids, which usually results in dramatic response with resolution of symptoms and radiologic manifestations. Whipple's procedure will be appropriate if malignancy cannot be ruled out. Celiac plexus neurolysis is used to treat pain in terminally ill patient with pancreatic carcinoma. Lateral pancreaticojejunostomy is a drainage procedure used for large duct chronic pancreatic. When indicated, ERCP can help evaluate the pancreatic duct in autoimmune pancreatitis, but given the risks associated with ERCP, MRCP is usually performed first.

46. **C** (S&F ch59)
Type 1 autoimmune pancreatitis represents the pancreatic manifestation of a systemic disease (IgG4-related disease). It is characterized by elevated IgG4 levels, and is associated with extrapancreatic manifestations, including sialoadenitits, retroperitoneal fibrosis, renal mass, biliary strictures, and lymphadenopathy. It is not typically associated with inflammatory bowel disease (IBD). However, type 2 disease is seen in association with IBD in up to 30% of cases. Type 1 is more common in males. Histology is characterized by a periductal lymphoplasmacytic infiltrate, obliterative phlebitis, storiform fibrosis, and >10 IgG4 cells/HPF. Options A, B, and D are all characteristic of type 2 autoimmune pancreatitis.

It commonly presents with painless jaundice and a pancreatic mass. If the patient has severe cachexia and pain, then pancreatic cancer should be strongly suspected. Type 2 autoimmune pancreatitis (idiopathic duct-centric pancreatitis) constitutes 20% of all cases of autoimmune pancreatitis and usually present at young age (mean age 40 to 50 years). Male and females are affected equally. Histology is characterized by neutrophilic infiltration with micro-abscesses.

47. C (S&F ch59)
Administration of 30,000 IU of lipase with each meal and snack should be sufficient to eliminate steatorrhea. This amount of lipase is equivalent to around 10% of the normal pancreatic enzyme output. The most common reason for pancreas enzyme therapy failure is suboptimal dosing. The supplements should be taken over the course of the meal (during and at the end of the meal).

48. C (S&F ch59)
The clinical presentation of abdominal pain, acute drop in hemoglobin, and a history of pancreatic pseudocyst should raise the suspicion of a pseudoaneurysm. If emergent upper endoscopy is negative, an emergent CT scan with IV contrast should be done (preferably without oral contrast). Positive findings of a pseudoaneurysm should be followed immediately by angiography and embolization. ERCP is unlikely to be helpful in this case. Technetium-99m–labeled red blood cell scan and capsule study would be indicated for evaluation of obscure GI bleeding.

49. D (S&F ch59)
Men are more likely to develop chronic alcoholic pancreatitis, which could be explained by more alcohol use and possibly genetic factors. Only 2% to 5% of chronic alcohol users eventually develop chronic pancreatitis. When activated by alcohol and other inflammatory cytokines, pancreatic stellate cells (not ductal cells) have a central role in secretion of extracellular matrix protein, eventually leading to fibrosis. After the diagnosis of alcoholic chronic pancreatitis, cessation of alcohol may slow down but does not stop the progression to exocrine and endocrine insufficiency.

50. D (S&F ch59)
EUS-guided drainage is the most appropriate therapy to offer this patient. Pseudocysts occurring in a chronic pancreatitis do not resolve as commonly as those occurring after acute pancreatitis. Conservative treatment is reasonable for patients with minimal or no symptoms. Symptomatic, large, and complicated pseudocysts typically require some form of treatment. Unlike pseudocysts after acute pancreatitis, pseudocysts associated with chronic pancreatitis are usually mature at the time of diagnosis. Percutaneous drainage is not the first-line treatment modality in the management of pseudocysts due to the risk of recurrence and fistula formation after removal of the drain. This occurs due to ductal obstruction downstream from the pseudocyst in most cases. Endoscopic and surgical drainage of pseudocysts are both very effective, but endoscopic treatment is preferred because it is associated with shorter hospital stay, better quality of life, and lower costs. Using the EUS-guided approach was found to reduce complications such as bleeding.

51. A (S&F ch59)
In type 2 autoimmune pancreatitis, the histologic pattern is referred to as idiopathic duct-centric pancreatitis. The pancreas demonstrates neutrophilic infiltration with microabscesses (granulocyte epithelial lesion [GEL]). The other answer choices are the histologic criteria for the diagnosis of type 1 autoimmune pancreatitis.

52. D (S&F ch59)
EUS features suggestive of chronic pancreatitis are shown in the table at end of the chapter. Hyperechoic foci, strands, lobularity of the pancreatic contour, and main pancreatic duct calculi are some of these features. Anechoic duct margins and a homogenous, granular parenchyma are normal findings.

53. B (S&F ch59)
This patient with chronic pancreatitis and pseudocyst formation is presenting with respiratory distress due to a rapidly reaccumulating left-sided pleural effusion. This presentation is suggestive of pancreatic pleural effusion. It is unlikely that a parapneumonic effusion would rapidly reaccumulate, especially if the pneumonia was properly treated. A high pleural fluid amylase level is diagnostic. Pleural effusions secondary to chronic pancreatitis usually occur after rupture of a pseudocyst. The fluid tracks into the pleural space, forming an internal fistula that leads to recurrent pleural effusions. Treatment consists of bowel rest, TPN, thoracentesis/chest tube placement, and octreotide. Evaluation of the pancreatic duct for leakage with an MRCP/MRI or ERCP should be considered. A therapeutic ERCP could be performed to bridge the site of pancreatic leak with stent placement. Pleural fluid cytology, cell count and culture, and bronchoscopy/lavage would not diagnose pancreatic pleural effusion. A chest CT scan would further evaluate the chest cavity and lung parenchyma but would not aid in establishing the pancreatic etiology of this pleural effusion.

54. C (S&F ch60)
Patients with Peutz-Jeghers syndrome with *STK11* gene mutations have an 11% to 36% cumulative risk of pancreatic cancer by age 65 to 70 years. The other syndromes are associated with an overall lower risk of pancreatic cancer compared to Peutz-Jeghers syndrome: hereditary breast/ovarian cancer syndrome, 1.2% to 3%; Lynch syndrome, 4%; familial pancreatic cancer (two or more first–degree relatives with pancreatic cancer) ~10%; and FAMMM, ~17%.

55. B (S&F ch60)
Because pancreatic cancer carries a dismal prognosis, screening options for high-risk individuals are being studied in an attempt to diagnose pancreatic cancer early. It is known that the number of first degree relatives with pancreatic cancer strongly influences individual cancer risk. Patients having two affected first-degree relatives have a 6.4-fold increased risk, and those having three or more have a 32-fold increased risk over the general population. Although there are no evidence-based guidelines, the International Cancer of the Pancreas Screening (CAPS) consortium recommends screening for pancreatic cancer in patients with two or more first-degree relatives, or those from familial pancreatic cancer kindreds. It is unclear if patients with just one first-degree relative with pancreatic cancer are at increased risk; however, based on current recommendations, the patient does not need screening. Screening is usually performed with MRI or EUS of the pancreas, and there is no consensus regarding the frequency of screening. Saliva-based genetic tests are being studied but are not routinely available.

56. **A** (S&F ch60)
New onset diabetes in a 65-year-old man with a strong smoking history, abdominal pain, and weight loss are very concerning for pancreatic adenocarcinoma. Jaundice in pancreatic adenocarcinoma is usually due to obstruction of common bile duct by tumor in the pancreatic head and leads to earlier diagnosis of these tumors when compared to tumors in the body and tail, which usually are asymptomatic in the early stage and then present with pain due to invasion of retroperitoneum or neural plexuses and weight loss as the tumor advances. Autoimmune pancreatitis can present with abdominal pain and weight loss, but severe weight loss is unusual. It is less common that pancreatic adenocarcinoma. Pancreatic neuroendocrine tumors (PNETs) frequently are diagnosed incidentally or if they grow very large in size due to their mass effect. Although patients with pancreatic neuroendocrine tumors may present as above, these symptoms in association with smoking and new onset diabetes after the age of 60 are very concerning for adenocarcinoma, which is by far more common than PNETs. Although this patient may also have chronic pancreatitis, chronic pancreatitis in itself is also a risk factor for pancreatic adenocarcinoma. Solid pseudopapillary tumors are rare heterogeneous neoplasms, most commonly seen in young women and not associated with significant weight loss.

57. **C** (S&F ch60)
The patient has presented with what appears to be mild diverticulitis and an incidental pancreatic cystic lesion. The imaging characteristics with numerous tiny cysts separated by delicate fibrous septa (honeycomb appearance) is consistent with serous cystadenoma. Mucinous cystic neoplasms are usually solitary cysts with few septations. Solid pseudopapillary neoplasms are solid tumors with a well-demarcated fibrous capsule. Pancreatic adenocarcinomas are solid lesions. Intraductal papillary mucinous neoplasms do not have the honeycomb appearance that is characteristic of serous cystadenomas.

58. **E** (S&F ch60)
The patient has obstructive jaundice with possible obstruction in the distal common bile duct (CBD) or the ampulla, based on the image and the CT report. The best option in this case would be to proceed to ERCP to endoscopically evaluate the ampulla, distal CBD, and to relieve the obstructive jaundice. Although an MR may help in better visualization of the head of pancreas, the etiology in this case may be in the ampulla or within the CBD because the pancreas has been visualized and reported as normal in the CT scan with no pancreatic ductal dilation. Continuous dilation of both intrahepatic and extrahepatic ducts with obstructive jaundice is not the classic presentation for a choledochal cyst. Therefore, cyst excision is not indicated. Liver biopsy is not appropriate for workup of extrahepatic obstructive jaundice and may lead to bile leak through the capsule of the liver.

59. **C** (S&F ch60)
The patient has a stage 1b (T2N0M0) lesion on imaging and therefore is an excellent candidate for curative resection, which in his case could be achieved by pancreaticoduodenectomy because the tumor is located in the head of the pancreas. EUS FNA is often done for tissue diagnosis when chemotherapy is planned or the diagnosis is unclear. However, tissue diagnosis is not required in this patient due to presence of localized, resectable disease. Neoadjuvant therapy is not indicated for resectable tumors. Routine preoperative ERCP and biliary stenting to relieve jaundice has not been shown to decrease postoperative morbidity and mortality and may increase the likelihood of surgical infectious complications.

60. **A** (S&F ch60)
Based on the MRI, the patient falls into the borderline resectable group of patients with pancreatic cancer. These are the patients who have localized disease but have relative contraindications to curative resection, which include venous involvement of the SMV/portal vein demonstrating tumor abutment with or without impingement and narrowing of lumen, encasement of the SMV/portal vein, tumor abutment of an SMA <180 degrees, and gastroduodenal artery encasement up to the hepatic artery. Neoadjuvant chemotherapy or chemoradiation is used in these patients in an attempt to downstage the tumor for resectability, although data for this approach is based on nonrandomized trials. Large multicenter trials are ongoing to better study this population. All patients undergoing neoadjuvant therapy need to have a tissue diagnosis prior to the start of therapy; therefore, this patient should undergo ERCP/EUS for cytology and drainage prior to referral to oncology. The patient is yet not unresectable and may get downstaged for a possible resection; therefore, placing a nonremovable, uncovered metal stent in the bile duct is not recommended and should be reserved for unresectable tumors.

61. **D** (S&F ch60)
This patient with metastatic pancreatic cancer would best be served by an ERCP with placement of an uncovered metal stent in the bile duct to achieve long-term biliary drainage. Chemotherapy has also been shown to decrease disease-related symptoms like pain and weight loss and also improve survival compared to controls. Surgery for combined biliary and duodenal bypass is very effective, but it is associated with greater morbidity and mortality than endoscopic procedures. Moreover, this gentleman does not exhibit any signs of gastric outlet obstruction and does not need duodenal diversion presently.

62. **C** (S&F ch60)
The patient is presenting with lipase hypersecretory syndrome, which is a feature of metastatic acinar carcinoma and manifests as subcutaneous nodules (which are due to peripheral fat necrosis), polyarthropathies, and elevated lipase levels. This may occur as the tumor arises from acinar cells and is associated with systemic release of pancreatic enzymes, including trypsin, chymotrypsin, amylase, and lipase. Pancreatic adenocarcinoma with liver metastasis is not associated with elevated lipase levels. Acute pancreatic fluid collections and IPMNs are more cystic on imaging, with IPMNs being frequently intrapancreatic. Solid pseudopapillary tumors are large heterogeneous encapsulated mass lesions classically seen in young females and often incidentally diagnosed on imaging performed for another reason.

63. **D** (S&F ch60)
The patient has primary pancreatic lymphoma (PPL), which is suggested by cytologic features of discohesive lymphocytes with large nuclei with prominent nucleoli and diagnosed by flow cytometry. Clinically, PPL may be difficult to distinguish from pancreatic adenocarcinoma but should be suspected in the setting of a large infiltrating mass, not associated with dilation of the pancreatic duct. These tumors are treated by chemoradiotherapy, not surgery, and have a much better prognosis than

adenocarcinoma. Nutritional support could be appropriate for acute necrotizing pancreatitis, which usually has a characteristic clinical presentation and is diagnosed by nonenhancing pancreatic parenchyma on contrast-enhanced CT scan.

64. **E** (S&F ch60)
A large heterogenous encapsulated mass arising from the pancreas in a young female is very suggestive of a solid pseudopapillary tumor. These tumors commonly present with abdominal pain or are diagnosed incidentally. Most of these tumors demonstrate benign behavior, although they have malignant potential and therefore should be resected. Serous cystadenomas usually present later in life and are characterized by numerous tiny cysts separated by delicate fibrous septa (honeycomb appearance). Pancreatic pseudocysts are thick-walled cystic lesions, typically with an antecedent history of pancreatitis, which this woman does not have. Acute trauma does not present with pancreatic fluid collections, which usually take days to weeks to accumulate. Acinar cell carcinomas present similar to pancreatic adenocarcinoma in the sixth decade and are more common in males.

65. **A** (S&F ch60)
The EUS appearance of honeycombing is due to numerous tiny cysts separated by delicate fibrous septae that are typical for serous cystadenoma. These cysts are filled with clear watery fluid and often arranged around a stellate scar that may be calcified. Unlike mucinous cystadenomas, serous cystadenomas are benign and can be followed with surveillance imaging if the patient is asymptomatic. Central calcification is pathognomonic of serous cystadenomas and is not a sign of malignant transformation. Surgical resection is only necessary for symptomatic patients. Serum chromogranin levels are useful for some neuroendocrine tumors. ERCP may be useful for evaluating ductal communication in pseudocysts but not for serous cystadenomas. PET scans are not helpful in benign pancreatic lesions because benign lesions do not accumulate fluorodeoxyglucose.

66. **D** (S&F ch60)
The endoscopic picture shows a patulous ampulla of Vater with dilated pancreatic orifice-extruding mucus ("fish-eye" ampulla), which is pathognomonic for main pancreatic duct intraductal papillary mucinous neoplasm.

67. **E** (S&F ch60)
The International Association of Pancreatology guidelines require the histologic presence of ovarian type stroma within the tumor to establish the diagnosis of MCN. MCNs are strongly female predominant with a 20:1 female-to-male ratio. MCNs and IPMNs are two distinct neoplasms with different genetics, biologic behaviors, and prognoses. They have a significant malignant potential, and therefore surgical resection is advocated for all cases, if possible. Serous cystadenomas, rather than MCNs, are characterized by numerous tiny cysts separated by delicate fibrous septa. Cyst ablation with varying percentages of alcohol remains experimental therapy and is not widely used.

68. **C** (S&F ch60)
The main differential diagnosis of the patient's pancreatic cystic lesion include a pseudocyst, and mucinous cystic neoplasms. Although chronic pseudocysts may have thick walls and septations, these patients often have a history of acute or chronic pancreatitis, or abdominal trauma, whereas most patients with cystic tumors lack such antecedent factors. EUS allows detailed characterization of the cyst wall, FNA of the cyst contents, and cyst fluid analysis. This helps in characterization of cystic neoplasms (see table at the end of the chapter).

69. **A** (S&F ch60)
Although the prognosis after resection of noninvasive IPMNs is excellent, disease recurrence in pancreatic remnant is often seen after resection of noninvasive IPMNs. After resection for benign IPMNs, the prevalence of both new IPMNs and invasive cancer increases over time. The American Gastroenterology Association recommends indefinite postoperative follow-up and surveillance with MRI every 2 years in patients with invasive cancer or dysplasia in a cyst that has been surgically resected. Repeat FNA of the remnant pancreas in the absence of a visualized lesion is not appropriate. Pancreatectomy should be reserved for patients with recurrent disease, which this patient does not have.

70. **D** (S&F ch60)
Incidental pancreatic cystic lesions are increasingly being recognized in cross-sectional imaging. Imaging and endosonographic criteria frequently help in classifying these cystic lesions into benign or malignant cystic lesions, or as pseudocysts, and are quite sensitive for diagnosing serous cystadenomas. CEA and amylase levels are frequently helpful in classifying cysts as pseudocysts (high amylase, low CEA), mucinous cystic neoplasms (low amylase, high CEA), or IPMN (high CEA, high amylase). However, sometimes small cystic lesions may not be satisfactorily classified even though imaging criteria may not suggest malignant transformation (lack of thick walls, mural nodules, large size, or wall calcifications). The optimal management of patients whose cystic lesions are not classified should be individualized. These cysts should be resected if they appear concerning for malignant transformation, or should be followed with serial imaging if they appear benign until their growth patterns have been established.

71. **C** (S&F ch61)
The patient has clinical gallstone pancreatitis and elevated bilirubin. She has a moderate likelihood of having choledocholithiasis, and an MRI/MRCP is indicated. Other options include endoscopic ultrasound or intraoperative cholangiogram during cholecystectomy. The indication for an early ERCP in patients with gallstone pancreatitis is suspected biliary obstruction with clinical cholangitis. Although there is some evidence that early laparoscopic cholecystectomy in mild biliary pancreatitis can improve outcomes and decrease need for ERCP, emergent cholecystectomy is not indicated in patients with mild biliary pancreatitis with no evidence of gangrenous or necrotizing cholecystitis. Intravenous antibiotics are not indicated for gallstone pancreatitis unless complicated by cholangitis or infected pancreatic necrosis. Abdominal CT scan is not indicated unless there is a suspicion of other intraabdominal pathology, complication, or in patients who do not improve in 48 to 72 hours.

72. **B** (S&F ch61)
Drainage for pseudocysts forming after a solitary acute attack of pancreatitis is indicated in symptomatic patients (abdominal pain, weight loss, nausea, and vomiting). Asymptomatic pseudocysts, especially in the absence of pancreatic ductal leaks, may resorb on their own. Progressive increase in the size of the pseudocyst or nonresolution

of large asymptomatic pseudocysts are suggested indications for drainage. At this time, this patient should be followed conservatively because he is asymptomatic and does not have a progressively enlarging pseudocyst. Both CT of the abdomen and MRI of the abdomen are very good imaging modalities for the pancreas, although some studies suggest that MRI is more sensitive for evaluation of pancreatic ducts. At this point, because this patient is asymptomatic with a simple pseudocyst, there is no need to repeat imaging immediately. Depending on local preference, he could get repeat imaging in a few months with either an MRI/MRCP or a CT of the pancreas.

73. **E** (S&F ch61)
Recurrent pseudocysts may occur in 5% to 20% of patients undergoing endoscopic drainage. In these cases, a persistent pancreatic duct leak should be suspected and investigated with an ERP. Pancreatic duct leak into the pseudocyst cavity may be missed on cross-sectional imaging due to the mass effect of a large pseudocyst. If a pancreatic duct leak is found, then the endoscopic drainage method of choice would be transpapillary drainage, with the goal of bridging the pancreatic duct leak. Surgical, endoscopic, or percutaneous drainage would decompress the pseudocyst but would not address a pancreatic duct leak, if present. Spontaneous resolution of the pseudocyst is unlikely after 3 months, and given that he is symptomatic, conservative management is not appropriate.

74. **A** (S&F ch61)
Pancreatic necrosis may occur on or after the fourth day of onset of pancreatitis and may manifest as lack of improvement or worsening in the patient's clinical status. Acute noninfected pancreatic necrosis is best managed conservatively with early introduction of nutritional support, preferably using the enteral route. Early surgical intervention in sterile necrosis has worse outcomes than conservative management. Antibiotic prophylaxis is no longer recommended for sterile necrosis because it has no survival advantage and may lead to development of antibiotic resistance or fungal infection.

75. **D** (S&F ch61)
Infected pancreatic necrosis should be suspected in patients with severe acute pancreatitis and deteriorating clinical status. Other sources of infection should be carefully ruled out. Once infected pancreatic necrosis is suspected, an attempt should be made to identify the organism by FNA (usually with a CT-guided approach) of the necrosis and provide targeted antibiotic therapy. If FNA is inconclusive, broad-spectrum antibiotic therapy (ofloxacin, meropenem) may be used. Antifungal therapy is not recommended at the time of initial diagnosis of infected pancreatic necrosis unless guided by FNA results. Although infected pancreatic necrosis is an indication for drainage, early surgery (<4 weeks from onset) prior to organization of necrosis is associated with worse outcomes when compared to delayed surgery (>4 weeks after onset) and therefore is not recommended. *Clostridium difficile* infection is unlikely in this patient without diarrhea or colonic dilation, and testing should be avoided.

76. **C** (S&F ch61)
Based on the above presentation, the patient is suspected to have recurrent acute pancreatitis secondary to pancreatic sphincter of Oddi dysfunction. This is manifested as recurrent abdominal pain, elevation of pancreatic enzymes, and dilation of pancreatic duct on imaging. The diagnosis of pancreatic sphincter of Oddi dysfunction is confirmed by pancreatic manometry and treated with sphincterotomy, which can be done at the time of manometry. Tramadol may help with short-term pain relief but does not address the primary etiologic cause of the patient's symptoms. Her biliary imaging and laboratory tests are within normal limits and do not suggest a biliary cause for her pancreatitis; therefore, ERCP and cholangiogram is not helpful. Ursodiol has been used in small studies for biliary microlithiasis and abdominal pain after cholecystectomy; however, it has no role in suspected recurrent pancreatitis in this setting. EUS of the pancreas is useful to look for occult malignancy. However, this patient has recurrent acute pancreatitis, is normal between episodes, and had an MRI/MRCP without evidence of a neoplasm. An EUS exam is unlikely to yield additional useful findings.

77. **E** (S&F ch61)
Pancreas divisum is a congenital anomaly that occurs due to failure of proper fusion of the dorsal and ventral pancreatic ducts and may be seen in 7% of the population. It is rarely a cause of symptoms, which may include recurrent pancreatitis or pancreatic pain. Pancreas divisum in this patient's case is an incidental finding. Similarly, her gallstones do not appear to be related to her symptoms. This patient appears to have nonbiliary and nonpancreatic pain and likely has irritable bowel syndrome (diarrhea-predominant subtype). Therefore, further workup for this patient should include colonoscopy with biopsy because she is older than 50 years, and biopsy will evaluate for microscopic colitis. ERCP with minor papillotomy is the treatment of choice in patients suspected to have recurrent pancreatitis due to pancreas divisum. ERCP with cholangiogram is useful in suspected choledocholithiasis. HIDA is considered in patients with suspected acalculous or acute cholecystitis and is not useful in this case. Cholecystectomy is indicated in cases of symptomatic gallstones.

78. **C** (S&F ch61)
The patient appears to have a pancreatic duct leak secondary to pancreatic trauma or due to pancreatic injury from pancreatic exploration. Endoscopic retrograde pancreatography is both diagnostic and therapeutic. Transpapillary pancreatic duct stent placement to bridge the area of leakage is minimally invasive and has a good success rate. The patient continues to have significant output despite 4 weeks of conservative management; therefore, continuing this approach is unlikely to be beneficial. MRCP would help confirm the clinically suspected pancreatic duct leak, which would still require an ERP or surgery for management. Distal pancreatectomy could be helpful in cases of a distal pancreatic duct leak that is not responding to transpapillary drainage. Lateral pancreaticojejunostomy is performed for pancreatic ductal decompression in patients with chronic obstructive pancreatitis and ductal dilation, and is not indicated for this patient.

79. **C** (S&F ch61)
The patient has pancreatic duct obstruction due to a pancreatic duct calculus and likely proximal stricture from chronic pancreatitis, which is resulting in this obstructive pattern of pain. Because he has a solitary calculus and likely a short proximal ductal stricture, he is a good candidate for endoscopic therapy. Weaning off opioid therapy will not be sufficient in this patient. Pancreatic enzyme supplementation is unlikely to result in consistent pain relief and will not resolve the pancreatic obstruction. Celiac plexus block results in temporary pain relief and will not

resolve the pancreatic obstruction. Distal pancreatectomy is an option for surgical management of chronic pancreatitis; however, in this patient, the ductal obstruction is in the head of the pancreas, and therefore he may not benefit from this procedure. Other surgical procedures (e.g., pancreaticojejunostomy) should also be considered in this patient if he is a good surgical candidate and is willing to undergo surgery.

80. **A** (S&F ch61)
This patient has multiple strictures and calculi in the distal pancreatic duct, along with parenchymal calcifications in the body and tail region of the pancreas. Patients with chronic constant pain, distal disease, multiple strictures with calculi, and parenchymal calcification are poor candidates for endoscopic therapy alone and may be best helped by surgery. ESWL helps in breakdown of tough ductal calculi and in conjunction with ERCP is the therapy of choice in large pancreatic calculi. Usually, patients undergoing ESWL need pancreatic ductal stenting to prevent blockage of the duct from stone fragments. In this case, because of the distal location and multiplicity of strictures, ESWL with endoscopic stricture dilation and stenting is challenging and unlikely to be successful. EUS-guided celiac blockade provides temporary relief of pain and is not the preferred treatment in this case. Percutaneous drainage is not feasible or beneficial in chronic calcific pancreatitis.

BOX FOR ANSWER 33 2012 Atlanta Classification Revision of Acute Pancreatitis

Definitions of Grades and Severity of Acute Pancreatitis

Mild Acute Pancreatitis
No organ failure
No local or systemic complications

Moderately Severe Acute Pancreatitis
Transient organ failure (<48 hours) and/or
Local or systemic complications* without persistent organ failure

Severe Acute Pancreatitis
Persistent organ failure (>48 hours) single organ or multiorgan

*Local complications are peripancreatic fluid collections, pancreatic necrosis and peripancreatic necrosis (sterile or infected), pseudocyst, and walled-off necrosis (sterile or infected).

BOX FOR ANSWER 34 Factors That Increase the Risk of Post-ERCP Pancreatitis

Patient Related
Young age, female gender, suspected sphincter of Oddi dysfunction, recurrent pancreatitis, history of post-ERCP pancreatitis, normal serum bilirubin level

Procedure Related
Pancreatic duct injection, difficult cannulation, pancreatic sphincterotomy, balloon dilation of intact sphincter

Operator or Technique Related
Trainee (fellow) participation, nonuse of a guidewire for cannulation, failure to use a pancreatic duct stent in a high-risk procedure

TABLE FOR ANSWER 52 Diagnosis of Chronic Pancreatitis on EUS

Standard EUS Grading System		Rosemont Criteria for EUS Diagnosis	
Parenchymal abnormalities	Hyperechoic foci Hyperechoic strands Lobularity of contour Cysts	Major features	Hyperechoic foci with shadowing (major A) Main pancreatic duct calculi (major A) Lobularity with honeycombing (major B)
Ductal abnormalities	Main-duct dilation Main-duct irregularity Hyperechoic ductal walls Visible side branches Calcification	Minor features	Lobularity without honeycombing Hyperechoic foci without shadowing Stranding Cysts Irregular main pancreatic duct contour Main pancreatic duct dilation Hyperechoic duct margin Dilated side branches

In the Standard EUS Grading System, Each Finding Counts Equally, and the Score is the Total Number of Findings. In the Rosemont System, the Diagnostic Strata are as Follows:

Most consistent with chronic pancreatitis	One major A feature and ≥3 minor features ***or*** One major A feature and major B feature ***or*** Two major A features
Suggestive of chronic pancreatitis	One major A feature and <3 minor features ***or*** One major B feature and ≥3 minor features ***or*** ≥5 minor features
Indeterminate for chronic pancreatitis	3-4 minor features ***or*** One major B feature with <3 minor features
Normal	≤2 minor features

TABLE FOR ANSWER 68 Analysis of Cyst Fluid in Various Cystic Lesions of the Pancreas

Parameter	Pseudocyst	Serous Cystadenoma	MCN-Benign	MCN-Malignant	IPMN
Viscosity	Low	Low	High	High	High
Amylase level	High	Low	Low	Low	High
CEA level	Low	Low	High	High	High
CA 72-4 level	Low	Low	Intermediate	High	Intermediate to high
Cytologic findings	Histiocytes	Cuboidal cells with glycogen-rich cytoplasm	Columnar mucinous epithelial cells with variable atypia	Adenocarcinoma cells	Columnar mucinous epithelial cells with variable atypia

CA, Cancer antigen; CEA, carcinoembryonic antigen; IPMN, intraductal papillary mucinous neoplasm; MCN, mucinous cystic neoplasm.

CHAPTER

8

Biliary Tract

Anthony Gamboa, Steven Keilin, and Emad Qayed

QUESTIONS

1. A 21-day-old female neonate presents with persistent jaundice. The infant's delivery was uneventful at full term. Her stools appear clay colored. On physical exam, the liver is palpable 4 cm below the right costal margin, and there is no splenomegaly. Serum bilirubin level is 10 mg/dL, with a direct bilirubin of 7 mg/dL. Imaging suggests biliary atresia. Exploratory laparotomy with intraoperative cholangiogram is performed and confirms obliteration of the proximal extrahepatic biliary tree. Which of the following is the most appropriate next step in management?
   A. Start glucocorticoids
   B. Start glucocorticoids and ursodeoxycholic acid
   C. Choledochoduodenostomy
   D. Hepatoportoenterostomy
   E. Begin evaluation for liver transplantation

2. An 8-week-old male infant presents with jaundice. He was born at full term after an uneventful pregnancy. Physical exam reveals a palpable mass in the right upper quadrant. Ultrasound of the abdomen shows diffuse fusiform dilation of the bile duct. What is the preferred management for this child?
   A. Serial imaging
   B. Endoscopic retrograde cholangiopancreatography (ERCP) with stent placement
   C. Percutaneous biliary drain placement
   D. Cyst excision and biliary reconstruction
   E. Liver transplantation

3. A 34-year-old female patient is referred to the gastroenterology clinic for evaluation of a dilated common bile duct (CBD). She had an abdominal ultrasound for evaluation of pelvic pain and was found to have a dilated CBD to 14 mm. She denies epigastric or right upper quadrant pain nausea, or vomiting. Abdominal exam reveals a soft, nontender abdomen and no organomegaly. Laboratory values are as follows:

ALT	18 U/L
AST	20 U/L
Alkaline phosphatase	130 U/L
Total bilirubin	1.2 mg/dL

A magnetic resonance cholangiopancreatography (MRCP) shows fusiform dilation of the bile duct extending from the ampulla to the common hepatic duct. There is no abnormality in the pancreaticobiliary junction, and no mass lesion is seen in the pancreas or distal bile duct. Which of the following is the most appropriate next step in management?
   A. Serial imaging
   B. ERCP with stent placement
   C. Percutaneous biliary drain placement
   D. Cyst excision and biliary reconstruction
   E. Observation

4. A 13-year-old girl is seen in clinic for evaluation of recurrent jaundice and cholangitis. She has required percutaneous biliary drainage four times over the last 5 years. A recent cholangiogram is shown (see figure). On physical exam, there is hepatomegaly and mild scleral icterus. Laboratory studies show bilirubin of 4 mg/dL. What is the most appropriate management?

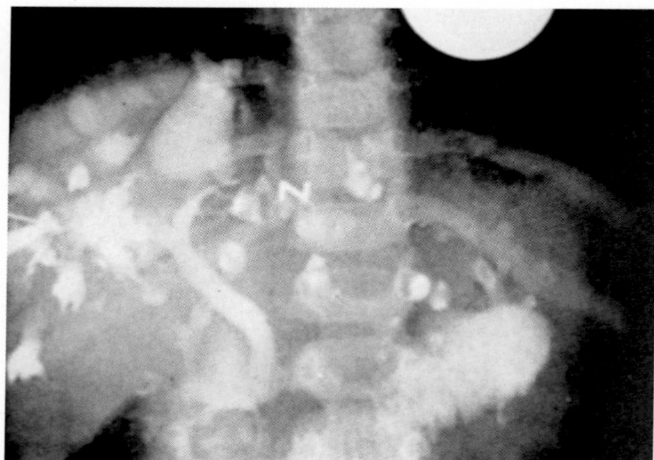

Figure for question 4.

   A. Start ursodeoxycholic acid
   B. Surgical resection of the affected bile ducts
   C. Serial biliary drain changes
   D. ERCP with cholangioscopy
   E. Begin workup for liver transplantation

5. Which of the following is true regarding primary sclerosing cholangitis (PSC) in pediatric populations?
   A. PSC in neonates is associated with ulcerative colitis
   B. Ursodeoxycholic acid has been shown to increase transplant-free survival
   C. 25% to 30% of children with PSC have an overlap syndrome with autoimmune hepatitis
   D. Prednisone and azathioprine have no role in children with PSC and autoimmune hepatitis overlap syndrome
   E. PSC recurs after liver transplantation in >50% of children

6. Which of the following is a risk factor for the development of gallstones in children?
   A. Trisomy 21
   B. Ulcerative colitis

C. Malnutrition
D. Jejunal tube feeds
E. Amoxicillin

7. A 15-year-old male with a history of type 2 diabetes and obesity presents to the emergency department with 3 days of right upper quadrant pain, nausea, and fevers. On presentation, his vital signs are as follows:

Temperature	103° F
Heart rate	120 bpm
Blood pressure	81/42 mm Hg

He is diaphoretic, lethargic, and is not answering questions appropriately. Physical exam reveals tenderness in the right upper quadrant with a positive Murphy sign. Laboratory values are as follows:

WBC	14,000/μL
ALT	50 U/L
AST	40 U/L
Alkaline phosphatase	150 U/L
Total bilirubin	1.2 mg/dL

Abdominal ultrasound shows a distended gallbladder, thickened gallbladder wall, and pericholecystic fluid. In addition to antibiotics, which of the following is the most appropriate management?
A. Watchful waiting
B. Laparoscopic cholecystectomy
C. Percutaneous cholecystostomy drain placement
D. Exploratory laparotomy
E. ERCP

8. An 11-year-old obese female presents with her parents for chronic abdominal pain. Her pain is in the right upper quadrant and is postprandial and intermittent. She is not taking any medications. Physical exam reveals no abdominal tenderness. Laboratory studies, including complete blood count and complete metabolic panel, are normal. Ultrasound of the abdomen reveals a normal-appearing gallbladder and liver with no gallstones. What is the next step in management?
A. Acetaminophen
B. MRI of the abdomen
C. Upper endoscopy
D. Hydroxy-iminodiacetic acid scan
E. Laparoscopic cholecystectomy

9. A 5-month-old infant is admitted to the hospital with worsening jaundice and abdominal distension of 6 weeks duration. She also has dark colored urine and light colored stool. The infant was a full-term baby delivered by normal vaginal delivery. Vitals signs are as follows:

Temperature	99° F
Heart rate	120 bpm
Respiratory rate	25 breaths/min

Physical examination reveals jaundice, abdominal distension, and no organomegaly. The liver and spleen are not enlarged. Laboratory values are as follows:

ALT	15 U/L
AST	17 U/L
Alkaline phosphatase	250 U/L
Total bilirubin is	2.8 mg/dL

Ultrasound reveals no dilation in the bile ducts. Which of the following is the most likely diagnosis?
A. Chronic cholecystitis
B. Choledocholithiasis
C. Biliary atresia
D. Bile leak
E. Cryptogenic cirrhosis

10. A 46-year-old female with intermittent right upper quadrant abdominal pain is found to have gallstones. She undergoes cholecystectomy for symptomatic gallstone disease. Two years later, she continues to have episodic epigastric and right upper quadrant abdominal pain. Her episodes last 1 to 2 hours. During a recent pain episode, she presented to the emergency department and was found to have an ALT of 82 U/L, AST of 72 U/L, and alkaline phosphatase of 120 U/L. Ultrasound at that time showed an 11 mm CBD. What is the appropriate management for this patient?
A. Observation
B. ERCP with sphincter of Oddi (SOD) manometry, followed by sphincterotomy if the basal pressure is elevated
C. ERCP with biliary stent placement
D. ERCP with sphincterotomy
E. Repeat ultrasound and laboratory tests in 6 months

11. A 55-year-old female is seen in clinic for evaluation of abdominal pain of 3 years duration. The pain occurs intermittently in the right upper quadrant, lasts for an hour, and then subsides slowly over the next few hours. She had a cholecystectomy 2 years ago for this type of pain, with minimal improvement. She denies a history of pancreatitis. Review of recent emergency department visits show normal liver enzymes during the pain episodes. Her ultrasound shows a dilated CBD to 11 mm. She had an upper endoscopy that was normal, and a computed tomography (CT) scan performed 6 months prior was unremarkable. The patient is referred for ERCP and manometry. An initial cholangiogram reveals biliary ductal dilation to 12 mm with no stones. A biliary manometry is performed next. Which of the following manometric findings predict pain improvement after biliary sphincterotomy?
A. Increased sphincter phasic contractions (>7/min)
B. Mean basal sphincter pressure >40 mm Hg
C. Peak sphincter pressure >200 mm Hg
D. Increased sphincter retrograde contractions (>50%)
E. Paradoxical response to cholecystokinin stimulation (stimulation instead of inhibition)

12. A 50-year-old female is seen in clinic for evaluation of abdominal pain of 2 years duration. The pain is located in the right upper quadrant, has an abrupt onset, and lasts for about an hour before it subsides slowly. It is often precipitated by food. She had a cholecystectomy 1 year ago for "gallbladder pain." Review of recent emergency department visits show elevated AST and ALT during the pain episodes, which always return to normal levels after the pain subsides. MRCP shows a dilated CBD to 13 mm, with no evidence of choledocholithiasis. The pancreas and liver appeared normal. She had an upper endoscopy 3 months ago that was normal. Which of the following is the most appropriate next step in management?
A. ERCP with SOD manometry, followed by sphincterotomy if increased sphincter basal pressure
B. ERCP with pancreatic sphincterotomy and stent placement
C. ERCP with biliary sphincterotomy
D. ERCP with bile examination for crystals
E. Treatment with ursodeoxycholic acid for 6 months

13. A 46-year-old female with intermittent right upper quadrant abdominal pain is found to have gallstones. She undergoes cholecystectomy for symptomatic gallstone disease. Two years later, she continues to have episodic epigastric and right upper quadrant abdominal pain. Her episodes last 1 to 2 hours. During a recent pain episode, she presented to the emergency department and was found to have the following laboratory values:

ALT	82 U/L
AST	72 U/L
Alkaline phosphatase	120 U/L

Ultrasound at that time showed a 5 mm CBD. What is the appropriate management for this patient?

A. Ursodeoxycholic acid
B. ERCP with SOD manometry, followed by sphincterotomy if the basal pressure is elevated
C. ERCP with biliary stent placement
D. ERCP with ampullary biopsies
E. Repeat ultrasound and laboratory tests in 6 months

14. A 32-year-old male with fibrostenotic ileocolonic Crohn's disease presents with abdominal pain, nausea, vomiting, obstipation, and abdominal distention. CT scan reveals a small bowel obstruction and a stricture in the distal ileum. He undergoes surgery, and 50 cm of ileum are resected. Which of the following is true about the consequences of this resection?

A. Decreased bile acid absorption and watery diarrhea
B. Decreased bile acid absorption and steatorrhea
C. Decreased bile acid content in stool
D. Normal bile acid absorption
E. Decreased total bile acid pool

15. A 26-year-old woman is scheduled to undergo cholecystectomy for biliary pain secondary to gallstones. She inquires about the effects of not having a gallbladder. She has read online that she might develop diarrhea, and she wonders where her bile will be stored. Which of the following is true about postcholecystectomy bile acid storage and diarrhea?

A. Bile is stored in the liver during fasting; diarrhea develops in a subset of patients
B. Bile is stored in the bile ducts during fasting; some patients develop diarrhea, which is treatable with a bile acid sequestrant
C. Bile will be stored in the small intestine during fasting; some patients develop diarrhea, which is treatable with a bile acid supplementation
D. The bile will be stored in the small intestine during fasting; some patients have diarrhea, which is treatable with a bile acid sequestrant
E. Bile will continuously flow into the intestine and the small bowel and the terminal ileum regardless of meals; diarrhea develops in a subset of patients

16. Which of the following is the most abundant solute in bile in healthy individuals?

A. Proteins
B. Bilirubin
C. Cholesterol
D. Phospholipids
E. Bile acids

17. Which of the following statements about the enterohepatic circulation of bile acids is true?

A. 15% of intestinal bile acids are normally excreted in feces
B. Bile acids enter the portal circulation by passive absorption in the distal ileum
C. During fasting, bile acids are concentrated in the gallbladder
D. Enterohepatic cycling of bile acids is accelerated during fasting and slows during a meal
E. Enterohepatic cycling of bile acids occurs 20 to 30 times per day

18. Which of the following is considered a risk factor for cholelithiasis?

A. Rapid weight gain
B. Ulcerative colitis
C. Octreotide
D. Gastrostomy tube feeding
E. Statins

19. A 12-year-old girl with a history of hereditary spherocytosis is found to have gallstones on an ultrasound that was performed to evaluate abdominal pain and abnormal liver enzyme levels. What is the most likely composition of the gallstones?

A. Calcium palmitate
B. Cholesterol
C. Bile salts
D. Calcium phosphate
E. Calcium bilirubinate

20. Which of the following symptoms is consistent with biliary pain secondary to gallstones (biliary "colic")?

A. Upper abdominal pain radiating through to the back
B. Persistent vomiting
C. Intermittent right upper quadrant pain
D. Pain lasting 1 to 6 hours
E. Fevers

21. In which of the following conditions is a prophylactic cholecystectomy recommended?

A. Anomalous pancreaticobiliary junction
B. Sickle cell disease with asymptomatic gallstones
C. Diabetes mellitus with asymptomatic gallstones
D. Primary sclerosing cholangitis with asymptomatic gallstones
E. Large asymptomatic gallstones

22. A 76-year-old white man with a history of hypertension and hypertriglyceridemia, presents with a 3-day history of right upper quadrant pain, nausea, abdominal distension, and constipation. He denies fevers or jaundice. Laboratory values are as follows:

WBC	13,000/μL
ALT	57 U/L
AST	64 U/L
Total bilirubin	1.5 mg/dL
Alkaline phosphatase	160 U/L
Lipase	80 U/L

CT scan of his abdomen shows gallstones, pneumobilia, and diffusely dilated loops of small bowel. Which of the following complications of gallstones is most likely to be found?

A. Pancreatitis
B. Small bowel obstruction
C. Cholangitis
D. Adynamic ileus
E. Mirizzi's syndrome

23. A 28-year-old obese Hispanic woman presents to the emergency department with acute right upper quadrant pain.

The pain is sharp and radiates to the back. She has never experienced similar pain in the past. Physical exam reveals tenderness in the right upper quadrant without Murphy's sign. Ultrasound shows gallstones without gallbladder wall thickening or pericholecystic fluid. Sonographic Murphy's sign is negative. The patient's pain subsides over the next several hours. If the patient does not have a cholecystectomy, what is the likelihood of not having any further episodes of pain?

A. 1%
B. 10%
C. 30%
D. 50%
E. 90%

24. A 53-year-old white male with a history of hypertension, alcohol abuse, and gallstones presents with a 3-day history of right upper quadrant pain, low-grade fevers, and nausea. On physical exam, he has a temperature of 101° F. Abdominal exam reveal tenderness in the epigastrium and right upper quadrant. Laboratory values are as follows:

WBC	13,000/µL
ALT	130 U/L
AST	270 U/L
Alkaline phosphatase	195 U/L
Total bilirubin	2.4 mg/dL

A HIDA scan shows tracer in the small intestine and nonvisualization of the gallbladder. Which of the following is the most likely diagnosis?

A. Acute pancreatitis
B. Cholangitis
C. Acute alcoholic hepatitis
D. Choledocholithiasis
E. Acute cholecystitis

25. A 12-year-old girl with a history of Henoch-Schönlein purpura presents with a 1-day history of crampy right upper quadrant and epigastric pain associated with nausea. On physical exam, she has a temperature of 99° F. Abdominal exam reveals tenderness to palpation in the right upper quadrant and epigastrium. She has a palpable purpuric rash on the lower extremities. Laboratory values are as follows:

WBC	8000/µL
ALT	25 U/L
AST	28 U/L
Alkaline phosphatase	120 U/L
Total bilirubin	1.2 mg/dL

She undergoes a right upper quadrant ultrasound, which shows an enlarged and distended gallbladder. There are no gallstones or gallbladder wall thickening. Which of the following is the most likely diagnosis?

A. Mesenteric vasculitis
B. Acute hydrops of the gallbladder
C. Acute acalculous cholecystitis
D. Pancreatic cancer
E. Biliary dyskinesia

26. A 64-year-old woman presents with acute right upper quadrant pain of 4 hours duration. She has a history of morbid obesity for which she underwent Roux-en-Y gastric bypass surgery and cholecystectomy 1 year prior. On physical exam, she has a temperature of 99° F. Abdominal exam reveals tenderness in the epigastrium and right upper quadrant. Laboratory values are as follows:

WBC	9000/µL
ALT	103 U/L
AST	86 U/L
Alkaline phosphatase	275 U/L
Total bilirubin	1.9 mg/dL

An MRI/MRCP demonstrates a dilated bile duct measuring 12 mm with a single 1 cm filling defect. Which of the following is the most appropriate next step in management?

A. ERCP
B. Surgery with open bile duct exploration
C. Ursodeoxycholic acid
D. Percutaneous transhepatic cholangiogram (PTC)
E. Conservative management

27. A 74-year-old woman present with right upper quadrant pain of 8 hours duration. On physical exam, she has a temperature of 100° F. Abdominal exam reveals tenderness in the epigastrium and right upper quadrant. Laboratory values are as follows:

WBC	13,000/µL
ALT	73 U/L
AST	56 U/L
Alkaline phosphatase	210 U/L
Total bilirubin	2.5 mg/dL

A CT scan of the abdomen is performed (see figure). Without treatment, this patient has a high risk of developing which of the following complications?

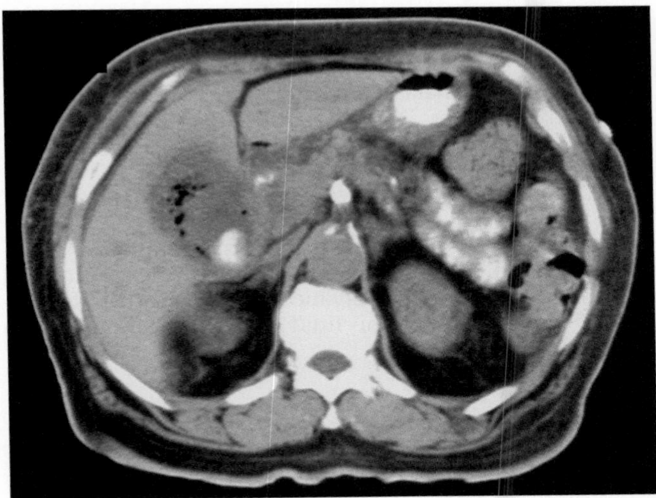

Figure for question 27.

A. Gallbladder perforation
B. Pancreatitis
C. Cholangitis
D. Gallbladder cancer
E. Choledocholithiasis

28. Which of the following ethnicities have the highest prevalence of gallstones?

A. U.S. Hispanics
B. U.S. blacks
C. U.S. whites
D. Native Americans
E. Asians

29. A 40-year-old woman is seen in clinic for evaluation of intermittent right upper quadrant and epigastric pain of 2 years duration. Her pain has a sudden onset, lasts for about an hour, and subsides slowly. She had two attacks of pain in the past 12 months. She is currently pain free. Her past history includes type 2 diabetes, hypertension, and dyslipidemia. She has a blood pressure of 138/74 mm Hg and a body mass index (BMI) of 28.0 kg/m². There is no abdominal tenderness on physical examination. Her fasting lipid panel shows a low-density lipoprotein (LDL) of 150 mg/dL and triglycerides 250 mg/dL. A right upper quadrant ultrasound reveals gallstones without gallbladder wall thickening. She is reluctant to undergo cholecystectomy. She is about to start treatment for dyslipidemia and wonders about the association of lipid-lowering drugs and gallstone formation. Which of the following drugs is associated with increased risk of gallstone formation?
A. Pravastatin
B. Ezetimibe
C. Clofibrate
D. Cholestyramine
E. Nicotinic acid

30. A 34-year-old woman is seen in clinic for evaluation of gallstones. She had an abdominal ultrasound performed for investigation of pelvic symptoms, which revealed incidental gallstones. Her past history includes hypertension, and dyslipidemia. She has a blood pressure of 144/74 mm Hg and a BMI of 32.0 kg/m². There is no abdominal tenderness on physical examination. Laboratory values are as follows:

WBC	9000/μL
ALT	18 U/L
AST	22 U/L
Alkaline phosphatase	120 U/L
Total bilirubin	1.4 mg/dL
LDL	162 mg/dL
Triglycerides	230 mg/dL
HDL	48 mg/dL

She is about to start treatment for dyslipidemia and wonders about the association of elevated cholesterol and gallstone formation. Elevation of which of the following components of the lipid panel is associated with gallstones?
A. LDL
B. VLDL
C. Triglyceride levels
D. HDL
E. Total cholesterol

31. A 32-year-old Korean man presents to the emergency department with acute right upper quadrant pain and fever. He denies prior history of liver or biliary disease. On physical exam, his vital signs are as follows:

Temperature	38.4° C
Heart rate	105 bpm
Blood pressure	110/58 mm Hg

He has an icteric sclera and normal mental status. There is right upper quadrant tenderness. There was no ascites and no stigmata of chronic liver disease. Laboratory values are as follows:

WBC	13,000/μL
ALT	408 U/L
AST	418 U/L
Alkaline phosphatase	220 U/L
Total bilirubin	5.8 mg/dL
Conjugated bilirubin	4 mg/dL

A right upper quadrant ultrasound showed a dilated CBD to 14 mm, with multiple filling defects. The gallbladder appeared normal without stones. He was started on intravenous fluids and broad-spectrum antibiotics. An ERCP was performed. Upon sphincterotomy, there was extrusion of numerous leaf shaped worms. Cholangiogram showed multiple CBD stones. Which of the following types of stones is associated with the patient's parasitic infestation?
A. Brown pigment stones
B. Black pigment stones
C. Cholesterol stones
D. Calcium carbonate stones
E. Fatty acid calcium stones

32. In which of the following clinical scenarios is prophylactic cholecystectomy recommended?
A. 10-year-old Hispanic girl on chronic total parenteral nutrition (TPN) and asymptomatic gallstones
B. 22-year-old black woman with sickle cell disease and asymptomatic pigment gallstones
C. 55-year-old Native-American man with asymptomatic gallstones and focal gallbladder calcification
D. 60-year-old black woman with a 10-year history of diabetes mellitus type 2 and asymptomatic gallstones
E. 68-year-old asymptomatic white woman with a 5 mm polyp of the gallbladder

33. A 22-year-old obese woman presents with sudden-onset right upper quadrant pain of 3 hours duration. She had a normal vaginal delivery 2 weeks prior to presentation. Physical examination shows the following:

Temperature	37.4° C
Heart rate	94 bpm
Blood pressure	112/68 mm Hg

She has no scleral icterus. Abdominal exam shows mild tenderness to deep palpation in the right upper quadrant. Murphy's sign is not present. Laboratory values are as follows:

WBC	9000/μL
ALT	208 U/L
AST	218 U/L
Alkaline phosphatase of	220 U/L,
Total bilirubin	1.4 mg/dL
Lipase	18 U/L

A right upper quadrant ultrasound shows cholelithiasis without signs of cholecystitis. The CBD measures 4 mm. Which of the following is the most appropriate next step in management?
A. ERCP
B. MRCP
C. Endoscopic ultrasound (EUS)
D. Laparoscopic cholecystectomy without cholangiography
E. Laparoscopic cholecystectomy with intraoperative ultrasound

34. A 24-year-old obese woman presents with sudden-onset right upper quadrant pain of 4 hours duration. Vital signs are as follows:

Temperature	37.2° C
Heart rate	98 bpm
Blood pressure	118/78 mm Hg

Physical examination shows scleral icterus. She has mild tenderness to deep palpation in the right upper quadrant.

Murphy's sign is not present. Laboratory values are as follows:

WBC	9000/µL
ALT	408 U/L
AST	418 U/L
Alkaline phosphatase of	250 U/L
Total bilirubin	5.4 mg/dL
Lipase	24 U/L

A right upper quadrant ultrasound shows cholelithiasis without signs of cholecystitis. The CBD measures 8 mm. The next morning her pain has improved. Laboratory studies reveal the following:

ALT	358 U/L
AST	328 U/L
Alkaline phosphatase	220 U/L
Total bilirubin	5.3 mg/dL

Which of the following is the most appropriate next step in management?

A. ERCP
B. MRCP
C. EUS
D. CT scan of the abdomen
E. Laparoscopic cholecystectomy without cholangiography

35. A 32-year-old female patient presents with sudden-onset right upper quadrant pain and fever. Her pain started 6 hours ago, described as severe, sharp, and radiates to the back. Vital signs are as follows:

Temperature	38.6° C
Heart rate	105 bpm
Blood pressure	144/84

Physical examination shows no scleral icterus. She has moderate tenderness to deep palpation in the right upper quadrant. Laboratory values are as follows:

WBC	13,000/µL
ALT	58 U/L
AST	68 U/L
Alkaline phosphatase	150 U/L
Total bilirubin	2 mg/dL
Lipase	28 U/L
Albumin of	4.2 g/dL

Ultrasound shows multiple gallstones. There is no ascites. Which of the following additional findings on ultrasound is the most predictive of acute cholecystitis?

A. Gallbladder wall thickness of 6 mm
B. Focal tenderness in the gallbladder area
C. Pericholecystic fluid
D. Presence of CBD stones
E. Gallbladder distension with sludge

36. An 83-year-old woman presents to the surgical clinic for evaluation of biliary pain secondary to gallstones. Her past medical history includes diabetes, coronary artery disease, and congestive heart failure. She is considered a poor surgical candidate, and the family inquires about medical therapy. Which of the following is true about oral dissolution therapy with ursodeoxycholic acid?

A. Small stones respond as quickly as large stones
B. Small radiolucent calcium bilirubinate stones respond to oral dissolution therapy
C. Nighttime dosing of ursodeoxycholic acid is more effective than mealtime dosing
D. Calcified stones are good targets for dissolution therapy
E. Oral dissolution therapy decreases gallbladder stasis

37. Which of the following characteristics of gallstones is considered an appropriate selection criteria for stone dissolution therapy?

A. Multiple stones
B. Cholesterol stones
C. Stones larger than 10 mm
D. Stones that are not radiolucent on conventional radiographs
E. Stones associated with acute cholecystitis

38. Which of the following is a true about external shock wave lithotripsy (ESWL) for treatment of gallstone disease?

A. ESWL is only effective against cholesterol stones
B. ESWL is safe in patients on anticoagulation
C. ESWL is safe in pregnancy
D. ESWL is reserved for patients with solitary stones less than 2 cm in size
E. Maintenance therapy with ursodeoxycholic acid is recommended after ESWL

39. A 38-year-old man presents with abdominal pain of 1 day duration. He underwent laparoscopic cholecystectomy for symptomatic gallstones 5 days ago. He reports low-grade fevers, nausea, and occasional vomiting. Laboratory values are as follows:

WBC	16,000/µL
ALT	208 U/L
AST	164 U/L
Total bilirubin	3.1 mg/dL

An ultrasound shows a dilated CBD to 7 mm. An ERCP is performed, and the cholangiogram is shown in the figure (see figure). What is the diagnosis?

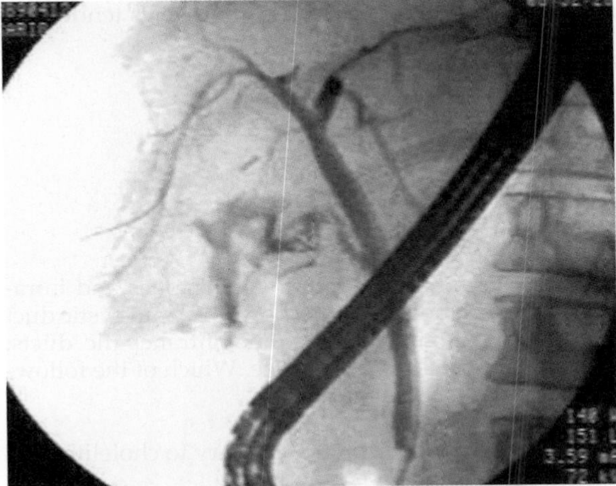

Figure for question 39.

A. Retained surgical item
B. Bile duct injury
C. Bile leak
D. Choledocholithiasis
E. Bile duct stricture

40. Which of the following is a risk factor for sepsis, gangrene, and perforation in patients with acute cholecystitis?

A. Chronic obstructive pulmonary disease
B. Leukopenia
C. Female gender
D. Diabetes
E. Age less than 20 years

41. A 72-year-old man presents to the emergency department with right upper quadrant pain, nausea, and fevers for the past 2 days. He has a history of type 2 diabetes mellitus, hypertension, and chronic kidney disease. On physical exam, his vital signs are as follows:

Temperature	103° F
Heart rate	99 bpm
Blood pressure	152/72 mm Hg

He is diaphoretic, but alert and oriented. Abdominal exam reveals tenderness in the right upper quadrant. Laboratory values are as follows:

WBC	14,000/μL
ALT	60 U/L
AST	50 U/L
Alkaline phosphatase	160 U/L
Total bilirubin is	1.8 mg/dL

Abdominal ultrasound shows a distended gallbladder, thickened gallbladder wall, and pericholecystic fluid. In addition to intravenous fluids and antibiotics, which of the following is the most appropriate management?

A. Early laparoscopic cholecystectomy
B. Delayed laparoscopic cholecystectomy
C. Percutaneous cholecystostomy drain placement
D. Exploratory laparotomy
E. HIDA scan

42. A 62-year-old man presents to the emergency department with right upper quadrant pain for the past 2 days. On physical exam, his vital signs are as follows:

Temperature	100° F
Heart rate	105 bpm
Blood pressure	132/62

He is alert and oriented. Abdominal exam reveals tenderness in the right upper quadrant.
Laboratory values are as follows:

WBC	5000/μL
ALT	278 U/L
AST	150 U/L
Alkaline phosphatase	290 U/L
Total bilirubin	4.8 mg/dL
Direct bilirubin	4 mg/dL

Abdominal ultrasound shows multiple gallstones and intrahepatic ductal dilation. CT scan shows a 12 mm cystic duct stone, dilated common hepatic, and intrahepatic ducts. The distal bile duct is normal in size. Which of the following is the most likely diagnosis?

A. Choledocholithiasis
B. Uncomplicated biliary pain secondary to cholelithiasis
C. Mirizzi's syndrome
D. Acute cholecystitis
E. Occult hilar cholangiocarcinoma

43. A 30-year-old female presents with intermittent right upper quadrant abdominal pain for the past year. The pain lasts for about 1 hour, then slowly subsides. She has had this pain three times over the past year. Physical exam reveals mild tenderness in the right upper quadrant without rebound or guarding. Liver tests, including bilirubin, AST, ALT, and alkaline phosphatase, are normal. Ultrasound shows a normal gallbladder wall, without gallstones or sludge. Which of the following is the best next step?

A. MRI
B. Conservative management
C. ERCP
D. Upper endoscopy
E. Stimulated cholescintigraphy

44. A 67-year-old female with a history of kidney transplant is admitted to the intensive care unit with pneumonia, septic shock, and heart failure exacerbation. She is intubated and requires two vasopressors. By the fourth day, her vasopressor and oxygen requirements increase. She has no diarrhea. On physical exam, she is febrile to 103.2° F, her abdomen is soft and mildly distended. There was pitting edema extending bilaterally from the ankles to the knees. Laboratory values are as follows:

WBC	19,000/μL
ALT	81 U/L
AST	100 U/L
Alkaline phosphatase	210 U/L
Total bilirubin	2.4 mg/dL
Conjugated bilirubin	1.2 mg/dL

Ultrasound of the right upper quadrant shows a 5 mm gallbladder wall and pericholecystic fluid but no gallstones. What is the best step in management?

A. Cholecystectomy
B. Percutaneous cholecystostomy tube
C. Continue current antibiotics and supportive care
D. Exploratory laparotomy
E. ERCP

45. Which of the following is characteristic of acute acalculous cholecystitis?

A. Female predominance
B. Predominance among younger and middle-aged patients
C. Mortality rate is less than 10%
D. Risk factors include hemodynamic instability, recent surgery, and atherosclerosis
E. Prognosis is better than acute calculous cholecystitis

46. A 41-year-old African-American woman is seen in clinic for evaluation of right upper quadrant of 2 years duration. Her pain starts suddenly and lasts 30 to 45 minutes before it slowly subsides. Physical exam reveals a healthy appearing female in no acute distress. Abdominal exam reveals no tenderness. Laboratory values are as follows:

WBC	8000/μL
ALT	21 U/L
AST	25 U/L
Alkaline phosphatase	120 U/L
Total bilirubin	2.4 mg/dL
Conjugated bilirubin	1.2 mg/dL

A right upper quadrant ultrasound reveals no gallstones. Hepatobiliary scintigraphy shows a gallbladder ejection fraction of 35%. She undergoes cholecystectomy for presumed acalculous biliary pain. The surgical pathology specimen reveals lipids deposited throughout the epithelial lining of the gallbladder, abruptly terminating at the cystic duct. The patient inquires about the significance of this finding. Which of the following is the best response?

A. Patients with this finding are more likely to have their pain resolve with cholecystectomy compared to those without this finding
B. This finding is associated with elevated serum cholesterol levels
C. This is a finding is found in most gallbladders that are removed

D. This finding is associated with elevated serum triglyceride levels
E. This finding is more common in African Americans

47. A 61-year-old otherwise healthy male is referred to you for evaluation. Previously, he had daily abdominal pain and bloating, but his symptoms have resolved with a lactose-free diet. As part of his workup, he had an abdominal ultrasound, which showed an 11 mm gallbladder polyp and no gallstones. What is the appropriate management?
A. Repeat ultrasound in 3 months
B. Repeat ultrasound in 6 months
C. Repeat ultrasound in 1 year
D. Laparoscopic cholecystectomy
E. Endoscopic ultrasound

48. Which of the following is true regarding gallbladder adenomas?
A. They are the most common type of gallbladder polyps
B. Open cholecystectomy is the preferred treatment for polyps larger than 18 mm
C. They have no malignant potential
D. They coexist with stones in >80% of cases
E. Multiple adenomas are present in >50% of cases

49. A 33-year-old woman with PSC presents for follow-up. She is asymptomatic. She has no encephalopathy, abdominal distension, or jaundice. Physical examination is unremarkable. Laboratory values are as follows:

ALT	81 U/L
AST	100 U/L
Alkaline phosphatase	410 U/L
Total bilirubin	2.4 mg/dL
Conjugated bilirubin	1.2 mg/dL
INR	1.3
Creatinine	1.2 mg/dL

A recent MRI of her abdomen shows an 8 mm polyp in the gallbladder, and this finding is corroborated by an abdominal ultrasound. Which of the following is the most appropriate management for this patient?
A. Repeat ultrasound in 3 months
B. Repeat ultrasound in 6 months
C. Laparoscopic cholecystectomy
D. Check cancer antigen (CA) 19.9
E. Start ursodeoxycholic acid

50. A 40-year-old obese woman is seen in clinic for intermittent abdominal pain of 1 year duration. The pain is located in the right upper quadrant, increases in intensity over 15 minutes, lasts for 30 to 60 minutes, then slowly subsides over several hours. The attacks are often precipitated by a meal. Her only medication is a calcium channel blocker for hypertension. Physical examination reveals a soft abdomen with no tenderness. Laboratory values are as follows:

WBC	3500/μL
Hemoglobin	13.1 gm/dL
ALT	18 U/L
AST	16 U/L
Alkaline phosphatase	120 U/L
Total bilirubin	1 mg/dL

A right upper quadrant ultrasound did not reveal any gallbladder stones. The CBD was 4 mm. You order a HIDA scan to check the gallbladder ejection fraction. Which of the following statements about the patient's condition is true?
A. A low gallbladder ejection fraction (<35%) can occur in patients taking calcium channel blockers
B. A low gallbladder ejection fraction (<35%) is a reliable predictor of the response to cholecystectomy
C. The majority of patients with this presentation have a low gallbladder ejection fraction
D. Bile sampling detects cholesterol crystals in the majority of patients with this presentation
E. Elective cholecystectomy is associated with poor long-term outcome

51. A patient is seen in clinic for chronic intermittent right upper quadrant abdominal pain. The pain increases in intensity over 20 minutes, lasts for 60 minutes, then slowly diminishes over 2 to 3 hours. A right upper quadrant ultrasound shows a normal gallbladder with no stones. You suspect that the patient is having acalculous biliary pain. Which of the following is true about this condition?
A. Females and males are affected equally
B. It commonly affects patients older than 50 years
C. Laboratory studies usually show minor elevation of ALT and AST
D. Physical examination reveals significant tenderness in the right upper quadrant
E. Attacks usually recur unless cholecystectomy is performed

52. Which of the following is true about adenomyomatosis of the gallbladder?
A. Adenomyomatosis refers to excessive cholesterol deposition in the epithelium leading to thickened mucosa
B. Rokitansky-Aschoff sinuses represent invaginations of the epithelium into the underlying muscularis mucosa
C. Generalized adenomyomatosis is the most common type
D. Segmental adenomyomatosis is associated with increased risk of malignancy
E. Segmental adenomyomatosis can present as a filling defect on oral cholecystography

53. A 32-year-old woman presents for evaluation of pruritus, fatigue, and abnormal liver function tests. She has no abdominal pain. Her medical history includes fibromyalgia and hypothyroidism. She has no family history of liver disease. She has had multiple sexual partners in the past. She takes levothyroxine and occasional ibuprofen. On physical exam, there is scleral icterus. Her abdominal exam shows no tenderness or distention. Her laboratory studies are as follows:

WBC	3300/μL
Hemoglobin	12.9 g/dL
Platelet count	165,000/μL
Alkaline phosphatase	329 U/L
Alanine aminotransferase	61 U/L
Aspartate aminotransferase	59 U/L
Total Bilirubin	3.2 mg/dL
Direct bilirubin	2.2 mg/dL

An MRI of her abdomen demonstrates diffuse stricturing and segmental dilations of the bile ducts. Which of the following is the most appropriate next step in management?
A. Inform the patient of her diagnosis of PSC
B. Start ursodeoxycholic acid
C. Liver biopsy

D. ERCP
E. Human immunodeficiency virus (HIV) antibody

54. Which of the following is true about PSC?
A. PSC is more common in females than males
B. Most patients are diagnosed between ages 25 and 45 years
C. Smokers are at higher risk for PSC than nonsmokers
D. First-degree relatives of patients with PSC are not at increased risk for PSC compared to the general population
E. 50% of patients with PSC have inflammatory bowel disease (IBD)

55. Which of the following is true of PSC and its relationship to IBD?
A. PSC is seen in patients with ulcerative colitis (UC), but there is no established relationship between PSC and Crohn's disease
B. Among patients with PSC and IBD, 85% to 90% have UC, and the remainder have Crohn's disease
C. A patient with UC and left-sided colitis has the same risk of having PSC as a patient with UC and pancolitis
D. PSC and IBD disease activity tend to progress in a parallel fashion
E. If a patient without UC undergoes liver transplantation for PSC, then the patient is no longer at risk for developing UC

56. A 36-year-old male with a history of primary sclerosing cholangitis is seen in clinic for follow-up. He reports bothersome pruritus and fatigue but otherwise feels well. Physical examination reveals soft abdomen with no ascites. Laboratory studies show the following:

Alkaline phosphatase	287 U/L
Alanine aminotransferase	42 U/L
Aspartate aminotransferase	44 U/L
Bilirubin	1.7 mg/dL
Direct bilirubin	1.2 mg/dL
WBC	6500/μL
Hemoglobin	13.9 g/dL
Platelet count	315,000/μL

His MRI shows no evidence of cirrhosis or a dominant stricture. What is the most appropriate medical management?
A. Ursodeoxycholic acid at 10 to 15 mg/kg/day
B. Ursodeoxycholic acid at 30 mg/kg/day
C. Cholestyramine
D. Glucocorticoids
E. Methotrexate

57. A 62-year-old man presents with intermittent right upper quadrant and epigastric pain for the past year. He has mild nausea but no vomiting. He denies diarrhea and rectal bleeding. His review of systems is significant for a 15-pound weight loss over the past year. His medication history includes omeprazole once daily for heartburn symptoms and occasional ibuprofen for knee pain. He denies any alcohol intake. Physical examination reveals scleral icterus, mild right upper quadrant and epigastric tenderness. Laboratory values are as follows:

ALT	88 U/L
AST	62 U/L
Alkaline phosphatase	320 U/L
Total bilirubin	3.2 mg/dL

A CT scan of the abdomen reveals bilateral intrahepatic biliary ductal dilation and possible stricture in the CBD. ERCP is performed and shows multifocal intrahepatic biliary strictures with beading and segmental dilation. There was mild, nonobstructive narrowing in the mid and distal CBD. Small stone fragments were extracted upon balloon sweep of the CBD. A colonoscopy and biopsy excludes the diagnosis of IBD. Which of the following is most appropriate next step?
A. Serum CA 19.9 measurement
B. Start ursodeoxycholic acid
C. Referral for cholecystectomy
D. IgG4 level measurements
E. Stool test for *Cryptosporidium*

58. A 40-year-old male with primary sclerosing cholangitis is seen in clinic for follow-up. He reports bothersome pruritus during the day and at night. Medical therapy thus far has included cholestyramine and a trial of rifampin, both of which have failed to relieve his pruritus. He has no jaundice, abdominal distension, or encephalopathy. Abdominal exam shows multiple scratch marks. Laboratory values are as follows:

ALT	70 U/L
AST	46 U/L
Alkaline phosphatase	440 U/L
Total bilirubin	2.2 mg/dL
INR	1.3
Creatinine	1.2 mg/dL

His last MRI/MRCP shows multifocal intrahepatic biliary strictures with beading and segmental dilation. Which of the following is the most appropriate next step in the treatment of the patient's pruritus?
A. Naloxone
B. Methadone
C. ERCP
D. Plasmapheresis
E. Liver transplantation

59. A 53-year-old female with PSC is admitted to the hospital with her third episode of cholangitis in 6 months. She also reports itching that is relieved by cholestyramine. She has no ascites. She has undergone three ERCPs with balloon dilation and stent placement over this time period for recurrent CBD stricture. Biliary brushings and biopsies are negative for cholangiocarcinoma. CA 19-9 shows no evidence of cholangiocarcinoma. She has no evidence of cirrhosis. Which of the following is appropriate management for her recurring cholangitis?
A. Liver transplantation
B. Long-term prophylaxis with daily ciprofloxacin
C. Long-term prophylaxis with daily trimethoprim-sulfamethoxazole
D. Long-term prophylaxis with weekly ciprofloxacin
E. Long-term prophylaxis with rotating cycles of different antibiotics given in 4-week cycles

60. A 35-year-old male patient with known ulcerative colitis is seen in clinic for routine follow up. His last colonoscopy 3 months ago showed diffuse mild colitis involving the rectum and extending to the mid-transverse colon. He is currently asymptomatic. His only medication is mesalamine. His vital signs are as follows:

Temperature is	97.2° F
Respiration rate	16 breaths/min
Heart rate	70 bpm

Physical exam reveals mild scleral icterus. There is no rash or joint swelling. The rest of the exam was unremarkable. Laboratory values are as follows:

ALT	80 U/L
AST	56 U/L
Alkaline phosphatase	350 U/L
Total bilirubin	2.2 mg/dL

Which of the following is most appropriate next step in management?

A. Abdominal ultrasound
B. Abdominal CT scan
C. Abdominal MRI/MRCP
D. ERCP
E. Liver biopsy

61. A 40-year-old man undergoes an ERCP for evaluation of elevated liver enzymes and abnormal MRCP findings. Which of the following conditions is the least associated with this appearance on cholangiogram (see figure)?

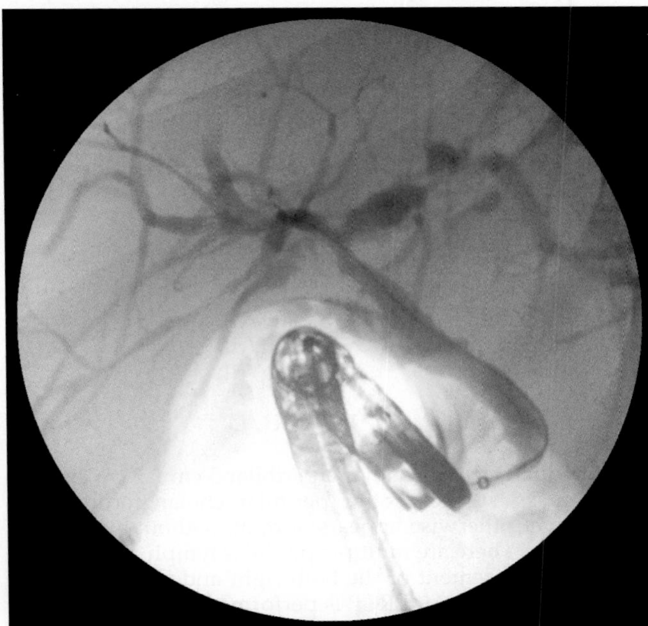

Figure for question 61.

A. Acquired immunodeficiency syndrome (AIDS) cholangiopathy
B. Primary biliary cirrhosis
C. IgG4-related cholangitis
D. Ischemic hepatic allograft injury
E. Intraductal formaldehyde therapy

62. Which of the following autoantibodies is the most prevalent in patients with primary sclerosing cholangitis?

A. Perinuclear antineutrophil cytoplasmic antibodies (p-ANCA)
B. Antinuclear antibodies (ANA)
C. Antimitochondrial antibodies
D. Anticardiolipin antibodies
E. Anti–smooth muscle antibodies

63. A 45-year-old woman is seen in clinic for evaluation of elevated liver enzymes. She has a history of hypertension and diabetes. Her medications include lisinopril, metformin, and once-daily aspirin. She denies excessive alcohol consumption. On physical examination, she is obese (BMI of 31 kg/m^2). Vital signs are unremarkable. She has no scleral icterus. Her abdominal exam is unremarkable. Laboratory values are as follows:

ALT	45 U/L
AST	35 U/L
Alkaline phosphatase	280 U/L
Total bilirubin	3.5 mg/dL

An abdominal MRI/MRCP was previously performed, which revealed a normal biliary tree without strictures or masses. You obtain a liver biopsy (see figure). Which of the following is the most likely diagnosis?

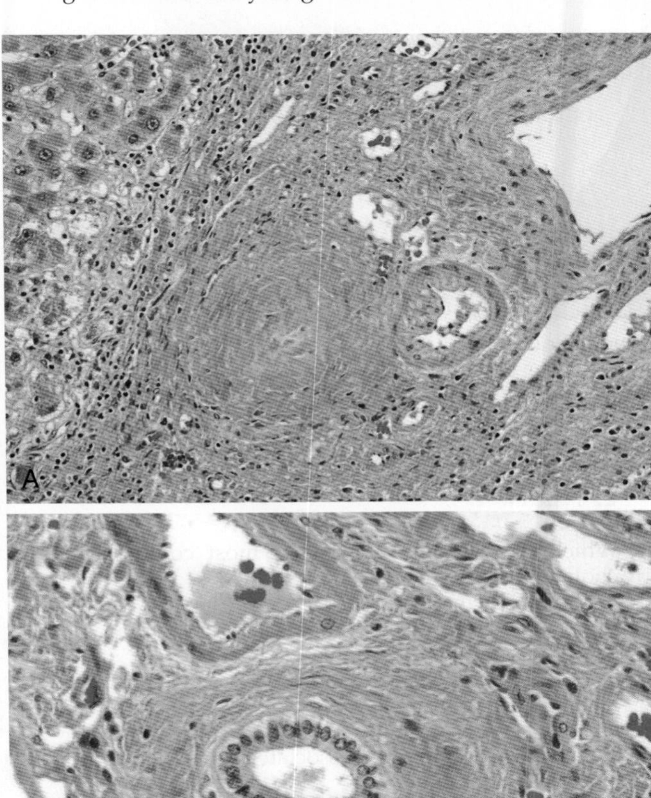

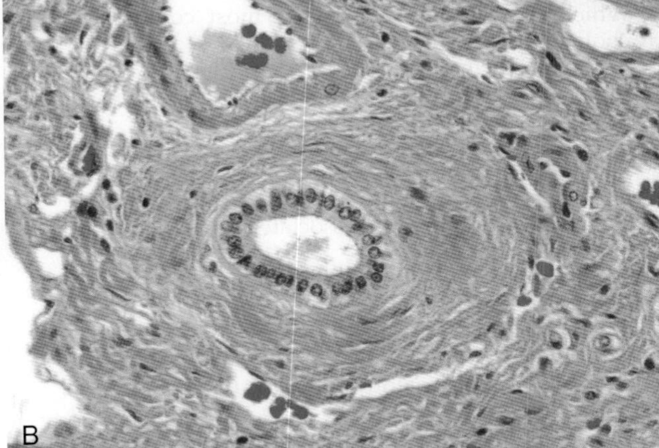

Figure for question 63.

A. Primary biliary cirrhosis
B. Nonalcoholic steatohepatitis
C. Drug-induced liver injury
D. IgG4-related cholangitis
E. Small duct PSC

64. A 58-year-old man presents with jaundice and clay-colored stools of 1 week duration. Physical exam reveals tenderness in the right upper quadrant. An abdominal CT scan shows a hilar mass with biliary obstruction, suspicious for perihilar cholangiocarcinoma. An ERCP is performed and a cholangiogram is obtained (see figure). What type of Bismuth-Corlette biliary stricture is seen on cholangiogram?

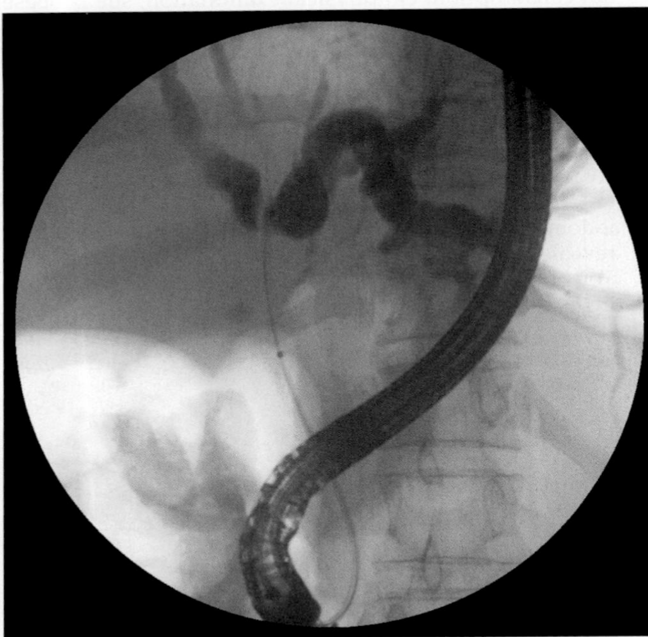

Figure for question 64.

A. Type I
B. Type II
C. Type IIIa
D. Type IIIB
E. Type IV

65. Which of the following is the most common type of cholangiocarcinoma?
A. Adenocarcinoma
B. Clear cell adenocarcinoma
C. Papillary adenocarcinoma
D. Adenosquamous carcinoma
E. Small cell carcinoma

66. Which of the following is associated with an increased risk of cholangiocarcinoma?
A. Cholelithiasis
B. Choledocholithiasis
C. Hepatolithiasis
D. *Echinococcus multilocularis*
E. Familiar adenomatous polyposis (FAP) syndrome

67. Which of the following viral hepatitides is associated with the highest risk of intrahepatic cholangiocarcinoma?
A. Hepatitis A
B. Hepatitis B
C. Hepatitis C
D. Hepatitis D
E. Hepatitis E

68. A 55-year-old woman was found on CT scan of the abdomen to have a 4 cm liver lesion located centrally in the right hepatic lobe. Which of the following is the typical CT appearance of intrahepatic cholangiocarcinoma?
A. Arterial enhancement and venous phase washout
B. Progressive contrast enhancement through the venous, arterial, and delayed venous phases
C. Peripheral arterial enhancement with gradual central filling of contrast
D. Hypodense or isodense lesion that enhances on arterial phase with a central scar
E. Well-demarcated homogenous lesion with peripheral enhancement

69. A 58-year-old man presents with painless jaundice and clay-colored stools of 2 weeks duration. Physical exam reveals tenderness in the right upper quadrant. An abdominal CT scan shows a perihilar mass, with biliary obstruction, suspicious for perihilar cholangiocarcinoma. An ERCP is performed that shows a hilar stricture that involves the confluence of the right and left hepatic duct. Brush cytology is obtained from the stricture. Which of the following significantly increases the sensitivity and specificity of cytology for diagnosing cholangiocarcinoma?
A. Obtaining multiple brush cytology specimens
B. Using a longer brush cytology
C. Dilation followed by brush cytology
D. Fluorescence in situ hybridization (FISH)
E. Obtaining samples from the right and left hepatic ducts

70. A 55-year-old woman presents with abdominal pain, jaundice and weight loss of 3 months duration. She also developed severe itching over the last 2 months. She is otherwise healthy and maintains an active lifestyle. Physical exam reveals tenderness in the right upper quadrant. Laboratory values are as follows:

WBC	5000/μL
Alkaline phosphatase	470 U/L
ALT	30 U/L
AST	60 U/L
Total bilirubin	8.2 mg/dL
Direct bilirubin	6.2 mg/dL
Creatinine	0.9 mg/dL
INR	1.1
Amylase	700 IU/L

An abdominal CT scan shows a perihilar 5 cm x 5 cm enhancing mass, suspicious for perihilar cholangiocarcinoma. The liver otherwise appears normal, without evidence of cirrhosis. There are multiple perihilar lymph nodes. There is also encasement of the both right and left branches of the portal vein. An ERCP is performed that shows a hilar stricture that involves the confluence of the right and left hepatic duct. Brush cytology and bile duct biopsy is obtained. Bilateral stenting is performed successfully. The patient's itching is improved, and bilirubin decreases to 2 mg/dL over the next week. Bile duct biopsy is positive for cholangiocarcinoma. Which of the following is the most appropriate next step in management?
A. Refer for surgical resection
B. Refer for radiation therapy
C. Refer for chemotherapy with gemcitabine
D. Refer for chemotherapy with gemcitabine and oxaliplatin
E. Refer for chemotherapy with gemcitabine and oxaliplatin combined with radiotherapy

71. Which of the following is true about gallbladder carcinoma?
A. It has a male preponderance
B. Global incidence rates parallel that of cholelithiasis
C. The majority of cases are diagnosed prior to surgical exploration

D. Radiotherapy is recommended in unresectable cases
E. Gallbladder carcinoma develops in 10% of patients with gallstones

72. Which of the following is true regarding the risk factors for gallbladder carcinoma?
A. Risk for gallbladder cancer is higher in patients with diffuse than in those with partial gallbladder calcification
B. Gallbladder surveillance with annual ultrasound is recommended in primary sclerosing cholangitis
C. 50% of patients with gallbladder cancer do not have associated gallstones
D. Cholesterol gallstones portend a higher risk of gallbladder cancer than pigment gallstones
E. Cholesterolosis is associated with increased risk of gallbladder cancer

73. A 55-year-old woman is seen in clinic with abdominal pain. Her pain occurs in the epigastric area, is burning in character, and associated with spicy food. It only responds partially to proton pump inhibitor (PPI) therapy. An esophagogastroduodenoscopy is performed and is normal. Biopsies are negative for *Helicobacter pylori* An MRI/MRCP ordered by the primary care physician shows a long common channel between the CBD and the pancreatic duct (measuring 2.5 cm). Otherwise, the scan did not show any abnormalities. Which of the following should be recommended?
A. ERCP
B. EUS
C. Cholecystectomy
D. Reassurance about the benign nature of MRI findings
E. Repeat MRI/MRCP in 6 to 12 months

74. A 55-year-old woman undergoes elective laparoscopic cholecystectomy for symptomatic gallstones. She has an uneventful recovery. On histopathologic examination of the gallbladder, a focus of adenocarcinoma is found in the mucosa of the gallbladder wall. The tumor invades the lamina propria. Margins are negative. A CT scan with intravenous contrast of the abdomen reveals postoperative changes without abdominal or liver lesions. Which of the following is the most appropriate next step in management?
A. No further intervention is needed
B. Surgical re-exploration for extended cholecystectomy
C. Surgical re-exploration for right extended hemihepatectomy
D. Surgical re-exploration for resection of segment IVb and V
E. Refer for adjuvant chemotherapy

75. A 50-year-old man undergoes elective laparoscopic cholecystectomy for symptomatic gallstones. He has an uneventful recovery. On histopathologic examination of the gallbladder, a focus of adenocarcinoma is found in the mucosa of the body of the gallbladder. The tumor invades into but not through the muscularis propria. Tumor margins are negative. A CT scan reveals postoperative changes without abdominal or liver lesions. Which of the following is the most appropriate next step in management?
A. No further intervention is needed
B. Surgical re-exploration and extended cholecystectomy
C. Surgical re-exploration and right extended hemihepatectomy
D. Surgical re-exploration and resection of segment IVb and V
E. Refer for adjuvant chemotherapy

76. Which of the following is true about ampullary adenocarcinoma?
A. It peaks in incidence in the fifth decade
B. It is associated with Lynch syndrome
C. It is the second most common cause of death in patients with FAP syndrome
D. In FAP patients, it usually develops before the diagnosis of colon cancer
E. It has a similar incidence in Gardener syndrome compared to the general population

77. A 61-year-old man presents with jaundice and clay-colored stool of 3 months duration. He denies abdominal pain, nausea, or vomiting. His past medical history is significant for hypertension, diabetes, and osteoarthritis. He is otherwise healthy and maintains an active lifestyle. On exam, he is afebrile. There is no abdominal tenderness or hepatomegaly. Laboratory values are as follows:

WBC	6200/μL
Hemoglobin	13.1 g/dL
Alkaline phosphatase	805 U/L
ALT	30 U/L
AST	60 U/L
Total bilirubin	6.9 mg/dL
Direct bilirubin	4.2 mg/dL
Creatinine	1.1 mg/dL
INR	1.0

An MRI of the abdomen shows intrahepatic and extrahepatic biliary ductal dilation with abrupt cutoff at the level of the ampulla. The pancreatic duct is also dilated. There are no abnormal masses or lymphadenopathy. An ERCP reveals irregular ampullary mucosa. Cannulation is achieved, and cholangiogram shows an ampullary stricture. A sphincterotomy is performed, and a plastic stent is placed across the ampulla. Biopsies are obtained from the ampullary mucosa, and pathology shows evidence of adenocarcinoma. Which of the following is the most appropriate next step in management?
A. Endoscopic ampullectomy
B. Limited surgical ampullectomy
C. Neoadjuvant chemotherapy
D. Pancreaticoduodenectomy
E. Chemoradiotherapy

78. A 28-year-old obese woman presents for evaluation of abdominal pain and jaundice of 1 day duration. On physical examination, she is afebrile. Her abdomen is tender in the right upper quadrant. Her laboratory values are as follows:

Platelet count	365,000/μL
Alkaline phosphatase	329 U/L
ALT	91 U/L
AST	110 U/L
Total bilirubin	8.2 mg/dL
Direct bilirubin	6.2 mg/dL
INR	1.2
Amylase	50 IU/L

Urine pregnancy test is negative. Ultrasound shows dilated CBD to 12 mm, with a possible stone in the distal CBD. An ERCP is performed, which shows a dilated CBD to 15 mm with smooth tapering to the ampulla. There is a 13 mm filling defect in the mid-CBD, consistent with a bile duct stone. A sphincterotomy is performed, and the cut is extended to the junction of the ampullary roof and the duodenal wall. Extraction of the stone with a 12 mm balloon tipped catheter is not successful, as the balloon and stone are constantly stuck at the ampulla. A stone extraction basket is inserted but could not capture the stone. Which of the following is the most appropriate next step in management?

A. Extend the sphincterotomy
B. Insert a plastic biliary stent and reattempt ERCP in 48 hours
C. Ampullary balloon dilation
D. Insert a plastic biliary stent and refer for PTC
E. Pancreatic stent insertion

79. A 65-year-old woman who was recently diagnosed with cholangiocarcinoma presents to the emergency department with jaundice and abdominal pain of 3 days duration. She is visiting her daughter from out of state. She denies fevers or chills. She noticed that her eyes are turning yellow, and her urine started turning dark 3 days ago. She mentions that her doctors found "cancer just below her liver" and was told it was cholangiocarcinoma. She has not received chemotherapy. On physical exam she is afebrile. She has tenderness in the right upper quadrant. There is no palpable mass and no hepatomegaly. Her laboratory values are as follows:

WBC	5000/μL
Alkaline phosphatase	659 U/L
ALT	140 U/L
AST	170 U/L
Total bilirubin	12.2 mg/dL
Direct bilirubin	10.2 mg/dL
Creatinine	1.3 mg/dL
INR	1.3
Amylase	80 IU/L

Ultrasound showed intrahepatic and extrahepatic biliary ductal dilation, with the CBD measuring 8 mm. There is no gallbladder wall thickening. Which of the following is the most appropriate next step in management?

A. CT scan of the abdomen with contrast
B. MRI/MRCP of the abdomen
C. ERCP
D. PTC
E. Intravenous antibiotics

80. A 68-year-old man presents with jaundice, abdominal pain, and fevers of 3 days duration. Physical exam reveals tenderness in the right upper quadrant. Laboratory values are as follows:

WBC	9000/μL
Alkaline phosphatase	870 U/L
ALT	130 U/L
AST	160 U/L
Total bilirubin	9.2 mg/dL
Direct bilirubin	7.2 mg/dL
Creatinine	1.1 mg/dL
INR	1.2
Amylase	50 IU/L

An abdominal CT scan shows biliary obstruction in the hilar area, without a clear mass. The intrahepatic ducts are dilated. An ERCP is performed and a cholangiogram is obtained (see figure). Brushings and endoscopic biopsy under fluoroscopy are obtained. Which of the following is the most appropriate next step in management?

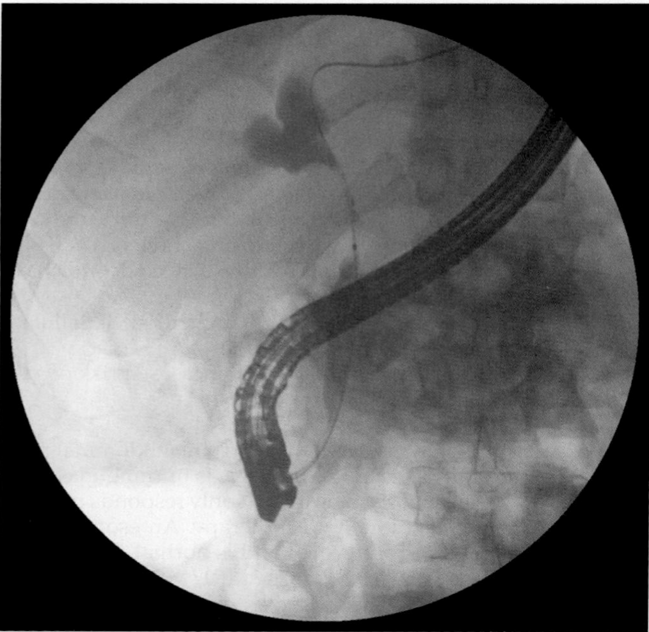

Figure for question 80.

A. Placement of bilateral fully covered metal stents
B. Placement of bilateral plastic stents
C. Placement of one plastic stent across the common hepatic duct
D. Placement of one uncovered stent across the common hepatic duct
E. Balloon dilation of the common hepatic duct without stent placement

81. Which of the following is associated with gadolinium-based intravenous contrast studies?

A. Lupus-like reaction
B. Dystonia
C. Contrast-induced nephropathy
D. Cholangiocarcinoma
E. Nephrogenic systemic fibrosis

82. A 32-year-old woman presents to the emergency department with dull right upper quadrant dull pain of 5 days duration. She has nausea but denies vomiting. One week ago she underwent laparoscopic cholecystectomy for symptomatic gallstones causing biliary pain. On exam, she is febrile with a temperature of 38.3° C. She is tender to palpation in the right upper quadrant. Laboratory values are as follows:

WBC	11,000/μL
Alkaline phosphatase	280 U/L
ALT	26 U/L
AST	30 U/L
Total bilirubin	4.1 mg/dL
Direct bilirubin	1.9 mg/dL
Creatinine	0.9 mg/dL
INR	1.2
Amylase	40 IU/L

An abdominal ultrasound shows moderate perihepatic and peripancreatic fluid. An ERCP is performed and the cholangiogram is shown (see figure). Which of the following is the most appropriate next step?

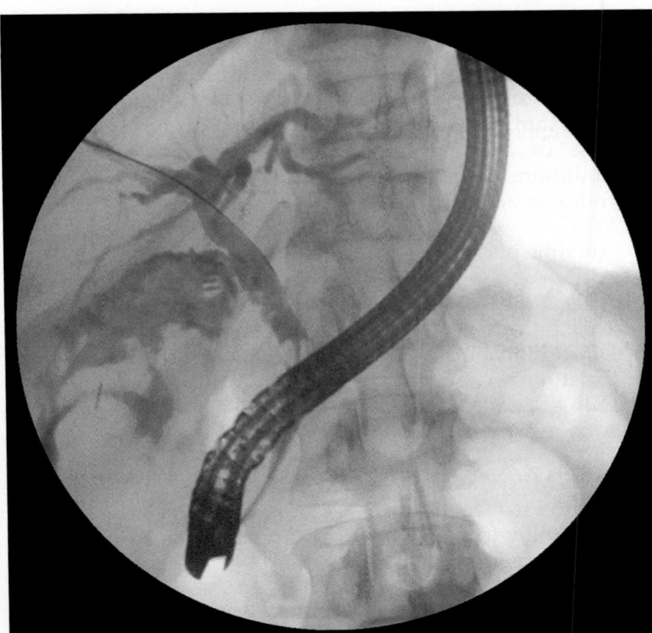

Figure for question 82.

A. Sphincterotomy
B. Sphincterotomy and biliary stent placement
C. Biliary stent placement
D. Surgical exploration
E. Sphincterotomy and ampullary balloon dilation

83. Which of the following is true about biliary strictures secondary to chronic pancreatitis?
A. Placement of one plastic stent provides similar response to placing multiple plastic stents simultaneously
B. These strictures are usually refractory to endoscopic management
C. Fully covered metal stents are not approved by the U.S. Food and Drug Administration (FDA) for chronic pancreatitis strictures
D. Strictures appear irregular with a shelflike cutoff on cholangiogram
E. Calcific chronic pancreatitis is associated with improved response rates to endoscopic therapy compared to noncalcific pancreatitis

84. A 55-year-old man with a known history of metastatic pancreatic cancer is admitted to the hospital with new-onset jaundice and pruritus. He is in relatively good health and maintains an active lifestyle. On physical examination, he is afebrile. He has icteric sclera. There is tenderness to deep palpation in the midepigastric area. A CT scan of the abdomen shows a pancreatic head mass with distal CBD stricture and upstream dilation. There are few hypodense lesions in the liver, consistent with metastatic disease. Laboratory values are as follows:

WBC	10,000/μL
Alkaline phosphatase	580 U/L
ALT	76 U/L
AST	60 U/L
Total bilirubin	6.1 mg/dL
Direct bilirubin	4.9 mg/dL
Creatinine	0.5 mg/dL
INR	1.3

Which of the following is true about the management of this patient?
A. ERCP is currently not indicated in this patient.
B. ERCP with placement of a CBD plastic stent is the preferred approach.
C. ERCP with placement of a CBD fully covered metal stent is associated with less stent migration compared to uncovered stent
D. ERCP with placement a CBD uncovered biliary stent is associated with less stent occlusion compared to a fully covered stent
E. Acute cholecystitis has been described in association with fully covered metal stent

85. A 54-year-old man presents with progressive painless jaundice and mild itching over the last 3 months. He reports a 20-pound weight loss but denies any fevers, chills, or abdominal pain. His past medical history is significant for hypertension and mild diabetes mellitus type 2. On physical examination, he appears thin but in no distress. He is afebrile. Abdomen is soft but tender to deep palpation in the epigastric area. Laboratory values are as follows:

WBC	4300/μL
ALT	84 U/L
AST	61 U/L
Alkaline phosphatase	320 U/L
Total bilirubin	8.2 mg/dL
Direct bilirubin	6.1 mg/dL

MRI of the abdomen shows a 2.5 cm solid mass lesion localized within the pancreatic head, causing obstruction of the distal CBD. The mass does not abut the portal and the superior mesenteric veins. It is not in contact with the celiac axis and the superior mesenteric artery. Which of the following is the most appropriate next step in management?
A. ERCP with brush cytology of CBD and stent placement
B. ERCP with brush cytology of CBD, stent placement and referral to chemotherapy
C. ERCP with brush cytology of CBD and referral for pancreaticoduodenectomy
D. Referral for pancreaticoduodenectomy
E. Check serum IgG4 levels

86. A 63-year-old man presents with jaundice, abdominal pain, and fevers of 4 days duration. On physical exam his vital signs are as follows:

Temperature	102° F
Blood pressure	100/50 mm Hg
Heart rate	110 bpm

Abdominal exam reveals tenderness in the epigastrium. Laboratory values are as follows:

WBC	11,000/μL
Alkaline phosphatase	770 U/L
ALT	120 U/L
AST	140 U/L
Total bilirubin	12.4 mg/dL
Direct bilirubin	9.2 mg/dL
Creatinine	1.1 mg/dL
INR	1.1

An abdominal CT scan shows a 4 cm mass in the hilum with biliary obstruction. There is narrowing of the hepatic duct that also involves the confluence of the right and left hepatic ducts. The left hepatic lobe appears atrophied. An ERCP is planned. Which of the following is the preferred endoscopic approach during ERCP?

A. Opacification of the left lobe, followed by drainage of the left lobe
B. Opacification of the right lobe, followed by drainage of the right lobe
C. Opacification of the right and left lobe, followed by stenting of the left lobe
D. Opacification of the right and left lobe, followed by stenting of the right lobe
E. Opacification of right and left lobes, followed by bilateral stenting

87. Which of the following is a risk factor for postsphincterotomy bleeding?
A. Resuming anticoagulation within 72 hours of the procedure
B. Large size sphincterotomy
C. Extension of a prior sphincterotomy
D. Extraction of large biliary stones
E. High bilirubin level

88. A 22-year-old obese woman presents to the emergency department with sharp right upper quadrant pain of 1 day duration. She has a history of deep vein thrombosis for which she is takes coumadin. On exam, she is febrile with a temperature of 39.3° C. She is tender to palpation in the right upper quadrant. Laboratory values are as follows:

WBC	13,000/μL
Alkaline phosphatase	680 U/L
ALT	126 U/L
AST	130 U/L
Total bilirubin	7.1 mg/dL
Direct bilirubin	5.9 mg/dL
Creatinine	0.9 mg/dL
INR	1.9
Amylase	60 IU/L

An abdominal ultrasound shows moderate perihepatic and peripancreatic fluid. An ultrasound shows a dilated bile duct to 10 mm with a distal CBD obstructing stone. An ERCP is performed, and the cholangiogram shows a dilated CBD to 12 mm with multiple, 4 mm to 6 mm filling defects in the distal CBD. Balloon dilation without prior sphincterotomy is performed at the biliary orifice to 6 mm. Stone extraction was successful. Which of the following complications is more common with dilation of the intact biliary sphincter compared to sphincterotomy?
A. Postsphincterotomy bleeding
B. Pancreatitis
C. Perforation
D. Distal CBD stricture formation
E. Chronic biliary pain

89. A 59-year-old man presents with painless jaundice and clay-colored stool of 2 months duration. He denies abdominal pain, nausea, or vomiting. He complains of bothersome itching not responsive to diphenhydramine. On exam, he is afebrile. There is no abdominal tenderness or hepatomegaly. He is otherwise healthy and maintains an active lifestyle. Laboratory values are as follows:

WBC	6000/μL
Alkaline phosphatase	630 U/L
ALT	146 U/L
AST	140 U/L
Total bilirubin	9.1 mg/dL
Direct bilirubin	5.9 mg/dL
Creatinine	0.9 mg/dL
INR	1.1
Amylase	60 IU/L

An MRI/MRCP is performed, and a representative image is shown (see figure). No masses are seen. Which of the following is the most appropriate next step in management?

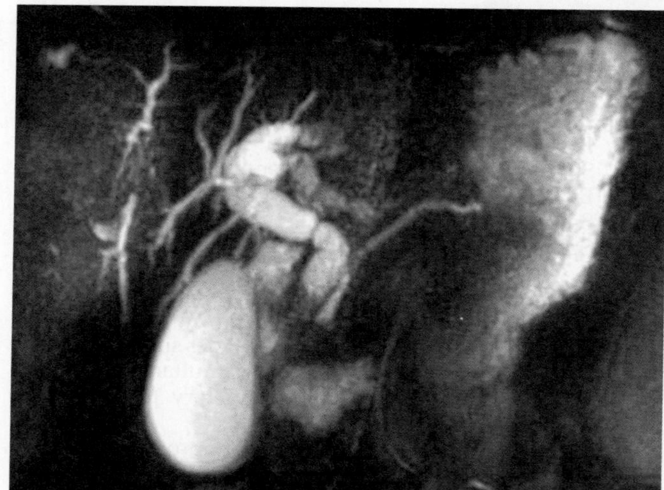

Figure for question 89.

A. EUS
B. ERCP
C. CT scan of the abdomen with contrast
D. Cholecystectomy
E. Cholecystectomy plus intraoperative cholangiogram

ANSWERS

1. **D** (S&F ch62)
A patient with biliary atresia should undergo exploratory laparotomy with intraoperative cholangiogram to confirm the site of obstruction. In patients with obliteration of the proximal extrahepatic biliary tree, the Kasai procedure (hepatoportoenterostomy) is the preferred treatment. A jejunal Roux-en-Y limb is anastomosed to the porta hepatis. Glucocorticoids and ursodeoxycholic acid are commonly given postoperatively. However, their use remains controversial due to lack of strong evidence for efficacy. A choledochoduodenostomy is not an appropriate treatment for biliary atresia. Liver transplantation may become necessary if the Kasai procedure fails.

2. **D** (S&F ch62)
The clinical presentation and imaging characteristics are consistent with a type 1 choledochal cyst. Surgical resection is accomplished by a choledocojejunostomy with a Roux-en-Y anastomosis, which reduces the risk of developing cancer or cholangitis. ERCP is not recommended, although most surgeons will perform an intraoperative cholangiogram to further define the anatomy of the biliary tree. Due to the risk of cancer, serial imaging or biliary drainage alone are not preferred options. Because surgical resection is feasible with choledochal cyst, liver transplantation is not indicated.

3. **D** (S&F ch62)
The cumulative lifetime risk of developing cancer with a type 1 choledochal cyst is 10% to 15%. Therefore, cyst excision with hepaticojejunostomy is the recommended treatment in otherwise healthy patients, regardless of the presence of symptoms. Serial imaging or observation could be appropriate if the patient is not a good surgical candidate. ERCP and percutaneous biliary drainage are not recommended.

4. **E** (S&F ch62)
This patient's history of recurrent cholangitis and the cholangiogram showing segmental saccular dilations of the intrahepatic bile ducts are consistent with a diagnosis of Caroli's disease. Note the normal extrahepatic ducts. Patients may be managed conservatively with biliary drainage, but if recurrent complications such as cholangitis occur, then liver transplant should be considered. Ursodeoxycholic acid may be useful to help dissolve stones in Caroli's disease, but it is not sufficient for a patient with recurrent cholangitis episodes. Surgical resection of affected ducts is only feasible if only one lobe of the liver is affected by the disease. Serial biliary drain changes are an option but not preferred due to potential for complications and the need for frequent drain changes. There is no role for cholangioscopy in Caroli's disease.

5. **C** (S&F ch62)
25% to 30% of children with PSC exhibit an overlap syndrome with autoimmune hepatitis. Both prednisone and azathioprine have been exhibited to offer some benefit for this overlap syndrome in uncontrolled studies in pediatric populations. In contrast to PSC in older children and adults, PSC in neonates is not associated with ulcerative colitis. Finally, PSC recurs in around 10% of pediatric patients who undergo liver transplantation.

6. **A** (S&F ch62)
Trisomy 21 (Down syndrome) is associated with an increased risk of gallstones. Unlike Crohn's disease, ulcerative colitis is not a risk factor for developing gallstones. Malnutrition is not associated with gallstones. Parenteral nutrition, not jejunal tube feeds, is associated with gallstone formation. Cephalosporins and diuretics have been linked to gallstones, but not amoxicillin.

7. **C** (S&F ch62)
The patient is presenting with acute cholecystitis. He is clinically unstable with septic shock and altered mental status. In addition to antibiotics, the most appropriate management is percutaneous cholecystostomy drain placement. Watchful waiting is inappropriate, as it does not address the source of sepsis. Laparotomy or laparoscopic cholecystectomy is associated with a higher risk of operative complications in unstable patients. Given the normal liver enzymes and bilirubin, there is no suspicion for cholangitis, and ERCP is not indicated.

8. **D** (S&F ch62)
The patient has typical biliary-type pain. She does not have gallstones, but she may have biliary dyskinesia as a cause of her pain. This is a recognized entity in children, and the diagnosis is made by HIDA scan. Gallbladder ejection fraction lower than 35% has been considered an indication for cholecystectomy.

9. **D** (S&F ch62)
The clinical presentation is consistent with bile leak secondary to spontaneous perforation of the bile duct. This is an uncommon condition of unclear etiology. The perforation usually occurs at the junction of the cystic and bile duct. Chronic cholecystitis is associated with normal liver biochemical tests and a thickened gallbladder on ultrasound. Choledocholithiasis presents more acutely and is associated with dilated CBD without ascites. Biliary atresia usually presents earlier in a neonate or infant with prolonged hyperbilirubinemia. Cirrhosis is less likely and is not associated with acholic stools and dark urine.

10. **D** (S&F ch63)
This patient meets criteria for SOD dysfunction type I. The criteria for this diagnosis are biliary-type pain; elevated AST, ALT, or alkaline phosphatase on one occasion; and bile duct diameter greater than 10 mm. In these cases, sphincterotomy provides pain relief in 90% to 95% of patients, regardless of the manometry findings. Stent placement is not necessary. Observation or repeating lab work in 6 months is inappropriate in this symptomatic patient.

11. **B** (S&F ch63)
The clinical presentation is consistent with type 2 SOD dysfunction (biliary-type pain with either elevated liver enzymes or biliary ductal dilation >10 mm). An elevated mean basal sphincter pressure >40 mm Hg is abnormal and was shown to predict improvement in symptoms after sphincterotomy compared to sham procedure. Increased sphincter phasic contraction, retrograde contractions, and a paradoxical response to cholecystokinin (CCK) are classified as sphincter "dyskinesia" but do not predict symptom improvement after sphincterotomy. Peak sphincter pressure is measured during manometry but is not useful clinically.

12. **C** (S&F ch63)
This clinical presentation is consistent with type 1 SOD. These patients have biliary-type pain with elevated liver enzymes and biliary ductal dilation greater than 10 mm. Biliary sphincterotomy results in pain relief in 90% to 95% of these patients, regardless of manometry results. Therefore, sphincterotomy can be performed empirically in these patients. ERCP with pancreatic sphincterotomy and stent placement is not indicated in type 1 SOD. ERCP with bile examination for crystals and/or treatment with ursodeoxycholic acid have been used to evaluate patients with biliary type pain postcholecystectomy, with normal ducts and liver enzymes (type 3 SOD). This is investigational and not recommended in type 1 SOD.

13. **B** (S&F ch63)
The patient meets criteria for type 2 SOD. The criteria for this diagnosis are biliary type pain plus elevated AST, ALT, or alkaline phosphatase on one occasion *or* bile duct diameter greater than 10 mm. In these cases, sphincterotomy provides pain relief in 85% of patients with elevated basal pressures on SOD manometry, and in 35% of patients with normal basal pressure. Some experts recommend performing a sphincterotomy regardless of manometry. Ursodeoxycholic acid has not been shown to relieve symptoms in SOD dysfunction. ERCP with biliary stent placement is not indicated in SOD. ERCP with ampullary biopsies for IgG4 immunostaining can help in making the diagnosis of autoimmune pancreatitis but is not indicated in this case. Repeating an ultrasound in 6 months does not address the patient's symptoms.

14. **A** (S&F ch64)
In general, resection of <100 cm of the terminal ileum results in decreased bile acid absorption and increased

fecal bile acid excretion. This results in watery diarrhea due to colonic irritation. Bile acid sequestrants such as cholestyramine are frequently successful in treating this diarrhea. Note that the total bile acid pool remains intact due to increased hepatic synthesis, which balances fecal loss. Resection of >100 cm of ileum greatly decreases the amount of bile acid absorption, which cannot be compensated by increased synthesis in the liver. This results in diminished bile acid pool and steatorrhea.

15. **D** (S&F ch64)
Bile acids are stored in the proximal small intestine in the absence of a gallbladder. After ingestion of a meal, they are propelled with small bowel contractions to the terminal ileum, where they are actively reabsorbed via the enterohepatic circulation. A subset of patients will have diarrhea following cholecystectomy if the terminal ileum is unable to absorb the increased bile acid load. Treatment with a bile acid sequestrant such as cholestyramine is usually effective for treating diarrhea.

16. **E** (S&F ch64)
Bile acids are the primary solute in bile (~67%). The other solutes are phospholipids (22%), cholesterol (4%), protein (4.5%), and bilirubin (0.3%) (see figure).

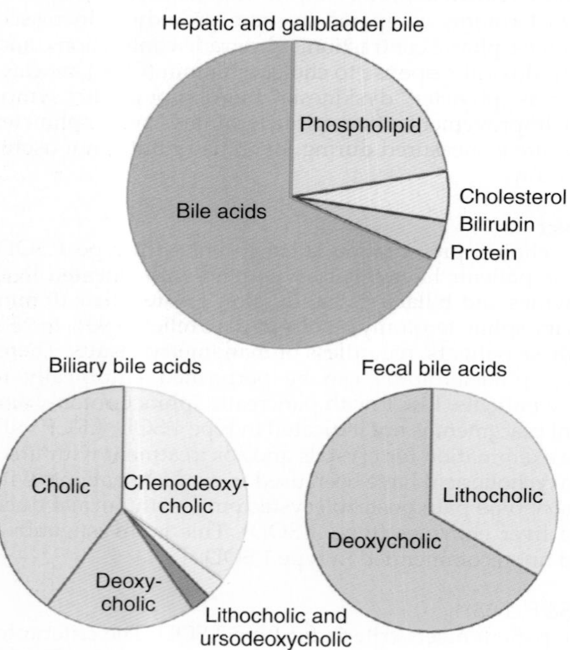

Figure for answer 16.

17. **C** (S&F ch64)
During fasting, bile acids are concentrated tenfold in the gallbladder. Less than 10% of intestinal bile acids are excreted in feces. Bile acids are actively absorbed in the distal ileum. Enterohepatic cycling of bile acids is accelerated during a meal and slows during fasting. The enterohepatic circulation of bile acids is completed 2 to 3 times per meal, or about 10 times per day.

18. **C** (S&F ch65)
Octreotide increases the prevalence of gallstones when used as treatment for acromegaly, which is likely due to decreased gallbladder motility. Cholelithiasis is not associated with feeding through a gastrostomy, but rather with total parenteral nutrition. Rapid weight loss, ulcerative colitis, and statins have not been shown to be associated with cholelithiasis. Other risk factors include obesity, ileal Crohn's disease, and treatment with octreotide.

19. **E** (S&F ch65)
Hereditary spherocytosis is associated with hemolytic anemia. Black-pigmented stones are common in patients with chronic hemolytic disorders. These stones are composed mainly of calcium bilirubinate, with lesser amounts of crystalline calcium carbonate and phosphate.

20. **D** (S&F ch65)
Symptoms of biliary pain due to cholelithiasis include right upper quadrant or epigastric pain that may radiate circumferentially to the back. Pain that radiates through to the back is more consistent with acute pancreatitis. The pain tends to intensify over 15 minutes and typically lasts 1 to 6 hours. It is constant, rather than intermittent (using the term colic is a misnomer). The associated symptoms include nausea with or without vomiting. Persistent vomiting is unusual. Fevers, gas, bloating, and jaundice are not symptoms commonly seen with gallstones.

21. **A** (S&F ch65)
Certain groups are at increased risk for gallbladder and bile duct cancer, and in these groups a prophylactic cholecystectomy should be considered. These include Caroli's disease, choledochal cysts, anomalous pancreaticobiliary junction, and porcelain gallbladder. Pigmented gallstones are commonly seen in patients with sickle cell disease, but the majority are asymptomatic. Prophylactic cholecystectomy is not recommended for this group. Asymptomatic stones are not an indication for cholecystectomy, regardless of the size.

22. **B** (S&F ch65, ch66)
The patient has evidence of gallstones and an ileus clinically. This is seen in patients that develop a cholecystenteric fistula with a gallstone eroding into the small intestine and leading to pneumobilia and mechanical small bowel obstruction. Adynamic ileus refers to nonmechanical obstruction. The patient does not have pancreatitis, based on normal lipase and imaging. He does not have cholangitis, because his bilirubin is not elevated and he does not have fevers. Mirizzi's syndrome results in biliary obstruction due to stones in the cystic duct compressing the common hepatic duct. There is no evidence of biliary obstruction with normal bilirubin and no ductal dilation.

23. **C** (S&F ch65)
After an initial attack of uncomplicated biliary pain due to gallstones, approximately 30% of patients will have no further symptoms. Symptoms develop in the other 70% at a rate of about 6% per year, and severe complications develop at a yearly rate of 1% to 2%.

24. **E** (S&F ch65)
Abdominal pain, fever, right upper quadrant tenderness and a positive HIDA scan with nonvisualization of the gallbladder is consistent with the diagnosis of acute cholecystitis. Cholescintigraphy or a HIDA scan is a nuclear medicine study that utilizes ^{99m}Tc-labeled hydroxy-iminodiacetic acid. This radiotracer is injected intravenously, taken up rapidly by the liver, and secreted into bile. Positive/abnormal findings associated with cholecystitis include nonvisualization of the gallbladder (due to cystic duct obstruction) and excretion of radiotracer into the bile duct and small intestine. Acute pancreatitis presents with epigastric and back pain, vomiting, elevated lipase, and normal HIDA scan. Alcoholic hepatitis is possible, although it would not lead to

abnormal HIDA scan. Choledocholithiasis and cholangitis are possible complications of gallstones but should not lead to nonvisualization of the gallbladder on HIDA scan.

25. **B** (S&F ch65)
This patient has acute hydrops of the gallbladder, which refers to an acute acalculous, noninflammatory distension of the gallbladder. This condition is often seen in children and infants and has been associated with Henoch-Schönlein purpura and Kawasaki's disease. It usually responds to conservative management. Acute cholecystitis is not likely, as there is no gallbladder wall thickening or edema on ultrasound. Biliary dyskinesia is diagnosed by demonstrating decreased gallbladder ejection fraction associated with acalculous biliary pain. Mesenteric vasculitis and intussusception are possible gastrointestinal complications of Henoch-Schönlein purpura, but the clinical presentation is not consistent with either of these conditions. Pancreatic cancer is rare at this age and should not be suspected.

26. **D** (S&F ch65)
This patient has a symptomatic CBD stone with elevated liver enzymes. Due to her postoperative anatomy, an ERCP is not feasible, and PTC is indicated. At some specialized centers, balloon-assisted ERCP can be performed successfully; however, this is not listed as an answer option. Ursodeoxycholic acid, has never been used as a primary therapy for treatment of bile duct stones. Surgery is an option but is more invasive than a PTC.

27. **A** (S&F ch65)
The figure shows the CT appearance of emphysematous cholecystitis. Pockets of air are seen in the gallbladder wall due to infection with gas-forming organisms. It often occurs in patients with diabetes or older men with atherosclerosis. The risk of gallbladder perforation is high if not treated with antibiotics and prompt cholecystectomy.

28. **D** (S&F ch65)
Native Americans have a 50% prevalence of gallstones by the age 50. The other ethnic groups have lower prevalence of gallstones (see figure).

29. **C** (S&F ch65)
Clofibrate increases cholesterol content in bile and decreases its bile salt content, resulting in increased lithogenicity and gallstone formation. Statins reduce cholesterol content in bile and are associated with a decreased the risk of gallstones. Ezetimibe reduces the risk of gallstones in animal studies. Cholestyramine and nicotinic acid have no association with gallstone formation or prevention.

30. **C** (S&F ch65)
Elevated triglyceride levels is associated with increased risk of gallstones. High-density lipoprotein (HDL) levels are inversely related to the risk of gallstones. High plasma total, LDL, and very-low-density lipoprotein (VLDL) cholesterol levels are not related to gallstone formation.

31. **A** (S&F ch65)
The patient presents with cholangitis secondary to infestation with *Clonorchis sinensis*, in addition to CBD obstruction from choledocholithiasis. Parasitic infestations are common in Asia and are associated with formation of brown pigment stones. The other types of stones are not related to biliary infections.

32. **C** (S&F ch65, ch67, ch69)
A Native-American patient with gallstones and incomplete calcification of the gallbladder (partial porcelain gallbladder) is at an increased risk of gallbladder carcinoma and should be offered prophylactic cholecystectomy. Cholecystectomy in asymptomatic patients with sickle cell disease, diabetes, and those on TPN is not recommended. Cholecystectomy is recommended in patients with gallbladder polyps ≥10 mm in size.

33. **D** (S&F ch65)
This patient most likely passed a stone and currently has a low risk of CBD stones (CBD <6 mm, bilirubin <1.8 mg/dL, no signs of cholangitis). Current guidelines recommend proceeding with cholecystectomy without cholangiography. If examination of the bile duct is performed as in cases of intermediate risk for choledocholithiasis,

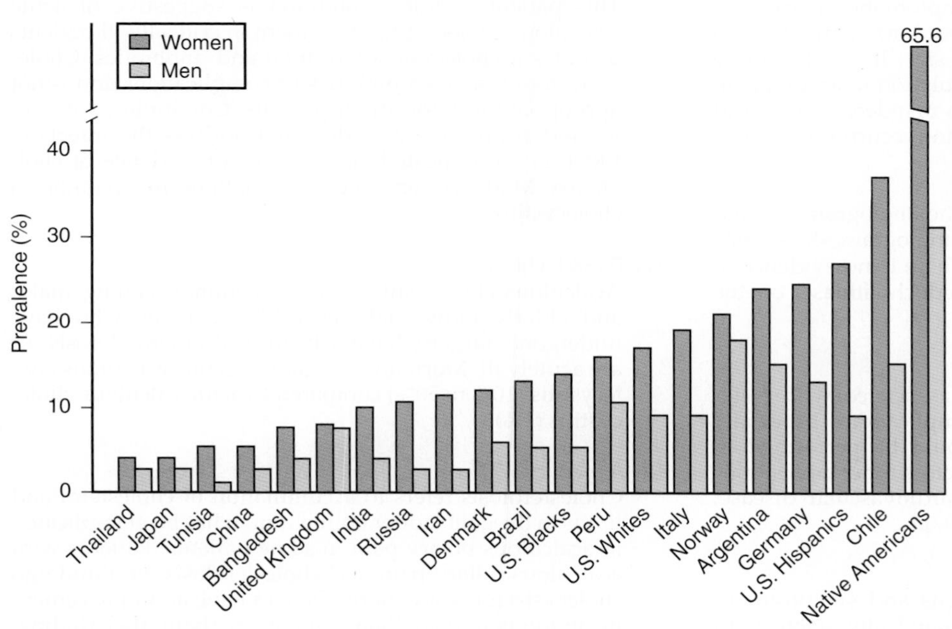

Figure for answer 28.

noninvasive studies should be performed. These include MRCP, EUS, and less commonly intraoperative ultrasound. ERCP is an invasive procedure that should only be performed if the likelihood of choledocholithiasis is high (bilirubin >4 mg/dL, cholangitis, and/or proven CBD stone on imaging studies).

34. **A** (S&F ch65)
This patient presents with biliary pain and choledocholithiasis. With a dilated bile duct to 8 mm and a persistently elevated bilirubin, the likelihood of persistent choledocholithiasis is high, and an ERCP is recommended for diagnostic and therapeutic purposes. Other imaging studies in this young patient with classic presentation of choledocholithiasis are not recommended. Laparoscopic cholecystectomy is recommended following clearance of CBD stones.

35. **B** (S&F ch65)
Focal tenderness above the gallbladder during ultrasound examination (sonographic Murphy's sign) has a positive predictive value of >90% for detecting acute cholecystitis when gallstones are present. Gallbladder wall thickening and pericholecystic fluid is suggestive but not specific of acute cholecystitis. Gallbladder distension with sludge is nonspecific. CBD stones are not predictive of acute cholecystitis.

36. **C** (S&F ch66)
Nighttime dosing of ursodeoxycholic acid is more effective and better tolerated than mealtime dosing. Oral dissolution therapy works only on cholesterol stones. Small stones respond more quickly than large stones. Calcified stones are not good targets for oral dissolution therapy. Gallbladder stasis is not affected by oral dissolution therapy.

37. **B** (S&F ch66)
Oral dissolution therapy works only for cholesterol stones. The selection criteria for oral bile acid dissolution therapy is listed in the box at end of the chapter.

38. **D** (S&F ch66)
ESWL is indicated in cases of symptomatic biliary pain without complications. It is reserved for patients with a single stone less than 20 mm in size. It should not be performed in patients on anticoagulation or in pregnant women. Maintenance therapy with ursodeoxycholic acid after ESWL is not effective in reducing recurrence rates.

39. **C** (S&F ch66)
The patient's presentation and cholangiogram is consistent with a bile leak. The cholangiogram shows bile leak from the cystic duct stump. There is no evidence of bile duct injury, stricture, or choledocholithiasis on the cholangiogram.

40. **D** (S&F ch66)
In diabetics, acute cholecystitis is associated with a significantly higher frequency of complications, especially sepsis. Early cholecystectomy should be performed in this group of patients. Other risk factors for complications include male gender, older age, cardiovascular disease, and leukocytosis with WBC >15,000/μL.

41. **A** (S&F ch66)
The patient is presenting with signs and symptoms of acute cholecystitis. He is hemodynamically stable with no contraindications for surgery. In diabetics and elderly patients, acute cholecystitis is associated with a significantly higher frequency of complications. Prompt cholecystectomy should be performed in this group of patients. Delayed cholecystectomy is associated with higher morbidity. Exploratory laparotomy is not indicated for acute cholecystitis. HIDA scan is helpful in patients with equivocal findings on ultrasound.

42. **C** (S&F ch66)
The patient's clinical presentation is most consistent with Mirizzi's syndrome, which refers to obstruction of the common hepatic duct due to compression by a stone impacted in the cystic duct. This results in common hepatic duct and intrahepatic ductal dilation, with a normal CBD below the level of the compression. Choledocholithiasis is less likely as there is no mention of such finding on ultrasound or CT scan. Furthermore, we would expect some degree of ductal dilation in the distal CBD. Acute cholecystitis is less likely due to absence of gallbladder wall thickening and pericholecystic fluid. Uncomplicated biliary pain does not lead to ductal dilation and abnormal liver enzymes. Hilar cholangiocarcinoma usually presents with obstructive jaundice of a more insidious onset over weeks to months.

43. **E** (S&F ch67)
The patient has classic biliary pain symptoms with no evidence of gallstones. Acalculous biliary pain is evaluated by either examination of the bile for cholesterol crystals (Meltzer-Lyon test) or by stimulated cholescintigraphy. The finding of a depressed ejection fraction may identify patients who are likely to improve after cholecystectomy. It is important to realize that some patients with normal ejection fraction can also improve with cholecystectomy. ERCP is not indicated in this patient. MRI might be of benefit if there were abnormal liver tests to rule out choledocholithiasis or choledochal cyst, but it is not indicated in this case. The patient does not have dyspeptic symptoms or alarm features, and an upper endoscopy is not indicated.

44. **B** (S&F ch67)
This patient's clinical condition is suggestive of acute acalculous cholecystitis. Treatment in critically ill patients includes a cholecystostomy tube and antibiotics. Cholecystectomy carries a high risk of complications and is not appropriate in critically ill patients. Continuing antibiotics and supportive care does not address the infection. ERCP is not indicated, as there is not evidence of cholangitis. Mild liver enzyme abnormalities are common in cholecystitis.

45. **D** (S&F ch67)
Acalculous cholecystitis is more common among males and elderly individuals, especially patients who have undergone surgery, have a history of atherosclerosis, or are acutely ill. Mortality is higher in acute acalculous cholecystitis (10% to 50%) compared to acute calculous cholecystitis (1%).

46. **A** (S&F ch67)
Cholesterolosis refers to accumulation of cholesterol and lipids in the gallbladder epithelium. It has been implicated in acalculous biliary pain in some patients. Patients with acalculous biliary pain and cholesterolosis who undergo cholecystectomy are more likely to have an improvement in abdominal pain than patients without this finding.

The condition is present in 12% of patients in autopsy studies and 18% in cholecystectomy specimens. There is no relationship between cholesterolosis of the gallbladder and hypercholesterolemia or hypertriglyceridemia. No racial difference in prevalence has been found.

47. **D** (S&F ch67)
Gallbladder polyps 10 mm or larger are associated with an increased risk of malignancy; therefore, cholecystectomy is recommended in these cases. Management of 6 mm to 9 mm polyps is more controversial, but most recommend repeating an ultrasound in 3 to 6 months, then at 6- to 12-month intervals to ensure stability. Endoscopic ultrasound may be helpful in characterizing gallbladder polyps, but in a polyp 10 mm or larger, cholecystectomy is the appropriate management.

48. **B** (S&F ch67)
Due to the high risk of invasive malignancy within gallbladder adenomas larger than 18 mm, open cholecystectomy should be considered because extended resection may be required in such cases. Adenomas comprise only 4% of gallbladder polyps. The majority of polyps in the gallbladder are either cholesterol polyps or adenomyomas. Gallbladder adenomas carry a risk of malignancy that increases with increasing size of the adenoma. Around half of adenomas coexist with gallstones. Two thirds of cases have only one adenoma, with the remainder having two to five adenomas in most cases.

49. **C** (S&F ch67)
Patients with primary sclerosing cholangitis are at increased risk for malignancy in the presence of gallbladder polyps. The risk of malignancy in polypoid lesions in the gallbladder is as high as 60% in patients with PSC. Therefore, cholecystectomy is recommended in all patients with PSC and gallbladder polyps, regardless of size (American Association for the Study of Liver Diseases [AASLD] recommendation, 2010). Follow-up imaging is reasonable in patients with high surgical risk. There is no role for ursodeoxycholic acid in managing gallbladder polyps. CA 19.9 does not add value to the management of this case because cholecystectomy is indicated regardless of CA 19.9 level.

50. **A** (S&F ch67)
This patient has a classic presentation of acalculous biliary pain. Calcium channel blockers and oral contraceptives can lead to a low gallbladder ejection fraction (GBEF). A low GBEF is not a reliable predictor of the response to cholecystectomy. Patients with typical acalculous biliary pain and a normal GBEF respond as well as those with depressed GBEF. Less than 50% of patients with acalculous biliary pain have a low GBEF, and one third of patients have cholesterol crystals upon bile sampling. The majority of patients with typical gallbladder pain experience long term symptom relief after cholecystectomy.

51. **E** (S&F ch67)
Pain attacks secondary to acalculous biliary pain usually recur until cholecystectomy is performed. Acalculous biliary pain is mainly a disease of young women. Physical exam and laboratory tests are usually normal.

52. **C** (S&F ch67)
Segmental adenomyomatosis appears as a circumferential narrowing of the gallbladder on oral cholecystogram (dumbbell gallbladder), and has been associated with increased risk of malignancy. Adenomyomatosis refers to excessive proliferation and invagination of the gallbladder epithelium into a thickened muscularis (propria) of the gallbladder. The gallbladder has no muscularis mucosa. These invaginations are called Rokitansky-Aschoff sinuses. The term adenomyomatosis is used when these invaginations are deep and branching. Fundal adenomyomatosis (adenomyoma) is the most common type and appears as a filling defect in the fundus (see figure).

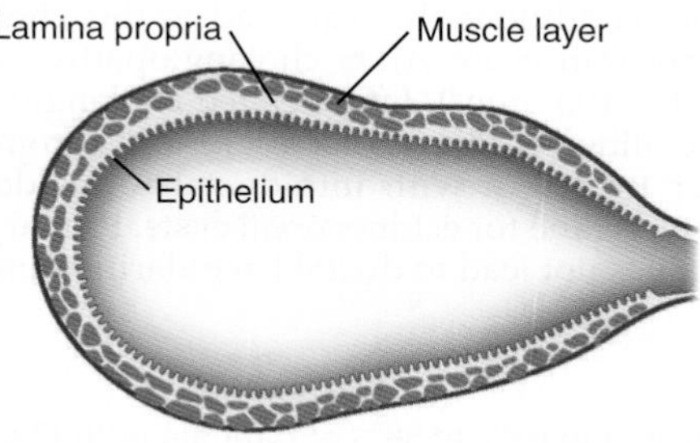

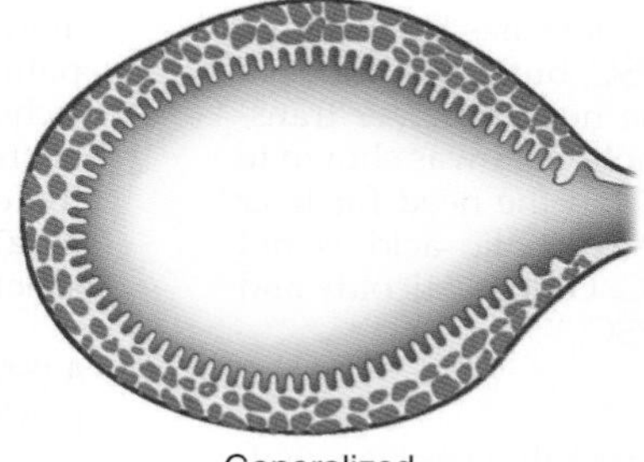

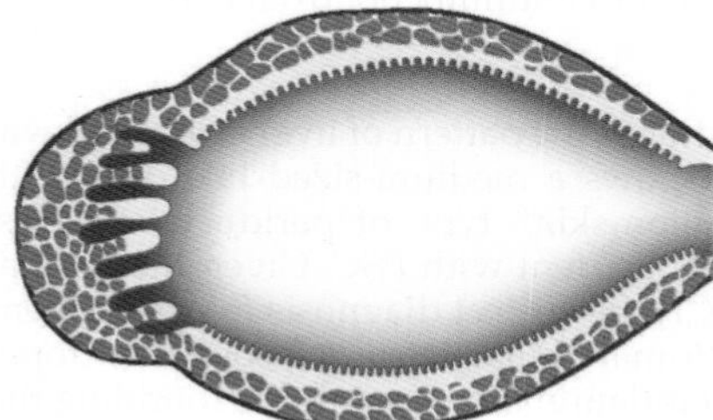

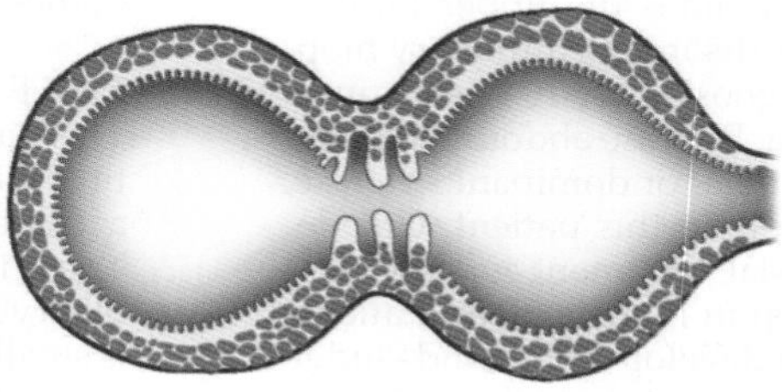

Figure for answer 52.

53. **E** (S&F ch68)
The patient's presentation and MRI are consistent with primary sclerosing cholangitis. However, secondary causes of sclerosing cholangitis must be excluded. Given the patient's history of high risk behavior and mild leukopenia, HIV should be checked. Patients with advanced HIV can develop AIDS cholangiopathy, an entity that closely resembles PSC on cholangiography. The diagnosis of PSC cannot be established without ruling out other etiologies of the abnormal biliary system. Ursodeoxycholic acid at any dose is not recommended for the treatment of PSC due to lack of clear benefit and potential adverse effects, including increased mortality with high doses. ERCP is not indicated in patients with classic findings of PSC without a dominant stricture. A liver biopsy is not required in patients with typical cholangiographic findings of PSC.

54. **B** (S&F ch68)
Most patients with PSC are diagnosed between ages 25 and 45 years, with a median age of 41 years. 70% of patients with PSC are males. Nonsmokers are at higher risk for PSC than smokers, and this relationship is not entirely explained by PSC's relationship to ulcerative colitis. PSC is seen more commonly among first-degree relatives of patients with PSC. IBD is present in 90% of patients with PSC. 85% to 90% of these patients with concomitant PSC and IBD have UC, and the remainder have Crohn's disease.

55. **B** (S&F ch68)
PSC is associated with both UC and Crohn's, but among patients with PSC and IBD, 85% to 90% have UC and the remainder have colonic or ileocolonic Crohn's disease. The risk of PSC increases with increased colonic involvement of IBD. PSC and IBD tend to progress independently. Liver transplantation for PSC does not obviate the risk of later developing IBD.

56. **C** (S&F ch68)
Cholestyramine is helpful in reducing pruritus in patients with PSC. It does not alter the course of the disease. Ursodeoxycholic acid at low to medium dose has been shown to improve liver function tests in PSC, but it has not been shown to decrease mortality or the need for liver transplantation. High-dose ursodeoxycholic acid was shown to increase the risk of death, varices, and the need for liver transplantation. Therefore, ursodeoxycholic acid is not recommended in patients with PSC. Glucocorticoids and methotrexate are not beneficial in PSC.

57. **D** (S&F ch68)
The clinical presentation is consistent with sclerosing cholangitis. In patients without IBD, this presentation should raise the suspicion for IgG4-associated cholangitis. IgG4 level elevation more than four times the upper limit of normal is 100% specific for this disorder. Ampullary biopsies can also establish the diagnosis. CA 19.9 is a tumor marker for cholangiocarcinoma. Because abdominal imaging and ERCP did not reveal a mass or dominant stricture, cholangiocarcinoma is less likely in this patient. Ursodeoxycholic acid is a controversial treatment for PSC and is not the appropriate next step in management. Patients with sclerosing cholangitis can develop stones and sludge of the biliary tract due to the presence of strictures. Cholecystectomy is not indicated in this patient at this time. HIV cholangiography can present with sclerosing cholangitis. An HIV test is appropriate in this case, rather than a stool test for *Cryptosporidium*.

58. **A** (S&F ch68)
Opioid antagonists such as naloxone or naltrexone may help pruritus in patients with PSC. These medications should be tried prior to plasmapheresis or liver transplantation, both of which are options for a patient with refractory pruritus if other options have been exhausted. There is no role for methadone or other opioids for pruritus in PSC. ERCP is not indicated in this patient because there is no stricture on MRI that may be addressed endoscopically.

59. **E** (S&F ch68)
For patients with PSC and recurrent cholangitis, prophylactic antibiotics are indicated. The preferred approach is rotating cycles of ciprofloxacin, trimethoprim-sulfamethoxazole, or amoxicillin-clavulanic acid given in 3- to 4-week cycles to reduce the risk of bacterial resistance. Liver transplantation may be necessary for recurrent cholangitis if antibiotic prophylaxis fails.

60. **C** (S&F ch68)
Primary sclerosing cholangitis should be suspected in patients with IBD presenting with liver enzyme elevation in a cholestatic pattern. MRCP is the best diagnostic test in this case because it has a high sensitivity (86%) and specificity (94%) for diagnosing PSC. Abdominal ultrasound and CT are generally considered insufficient for diagnosis because negative results do not exclude the diagnosis of PSC. ERCP is the standard test for diagnosis of PSC; however, it is associated with complications such as pancreatitis and infection. In a patient with mild elevation of liver enzymes who is unlikely to require a therapeutic intervention, MRCP should be performed first. If imaging of the biliary tract reveals no abnormalities, then liver biopsy is helpful to diagnose small duct PSC and other cholestatic liver disorders.

61. **B** (S&F ch68)
The cholangiogram shows multiple strictures and segmental dilations consistent with sclerosing cholangitis. This appearance is commonly due to primary sclerosing cholangitis. Other conditions that can lead to this cholangiographic appearance are AIDS cholangiopathy (in patients with CD4 <100/mm^3), IgG4-related cholangitis, ischemic hepatic allograft injury (hepatic artery thrombosis), and prior treatment with intraductal formaldehyde or hypertonic saline for echinococcal cysts. Primary biliary cirrhosis does not lead to ductal irregularities and stricturing.

62. **A** (S&F ch68)
p-ANCAs are present in 65% to 88% of patients with PSC. ANAs are present in low titers in 24% to 53% of patients. The other antibodies are less common: anticardiolipin antibodies (66%), ANA (24% to 53%), smooth muscle antibodies (13% to 20%), and antimitochondrial (<10%).

63. **E** (S&F ch68)
This patient has a cholestatic pattern of liver enzyme elevation. Liver biopsy shows a medium-sized bile duct with a characteristic "onion-skin" type of periductal fibrosis. These findings are consistent with PSC. Given the normal biliary tree on MRCP, the correct diagnosis for this patient is small duct PSC. Primary biliary cirrhosis shows ductopenia and portal tract inflammation, mainly surrounding the bile ducts. IgG4-related cholangitis shows IgG4-positive lymphoplasmacytic portal infiltrate. Nonalcoholic steatohepatitis shows steatosis, necroinflammation, and Mallory bodies.

64. B (S&F ch69)
The Bismuth-Corlette classification of hilar cholangiocarcinoma is useful in classifying hilar strictures and devising further endoscopic management. It can also be used to classify benign hilar strictures. Type I is a stricture that is limited to the common hepatic duct below the confluence of the right and left hepatic duct. Type I strictures can be treated with a single traversing stent. The stricture shown in the cholangiogram is type II, where the obstruction involves the confluence of the right and left hepatic duct. Type III strictures are an extension of type II, in which the tumor also involves the bifurcation of the right (IIIb) and left (IIIa) hepatic ducts. Type IV strictures are complex and extend to the right and left hepatic duct and their bifurcation, or are multifocal strictures (see figure).

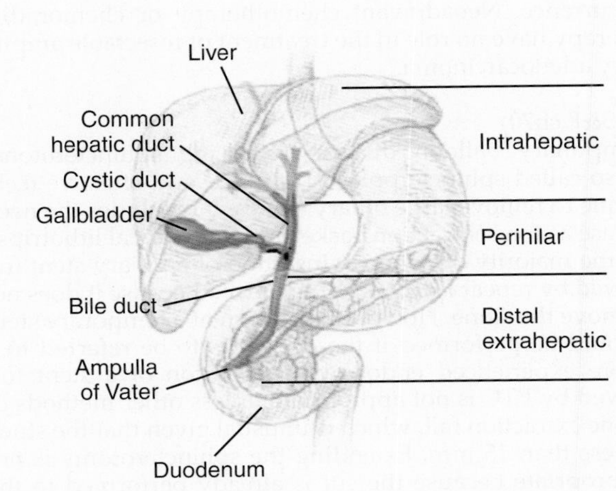

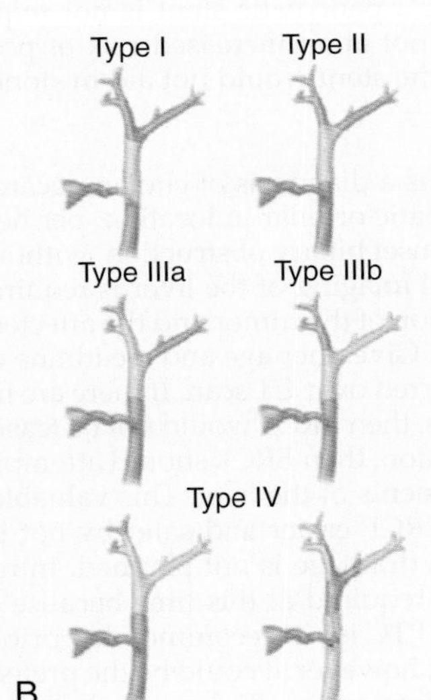

Figure for answer 64.

65. A (S&F ch69)
Adenocarcinoma is the most common type of cholangiocarcinomas, comprising more than 90% of cases. The other subtypes that are listed are much less common.

66. C (S&F ch69)
Hepatolithiasis is a risk factor for cholangiocarcinoma, especially in the setting of recurrent pyogenic cholangitis. Cholelithiasis and choledocholithiasis are not risk factors for cholangiocarcinoma. *Opisthorchis viverrini* (not *Echinococcus multilocularis*) is associated with increased risk of cholangiocarcinoma. Lynch syndrome and Peutz-Jeghers syndrome are associated with increased risk of cholangiocarcinoma, but not FAP.

67. C (S&F ch69)
Both hepatitis B and C have been associated with a higher risk of intrahepatic cholangiocarcinoma, and the risk with chronic hepatitis C is much higher than hepatitis B. The other viral infections have not been associated with intrahepatic cholangiocarcinoma.

68. B (S&F ch69)
Progressive contrast enhancement through the venous, arterial, and delayed venous phases is characteristic of cholangiocarcinoma, compared to the arterial enhancement and venous phase washout that is characteristic of hepatocellular carcinoma. Peripheral arterial enhancement with gradual filling of contrast is seen in hemangiomas. Focal nodular hyperplasia is usually a hypodense or isodense lesion, enhances on arterial phase, and may have a central scar. Hepatocellular adenomas are usually well-demarcated homogenous lesions with peripheral enhancement.

69. D (S&F ch69)
FISH is a DNA proliferation method that increases the sensitivity and specificity for diagnosing cholangiocarcinoma in patients with or without PSC. DNA changes such as trisomy 7, tetrasomy, and polysomy are detected using this method. The other methods in the question are not associated with a significant increase in the diagnostic yield of brush cytology.

70. D (S&F ch69)
The patient has locally advanced cholangiocarcinoma with bilateral portal vein involvement. Therefore, she is not a candidate for resection. Chemotherapy with gemcitabine and oxaliplatin is currently the standard of care in patients with unresectable cholangiocarcinoma without cirrhosis. Radiotherapy is not recommended for treatment due to lack of sufficient evidence for efficacy.

71. B (S&F ch69)
Cholelithiasis is the most important risk factor for gallbladder carcinoma; therefore, incidence rates of gallbladder cancer parallel that of cholelithiasis. However, gallbladder cancer occurs in 1% to 3% of those with gallstones. Given this low risk, prophylactic cholecystectomy in asymptomatic patients with gallstones is not recommended. Globally, gallbladder carcinoma has a female preponderance. Only one third of patients are diagnosed before surgical exploration. Surgical resection is the only potentially curative treatment. Unresectable cases should receive chemotherapy with gemcitabine and oxaliplatin. There is no role for radiotherapy in gallbladder carcinoma.

72. B (S&F ch69)
Patients with primary sclerosing cholangitis have an increased risk of gallbladder carcinoma. Yearly gallbladder ultrasound is recommended by the AASLD to detect mass lesions. Porcelain gallbladder is associated with increased risk of gallbladder cancer; however, the risk may be limited to cases of partial calcification rather than diffuse calcification of the gallbladder wall. 20% of patients with gallbladder cancer do not have associated gallstones. There is no difference in the risk of malignancy among the

different types of gallstones. Segmental adenomyomatosis (not cholesterolosis) is associated with increased risk of gallbladder cancer.

73. **C** (S&F ch69)
This patient most likely has functional dyspepsia, but the MRCP shows an incidental finding of abnormal union of the pancreaticobiliary ductal system (AUPBD). This lesion can be found incidentally and leads to the reflux of pancreatic secretions into the gallbladder and chronic inflammation of its mucosa. There are many versions of AUPBD. In this patient there is a long common channel between the CBD and the pancreatic duct (>15 mm). There is an increased risk of gallbladder carcinoma, and therefore cholecystectomy is recommended. ERCP and EUS would not add any additional diagnostic or therapeutic value. Repeat imaging would not be appropriate.

74. **A** (S&F ch69)
This patient is diagnosed incidentally with gallbladder cancer following cholecystectomy. The tumor invades the lamina propria, consistent with a T1a tumor. For these early tumors, simple cholecystectomy is sufficient. The other surgical procedures listed are indicated for more advanced tumors. Adjuvant (or neoadjuvant) chemotherapy is not recommended, as it does not provide any survival advantage (see figure and see table at end of chapter).

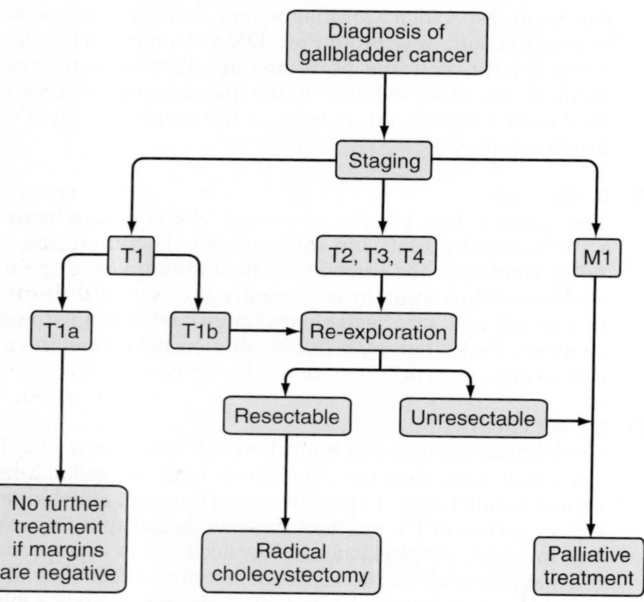

Figure for answer 74.

75. **B** (S&F ch69)
This patient is diagnosed incidentally with gallbladder cancer following cholecystectomy. The tumor invades the muscularis propria, which is consistent with a T1b tumor. For these tumors, it is recommended to re-explore the abdomen and extend the cholecystectomy. This may include resection of part of the liver around the gallbladder fossa and lymph node dissection. It would be inappropriate not to recommend further surgery, as T1b tumors have a higher risk of recurrence after simple cholecystectomy compared to extended cholecystectomy. Extended hemihepatectomy or liver resection is not indicated in T1b tumors. Adjuvant (or neoadjuvant) chemotherapy is not recommended as it does not provide any survival advantage.

76. **C** (S&F ch69)
Ampullary adenocarcinoma is the second most common cause of death (after colon cancer) in FAP patients. It is not associated with Lynch syndrome, which is increased in incidence in patients with Gardener syndrome (FAP variant). It peaks in incidence in the sixth decade. In FAP patients, it arises after the diagnosis of colon cancer, but the age of onset is earlier than in cases of sporadic ampullary carcinoma.

77. **D** (S&F ch69)
This patient has ampullary adenocarcinoma that appears resectable. Pancreaticoduodenectomy is the treatment of choice for resectable ampullary adenocarcinomas. Endoscopic or surgical ampullectomy is appropriate for small, benign diseases of the ampulla (e.g., adenoma) but is not recommended for adenocarcinoma due to the high rate of recurrence. Neoadjuvant chemotherapy or chemoradiotherapy have no role in the treatment of resectable ampullary adenocarcinoma.

78. **C** (S&F ch70)
Ampullary balloon dilation following sphincterotomy (also called sphincteroplasty) is a safe and effective technique to remove large biliary stones. It precludes the need to use a stone extraction basket and mechanical lithotripsy in the majority of patients. Insertion of a biliary stent followed by repeat ERCP is not preferred because it does not remove the stone. However, insertion of a temporary stent should be performed if the patient is to be referred to a more experienced endoscopist. Insertion of a stent followed by PTC is not appropriate unless other methods of stone extraction fail, which is unusual given that the stone is less than 15 mm. Extending the sphincterotomy is not appropriate because the cut is already performed to the maximal extent. Further extension may lead to perforation. Inserting a pancreatic stent is not required because the patient is not at an increased risk of post-ERCP pancreatitis, and the stent would not aid in stone extraction.

79. **B** (S&F ch70)
This patient has a diagnosis of cholangiocarcinoma that is likely intrahepatic or hilar in location, per her description. She has new-onset biliary obstruction, without cholangitis. Cross sectional imaging of the liver is required to find out the exact location of the tumor and the affected bile ducts to plan for ERCP. Given her age and creatinine of 1.4 mg/dL, MRCP is preferred over CT scan. If there are multiple intrahepatic masses, then ERCP would not be feasible. If there is a hilar obstruction, then ERCP should attempt to stent nonatrophied segments of the liver. This valuable information would make ERCP easier and safer by not injecting liver lobes in which drainage is not planned. Intravenous antibiotics are not required at this time because cholangitis is not suspected. PTC is not recommended prior to cross sectional imaging; however, it could be the preferred drainage procedure if there are multiple occluded segments of the biliary tract that cannot be reached or stented with ERCP.

80. **C** (S&F ch70)
This patient has a severe stricture in the common hepatic duct that does not involve the bifurcation (type 1 Bismuth-Corlette hilar stricture). A single stent is sufficient to treat the stricture. Given that the diagnosis of malignancy has not been established, and resectability (if this proves to be malignant) has not been considered, a single plastic stent is the best option to achieve biliary drainage at this time. Bilateral stenting is not necessary given that the stricture

does not involve the bifurcation. Placement of an uncovered stent could be considered if the stricture proves to be malignant and the tumor is not resectable. Balloon dilation without stent placement could be appropriate for mild benign strictures but is not appropriate for severe tight strictures with a high likelihood of malignancy.

81. **E** (S&F ch70)
Gadolinium-based intravenous contrast studies, such as MRI, have been associated with development of nephrogenic systemic fibrosis (NSF). This condition leads to thickening of the skin with erythematous plaques and nodules in all patients. Some patients develop fibrosis of other organs such as skeletal muscles, lung, and myocardium. The other conditions listed in the answer choices are not known to be associated with gadolinium-based intravenous contrast agents.

82. **B** (S&F ch70)
The clinical presentation (dull pain after cholecystectomy, fevers, fluid collections seen on ultrasound) is suspicious for a bile leak. The cholangiogram shows a large-volume leak of contrast in the gallbladder area. Treatment of such a large leak is best managed with both sphincterotomy and biliary stent placement, which will divert the bile to the duodenum away from the leak site. Smaller leaks respond to either sphincterotomy or stent placement alone. Surgical exploration is not required at this time, as most leaks respond to endoscopic management. Sphincterotomy and ampullary balloon dilation (sphincteroplasty) are not indicated as there are no large stones on cholangiogram.

83. **C** (S&F ch70)
CBD obstruction secondary to inflammatory strictures occurs in up to 10% of patients with chronic pancreatitis. Placing a fully covered metal stent has been shown to improve stricture resolution compared to single plastic stents. However, metal stents are not approved by the FDA for benign indications. These strictures are usually refractory to endoscopic treatment and may require multiple ERCPs with stenting. This is especially true in cases of chronic calcific pancreatitis where there are hard calcifications leading to stricture formation. Placing multiple plastic stents simultaneously improves the chances of stricture resolution compared to placing a single stent. Biliary strictures related to chronic pancreatitis are benign and appear smooth and tapered. A shelf-like cutoff in the bile duct should raise the suspicion of a malignant stricture.

84. **E** (S&F ch70)
The patient has malignant symptomatic CBD obstruction. Because he is not a surgical candidate due to metastatic disease, biliary drainage with ERCP is indicated. Given that the patient's performance status seems acceptable, a metal stent, rather than a plastic one, is the preferred approach. Metal stents have higher patency rates and are cost effective if placed in patients with life expectancy of more than 3 months. Fully covered metal stents are associated with higher migration rate and have been occasionally associated with acute cholecystitis (presumably due to blockage of the cystic duct take-off). The advantage of covered stents is that they may prevent tumor ingrowth; however, studies have provided mixed results regarding whether covered stent provide better patency than uncovered stents. Uncovered stents are not associated with less occlusion rates than covered ones.

85. **D** (S&F ch70)
The patient has a resectable pancreatic head lesion on CT scan, and he is an excellent candidate for curative resection by pancreaticoduodenectomy. Routine preoperative drainage is not indicated in this case with mild itching. Indications for preoperative drainage are cholangitis, severe itching, or locally advanced disease prior to chemotherapy. This patient is a surgical candidate and should proceed to surgery. Chemotherapy is not indicated given that the disease is not locally advanced. This patient has severe weight loss without imaging findings suggestive of autoimmune pancreatitis. Therefore, checking IgG4 levels is not indicated in this case.

86. **B** (S&F ch70)
The patient has a Bismuth type 2 stricture, which involves the confluence of the right and left hepatic ducts. Given that the left lobe appears atrophied, opacification of that lobe should be avoided as it will not improve biliary drainage. Attempts should be made to opacify and drain the right lobe. If the left lobe is inadvertently injected with contrast, then it should be drained to prevent the development of cholangitis.

87. **A** (S&F ch70)
Postsphincterotomy bleeding occurs in 1% to 2% of ERCPs. Risk factors include coagulopathy and restarting anticoagulation within 72 hours postprocedure. The presence of cholangitis also appears to be a risk factor for bleeding. The size of the sphincterotomy, extension of prior sphincterotomy, high bilirubin levels, and extraction of large biliary stones are not associated with increased risk of bleeding.

88. **B** (S&F ch70)
Balloon dilation of the intact papilla has largely fallen out of favor due to the risk of pancreatitis. In the only U.S. randomized trial that compared balloon dilation with sphincterotomy, two patients in the dilation group died due to severe pancreatitis, and the trial was stopped early. Bleeding is less common after dilation compared to sphincterotomy. Perforation is uncommon with both procedures. Distal CBD stricture formation and chronic biliary pain are not associated with either procedure. In this patient, an alternative (probably safer) approach would have been to insert a plastic biliary stent to achieve drainage and repeat the procedure once cholangitis has subsided and INR corrected. A sphincterotomy and regular stone extraction can be performed during the repeat ERCP.

89. **B** (S&F ch70)
This patient is presenting with painless obstructive jaundice, with intrahepatic and extrahepatic biliary dilation on MRCP. Without a history of pain to suggest choledocholithiasis, malignancy should be suspected. He is symptomatic with bothersome itching. Small ampullary carcinoma or occult cholangiocarcinomas may not show on cross sectional imaging. ERCP for examination of the ampulla and the distal bile duct would be diagnostic and therapeutic (stent insertion). Endoscopic ultrasound could be a complementary test to look for occult masses of pancreas and distal bile duct but would not be the first choice in this patient with symptomatic biliary obstruction. CT scan of the abdomen would not add much to the current information obtained from MRI/MRCP. Cholecystectomy (with or without a cholangiogram) is inappropriate, because the diagnosis of choledocholithiasis is unlikely and has not been confirmed.

BOX FOR ANSWER 37 Selection Criteria for Oral Bile Acid Dissolution Therapy

Stage of Gallstone Disease
Symptomatic (biliary pain) without complications

Gallbladder Function
Opacification of gallbladder on oral cholecystography (patent cystic duct)
Normal result of stimulated cholescintigraphy (normal gallbladder emptying)
Normal result of functional ultrasound (normal gallbladder emptying after a test meal)

Stone Characteristics
Radiolucent
Isodense or hypodense to bile and absence of calcification on CT
Diameter ≤ 10 mm (<6 mm optimal)

TABLE FOR ANSWER 74 TNM and American Joint Committee on Cancer (AJCC)/International Union Against Cancer (UICC) Staging Systems for Gallbladder Carcinoma

TNM stage	Criteria		
Tx	Primary tumor cannot be assessed		
T0	No evidence of primary tumor		
Tis	Carcinoma in situ		
T1a	Tumor invades lamina propria		
T1b	Tumor invades muscularis propria		
T2	Tumor invades perimuscular connective tissue without extension beyond serosa or into liver		
T3	Tumor perforates the serosa *and/or* Tumor directly invades the liver *and/or* Tumor invades one other adjacent organ (e.g., stomach, duodenum, colon, pancreas, omentum, extrahepatic bile ducts)		
T4	Tumor invades the portal vein or hepatic artery *or* Tumor invades ≥2 extrahepatic organs or structures		
Nx	Regional lymph nodes cannot be assessed		
N0	No regional lymph node metastases		
N1	Lymph node metastases along the cystic duct, bile duct, hepatic artery, *and/or* portal vein		
N2	Metastases to periaortic, pericaval, superior mesenteric artery, *and/or* celiac artery lymph nodes		
M0	No distant metastases		
M1	Distant metastases		
AJCC/UICC stage	**Tumor**	**Node**	**Metastasis**
0	Tis	N0	M0
I	T1	N0	M0
II	T2	N0	M0
III A	T3	N0	M0
III B	T1-3	N1	M0
IV A	T4	N0-1	M0
IV B	Any T Any T	N2 Any N	M0 M1

TNM, Tumor, node, metastasis.

CHAPTER

9

Liver

Nader Dbouk, Anjana Pillai, Brett Mendel, José Rivera-Acosta, Joel P. Wedd, Samir Parekh, John Paul Norvell, William Joseph Goldkamp, Kanak Das, Matthew Barnes, and Jeffrey Nadelson

QUESTIONS

1. At what age does the development of the liver start?
A. First week of gestation
B. Sixth week of gestation
C. Third week of gestation
D. Tenth week of gestation
E. Twentieth week of gestation

2. Which of the following statements is true regarding Riedel's lobe?
A. It is an accessory lobe arising from the left hepatic lobe
B. It is more common in males
C. It is usually associated with elevated liver enzymes
D. It is often mistaken for a mass on imaging
E. It is associated with increased risk of malignancy

3. Which of the following statements is correct regarding Abernethy's malformation?
A. This is a congenital intrahepatic portocaval shunt
B. Type 1 Abernethy malformation may be complicated by focal nodular hyperplasia
C. In type 2 malformation, the portal vein is absent
D. Type 1 malformation is more common in boys
E. Type 2 malformation is associated with cardiac defects or biliary atresia

4. What is the most common origin of the hepatic artery?
A. Superior mesenteric artery (SMA)
B. Celiac trunk
C. Gastroduodenal artery
D. Inferior mesenteric artery (IMA)
E. Splenic artery

5. Which of these statements is true regarding hepatoblasts?
A. They can only give rise to hepatocytes
B. Their numbers increase with increasing age
C. They are present throughout the parenchyma of fetal livers
D. They are present in the canal of Luschka in adults
E. They arise from Kupffer cells

6. Which of the following cells function as macrophages in the hepatic parenchyma?
A. Stellate cells
B. Cholangiocytes
C. Kupffer cells
D. Natural killer (NK) cells
E. Sinusoidal endothelial cells

7. Expression of which of the following genes is responsible for extrahepatic biliary development?
A. *SOX17*
B. *Wnt/β-catenin*
C. *HNF1B*
D. *FOXA2*
E. *HNF6*

8. A 9-month-old boy underwent liver biopsy after manifesting jaundice, clay-colored stool, and organomegaly for 2 months. Liver histology shows bile duct injury, cellular infiltration of portal tracts, lymphocytic infiltration, and periductal fibrosis, in addition to paucity of bile ducts. He was diagnosed with Alagille syndrome. Which of the following is correct regarding this patient's condition?
A. It is an autosomal dominant disorder with 100% penetrance rate
B. Mutations in the *JAG1* gene are detected in more than 90% of patients
C. The hallmark of this syndrome is the absence of extrahepatic bile ducts
D. Severe mental retardation is seen in more than 80% of the affected patients
E. None of these patients survive to the age of 2 years

9. A 60-year-old former intravenous drug user was found to have elevated liver enzymes. Further testing revealed he was positive for hepatitis C. A liver biopsy showed bridging fibrosis and nodule formation. Which type of cell is activated in fibrosis progression?
A. Kupffer cells
B. Stellate cells
C. Pit cells
D. Cholangiocytes
E. Sinusoidal cells

10. A 25-year-old man with primary sclerosing cholangitis presents with worsening jaundice, esophageal variceal bleeding, and ascites. He undergoes a liver transplant evaluation and his brother is identified as a suitable donor for living donor liver transplantation and donates the right lobe of the liver. Which cells play a central role in hepatic regeneration after a partial hepatectomy?
A. Adult hepatocytes
B. Liver progenitor cells
C. Oval cells
D. Stellate cells
E. Pit cells

11. Which of these proteins produced in the liver inhibits elastin?
A. α1-Acid glycoprotein
B. α1-Antichymotrypisn
C. Serum amyloid A
D. α1-Antitrypsin
E. Transferrin

12. Which of the following apolipoproteins synthesized in the liver are instrumental for triglyceride transport and is the predominant transport carrier in very low density lipoprotein (VLDL)?
A. Apo-E
B. ApoB-100
C. ApoB-48
D. ApoA-1
E. Apo-C

13. A 30-year-old woman was noted to have extremely low HDL levels on a routine physical exam. Her only other pertinent history was having orange-colored tonsils removed at age 6. She was told her risk of atherosclerotic heart disease is four- to sixfold higher than the general population. Which gene mutation is responsible for the above scenario?
A. Lecithin-cholesterol acyltransferase
B. Hepatic TG lipase
C. Cholesteryl ester transfer protein
D. ATP-binding cassette transporter A1
E. HMG-CoA reductase

14. On routine physical exam, a 25-year-old man is found to have laboratory values as follows:

Total bilirubin 15 mg/dL
Unconjugated bilirubin 0.8 mg/dL
ALT 18 U/L
AST 25 U/L
Alkaline phosphatase 80 U/L

A liver biopsy is performed and the tissue obtained is black in appearance. Which of the following disorders is the cause of the above condition?
A. Rotor's syndrome
B. Gilbert's syndrome
C. Crigler-Najjar syndrome type 1
D. Dubin Johnson syndrome
E. Crigler-Najjar syndrome type 2

15. A 55-year-old obese man with a past medical history of hypertriglyceridemia, diabetes and daily alcohol consumption presents with laboratory values as follows:

ALT 200 U/L
AST 120 U/L
Alkaline phosphatase 150 U/L
Total bilirubin 1.5 mg/dL
Glucose 250 mg/dL
Platelet count 200,000/μL

Liver biopsy shows significant macrovesicular steatosis, ballooning, and mild inflammation. What is the most likely cause of his liver disease?
A. Alcoholic hepatitis
B. Nonalcoholic fatty liver disease
C. Autoimmune hepatitis
D. Wilson's disease
E. Ischemic hepatitis

16. What causes the AST to ALT ratio to be greater than 2 in alcoholic liver disease?
A. Deficiency of 5′-nucleotidase
B. Increased synthesis of AST
C. Deficiency of pyridoxal-5′-phosphate
D. Increased synthesis of pyridoxal-5′-phosphate
E. Deficiency of tissue transglutaminase

17. A 50-year-old Caucasian woman presents with generalized pruritus and mild scleral icterus, which was initially noted by her husband 3 weeks ago. Laboratory values are as follows:

ALT 125 U/L
AST 150 U/L
Alkaline phosphatase 300 U/L
Total bilirubin 3.5 mg/dL
Platelet count 70,000/μL

Physical exam reveals spider angiomas on her chest and face in addition to palmar erythema. Chest x-ray is normal and an ultrasound of the abdomen reveals a cirrhotic liver. Which of the following tests would confirm the diagnosis?
A. Angiotensin converting enzymes (ACE) level
B. Anti–smooth muscle antibodies (ASMA)
C. Antimitochondrial antibodies (AMA)
D. Ferritin
E. Serum copper

18. Which one of the following clotting factors is produced by vascular endothelial cells?
A. Factor V
B. Factor VII
C. Factor IX
D. Factor X
E. Factor VIII

19. A 49-year-old Chinese man is referred for evaluation of hepatitis B virus (HBV). He is asymptomatic. He notes a family history of viral hepatitis and his father was treated for hepatocellular carcinoma (HCC). Physical exam is significant for anicteric sclera, soft and nontender abdomen with no hepatosplenomegaly. No spider nevi or jaundice noted. Laboratory values are as follows:

ALT 21 U/L
AST 23 U/L
Bilirubin 0.6 mg/dL
ALP 76 U/L
WBC 4500/μL
Hematocrit 43%
Platelet count 230,000/μL
HBsAg positive
HBeAg negative
HBe antibody positive
HBV DNA 80 IU/mL
Hepatitis C virus (HCV) antibody negative

Abdominal ultrasound shows normal-appearing liver. Which of the following would you recommend?
A. Liver biopsy
B. Entecavir
C. Tenofovir
D. Pegylated interferon (IFN)
E. Abdominal ultrasound every 6 months

20. A 57-year-old man with alcoholic cirrhosis presents for evaluation. He has been abstinent for 18 months and is engaged in Alcoholics Anonymous (AA). Complications of liver disease are fatigue and mild ascites controlled with diuretics. Pertinent physical findings on exam include muscle wasting and splenomegaly. Laboratory values are as follows:

INR	1.5
Albumin	3 mg/dL
Bilirubin	3.5 mg/dL
Creatinine	0.9 mg/dL
AFP	6 ng/mL
Hematocrit	38%

Serology studies for autoimmune hepatitis or viral hepatitis are negative. PaO2 on room air is 80 mm Hg. Abdominal ultrasound shows coarse echotexture, splenomegaly but no suspicious mass. An EGD done last month revealed severe portal hypertensive gastropathy. Cardiac echo last week showed positive bubble study. The patient is listed for liver transplantation. Which additional evaluation would you recommend at this time?

A. Liver biopsy
B. Contrast-enhanced MRI of the liver
C. Bone densitometry
D. Macroaggregated albumin perfusion scan
E. Nadolol

21. A patient with alcoholic cirrhosis presents to the emergency department with abdominal pain in the last 3 days. On exam his abdomen is markedly distended and diffusely tender. He is afebrile. He admits ongoing alcohol abuse. An abdominal ultrasound shows a cirrhotic liver, splenomegaly, and large volume ascites. No suspicious mass is noted. You perform a diagnostic paracentesis and the cell count shows the following:

WBC	1000/μL
Neutrophils	76%
Gram stain	negative

You diagnose spontaneous bacterial peritonitis and admit him to the hospital for intravenous antibiotics and fluids. The patient completes 7 days of intravenous antibiotics and is ready for discharge. What is the most appropriate recommendation at this time?

A. Start daily norfloxacin and continue indefinitely
B. Refer for a liver transplant evaluation
C. Schedule an urgent EGD for variceal screening
D. Schedule a weekly paracentesis to relieve symptoms
E. Schedule an abdominal MRI for hepatocellular carcinoma screening

22. A 65-year-old Asian man with chronic HBV and cirrhosis is referred to your clinic. He is not currently on HBV treatment. A recent abdominal ultrasound did not show any suspicious lesion in the liver. His laboratory values are as follows:

AST	45 U/L
ALT	34 U/L
HBeAg	negative
HBeAb	positive
HBV DNA	3000 IU/mL
INR	1.3
Total bilirubin	1 mg/dL

What is the most appropriate recommendation at this time?

A. A liver biopsy to assess for inflammation
B. An abdominal MRI
C. Initiating antiviral treatment with tenofovir
D. Holding antiviral treatment for now and monitor liver function tests every 6 months
E. Treatment with interferon

23. A 60-year-old man with chronic HCV and cirrhosis is referred to your clinic for further evaluation. A recent MRI showed a new 2 cm lesion with imaging characteristics typical for hepatocellular carcinoma. AFP level is 230 ng/mL. The patient's liver disease has been complicated by ascites and encephalopathy. He does not have significant medical comorbidities and has good social support. What is the most appropriate next step?

A. Refer for a transplant evaluation
B. Refer to oncology
C. Refer to surgery for resection
D. Observation with serial imaging every 3 months
E. Start antiviral therapy for HCV

24. A 54-year-old woman with autoimmune hepatitis and cirrhosis presents for follow-up. She is maintained on a low dose of prednisone. Her liver disease has been complicated by ascites and she requires a paracentesis once every 2 to 3 months. She states that she feels more fatigued recently. Physical exam shows the following:

Blood pressure	100/56 mm Hg
Heart rate	94 bpm
Temperature	36° C

Sclera is icteric, mild temporal wasting is present, and moderate ascites on abdominal exam is noted. Her laboratory values are as follows:

AST	65 U/L
ALT	57 U/L
Total bilirubin	2.4 mg/dL
INR	1.7
Creatinine	3.5 mg/dL (Baseline creatinine is 0.8 mg/dL)

Urinalysis shows no pyuria, proteinuria, or hematuria. You admit her to the hospital. Diuretics are held and the she is started on intravenous fluids and empiric antibiotics, pending culture results. Ascitic fluid cell count is 100/μL and gram stain is negative. Repeat labs after 48 hours show the following:

Creatinine	5.6 mg/dL
Sodium	128 mEq/dL
Postassium	4.3 mEq/dL
Bicarbonate	21 mEq/dL

The patient is breathing comfortably on room air. What is the most appropriate next step at this time?

A. Urgent evaluation for a kidney transplant
B. Urgent evaluation for a combined liver-kidney transplant
C. Nephrology consult to initiate dialysis
D. Aggressive intravenous fluids
E. Urgent evaluation for a liver transplant

25. A 38-year-old woman with autoimmune hepatitis and cirrhosis is referred to your clinic. She complains of dyspnea on exertion, which has been present for several months. She denies any history of tobacco use. A chest x-ray is normal. Room air arterial blood gas shows a PaO2 of 58 mm Hg. What is the next most appropriate step in her evaluation?

A. An exercise stress test
B. A chest CT with intravenous contrast

C. Pulmonary function tests
D. An echocardiogram with bubble study
E. A bronchoscopy

26. A 45-year-old man with primary sclerosing cholangitis (PSC) and cirrhosis presents with worsening pruritus and new onset jaundice. He reports weight loss of about 15 pounds over the past month. He is afebrile and denies any significant abdominal pain. His laboratory values are as follows:

ALP	644 U/L
Total bilirubin	5.8 mg/dL
AST	122 U/L
ALT	120 U/L
INR	1.3
Hematocrit	32%
WBC	5000/μL
CA 19-9	533 U/mL
AFP	23 ng/mL

What is the most appropriate next step in his management?
A. Proceed with a liver biopsy
B. Start intravenous antibiotics
C. Refer for a transplant evaluation
D. MRI/MRCP
E. ERCP

27. What is the most common cause of death in patients with compensated cirrhosis?
A. Cardiovascular disease
B. Hepatocellular carcinoma
C. Stroke
D. End-stage renal disease
E. Sepsis

28. A 30-year-old Caucasian woman with no past medical history is referred to your office for anemia. On a routine physical, her primary care doctor noted a hemoglobin of 10.0 g/dL with an MCV of 78 fL. She has no history of gastrointestinal bleeding, pregnancy, heavy menses, diarrhea, or weight loss. She does not drink alcohol. Her father and his brother were both said to have some kind of liver problem due to iron. Her mother was told she does not carry any mutations associated with iron storage diseases. Her physical examination is normal. Stool studies for occult blood were negative. Her fasting serum iron (51 mcg/dL) and total iron- binding capacity (302 mcg/dL) both were normal, but her serum ferritin is 1121 ng/mL. Other laboratory values are as follows:

Alkaline phosphatase	78 U/L
ALT	28 U/L
AST	35 U/L
Total bilirubin	1.0 g/dL
LDH	160 U/L

Thyroid function tests and celiac serology all were normal. There is no evidence of hemolysis. Which of the following findings would be most likely?
A. She has a mutation in the *HAMP* gene
B. She is a homozygote for the *C282Y* mutation
C. She is a *C282Y/H63D* compound heterozygote
D. She has a transferrin receptor 2 mutation
E. Her liver biopsy demonstrates increased iron predominantly in Kupffer cells

29. A 40-year-old Caucasian woman presents to your office for consultation. Her brother was recently diagnosed with hereditary hemochromatosis requiring weekly phlebotomy. She reports no history of anemia, abnormal menses, unusual skin color changes or diabetes. Her parents recently saw a geneticist, and were both informed that they are heterozygous for the *C282Y* mutation. She is very concerned about developing symptomatic hemochromatosis. Her genetic testing is still pending. Including her risk of inheriting the genotype, what is her risk of developing iron overload–related disease?
A. 1/4
B. 1/15
C. 1/100
D. 1/200
E. 1/400

30. A 45-year-old man comes to your office for a follow-up visit. One year ago he was diagnosed with hereditary hemochromatosis after routine blood work found elevated ferritin and genetic testing revealed he had a *C282Y/H63D* genotype. He has been treated by phlebotomy with one unit of blood removed every week for the past year. His most recent laboratory results include the following:

Hemoglobin	12.0 g/dL
Hematocrit	36%
Serum ferritin	50 ng/mL
Serum iron	100 ug/dL
Serum total IBC	260 mg/dL

What is the most appropriate next step in his therapy?
A. Phlebotomy 1 unit every 3 months
B. A low iron diet
C. Phlebotomy 1 unit every 2 weeks until the hemoglobin concentration is less than 10.0 g/dL
D. Liver biopsy to assess hepatic iron overload
E. Phlebotomy 1 unit every 2 weeks until the serum iron level is less than 20 ug/dL

31. A 30-year-old man is referred to you after his brother is found to have *C282Y* homozygous hereditary hemochromatosis. The patient feels well and has no medical problems. The physical examination reveals a healthy, muscular white male in no distress. Serum iron, total iron binding capacity, ferritin, and transferrin saturation are normal. Which of the following should you order now?
A. HLA typing
B. Genetic testing for *C282Y* mutation
C. MRI of the liver with gadolinium
D. Liver biopsy with quantitative iron studies
E. No further diagnostic testing at this time

32. A 45-year-old man presents to the clinic one week after an emergency department visit for palpitations. He was diagnosed with supraventricular tachycardia that resolved after cardioversion. His primary care doctor recently diagnosed him with diabetes. He reports that his brother died of liver failure 1 year ago. In the office, review of systems reveals 1 year of progressively worsening fatigue, darkening of his skin, and arthralgia. He has recently noticed difficulty keeping an erection. On cardiac exam, he has a laterally displaced point of maximal impulse (PMI). Abdominal exam reveals hepatomegaly with mild right upper quadant tenderness. Joint exam reveals bony enlargement of the second and third metacarpophalangeal joints in both hands with limited extension secondary to pain. Laboratory examination reveals the following:

Hemoglobin	15.0 g/dL
Hematocrit	45%
Serum ferritin	2000 ng/mL
Serum iron	100 mg/dL
Serum total IBC	150 mg/dL
Transferrin saturation	70%
AST	80 U/L
ALT	75 U/L
ALP	80 U/L

Testing for *HFE* mutations reveals the patient is homozygous for the *C282Y* mutation. Which of the following is unlikely to improve with proper therapy?

A. Cardiomyopathy
B. Joint space changes
C. Hepatomegaly
D. Diabetes
E. Skin discoloration

33. A 42-year-old Caucasian man with a normal physical examination and normal liver function tests comes to your office for evaluation. Routine blood work recently revealed an iron saturation of 55%. The patient's brother died at the age 52 of cirrhosis complicated by hepatocellular carcinoma. Which of the following is the next best step in evaluating this patient for hemochromatosis?

A. Perform genetic testing for the *C282Y* mutation
B. Measure serum ferritin
C. Obtain HLA typing of the remaining siblings
D. Measure liver iron by performing MRI
E. Determine response to phlebotomy

34. A 50-year-old Caucasian woman with a history of rheumatoid arthritis presents to your office for evaluation of chronic anemia. Her rheumatic disease has been well controlled on adalimumab for the past 5 years. Her primary care doctor, however, noticed a lower hemoglobin on a recent physical. She has no history of abnormal menses or GI bleeding. Her most recent laboratory values include the following:

Hemoglobin	11.0 g/dL
Hematocrit	32%
MCV	83 fL
Serum ferritin	195 ng/mL
Serum total IBC	225 mg/dL
Transferrin Saturation	25%

Abnormal expression of which of the following genes is most likely the cause of her anemia?

A. *HFE*
B. *Hepcidin*
C. *Ferroportin*
D. *BMP*
E. *HAMP*

35. A 33-year-old man presents to your office for evaluation after his father was diagnosed with hereditary hemochromatosis. His mother underwent genetic testing, and was found to be a heterozygous carrier of the *H63D* mutation. The patient is worried about developing hemochromatosis. Which of the following laboratory values would be the most sensitive and specific finding that would predict the development of symptomatic iron overload?

A. Genetic testing showing a *C282Y/H63D* genotype
B. ALT elevation
C. Elevated transferrin saturation
D. Elevated serum ferritin
E. Elevated iron binding capacity

36. A 46-year-old man is found to have an iron saturation of 90% and a serum ferritin of 1000 ng/mL. Genetic testing for *HFE* confirms that he is homozygous for the *C282Y* mutation. His wife asks about screening their three sons. What is the best test to predict their children's risk of developing hemochromatosis?

A. Measure serum iron and total iron binding capacity (TIBC) in all three sons
B. Measure serum ferritin only in all three sons
C. Test all three sons for the *HFE* mutation
D. Measure serum iron, TIBC, ferritin and screen for the *HFE* in all three sons
E. Test the wife for the *HFE* mutation

37. A 67-year-old man is referred to you from his hematologist. He has a history of myelodysplastic syndrome requiring frequent blood transfusions. Recent blood work revealed a ferritin level of 1050 ng/mL. An echocardiogram revealed biventricular dilation and early diastolic dysfunction. You inform the patient that he will need to start iron chelation therapy. Which of the following is a possible side effect of oral iron chelation therapy with deferasirox?

A. Skin discoloration
B. Pulmonary fibrosis
C. Neuropathy
D. Gastrointestinal bleeding
E. Heart failure

38. A 14-year-old Caucasian boy was referred for evaluation after elevated liver enzymes were identified on a routine laboratory workup. The patient is asymptomatic and does not have other systemic diseases.. He reports a healthy lifestyle with no previous use of alcohol or any other drugs and is physically active and involved in his school basketball team. Patient has two younger siblings who are healthy. His father died of fulminate hepatic failure at the age 25. The patient is 5 feet 5 inches and weighs 125 pounds. The physical exam is unremarkable. Laboratories revealed the following values:

ALT	63 U/L
AST	140 U/L
Total bilirubin	0.7 mg/dL
Alkaline phosphatase	27 IU/L
Hemoglobin	14.0 g/dL

A workup for most common causes of chronic and acute viral hepatitis is negative. Liver biopsy reveals steatosis, focal necrosis, glycogenated nuclei in hepatocytes and scattered apoptotic bodies. Electron microscopy of the specimen is remarkable for mitochondria of variable size with dilatation of the tips of the cristae. What will be the most expected laboratory results in this patient?

A. Insulin resistance calculated with homeostasis model (HOMA-IR)
B. High concentration of urinary copper
C. Elevated ferritin levels
D. Elevated anti–smooth muscle antibodies titers
E. Low serum alpha1-antitrypsin levels

39. A 14-year-old Japanese boy is brought to the hospital after he developed abdominal discomfort for duration of 2 days. The patient's mother reports that he developed yellow discoloration of skin and increase of the abdominal girth in the last 3 months. He had previous episodes of discoloration of skin that resolved with no medical treatment. On physical exam the patient is alert and oriented with an unremarkable neurological exam. Abdomen is mildly distended with a positive fluid wave and no rebound tenderness. Abdominal sonogram revealed a normal size liver with coarsened echotexture and moderate ascites. Laboratories revealed the following:

ALT	135 IU/L
Alkaline phosphatase	30 IU/L
Total bilirubin	3.4 mg/dL
Indirect bilirubin	2.2 mg/dL
Prothrombin time	17 seconds
Creatinine	1.7 mg/dL

Which of the following is the best next step to confirm the diagnosis?

A. Slit-lamp exam
B. Serum ceruloplasmin by immunologic method
C. 24-hour urine collection for copper
D. *ATP7B* gene mutation analysis
E. Percutaneous liver biopsy

40. A 13-year-old girl presents to your clinic to establish medical care. Her family recently moved from her hometown in California to Florida. She was diagnosed with Wilson disease 2 years ago after she developed elevated liver enzymes and mild hyperbilirubinemia. She was started on D-penicillamine and the last biochemical test performed 1 month ago demonstrated normalization of liver enzymes and bilirubin levels. She has two brothers and one sister all less than 18 years old. Her father is 33 years old and mother is 32 years old; both are alive and have no diagnosed systemic disease. What should be your next recommendation to this patient and her relatives?

A. Screening ceruloplasmin levels of all siblings
B. Screening serum ceruloplasmin of all first-degree relatives
C. Gene mutation analysis of the patient, followed by gene screening of siblings
D. Gene mutation analysis of the patient, followed by gene screening of all first-degree relatives
E. Careful slit-lamp examination of all siblings

41. A 22-year-old woman with no previous systemic illness is brought by her fiancé to the emergency department with new onset altered mental status, associated with jaundice. The fiancé reports that the patient started turning yellow approximately 1 week ago and complained of dark urine. Symptoms progressed during the week, with general malaise, arthralgia, abdominal bloating, and lower extremity swelling. This morning she became disoriented. Her fiancé reports she is a healthy person that exercises regularly, with no toxic habits and no recent use of herbal supplements. She used 1 gm of acetaminophen yesterday for what she described as "mild pounding headaches." The fiancé does not know her family medical history, but he reports that her stepbrother had a liver transplant when he was a child. Her vital signs are as follows:

Temperature	37.7° C
Blood pressure	101/74 mm Hg
Heart rate	107 bpm
Respiratory rate	23 breaths/min

During physical exam the patient is disoriented and with incoherent thinking. She has scleral jaundice, decreased breath sounds on lung bases, a distended abdomen with positive fluid wave and shifting dullness. She has lower extremity pitting edema and flapping tremors on upper extremities. Laboratory values are as follows:

Sodium	134 mmol/L
Potassium	5.8 mmol/L
Chloride	102 mmol/L
CO2	125 mmol/L
BUN	40 mg/dL
Creatinine	1.8 mg/dL
Glucose	54 mg/dL
Phosphate	5.4 mg/dL
WBC	11,400/μL
Hemoglobin	8.0 g/dL
Platelets	120,000/μL
PT	25 sec
Total bilirubin	8.0 mg/dL
Indirect bilirubin	5.7 mg/dL
ALT	240 IU/L
AST	552 IU/L
ALP	30 IU/L
ANA	1:120
Lactic acid	2.2 mmol/L
LDH	380 U/L (elevated)
Hepatitis B surface antigen	negative
Hepatitis B surface antibody	positive
Hep B core IgM	negative
Hep B core IgG	negative
Hepatitis A total antibody	negative

The patient is transferred to the intensive care unit, started on intravenous fluids and empiric antibiotics, and your service is consulted for recommendations. What is the best next step in the management?

A. Start methylprednisolone 1gm intravenously daily for 3 days
B. Prednisolone 40 mg orally daily
C. Transfer to liver transplant center for emergent orthotropic liver transplant
D. Start acetylcysteine 140 mg/kg by nasogastric tube followed by 70 mg/kg every 4 hours until you have the results of acetaminophen levels in serum
E. Start tenofovir 300 mg orally daily

42. A 10-year-old girl was diagnosed with Wilson disease 3 weeks ago after being found with elevated liver enzymes, anemia, and mild jaundice. The patient is shorter than her same age classmates. A serum ceruloplasmin level was 5 and 24-hour urine collection for copper was 250 microgram/day. A liver biopsy was performed that revealed moderate steatosis, glycogenated nuclei of hepatocytes, mild lobular inflammation, and mild periportal fibrosis. She was started on D-penicillamine at 20 mg/kg/day and pyridoxine 25mg daily, and was referred for evaluation with you in 3 weeks. She returns to your clinic today reporting no complaints. Physical exam is unremarkable with no rashes. Today's laboratories results are as follows:

Sodium	145 mmol/LU/A
Potassium	3.0 mmol/L
Chloride	120 mmol/L
CO2	18 mmol/L
BUN	15 mg/dL
Creatinine	1.6 mg/dL
Glucose	60 mg/dL
Phosphate	1.9 mg/dL
Albumin	3.2 mg/dL
WBC	5400/μL
Hemoglobin	9.9 gm/dL
Platelets	180,000/μL

Urinalysis:	
WBC	0/HPF
RBC	2-4/HPF
Protein	+
No cast	
pH	5.3
Urine phosphate	high
24-hr copper	400 microgram/day

What is the most probable cause of patient's eleveted creatinine level?
A. Adverse effect of penicillamine
B. Hepatorenal syndrome
C. Interstitial nephritis
D. Fanconi syndrome
E. Severe prerenal state

43. A 13-year-old patient was diagnosed with Wilson disease 9 days ago after elevated liver enzymes were found on a routine well-being evaluation. A serum ceruloplasmin level was 10 mg/dL and 24-hour urine collection for cooper was 300 microgram/day. A liver biopsy was performed that revealed a copper concentration of 200 microgram/gram of dry weight. Patient was started on D-penicillamine at 20 mg/kg/day and pyridoxine 25mg orally daily. The Patient presents to the emergency department with complaint of fever spikes that started this morning. The Patient reports general malaise but denies sore throat, earache, abdominal pain, dysuria, shortness of breath, or diarrheas. He reports foamy urine since yesterday. Vital signs reveal a Temperature 39.3° C. Physical exam is remarkable for a macular rash on the thorax in addition to edema in the upper and lower extremities. Today's laboratory results are as follows:

Sodium	143 mmol/LU/A
Potassium	4.5 mmol/L
Chloride	109 mmol/L
CO2	24 mmol/L
BUN	21 mg/dL
Creatinine	0.9 mg/dL
WBC	2500/μL
Hemoglobin	10 gm/dL
Platelets	124,000/μL
Urinalysis:	
WBC	0/HPF
RBC	2-4/HPF
Leukocyte esterase	negative
Protein	2+

What is the most appropriate next step in the management of this patient?
A. Perform blood cultures and start the patient on vancomycin and cefepime
B. Decrease D-penicillamine dose to half
C. Increase D-penicillamine dose to 25 mg/kg/day
D. Discontinue D-penicillamine and start trientine 250 mg orally four times daily
E. Start furosemide 20 mg orally daily in combination with spironolactone 100 mg once daily

44. A 22-year-old nullipara woman with Wilson disease, currently on her 20 weeks of gestation is referred for your evaluation. She has been using penicillamine 1 gm orally divided four times daily for the last 2 years. She reports no complications related to her liver disease since starting penicillamine. She is also using prenatal vitamins including pyridoxine 25 mg orally daily. Her last liver biochemical tests 1 week ago were completely unremarkable. However, CBC was remarkable for mild anemia with hemoglobin of 11.0 gm/dL. She reports that the pregnancy was unplanned and is concerned about the teratogenic risk of penicillamine. Last obstetric sonogram 1 week ago revealed a normal intrauterine pregnancy and adequate for gestational age. What is the most appropriate recommendation for this patient?
A. Pregnancy termination in view of the teratogenic risk of penicillamine
B. Reduce penicillamine dose to 750 mg orally daily and close follow-up of liver function test
C. Discontinue penicillamine and start patient on trientine
D. Discontinue penicillamine and continue close follow-up of liver function test
E. Increase penicillamine dose to 1.5 gram daily divided in four doses daily

45. A 13-year-old boy, with no systemic illness, is referred to you for evaluation after developing acute cholecystitis. He reports that approximately 1 month ago he suffered a severe acute right upper quadrant pain associated with chills and fever. He was admitted to the hospital, and an abdominal sonogram was remarkable for an enlarged liver with increase parenchymal echogenicity consistent with fatty infiltration, and multiple internal hyperechoic structures inside the gallbladder with acoustic shadow and diffuse wall edema. He received 1 week of intravenous antibiotics and underwent a laparoscopic cholecystectomy. Surgery was successful and was remarkable for an enlarged liver. Multiple, small, black pigmented stones were found in the gallbladder specimen. Her laboratories values were also remarkable for mild anemia, an elevated indirect bilirubin, and mildly elevated ALT levels (80 IU/L). Which of the following is most probable to be abnormal in this patient?
A. Iron transferrin saturation
B. Serum ceruloplasmin and 24-hour urine copper concentration
C. Hemoblobin A1C levels
D. Serum cholesterol levels
E. Serum triglycerides levels

46. Which of the following is associated with elevated ceruloplasmin levels?
A. Wilson disease
B. Pregnancy
C. Nephrotic syndrome
D. Menkes disease
E. Intestinal malabsortion

47. Which one of the following neurologic presentation tends to occur earlier in patients with Wilson disease?
A. Seizure
B. Mental retardation
C. Loss of fine motor control
D. Rigidity
E. Dysarthria

48. A 5-week-old, previously healthy female infant develops irritability, poor feeding, vomiting, lethargy, hypotonia, seizures, and coma. Five days previously, her parents noted some diarrhea. She is seen in the emergency department and rapidly moved to the neonatal intensive care unit where she requires intubation. She is noted to be hyperventilating on the ventilator. Her heart rate is 130 and her temperature is 37.1° C. A diagnostic test is performed. Which of the following is likely to be diagnostic?
A. Bacterial blood cultures
B. Quantitative urine delta-aminolevulinic acid (ALA) and porphobilinogen (PBG)

C. Serum ammonia level
D. Arterial blood gas analysis
E. Serum phenylalanine

49. Which one of the following disorders has proven dietary treatment options?
A. Congenital disorder of glycosylation type II
B. Congenital disorder of glycosylation type Ia
C. Mitochondrial respiratory chain disorders
D. Congenital disorder of glycosylation type Ib
E. Congenital disorder of glycosylation type Ic

50. A 53-year-old man with a past medical history of asthma and hypertension presents to the emergency department with 2 weeks of progressive abdominal distension. Imaging showed ascites and a nodular liver. He was treated with paracentesis and diuretics. He followed up with a gastroenterologist who checked his *SERPINA1* genotype and documented a *PiZZ* genotype. Which of the following is the mechanism of liver disease in this patient?
A. Increased fatty acid influx into the liver
B. Aberrant retention of a mutant protein in the hepatocyte endoplasmic reticulum
C. Uninhibited neutrophil elastase activity
D. Accumulation of fumarylacetoacetate and maleylacetoacetate in the liver
E. Obstruction of small bile ducts leading to chronic inflammatory changes

51. Which of the following is most likely to be seen in the liver biopsy of a patient with alpha1-antitrypsin deficiency?
A. Myelosomes on electron microscopy
B. Micronodular cirrhosis, bile duct plugging, steatosis, and giant cell transformation
C. Steatosis and iron deposition
D. Hepatocyte pallor and minimal fatty infiltration
E. Bile duct proliferation, intracellular cholestasis, and PAS-positive, diastase-resistant globules

52. A newborn is found to have hypertelorism, deformed earlobes, hypotonia, and subsequently suffers from difficult-to-treat seizures. Which of the following is this infant also likely to have?
A. Hepatomegaly
B. Mutation of the *CFTR* gene
C. Requirement for strict protein avoidance
D. Cutaneous vesicles and bullae in light exposed areas
E. Requirement for continuous nighttime tube feeding

53. A 50-year-old businessman recently returned after a 3-day stay in Asia. Several weeks later, he was noted to have symptoms of fever, malaise, decreased appetite, and scleral icterus. His two children who are in daycare have recently been sick with a diarrheal illness. What is the most common risk factor for acquiring hepatitis A virus (HAV) infection in this patient?
A. Household contact of an infected person
B. Travel to endemic countries
C. Children in a daycare setting
D. Exposure during food or waterborne outbreak
E. Illicit drug use

54. An 18-year-old college student presents with malaise, scleral icterus, and dark, tea-colored urine for 3 days. Further testing reveals anti-HAV IgG negative, anti-HAV IgM positive, HBsAg negative and anti-HCV antibody negative. What is the most appropriate treatment for this patient?
A. Administration of one dose of HAV vaccine
B. Administration of serum immune globulin (IG)
C. Administration of one dose of HAV vaccine and vaccination of household contacts
D. No treatment necessary
E. Administration of serum immune globulin and vaccination of household contacts

55. A 36-year-old woman presents to your clinic with 2-month history of jaundice. She was diagnosed with acute hepatitis A infection 8 weeks ago after returning from India. She complains about malaise, pruritus, and dark color of her urine that has been going on since the diagnosis. She is mainly concerned about prolonged jaundice. On physical exam, her vital signs are as follows:

Temperature	37° C
Blood pressure	110/65 mm Hg
Heart rate	80 bpm

Significant scleral icterus is noted. Abdominal exam is soft and nontender without any evidence of organomegaly. She is alert and oriented to time, place, and person. No asterixis was noted. She brought the studies ordered by her primary care physician last week to your office. Laboratory values are as follows:

Hemoglobin	12 g/dL
WBC	9000/μL
Total bilirubin	10.2 g/dL
Direct bilirubin	8.0 g/dL
Alkaline phosphatase	478 U/L
ALT	218 U/L
AST	165 U/L
INR	1.1

Anti-HAV IgM and IgG are both detectable. Recent abdominal ultrasound showed normal liver size and texture without any evidence of intrahepatic or extrahepatic bile ducts dilation. What would be the best next step at this time?
A. Liver biopsy
B. ERCP
C. Abdominal MRI
D. Referral for liver transplant evaluation
E. Reassurance

56. A 50-year-old Caucasian woman with chronic hepatitis C infection recently came back from a trip to Mexico with significant jaundice and altered mental status. Further studies showed a cirrhotic liver, total bilirubin of 10 mg/dL, creatinine of 1.5 mg/dL, and INR of 2.5. The patient was diagnosed with acute liver failure due to hepatitis A infection. Which of the following features is a known risk factor for this patient's fulminant course?
A. Gender
B. Mode of transmission of virus
C. Chronic hepatitis C infection
D. Race
E. Age

57. What is the primary route of transmission of hepatitis A?
A. Direct contact with blood or body fluids
B. Sexual contact
C. Illicit drug use
D. Fecal-oral contact
E. Parenteral route

58. A 48-year-old man presents to your clinic with new onset jaundice and malaise in the last 2 days. He had an

episode of acute hepatitis A infection 6 months ago with clinical and biochemical full recovery after 8 weeks. He denies any recent travel or risky behavior since recovery. His physical exam is only remarkable for scleral icterus. Laboratory values are as follows:

Hemoglobin	14 g/dL
WBC	10,000/μL
Total bilirubin	6.4 g/dL
Alkaline phosphatase	178 U/L
ALT	138 U/L
AST	115 U/L
INR	1.1

Right upper quadrant abdominal ultrasound shows normal liver and bile ducts. Which statement is correct for this patient's condition?

A. Mortality rate is about 20%
B. Patient may be infectious for hepatitis A
C. Patient may develop chronic hepatitis A infection
D. Anti-HAV IgM is usually undetectable
E. Liver biopsy is indicated

59. What is the most common mode of infection of hepatitis B in the United States?

A. Hemodialysis
B. Vertical transmission
C. Homosexual contact
D. Heterosexual contact
E. "Street" tattoos

60. What is the most common mode of infection of hepatitis B in China?

A. Injection drug use
B. Vertical transmission
C. Heterosexual contact
D. Homosexual contact
E. "Street" tattoos

61. Hepatocellular Carcinoma (HCC) surveillance is recommended in which of the following patients with hepatitis B?

A. A 43-year-old Taiwanese woman with chronic hepatitis B
B. A 35-year-old Korean man with vertically transmitted HBV infection
C. A 45-year-old Caucasian male intravenous drug abuser with HIV and HBV coinfection and undetectable viral loads for both infections on antiviral therapy
D. A 22-year-old nursing student from Turkey with normal liver enzymes and a very high HBV viral load
E. A 25-year-old Sudanese man with chronic hepatitis B

62. A 20-year-old Taiwanese nursing student tested positive for hepatitis B infection on routine health screening labs. She and her family moved to the Unites States when she was 5 and she cannot recall if she was ever vaccinated for the virus. What is the lifetime risk of chronicity for this patient if her hepatitis B was acquired via vertical transmission?

A. 1%
B. 5%
C. 30%
D. 70%
E. 95%

63. A 45-year-old man with long-standing history of injection drug use and high-risk sexual behavior is admitted with severe jaundice, scleral icterus and dark, tea-colored urine. Laboratory values reveal the following:

Total bilirubin	7 mg/dL
ALT	2000 U/L
AST	1500 U/L
INR	1.5
HBV DNA	> 1,000,000 IU/mL

What is the risk of acute liver failure in this patient?

A. 1%
B. 20%
C. 30%
D. 50%
E. 95%

64. A 25-year-old medical student with no history of exposure to hepatitis B has recently been vaccinated for the virus. Which of the following choices below represent his status?

A. HBsAg negative, anti-HBc positive, IgM anti-HBc negative, anti-HBs positive
B. HBsAg negative, anti-HBc negative, IgM anti-HBc negative, anti-HBs positive
C. HBsAg positive, anti-HBc positive, IgM anti-HBc positive, anti-HBs negative
D. HBsAg negative, anti-HBc negative, IgM anti-HBc negative, anti-HBs negative
E. HBsAg positive, anti-HBc positive, IgM anti-HBc negative, anti-HBs negative

65. A 39-year-old Chinese woman presents for a routine physical exam to her primary care physician for the first time. Family history is pertinent for father with "liver tumor" and two grandparents who died of "liver infection" in China. Laboratory values are as follows:

HBsAg	positive
anti-HBc	positive
anti-HBs	negative
HBeAg	positive
ALT	15 U/L
AST	10 U/L
Total bilirubin	0.5 mg/dL
Alkaline phosphatase	80 U/L
HBV viral load	2.5 million IU/mL

What is the next step in her management?

A. Observe
B. Treat with entecavir
C. Liver biopsy
D. Treat with lamivudine
E. Start hepatocellular carcinoma surveillance

66. A 25-year-old African-American man who was recently diagnosed with large B-cell lymphoma needs rituxan-based chemotherapy. Laboratory values reveal the following: HBsAg positive, anti-HBc positive, anti-HBs negative. You start treatment with tenofovir 2 weeks prior to initiation of chemotherapy to prevent HBV reactivation. How long do you continue the tenofovir?

A. Indefinitely, he needs lifelong treatment
B. Discontinue 1 month after chemotherapy ends
C. Discontinue 3 months after chemotherapy ends
D. Discontinue 6 to 12 months after chemotherapy ends
E. Discontinue same time as last day of chemotherapy

67. A 45-year-old woman with known hepatitis B had the following laboratory values:

Total bilirubin	0.5 mg/dL
ALT	120 U/L

AST	100 U/L
ALP	90 U/L
HBeAg	positive
HBeAb	negative
Hepatitis B viral load	510,000 IU/mL

She believes she was treated 5 years ago with lamivudine and had excellent response in her viral load but stopped the medication when she ran out. A liver biopsy showed necroinflammatory activity and stage 3 fibrosis. You decide that she should start antiviral therapy. What is the best treatment option for this patient?

A. pegylated interferon (pegIFN)
B. Entecavir
C. Lamivudine
D. Adefovir
E. Telbivudine

68. A 33-year-old Filipino woman is pregnant with her first child. She has known hepatitis B infection and has never been on treatment. Her laboratory values are as follows:

Total bilirubin	1 mg/dL
ALT	30 U/L
AST	25 U/L
ALP	120 U/L
HBeAg	negative
HBeAb	positive
HBV viral load	20,000,000 IU/mL

What is the appropriate regimen and duration of therapy for her?

A. Lamivudine alone, start third trimester and stop 4 weeks postpartum
B. Adefovir alone, start first trimester and stop at delivery
C. Lamivudine alone, start first trimester and stop 4 weeks postpartum
D. Adefovir + Lamivudine, start third trimester and stop 4 weeks postpartum
E. pegIFN, start second trimester and complete 48 weeks of treatment.

69. In which of the following scenarios is close observation rather than HBV treatment indicated?

A. A 45-year-old HIV-HBV coinfected patient with CD4 count of 500 cells/mm^3, HIV viral load undetectable and HBV viral load of 80,000 IU/mL
B. A 55-year-old man with compensated hepatitis B cirrhosis and hepatitis B viral load of 5000 IU/mL
C. A 65-year-old woman with hepatitis B cirrhosis, decompensated by ascites and hepatic encephalopathy with a hepatitis B viral load of 100 IU/mL
D. A 25-year-old intravenous drug user with new onset jaundice and labs as follow: ALT 2000 U/L, AST 1500 U/L, INR 1.0, total bilirubin 3.0 mg/dL, positive HBsAg, hepatitis B viral load of 1800,000 IU/mL and hepatitis C virus antibody negative.
E. A 40-year-old Chinese man with known chronic hepatitis B with HBsAg positive, HBeAg positive, HBeAb negative, HBV viral load of 40,000 IU/mL and stage 2 fibrosis on liver biopsy

70. Which of the following proteins is a serine protease responsible for cleavage of the HCV polyprotein?

A. p7
B. NS2
C. NS3
D. NS4B
E. NS5B

71. A 65-year-old man from Egypt immigrated to the United States in 2002. During his annual physical he is found to have an elevated ALT and subsequent testing was positive for hepatitis C antibody. He denies any known risk factors. HCV PCR confirmed active infection with a viral load of 2,300,000 IU/mL. This patient is most likely infected with which of the following HCV genotypes?

A. Genotype 1a
B. Genotype 1b
C. Genotype 2
D. Genotype 4
E. Genotype 6

72. Which of the following is true about the incidence and prevalence of hepatitis C?

A. The worldwide prevalence of hepatitis C is declining
B. The age group with the highest prevalence of hepatitis C is 35-44 years
C. The incidence of acute hepatitis C is declining
D. There is a higher prevalence of hepatitis C in females compared to males
E. There is a higher prevalence of hepatitis C in whites compared to African Americans

73. A 60-year-old man presents for his routine annual physical. His past medical history includes hypertension and stage 2 chronic kidney disease. In 1998 he received a blood transfusion after suffering trauma from a motor vehicle accident. He drinks three beers daily and does not smoke tobacco. He denies intravenous drug use but did smoke crack and marijuana from age 35 to 40. His physical exam is unremarkable and his liver enzymes are normal. Which of the following is an indication for hepatitis C antibody testing?

A. Age 60 years
B. History of blood transfusion
C. History of illicit drug use
D. History of alcohol use
E. He has no risk factors and his liver enzymes are normal. Therefore, there is no indication for HCV testing

74. A 25-year-old African American female medical student suffers a needle stick while caring for a patient with hepatitis C. One month later, the medical student remains asymptomatic, however, she tests positive for hepatitis C by PCR. Laboratory values are as follows:

ALT is	250 U/L
Bilirubin	0.9mg/dL
Hepatitis C virus (HCV) viral load is	840,000 IU/mL
Genotype	1
Interleukin 28B polymorphism	TT

Which one of the following factors may increase the likelihood of spontaneous clearance of hepatitis C?

A. Asymptomatic infection
B. Age and gender
C. Genotype
D. TT interleukin 28B polymorphism
E. Race

75. A 46-year-old man with chronic hepatitis C presents with a 2-month history of worsening fatigue, arthralgia, and a skin rash involving his legs (see figure). Laboratory testing is as follows:

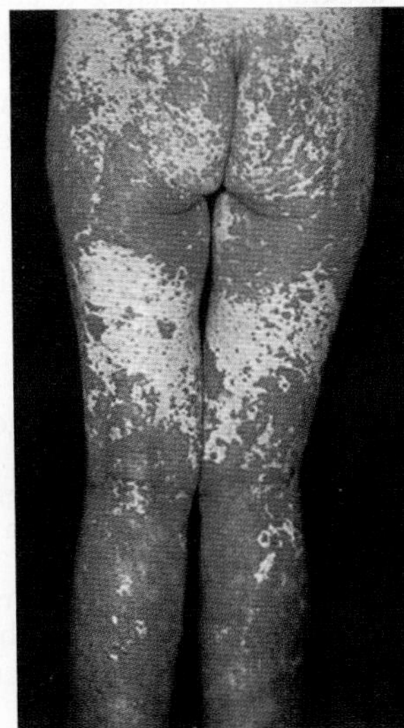

Figure for question 75.

ALT	67 U/L
Creatinine	1.2 mg/dL
HCV PCR	2,456,000 IU/mL
Genotype	1b
Rheumatoid factor	positive
Complement factors low	

Which of the following treatments is most appropriate?

A. Prednisone
B. Rituximab
C. Cyclophosphamide
D. Plasmapheresis
E. HCV treatment

76. A 54-year-old African American woman with end-stage renal disease on hemodialysis is being evaluated for an elevated ALT of 81 U/L. She is asymptomatic. Her laboratory workup includes the following:

Hepatitis C antibody	negative
Hepatitis B surface antigen	negative
Hepatitis B core IgG	positive,
Hepatitis B surface antibody	positive
Hepatitis A IgG	positive
Antinuclear antibody (ANA)	1:40

Which of the following is the next most appropriate step in her care?

A. Perform a liver biopsy for suspected autoimmune hepatitis
B. Order a hepatitis B PCR
C. Order a hepatitis C PCR
D. Notify the health department of the positive hepatitis A testing
E. Order a tissue transglutaminase IgA

77. A 58-year-old male is diagnosed with chronic hepatitis C. He is asymptomatic. His past medical history also includes type 2 diabetes. A liver biopsy is performed and demonstrates cirrhosis. The patient inquires about his risk of hepatocellular carcinoma (HCC). You should inform him which of the following?

A. Since he is a male, he is at a lower risk of developing HCC
B. He has a 10% per year risk of hepatocellular carcinoma
C. Drinking 2 glasses of wine per day may reduce his risk of HCC
D. Diabetes is a risk factor of HCC
E. Excessive coffee consumption may increase his risk of HCC

78. A 35-year-old African-American woman with hepatitis C and past medical history, including obesity and diabetes is seen in your clinic for consultation. She drinks coffee regularly and denies alcohol consumption. She has genotype 1a infection and a HCV PCR of 4,500,000 IU/mL. Which of the following factors is associated with progression of hepatic fibrosis in this patient?

A. Age
B. Viral load
C. Genotype
D. Gender
E. Obesity

79. Which of the following class of hepatitis C direct acting antiviral drugs is potent, pan-genotypic, and has a high barrier to resistance?

A. Protease inhibitors (second generation)
B. Non-nucleos(t)ide polymerase inhibitors
C. Nucleos(t)ide polymerase inhibitors
D. NS5A inhibitors
E. Interferon lamda

80 Which of the following is true of a sustained viral response (SVR) after hepatitis C treatment?

A. The risk of hepatitis C viral relapse after achieving a sustained viral response is 10%
B. An improvement in quality of life is not associated with a sustained viral response
C. In patients with cirrhosis, sustained viral response eliminates the risk of developing hepatocellular carcinoma
D. Sustained viral response is defined as the absence of detectable virus in the blood 48 weeks after completion of therapy
E. Sustained viral response may lead to regression of fibrosis

81 A 61-year-old man with hepatitis C and hepatocellular carcinoma undergoes a deceased donor liver transplant. He has genotype 1a infection with a viral load of 132,000 IU/mL. The donor's age was 25. Following liver transplant, he develops moderate acute cellular rejection and requires high-dose intravenous corticosteroids. Subsequently, his HCV viral load was 12,675,000 IU/mL. Which one of the following statements is true?

A. Due to donor age, the patient is at increased risk for graft loss
B. This patient's post transplant hepatitis C viral load may result in an increased severity of HCV recurrence and graft loss
C. The corticosteroids this patient received will have no effect on fibrosis progression
D. This patient has a 5% chance of developing graft cirrhosis within 5 years after liver transplantation
E. Even low dose corticosteroids must be avoided in patients with HCV infection after liver transplantation

82. A 41-year-old man who is known to be a hepatitis B carrier presents to the emergency department with a 1-week history of fatigue, nausea, and jaundice. He admits to active intravenous drug use. His vital signs are as follows:

Temperature	36.5° C
Heart rate	80 bpm
Blood pressure	100/50 mm Hg

Physical exam is significant for icterus, mild ascites without tenderness, and mild confusion without asterixis. In reviewing his labs, one month ago, his liver enzymes and bilirubin were normal and HBV DNA PCR was 410 IU/mL. His current laboratory values are significant for the following:

ALT	1087 U/L
AST	980 U/L
Total bilirubin	4.2 mg/dL
Hepatitis B surface antigen	positive
Hepatitis B DNA PCR	105 IU/mL
HIV testing	negative

Which of the following tests is most likely to lead to the diagnosis in this patient?

A. Cytomegalovirus IgM
B. Hepatitis A IgG
C. Hepatitis C antibody
D. Serum hepatitis D antigen
E. Hepatitis D IgM

83. Which of the following statements is correct regarding hepatitis B and D coinfection compared to hepatitis D superinfection?

A. Coinfection is more likely to lead to resolution of infection
B. Coinfection often presents with negative hepatitis B core IgM
C. Coinfection carries a higher risk for hepatocellular carcinoma
D. Coinfection more often leads to rapid disease progression to end-stage liver disease
E. Double peak pattern of ALT level is a typical manifestation in hepatitis D superinfection

84. A 60-year-old man with 15-year history of hepatitis B and hepatitis D coinfection presents to your clinic to seek your opinion about treatment options. He is asymptomatic. His vital signs are as follows:

Temperature is	36.9° C
Blood pressure	110/60 mm Hg
Heart rate	76 bpm

Exam is significant for mild icterus but is negative for ascites, asterixis, or any change in mental status. Most recent laboratory values are as follows:

Hemoglobin	12 g/dl
Platelet count	135,000/µL
WBC	4000/µL
Total bilirubin	1.9 mg/dL
Albumin	2.8 g/dL
Alkaline phosphatase	129 U/L
ALT	69 U/L
AST	76 U/L
Creatinine	1.1 mg/dL
INR	1.3

Abdominal MRI last month showed evidence of cirrhosis without any suspicious mass. Which of the following statements is correct regarding the treatment options and prognosis in this patient?

A. Long duration of his disease increases the likelihood of treatment response
B. There is more than 70% chance to achieve a sustained viral response in this patient after a 6-month treatment course
C. The only therapeutic option available has side effects that include flu-like symptoms, cytopenias, and depression
D. Treatment of his hepatitis B with tenofovir will lead to eradication of his hepatitis D
E. Combination therapy with lamivudine will improve response rates

85. Which of the following statements is true concerning hepatitis E virus (HEV) infection with genotype 1 versus genotype 3 infection?

A. Genotype 1 infection occurs in young, healthy persons while genotype 3 infection results in large epidemics and frequent sporadic cases
B. Genotype 1 infection does not have documented animal-to-human transmission while genotype 3 infection is likely via consumption of undercooked meat
C. Genotype 1 infection has an animal reservoir while genotype 3 infection does not
D. Genotype 1 results in chronic infection while genotype 3 does not
E. Genotype 1 infection occurs in immunosuppressed persons while genotype 3 does not

86. A 25-year-old Malaysian woman in her second trimester of pregnancy complains of malaise, fever, and scleral icterus for one week. She does not have any other significant past medical history. Her vital signs are as follows:

Temperature	38.1° C
Blood pressure	110/62 mm Hg
Heart rate	86 bpm

Exam is significant for scleral icterus, and mild right upper quadrant abdominal tenderness without rebound or guarding. She is alert and oriented. Laboratory values are as follows:

Hemoglobin	11.4 g/dL
WBC	12,000/µL
Total bilirubin	5.0 g/d
Alkaline phosphatase	208 U/L
ALT	845 U/L
AST	921 U/L
INR	1.1
Albumin	3.2 g/dL
Viral serology shows	
HBs antigen	negative
HBs antibody	positive
HBc antibody	negative
HCV antibody	negative
HAV IgG	positive
HAV IgM	negative
HEV IgM	positive

Ultrasound of the liver only demonstrated mild hepatomegaly. What is the mortality rate for this patient?

A. 0.1% to 0.6%
B. 1% to 3%
C. 5% to 25%
D. 50%
E. 95% to 100%

87. A 35-year-old kidney transplant recipient is in her first trimester of pregnancy and presents with malaise and dark, tea-colored urine for 1 week. Her laboratory values are as follows:

ALT	670 U/L
AST	700 U/L
Total bilirubin	3.8 mg/dL

She had similar symptoms in the early years after her transplant about 5 years ago. She is suspected to have chronic hepatitis E infection. What is the best treatment option for this patient?

A. Termination of pregnancy
B. Pegylated interferon α-2a for 6 months
C. Ribavirin for 6 months
D. Reduction in dose of immunosuppressive medication
E. Supportive therapy and close monitoring

88. What is the predominant route of transmission for HEV infection?

A. Person-to-person contact
B. Consumption of contaminated drinking water
C. Vertical transmission from mother to child
D. Parenteral route of infection
E. Transmission by blood transfusion

89. Compared to hepatitis C, which of the following is true about hepatitis G virus (GBV-C)?

A. GBV-C is transmitted via fecal-oral route
B. GBV-C infection is not associated with clinical liver disease
C. The rate of natural clearance of GBV-C is similar to HCV
D. HCV–GBV-C coinfection is uncommon
E. Similar to HCV, patients with HIV—GBV-C coinfection have a worse prognosis that HIV-monoinfected patients.

90. A 45-year-old homeless man presents to the emergency department complaining of pruritus for 1 month. On exam he is cachectic and has jaundice. Oropharyngeal exam is consistent with thrush. He has excoriations but no skin rash. Laboratory values are as follows:

ALT	76 U/L
AST	89 U/L
Alkaline phosphatase	455 U/L
Total bilirubin	8.4 mg/dL
WBC count	1500/μL
HIV antibody	positive

A right upper quadrant ultrasound reveals cholelithiasis, dilated common bile duct, and irregular intrahepatic ducts. The patient is admitted to the hospital for further workup and treatment. Which of the following interventions is most likely to improve jaundice in this patient?

A. ERCP
B. Cholecystectomy
C. Fluconazole
D. Valgancyclovir
E. Liver transplant evaluation

91. A 26-year-old woman is referred to hepatology clinic in week 32 of gestation with severe elevation of liver enzymes. Her only complaint includes mild fatigue. Her vital signs are as follows:

Blood pressure	100/50 mm Hg
Temperature	37.2° C
Heart rate	78 bpm

Mental status is normal. Skin and mucosal exam is unremarkable. She has mild icterus and the rest of the physical exam is unremarkable. Pertinent laboratory values are as follows:

Hemoglobin	10.5 g/L
WBC	10,000/μL
Platelet count	150,000/μL
ALT	9000 U/L
AST	10,110 U/L
Alkaline phosphatase	277 U/L
Total bilirubin	3.4 mg/dL
INR	1.4
HCV antibody	negative
, HAV antibody	negative
HBs antigen	negative
HBs antibody	positive.

A transjugular liver biopsy is performed (see figure). Which of the following is the most appropriate treatment for this patient?

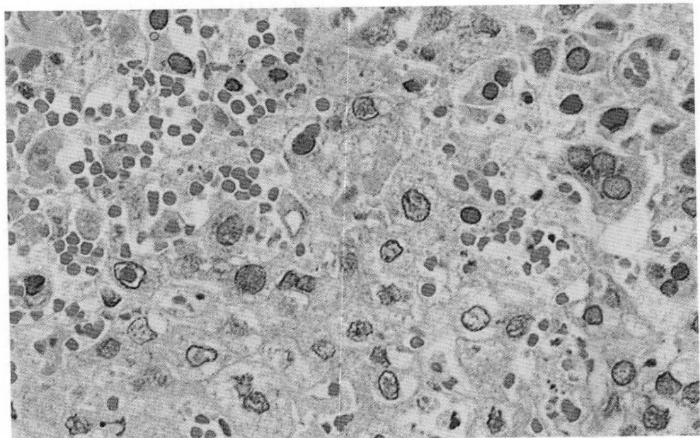

Figure for question 91.

A. Corticosteroids
B. Sofosbuvir and ribavirin
C. Intravenous acyclovir
D. Liver transplantation
E. Emergent delivery

92. Which of the following is true about TT virus (TTV)?

A. TTV is a single-stranded RNA virus
B. TTV is relatively uncommon
C. TTV can be transmitted by both parenteral and fecal-oral routes
D. Most patients with TTV present with elevated liver enzymes
E. It is only seen in Sub-Saharan Africa

93. A 20-year-old female college student presents with a 1-week history of fever and sore throat. Her roommate recently had a similar illness. On exam she has evidence of pharyngitis and cervical lymphadenopathy. Laboratory values are significant for the following:

ALT	202 U/L
AST	186 U/L
Alkaline phosphatase	155 U/L
Total bilirubin	1.0 mg/dL

An abdominal ultrasound reveals hepatosplenomegaly. What test is most likely to confirm the diagnosis?

A. Hepatitis A IgM
B. Cytomegalovirus (CMV) IgG

C. Herpes simplex virus (HSV) PCR
D. Liver biopsy
E. Epstein-Barr (EBV) IgM

94. An infant presents with jaundice, hepatosplenomegaly, thrombocytopenic purpura, and severe neurologic impairment. A liver biopsy is most likely to show which of the following features?
A. Hepatocyte nuclei containing eosinophilic viral inclusions
B. Hepatocyte nuclei containing large "owl's eye" viral inclusions
C. Severe microvesicular steatosis
D. Lymphoplasmacytic interface activity
E. Minimal nonspecific mixed inflammation

95. Which of the following statements is true regarding HIV–hepatitis G virus (GBV-C) coinfection?
A. Patients with HIV–GBV-C coinfection have worse prognosis than patients with HIV monoinfection
B. Children infected with GBV-C at birth have an increased risk of contracting HIV via vertical transmission
C. Patients with HIV–GBV-C coinfection have an improved response to HIV antiviral therapy
D. Treatment with pegylated interferon and ribavirin is an important part of the therapy in these cases
E. HIV antiviral therapy has been shown to decrease GBV-C viral titers

96. A 28-year-old man without significant past medical history has been admitted in the intensive care unit with 3-day history of high-grade fever, bleeding from the gums, and change in the mental status. His vital signs are as follows:

Temperature	38.5° C
Blood pressure	100/60 mm Hg
Heart rate	105 bpm

Physical exam is significant for marked hepatosplenomegaly in the abdominal exam. Laboratory values are as follows:

Hemoglobin	9 g/dL
WBC	2200/μL
Platelet count	93,000/μL
INR	2.8
Total bilirubin	3.0 g/dL
Alkaline phosphatase	138 U/L
ALT	158 U/L
AST	170 U/L
Ferritin	12,000 mcg/L

Blood cultures have been negative after 48 hours. Which of the following viral infections is usually associated with this condition?
A. EBV
B. CMV
C. HSV
D. SEN virus (SENV)
E. TTV

97. A 20-year-old woman with a past history of pelvic inflammatory disease presents with severe right upper quadrant pain. Laboratory values are as follows:

AST	500 U/L
ALT	200 U/L
Alkaline phosphatase	450 U/L
Total bilirubin	0.6 mg/dL

On physical exam, the patient is afebrile. A friction rub is heard over the liver. The rest of the exam is unremarkable. All cultures are negative and an abdominal ultrasound is unremarkable except for the presence of gallstones. What is the likely cause of the patient's symptoms?
A. Acute cholecystitis
B. *Yersinia enterocolitica*
C. *Legionella pneumophila*
D. Gonococcal infection
E. *Salmonella typhi*

98. A 30-year-old man with long-standing HIV and hepatitis C is admitted with fever, blood-red papular skin lesions, shortness of breath, hypotension, and elevated liver enzymes. An abdominal ultrasound is unremarkable. He denies any recent travel and lives in a townhome in the city. A liver biopsy and skin biopsy are done. The liver biopsy shows peliosis hepatis. What is the most likely diagnosis?
A. *Coxiella Burnetti* infection
B. *Bartonella henselae* infection
C. Fitz-Hugh-Curtis Syndrome
D. Brucellosis
E. *Bartonella bacilliformis* infection

99. A 25-year-old farmer who lives with his parents presents with worsening jaundice for 3 weeks. He now has persistent fevers of 102 °F to 103°F, malaise, conjunctival hemorrhage, and dark, tea-colored urine. Laboratory values are as follows:

Total bilirubin	25 mg/dL
Unconjugated bilirubin	7 mg/dL
Creatinine	2.5 mg/dL
ALT	200 U/L and
AST	180 U/L

Urinalysis shows muddy casts. Which of the following is the drug of choice for treatment of this infection?
A. Penicillin
B. Gentamicin
C. Doxycycline
D. Trimethoprim-sulfamethoxazole
E. Vancomycin

100. A 40-year-old Sudanese man with hemophilia presents with tender hepatomegaly, splenomegaly, jaundice, and fevers. Malarial infection is suspected. Which of the following is the best test to diagnose this infection?
A. Peripheral blood smear
B. Blood cultures
C. Liver biopsy
D. Abdominal ultrasound
E. Stool antigen

101. A 45-year-old Pakistani man who works as a cook in a fast food restaurant was noted to have dark pigmented spots on his face and arms by his coworkers. At the urging of his coworkers he sought medical attention and, upon further exam, revealed a 20-pound weight loss, intermittent fevers, and diarrhea. Physical exam revealed dark hyperpigmented spots throughout the body, generalized lymphadenopathy, and tenderness over the liver and spleen. The spleen was palpated down to the pelvis and extending across to the midabdomen. Abdominal ultrasound confirmed hepatosplenomegaly and ascites. What is the most likely diagnosis?

A. *Plasmodium falciparum* infection
B. *Leishmania donovani* infection
C. Babesiosis
D. *Entamoeba histolytica* infection
E. *Toxoplasma gondii* infection

102. A 10-year-old boy with fever, hepatomegaly, persistent eosinophilia, and history of pica is admitted to the hospital. Infection with visceral larva migrans is suspected. Which of the following is the best test to diagnose this infection?
A. Blood culture
B. Stool ova and parasite exam
C. Liver biopsy
D. Urine culture
E. Enzyme-linked immunosorbent assay (ELISA)

103. Which of the following statements accurately depicts the *Schistosoma* species life cycle?
A. Sandfly bite → schistosomes migrate to liver and fertilize → adult worms migrate to mesenteric vessels → fertilized eggs pass into small intestine → eggs pass into feces and deposit in fresh water
B. Miracidia infect snail → Cercariae enter skin of human host → fertilization occurs in the liver → adult worms migrate to mesenteric vessels → fertilized eggs pass into small intestine
C. Eggs ingested by sheep → Cercariae enter skin of human host → fertilization occurs in liver → adult worms migrate into mesenteric vessels → fertilized eggs pass into small intestine
D. Eggs ingested by cattle → human host ingests eggs → eggs fertilized in liver → adult worms migrate to mesenteric vessels → fertilized eggs pass into small intestine
E. Miracidia infects snail → Cercariae enter skin of human host → fertilization occurs in lung → adult worms migrate into the liver → eggs are deposited in mesenteric vessels and pass into small intestine

104. A 55-year-old Egyptian man presents with anemia, worsening shortness of breath, and abdominal distension. Abdominal ultrasound reveals cirrhosis and ascites. A chest x-ray is normal. Further workup reveals large nonbleeding esophageal varices and pulmonary hypertension. What is the likely cause of this patient's symptoms and what is the appropriate treatment?
A. *Echinococcus granulosus*, surgery
B. *Histoplasma capsulatum*, fluconazole
C. *Strongyloidiasis stercoralis*, ivermectin
D. *Trichinella spiralis*, praziquantel
E. *Schistosoma japonicum*, praziquantel

105. Which of the following accurately depicts the *Echinococcus* life cycle?
A. dogs ingest eggs (intermediate host) → sheep ingest cysts (definitive host) → human hosts ingest contaminated eggs → eggs release oncospheres into the small intestine → oncospheres migrate into circulation and produce hydatid cysts in liver
B. sheep ingest eggs (definitive host) → *Cercariae* enter skin of human host → fertilization occurs in liver → adult worms migrate into mesenteric vessels → fertilized eggs pass into small intestine
C. Sheep ingest eggs (intermediate host) → dogs ingest cysts (definitive host) → human hosts ingest contaminated eggs → eggs release oncospheres into the small intestine → oncospheres migrate into circulation and produce hydatid cysts in liver or lungs
D. *Miracidia* infect snail → *Cercariae* enter skin of human host → fertilization occurs in the liver → adult worms migrate to mesenteric vessels → fertilized eggs pass into small intestine
E. Cattle ingest eggs → human hosts ingest eggs → eggs fertilized in the liver → adult worms migrate to mesenteric vessels → fertilized eggs pass into small intestine

106. Which of the following is the correct treatment for the given infection?
A. *Histoplasma capsulatum*, ivermectin
B. *Trichinella spiralis*, prednisone
C. *Entamoeba histolytica*, metronidazole and paromomycin
D. *Salmonella typhi*, paromomycin
E. *Entamoeba histolytica*, metronidazole

107. A 38-year-old woman presents with 2 days history of abdominal pain. On physical exam, vital signs are within normal range; she has tender hepatomegaly but the exam is otherwise unremarkable. Past medical history is significant for alcohol abuse. She takes oral contraceptives. Laboratory values are as follows:

WBC	7500/μL
Hematocrit	40%
Platelet count	300,000/μL
INR	0.9
ALT	86 U/L
AST	80 U/L
Total bilirubin	1.1 mg/dL
Creatinine	0.9 mg/dL

Abdominal Doppler ultrasound is remarkable for hepatomegaly, steatosis, and cholelithiasis but absence of gallbladder wall thickening or pericholecystic fluid. The common bile duct (CBD) is 4 mm. Portal vein is patent and flow in the hepatic veins is absent. What is the most likely diagnosis?
A. Alcoholic hepatitis
B. Cholecystitis
C. Budd-Chiari syndrome (BCS)
D. Ruptured hepatic adenoma
E. Choledocholithiasis

108. A 23-year-old African-American woman with systemic lupus erythematosus (SLE) presents to the emergency department with abdominal pain for one day. She takes oral contraceptives. Her abdominal CT scan demonstrates hepatic artery aneurysm. What is the next best step in the management?
A. Refer for surgical resection
B. CT-guided biopsy
C. Refer to a transplant center
D. Angiogram with coil embolization
E. Discontinue oral contraceptives and repeat imaging in 3 months

109. A 24-year-old woman with acute lymphoblastic leukemia (ALL) who recently underwent bone marrow transplantation develops abdominal distention. Vital signs on physical exam are as follows:

Heart rate	100 bpm
Blood pressure	96/60 mm Hg
Temperature	37.2° C

On abdominal exam she has tense ascites, hepatomegaly, and diffuse abdominal tenderness. An abdominal Doppler ultrasound shows a large amount of ascites. There is normal flow in the hepatic veins and portal vein. Laboratory values are as follows:

WBC	2500/μL
Hematocrit	26%
Platelet count	56,000/μL
Bilirubin	4.8 mg/dL
AST	133 U/L
ALT	154 U/L
ALP	88 U/L
Creatinine	1.7 mg/dL

You diagnose the patient with sinusoidal obstruction syndrome (SOS). What is the next step in management?

A. Start anticoagulation with heparin
B. Refer to interventional radiology for angioplasty
C. Urgent evaluation for a liver transplant
D. Refer to interventional radiology for transjugular intrahepatic portosystemic shunt
E. Symptomatic treatment with diuretics, and paracentesis as needed

110. A 25-year-old man who is a professional body builder presents with abdominal pain and new-onset jaundice. Exam reveals scleral icterus and hepatomegaly with abdominal tenderness. Abdominal ultrasound shows hepatomegaly but is otherwise unremarkable. A Liver biopsy shows multiple blood-filled cysts (see figure). What is the correct diagnosis?

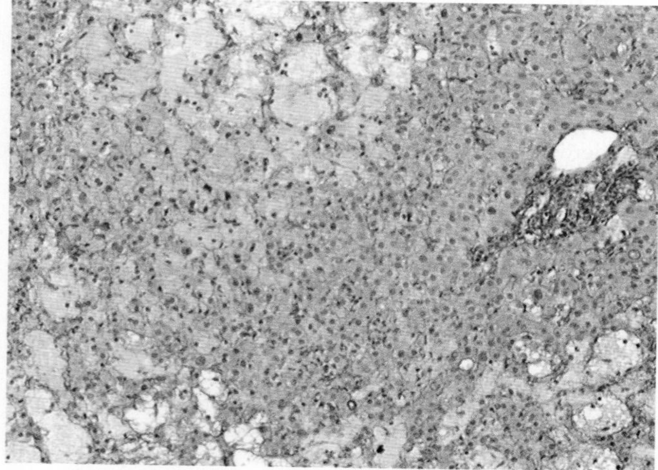

Figure for question 110.

A. Budd-Chiari syndrome
B. Portal vein thrombosis
C. Hepatic artery thrombosis
D. Peliosis hepatis
E. Hepatic hemangiomas

111. A 19-year-old woman is referred to your clinic for evaluation due to recurrent episodes of confusion associated with increased serum ammonia levels. Evaluation by her primary gastroenterologist includes abdominal ultrasound and a liver biopsy that did not reveal any evidence of cirrhosis or portal hypertension. On exam, vital signs are stable, abdomen is soft and nontender with no appreciable ascites, no scleral icterus, spider nevi or jaundice noted; she is alert and oriented to time, person, and place but has asterixis. Laboratory studies are as follows:

AST	35 U/L
ALT	22 U/L
Bilirubin	1.2 mg/dL
ALP	97 U/L
Platelet count	167,000/μL
Hematocrit	34%
WBC	6500/μL

You request a triple-phase CT scan, which shows an intrahepatic porto-systemic shunt. She is already on lactulose and having at least three bowel movements daily, however, symptoms are not well controlled. What is the most appropriate next step in the management?

A. Add rifaximin
B. Refer to interventional radiology for embolization
C. Refer for a liver transplant evaluation
D. Evaluate for urea cycle defects
E. Increase her lactulose dose

112. A 24-year-old pregnant woman at 14 weeks of gestation is brought to the emergency department due to altered mental status. Her husband reports that the patient started complaining of abdominal pain and worsening abdominal distention over the preceding day. Her past medical history is significant for factor V Leiden deficiency and a prior history of deep vein thrombosis (DVT). On exam she has tense ascites, hepatomegaly, and scleral icterus. Her laboratory values are as follows

ALT	1200 U/L
AST	1329 U/L
Bilirubin	5 mg/dL
INR	2.8
Ammonia level	154 mcg/dL
WBC	8700/μL
Hematocrit	32%

A Doppler ultrasound shows absence of flow in all hepatic veins. You determine that this is a fulminant presentation of Budd-Chiari syndrome. What is the next most appropriate step in the management?

A. Start anticoagulation with heparin
B. Urgent transjugular intrahepatic portosystemic shunt
C. Surgery to create a porto-systemic shunt
D. Urgent liver transplant evaluation
E. Symptomatic treatment with lactulose and diuretics

113. A 32-year-old man with ulcerative colitis presents with new onset ascites. He has no prior history of liver disease. He is on azathioprine and mesalamine and a recent colonoscopy showed that his colitis was in remission. An abdominal MRI shows hepatomegaly but no evidence of cirrhosis. His portal vein appears patent. MRCP shows normal appearing bile ducts. His laboratory values are as follows:

AST	67 U/L
ALT	56 U/L
Bilirubin	3 mg/d
INR	1.1
WBC	6500/μL
Hematocrit	35%
Platelet count	187,000/μL

You perform a transjugular liver biopsy and this shows sinusoidal dilation and hepatic congestion. What is the most likely diagnosis in this patient?

A. sinusoidal obstruction syndrome
B. Small duct primary sclerosing cholangitis

C. Congestive heart failure
D. Budd-Chiari syndrome
E. Allergic reaction to mesalamine

114. A 60-year-old man with chronic HCV and cirrhosis presents to your clinic for a follow-up visit. He notes progressive abdominal distention over the past few weeks. His liver disease has so far been compensated and he does not have a history of ascites. Vital signs are normal. Pertinent exam findings include scleral icterus, spider nevi and tense ascites. His laboratory values are as follows:

ALT	87 U/L
AST	66 U/L
Bilirubin	2.8 mg/dL
INR	1.4
Platelet count	100,000/μL
Hematocrit	36%
Creatinine	0.6 mg/dL
INR	1
Model for End-Stage Liver Disease (MELD) score is	10

You perform an abdominal CT scan and find an occlusive thrombus in the main portal vein. A recent CT scan 3 months earlier showed a patent portal vein. What is the best next step in his management?

A. Refer to surgery for an urgent thrombectomy
B. Refer to interventional radiology for a transjugular intrahepatic portosystemic shunt procedure (TIPS)
C. Perform an EGD to band any varices then start anticoagulation
D. Urgent thrombolysis
E. Refer for a liver transplant evaluation

115. A 62-year-old man with chronic HCV and newly diagnosed cirrhosis is referred to your clinic for a liver transplant evaluation. Vital signs are stable. Physical exam is significant for scleral icterus but abdomen is soft and nontender with no appreciable ascites. Laboratory studies are as follows:

AST	65 U/L
ALT	44 U/L
Bilirubin	3.6 U/L
ALP	110 U/L
WBC	5500/μL
Hematocrit	33%
Platelet count	59,000/μL
INR	1.5
Creatinine	0.8 mg/dL
MELD score	16

You order an abdominal MRI for routine hepatocellular carcinoma screening and this reveals a portal vein thrombus with cavernous transformation and extensive collaterals. What is the most appropriate next step in the management of this patient?

A. Referral to surgery for a thrombectomy
B. Admission for intravenous heparin
C. Initiatie oral anticoagulation with Coumadin
D. An EGD to screen for varices
E. Referral to interventional radiology (IR) for transjugular intrahepatic portosystemic shunt placement

116. A 64-year-old man with arterial hypertension is admitted to the hospital after developing acute renal failure. He reports lower extremity swelling in the last 6 months and weakness. He is a lawyer with a sedentary life and high carbohydrate diet. He endorses a consumption of two to three cocktails of bourbon whiskey daily, with a slightly higher intake during weekends. Physical exam is remarkable for an obese man with a BMI of 32 kg/m2, mild yellow discoloration of skin, scattered spider telangiectasias on the upper thorax, clear pulmonary sound to auscultation, a displaced point of maximum input laterally to the left mid-axillary line, enlarged liver size by percussion, no shifting dullness, easily palpable spleen below the left inferior costal margin, palmar erythema, and lower extremity pitting edema. Which of the above findings is most common in patients with alcoholic hepatitis?

A. Scleral jaundice
B. Spider telangiectasias
C. Displaced point of maximun impulse (PMI) on cardiac exam
D. Hepatomegaly
E. Splenomegaly

117. A 40-year-old homeless man is brought to the emergency department after being found unresponsive in the street. The Patient is obtunded and unable to provide medical history. Vital signs are remarkable for the following:

Temperature	38.8° C
Blood pressure of	99/69 mm Hg
Heart rate	105 bpm
Respiratory rate	19 breaths/min

On physical exam, he has scleral jaundice, bitemporal wasting, decreased breath sounds on lung bases bilaterally, a soft and distended abdomen with a positive shifting dullness and fluid wave, needles tracks on upper extremities and pitting lower extremity edema. Rectal exam reveals an empty fecal vault with traces of brown stool. The Patient is started on intravenous fluid, empiric broad-spectrum antibiotics and admitted to the hospital. Laboratory values are as follows:

Sodium	148 mmol/L
WBC	12,000/μL
Potassium	2.8 mmol/L
Hemoglobin	13.8 g/dL
Chloride	118 mmol/L
Platelet count	110,000/μL
CO2	32 mmol/L
Blood culture Negative in	24 hours
BUN	25 mg/dL
Acetaminophen level	0
Creatinine	1.0 mg/dL
AST	330 U/L
Alb	2.2 g/dL
ALT	100 U/L
Total Bilirubin	22.5 mg/dL
Hepatitis A IgG	positive
Alkaline phosphatase	200 U/L
Hepatitis B surface antigen	negative
INR	1.9
Hepatitis B surface antibody	positive
Prothrombin time	20.7 sec
Hepatitis B core antibody	positive
Hepatitis C antibody	positive

What is the most appropriate management in this patient?

A. Start N-acetylcysteine 150 mg/kg orally followed by 70 mg/kg every 4 hours for 17 doses
B. Prednisolone 32 mg orally daily
C. Prednisolone 32 mg orally daily plus pentoxifylline 400 mg orally three times daily
D. Tenofovir 300 mg orally once daily
E. Sofosbuvir 400 mg orally daily in combination with simeprevir 150 mg orally daily

118. A 53-year-old man came to the emergency department after complaining of anorexia, nausea, vomiting, and fatigue for the last 4 days. He is an accountant with long history of alcohol and cocaine abuse. One week ago, he and his friends went to Las Vegas for a bachelor party. He used marijuana, intravenous heroin, and had unprotected sex with prostitutes. He used acetaminophen a "couple of times" during the last three days for abdominal pain, however, cannot remember the amount of pills. He has no family history of chronic liver disease. On evaluation, vital signs are as follows:

Temperature	39.0° C
Blood pressure	100/75 mm Hg
Heart rate	102 bpm
Respiratory rate	19 breaths/min

On physical exam, the patient has scleral jaundice, lungs clear to auscultation, a soft and depressive distended abdomen with a positive shifting dullness and a palpable liver, needle tracks on upper extremities and pitting lower extremity edema. The Patient is started on intravenous fluid and admitted to the hospital. Laboratory values are as follows:

Sodium	144 mmol/L
WBC	14,000/μL
Potassium	3.4 mmol/L
Hemoglobin	13.8 g/dL
Chloride	118 mmol/L
Platelet count	145,000/μL
CO2	28 mmol/L
Blood culture negative in	24 hours
BUN	20 mg/dL
Acetaminophen level	undetectable
Creatinine	1.3 mg/dL
AST	230 U/L
Albumin	3.2 mg/dL
ALT	101 U/L
Total Bilirubin	18.5 mg/dL
Hepatitis A IgG	positive
Alkaline phosphatase	180 U/L
Hepatitis B surface antigen	negative
INR	1.4
Ferritin	400 ng/mL
Hepatitis B surface IgG Antibody	positive
Transferrin saturation	60%
Hepatitis B core IgG antibody	positive
Hepatitis C antibody	positive
HFE gene *C282Y*	heterozygous
HFE gene *H63D*	wild type

Which of the following is the most probable diagnosis?

A. Acute hepatitis B infection
B. Acute hepatitis C infection
C. Acetaminophen intoxication
D. Alcoholic hepatitis
E. Hereditary hemochromatosis

119. A 60-year-old woman presents to your clinic, referred by her primary care physician for evaluation of chronic hepatitis C. She was diagnosed with hepatitis C around 20 years ago after elevated serum aminotransferases were identified on a routine laboratory workup. Her only risk factor was a blood transfusion received in 1983 during a complicated delivery of her only son. She underwent therapy with pegylated interferon and ribavirin for 48 weeks in 2002 with relapse. She also has hypertension, diabetes mellitus type 2, hypercholesterolemia, and hypothyroidism. Despite her systemic conditions, she is an active women who goes daily to the gym and is compliant with a low calorie, low carbohydrate diet. She consumes 8 ounces of coffee every morning and 4 glasses wine, of 5 ounces each, daily with supper. On evaluation vital signs are remarkable for the following:

Temperature	37.0° C
Blood pressure	110/75 mm Hg
Heart rate	72 bpm
Respiratory rate	19 breaths/min

Physical exam is unremarkable otherwise. Laboratory values are as follows:

Sodium	144 mmol/L
WBC	5000/μL
Potassium	3.8 mmol/L
Hemoglobin:	13.8 g/dL
Chloride	118 mmol/L
Platelet count	200,000/μL
CO2	28 mmol/L
Cholesterol	220 mg/dL
BUN	8 mg/dL
Acetaminophen level	undetectable
Creatinine	0.9 mg/dL
AST	48 U/L
Albumin	3.9 g/dL
ALT	75 U/L
Total Bilirubin	1.2 mg/dL
Hepatitis A IgG	positive
Alkaline phosphatase	110 U/L
Hepatitis B surface antigen	negative
INR	1.4
Ferritin	400 ng/mL
Hepatitis B surface IgG antibody	positive
Transferrin saturation:	60%
Hepatitis B core IgG antibody	positive
Fasting glucose	145 mg/dL
Hepatitis C	positive
Hepatitis C viral load	2,000,000 IU/mL

Which one of the following is the most important risk factor in this patient for the development of liver cirrhosis?

A. High cholesterol levels
B. Consumption of 20 ounces of wine daily
C. Positive hepatitis B core antibody serology
D. Consumption of 8 ounces of coffee daily
E. Insulin resistance

120. A 65-year-old man presents to your clinic for evaluation of chronic hepatitis C infection. He was diagnosed with hepatitis C around 12 years ago after elevated serum aminotransferases were noted on a routine laboratory workup. He was an intravenous drug user 30 years ago. He underwent therapy with pegylated interferon and ribavirin for 48 weeks, 11 years ago, with no response. He also has hypertension, hypercholesterolemia, and diabetes mellitus type 2. He consumes four cocktails daily and smokes one pack of cigarettes daily for the last 14 years. A liver biopsy performed 11 years ago was remarkable for active portal inflammation with interface hepatitis, centrilobular and perivenular fatty infiltration, ballooning degeneration of hepatocytes, hyaline Mallory bodies on hepatocytes, and hepatic micronodules surrounded by fibrous tissue. On evaluation vital signs are remarkable for the following:

Temperature	37.0° C
Blood pressure	165/85 mm Hg
Heart rate	72 bpm
Respiratory rate	19 breaths/min
Body mass index (BMI)	40 kg/m²

Physical exam is remarkable for central obesity and lower extremity edema. You order serology for chronic viral hepatitis before starting therapy for chronic hepatitis C. The Patient has a positive hepatitis A IgG, positive Hepatitis B surface IgG antibody, positive hepatitis B core IgG antibody, hepatitis C positive antibody, hepatitis C viral load with 1,500,000 IU/mL, and genotype 1a. Which of the following findings in this patient is the most important risk factor for the development of hepatocellular carcinoma?

A. Obesity
B. Hypercholesterolemia
C. Diabetes mellitus type II
D. Age
E. Hepatitis B serology

121. A 54-year-old alcoholic man is brought to the emergency department after being found unresponsive in the street. The patient is obtunded and unable to provide medical history. Vital signs are remarkable for the following:

Temperature	39.8° C
Blood pressure	100/68 mm Hg
Heart rate	110 bpm
Respiratory rate	19 breaths/min

On physical exam, the patient has scleral jaundice, bitemporal wasting, decrease breath sounds on lung bases bilaterally, a soft and depressive distended abdomen with a positive shifting dullness and fluid wave, and pitting lower extremity edema. Laboratory values are as follows:

Sodium	149 mmol/L
WBC	18,000/μL
Potassium	3.0 mmol/L
Hemoglobin	9.8 g/dL
Chloride	118 mmol/L
Platelet count	110,000/μL
CO2	20 mmol/L
Blood culture negative in	24 hours
BUN	30 mg/dL
Acetaminophen level	negative
Creatinine	2.1 mg/dL
AST	450 U/L
Albumin	2.2 gm/dL
ALT	200 U/L
Total Bilirubin	25.5 mg/dL
Hepatitis A IgG	positive
Alkaline phosphatase	214 U/L
Hepatitis B surface antigen	negative
INR	2.1
Hepatitis B surface antibody	positive
Hepatitis B core antibody	negative
Hepatitis C antibody	positive

Which of the following has been associated with severe disease in patients with this condition?

A. AST/ALT ratio >2
B. Platelet count <140,000/μL
C. Hypokalemia
D. WBC >15,000/μL
E. Hemoglobin <10 g/dL

122. Which of the following patients has the highest 1-year mortality?

A. An asymptomatic 67-year-old man, with an uncomplicated medical history, diagnosed with alcoholic cirrhosis after a comprehensive health maintenance evaluation
B. A 66-year-old man diagnosed with alcoholic cirrhosis after presenting with hepatic encephalopathy
C. A 62-year-old man diagnosed with alcoholic cirrhosis after being found with esophageal varices on a upper endoscopy performed for GERD
D. A 63-year-old man diagnosed with alcoholic cirrhosis after presenting with new-onset ascites
E. A 65-year-old man diagnosed with alcoholic cirrhosis after presenting with new-onset ascites and esophageal varices

123. A 70-year-old woman came to the emergency department after complaining of anorexia, nausea, vomiting, abdominal pain, and fatigue for the last 2 days. She is a retired nurse that worked for 30 years, and reports several needle-sticks in the past. One week ago she had a tooth extraction and started to use acetaminophen daily for pain. She reports using 2 tablets of 500 mg every 6 hours and cannot remember when she took the last dose. She is a chronic smoker of 1 pack of cigarettes daily and consumes 3 to 4 glasses of wine daily. She has no family history of chronic liver disease. On evaluation vital signs are remarkable for the following:

Temperature	36.9° C
Blood pressure	98/69 mm Hg
Heart rate	105 bpm
Respiratory rate	19 breaths/per
Weight	102 pounds
Height	64 inches

On physical exam, the patient has scleral jaundice, lungs are clear to auscultation, a soft and depressive abdomen with a palpable liver, and mild lower extremity pitting edema. Laboratory values are as follows:

Sodium	146 mmol/L
WBC	14,000/μL
Potassium	5.4 mmol/L
Hemoglobin	9.8 g/dL
Chloride	118 mmol/L
Platelet count	100,000/μL
CO2	20 mmol/L
MCV	100 fL
BUN	29 mg/dL
Blood culture negative in	24 hours
Creatinine	1.5 mmol/L
Acetaminophen level	undetectable
Albumin	3.0 gm/dL
AST	2300 U/L
Total Bilirubin	19.5 mg/dL
ALT	1010 U/L
Alkaline phosphatase	180 U/L
Hepatitis A IgG	positive
GGT	89 U/L
Hepatitis B surface antigen	negative
INR	2.0
Ferritin	350 ng/dL
Hepatitis B surface IgG antigen	positive
Transferrin saturation	70%
Hepatitis B core IgG antibody	positive
HFE gene *C282Y* wild-type	
Hepatitis C antibody	positive
HFE gene *H63D* heterozygous	

Which of the following is the most probable diagnosis?

A. Reactivation of hepatitis B infection
B. Acute hepatitis B
C. Acute hepatitis C infection
D. Acetaminophen intoxication
E. Hereditary hemochromatosis

124. A 67-year-old man presents to your clinic for consultation. He has hypertension, diabetes mellitus type 2, and dyslipidemia. He is a chronic smoker and consumes 3 to 4 cocktails daily with supper for the last 13 years. On evaluation vital signs are remarkable for the following:

Temperature	37.0° C
Blood pressure	147/85 mm Hg
Heart rate	72 bpm
Respiratory rate	19 breaths/min

Physical exam is remarkable for hepatosplenomegaly. Laboratory studies reveal the following:

Platelet count	105,000/µL
Hemoglobin	11.5 g/dL
MCV	104 fl/cell
ALT	45 U/L
AST	98 U/L.

An abdominal sonogram shows a liver with a nodular contour and mild splenomegaly. In addition to alcohol abstinence, what additional measure will decrease his risks of alcoholic liver disease progression and hepatocellular carcinoma in this patient?

A. Smoking cessation
B. Vitamin B_{12} supplementation
C. Folic acid supplementation
D. Silymarin
E. Pentoxifylline

125. A 62-year-old man with alcoholic cirrhosis was admitted to the hospital after he developed acute renal failure and tense ascites. He reports that his symptoms worsened in the last 3 weeks. Physical exam is remarkable for a debilitated man with a weight of 167 pounds and height of 66 inches, bitemporal wasting, mild yellow discoloration of skin, scattered spider telangiectasias on the upper thorax, decrease pulmonary sound to auscultation, tense ascites with marked shifting dullness, easily palpable spleen below the left inferior costal margin, palmar erythema and severe lower extremity pitting edema. Which of the following is most useful to assess patient nutritional status?

A. Albumin levels
B. Pre-albumin levels
C. BMI
D. Creatinine-height index
E. Subjective global assessment (SGA) of protein malnutrition

126. A 52-year-old man with alcoholic cirrhosis is admitted to the hospital after developing tense ascites and altered mental status. The patient is oriented only to person, but can cooperate with the medical evaluation. Caregiver reports that patient has continued drinking alcohol daily. Patient has been irritable lately and is not eating much and complaints that food "does not smell and taste like before." He is having four to five episodes of loose to watery nonbloody stools daily. Patient reports difficulty reading at night. He reports symptoms have worsened in the last 3 weeks. Physical exam is remarkable for a debilitated man with a weight of 120 pounds and height of 66 inches, bitemporal wasting, alopecia with areas of thin sparse hair, mild yellow discoloration of skin, scattered spider telangiectasias, ascites, palmar erythema, lower extremity pitting edema and red inflamed areas of dry skin with scattered blisters on buttocks. Which of the following will be more effective to resolve the patient's symptoms?

A. Lactulose 30 mL orally twice daily
B. Rifaximin 550 mg orally twice daily
C. Vitamin B_{12} supplementation
D. Zinc supplementation
E. Vitamin A supplementation

127. A 40-year-old man is brought to the emergency department after being found unresponsive at his home. Several empty bottles of medications and liquor were found in his apartment. The patient is obtunded and unable to provide medical history. Vital signs are remarkable for the following:

Temperature	38.1° C
Blood pressure	98/69 mm Hg
Heart rate	110 bpm
Respiratory rate	19 breaths/min

On physical exam, the patient has scleral jaundice, bitemporal wasting, decreased breath sounds on lung bases bilaterally, a soft and depressive distended abdomen consistent with tense ascites, and severe pitting lower extremity edema. Rectal exam reveals an empty fecal vault with traces of brown stool. Patient is started on intravenous fluid, empiric broad-spectrum antibiotics and admitted to the hospital. Laboratory values are as follows:

Sodium	149 mmol/L
WBC	18,000/µL
Potassium	2.8 mmol/L
Hemoglobin	10.8 g/dL
Chloride	118 mmol/L
Platelet count	100,000/µL
CO2	19 mmol/L
Blood culture negative in	24 hours
BUN	35 mg/dL
Acetaminophen levels	negative
Creatinine	2.2 mg/dL
AST	350 U/L
Albumin	2.2 gm/dL
ALT	120 U/L
Total Bilirubin	28.3 mg/dL
Hepatitis A IgG	positive
Alkaline phosphatase	210 U/L
Hepatitis B surface antigen	negative
INR:	1.9
Hepatitis B surface antibody	positive
Hepatitis B core antibody	positive
Hepatitis C antibody	positive

What is the most appropriate management in this patient?

A. Start N-acetylcysteine 150 mg/kg orally followed by 70 mg/kg every 4 hours for 17 doses
B. Prednisolone 32 mg orally daily
C. Prednisolone 32 mg orally daily plus pentoxifylline 400 mg orally three times daily
D. Pentoxifylline 400 mg orally three times daily
E. Tenofovir 300 mg orally once daily

128. A 64-year-old man is brought to the emergency department by his caregiver after being found unresponsive at his home. The patient is an alcoholic who consumes a pint of vodka daily and smokes 2 packs of cigarettes daily. The patient is obtunded and unable to provide medical history. Vital signs are remarkable for the following:

Temperature	40.1° C
Blood pressure	88/59 mm Hg
Heart rate	120 per minute
Respiratory rate	25 breaths/min
Oxygen saturation	88% on room air

On physical exam, the patient has scleral jaundice, bitemporal wasting, decreased breath sounds on lung bases bilaterally, a soft and depressive distended abdomen consistent with tense ascites, and severe pitting lower extremity edema. Rectal exam reveals an empty fecal vault with traces of black stools. The patient is placed on mechanical ventilation, started on intravenous vasopressors, empiric broad-spectrum antibiotics, and is admitted to the intensive care unit (intensive care unit). The patient's urinary output in the last 4 hours has been only 10 mL. The patient has the following laboratories the second day after admission:

Sodium	154 mmol/L
WBC	20,000/μL
Potassium	2.8 mmol/L
Hemoglobin	8.8 g/dL
Chloride	118 mmol/L
Platelet count	80,000/μL
CO2	15 mmol/L
Blood culture: gram negative cocci in cluster	
BUN	45 mg/dL
Acetaminophen levels	negative
Creatinine	3.14 mg/dL
AST	250 U/L
Albumin	2.2 gm/dL
ALT	110 U/L
Total Bilirubin	30.3 mg/dL
Hepatitis A IgG	positive
Alkaline phosphatase	210 U/L
Hepatitis B surface antigen	negative
INR	2.5
Hepatitis B surface antibody	positive
Hepatitis B core antibody	negative

Which of the following is the most appropriate next step in the management of this patient?

A. Liver transplantation evaluation
B. Prednisolone 32 mg orally daily
C. Prednisolone 32 mg orally daily and pentoxifylline 400 mg orally three times daily
D. Palliative care service consult
E. Molecular adsorbent recirculating system (MARS)

129. All of the following pathophysiologic mechanisms are involved in the development of alcoholic liver disease, *except*:

A. Intestinal barrier dysfunction ad endotoxemia
B. Increased NADH/NAD+ ratio causing superoxide generation
C. Deficiency in S-adenosylmethionine (SAMe)
D. Augmented biliary production of endothelin-1 and increased nitric oxide production
E. TNF-mediated destruction of sensitized hepatocytes

130. A 48-year-old man comes to the emergency department for evaluation of increase in the abdominal girth, abdominal pain, and lower extremity edema for the last 2 days. He is a salesman with history of daily alcohol use with binge drinking on the weekends. He reports consumption of 2 to 3 beers daily with a 12-pack of beers in combination with a couple of cocktails on the weekends. He has no family history of chronic liver disease. On evaluation vital signs are remarkable for the following:

Temperature	38.5° C
Blood pressure	120/75 mm Hg
Heart rate	103 bpm
Respiratory rate	19 breaths/min

On physical exam, the patient has scleral jaundice, lungs are clear to auscultation, a distended abdomen with a positive shifting dullness and a palpable liver, and pitting lower extremity edema. Laboratory values are as follows:

Sodium	144 mmol/L
WBC	14,000/μL
Potassium	3.6 mmol/L
Hemoglobin	13.8 g/dL
Chloride	118 mmol/L
Platelet count	250,000/μL
CO2	28 mmol/L
Blood culture negative in	24 hours
BUN	20 mg/dL
Hepatitis A IgG antibody	positive
Creatinine	0.6 mg/dL
AST	130 U/L
Albumin	3.4 gm/dL
ALT	65 U/L
Total bilirubin	4.5 mg/dL
Alkaline phosphatase	190 U/L
Prothrombin time	15 sec

Abdominal CT revealed marked hepatomegaly with caudate lobe hypertrophy. Abdominal Doppler ultrasound failed to visualize the hepatic veins. Which of the following is the most appropriate therapeutic approach?

A. Start enoxaparin 1 mg/kg subcutaneously once daily
B. Start thrombolytic therapy with tenecteplase 40 mg intravenously
C. Start prednisolone 32 mg orally daily
D. Transjugular intrahepatic portosystemic shunt (TIPS)
E. Optimize nutrition, fluids, and electrolytes

131. A 48-year-old woman is referred to your GI office by her primary care provider. She has gained 23 pounds in the last 2 years and has a BMI of 38 kg/m^2. She works long hours at an administrative job and is relatively sedentary. She has no specific complaints. A comprehensive metabolic panel is checked and notable for the following:

Creatinine	0.8 mg/dL
AST	46 U/L
ALT	59 U/L
Total bilirubin	1.1 mg/dL
Platelet count	247,000/μL
WBC	9900/μL
INR of	0.9
Hemoglobin A1c	5.7%
Iron saturation of	44%

Which of the following is the next best step in evaluation?

A. Check a FibroSURE Test
B. Order a right upper quadrant ultrasound
C. Refer for bariatric surgery
C. Obtain a liver biopsy
D. Order a CT of the abdomen

132. A 48-year-old woman is referred to your GI office by her primary care provider. She has gained 23 pounds in the last 2 years and has a BMI of 38 kg/m^2. She works long hours at an administrative job and is relatively sedentary. She has no specific complaints. Upon further questioning, she admits to drinking 3 to 4 glasses of wine about twice per week. A comprehensive metabolic panel is checked and notable for the following:

Creatinine normal	
AST	46 U/L
ALT	59 U/L

Total bilirubin	1.1 mg/dL
Platelet count	247,000/μL
WBC	9900/μL
INR of	0.9
Hemoglobin A1c	5.7%
Iron saturation	44%

Which of the following could distinguish alcoholic steatohepatitis from nonalcoholic steatohepatitis on biopsy?

A. These two entities are histopathologically indistinguishable
B. Presence of Mallory-Denk bodies
C. Presence of macrovescicular fat
D. Presence of ballooning hepatocytes
E. Acidophil bodies

133. A 48-year-old woman is referred to your GI office by her primary care provider. She has gained 23 pounds in the last 2 years and has a BMI of 38 kg/m². She works long hours at an administrative job and is relatively sedentary. She has no specific complaints. A comprehensive metabolic panel is checked and notable for the following:

Creatinine normal	
AST	46 U/L
ALT	59 U/L
Total bilirubin	1.1 mg/dL
Platelet count	247,000/μL
WBC	9900/μL
INR	0.9
Hemoglobin A1c	5.7%
Iron saturation	44%

Abdominal ultrasound confirms your suspicion of steatosis. What is the next best step in management?

A. Start vitamin E, 800 IU daily
B. Start vitamin E, 400 IU daily
C. Start pioglitozone
D. Start atorvastatin
E. Initiate a trial of diet and exercise

134. Which of the following conditions has been demonstrated to be associated with nonalcoholic fatty liver disease (NAFLD)?

A. Colonic adenomas
B. Carcinoid lung tumors
C. Eczema
D. Dental carries
E. Mitral valve disease

135. A 52-year-old woman is referred to your clinic by her primary care provider. Her BMI is 38 kg/m². She works long hours at an administrative job and is relatively sedentary. She has no specific complaints. A comprehensive metabolic panel is checked and notable for the following:

AST	59 U/L
ALT	86 U/L
Total bilirubin	1.2 mg/dL
Platelet count	182,000/μL
INR	1.2
Hemglobin A1c	6.3%

Which of the following is the primary risk for mortality in this patient?

A. Variceal bleeding
B. Cardiovascular disease
C. Spontaneous bacterial peritonitis
D. Hepatocellular carcinoma
E. Ovarian cancer

136. A 57-year-old woman returns to your clinic 1 year after being diagnosed with NAFLD. In the last visit, you counseled her to increase her level of activity and lose about 10% of her weight. Today, she reports to you that she remains overall sedentary. She does not drink alcohol. Her BMI is now 42 kg/m². Her primary care provider started her on metformin roughly 9 months ago when her Hemoglobin A1c was 7.3%. She is also on hydrochlorothiazide, metoprolol, and atorvastatin.

AST	59 U/L
ALT	86 U/L
Total bilirubin	1.2 mg/dL
Platelet count	182,000/μL
INR	1.2

You consider adding vitamin E to her regimen. Which of the following should concern you about the use of vitamin E in this patient?

A. Her age
B. Her gender
C. Her use of atorvastatin
D. Her diabetes
E. Her use of hydrochlorothiazide

137. A 44-year-old Chinese man without a history of known liver disease or malignancy undergoes an abdominal CT during a self-limited episode of nausea, vomiting, diarrhea, and abdominal pain. It showed a nonspherical lesion without mass affect (see figure). Its attenuation was similar to that of soft tissue and did not show arterial enhancement. Which of the following is possibly the pathogenesis of this lesion?

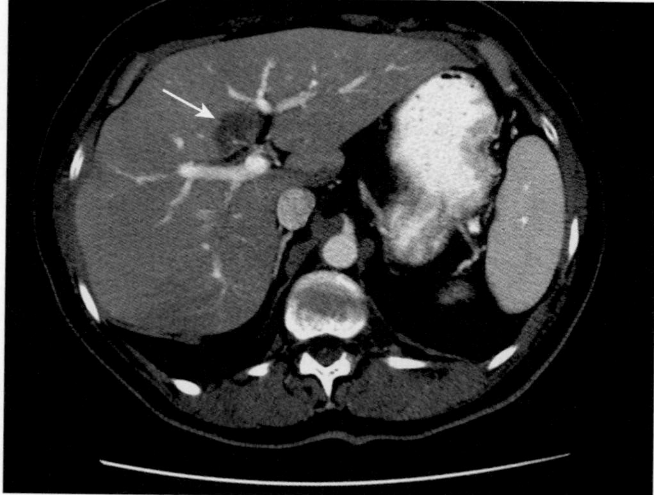

Figure for Question 137.

A. Dysplastic growth of hepatocytes
B. Altered venous flow to the liver
C. Hepatitis B virus
D. Angiogenesis
E. Trauma

138. A 44-year-old Chinese man without a history of known liver disease or malignancy undergoes an abdominal

CT during a self-limited episode of nausea, vomiting, diarrhea, and abdominal pain. It showed a 2.5 cm nonspherical lesion without mass affect. Its attenuation was similar to that of soft tissue and did not show arterial enhancement. Which is the next best step in management?
A. Reassurance
B. Biopsy of the lesion
C. Transarterial chemoembolization (TACE)
D. Liver transplantation evaluation
E. Referral to an oncologist

139. Significant steatosis in a donor liver has been associated with increased risk of which of the following in the recipient?
A. Posttransplant malignancies
B. Posttransplant weight gain
C. Primary nonfunction of the liver graft
D. Posttransplant hepatitis C recurrence
E. Posttransplant alcohol use

140. Which of the following findings should prompt consideration for other causes of liver injury rather than nonalcoholic steatohepatitis (NASH)?
A. ALT greater than AST
B. ALT >500 U/L
C. Low positive ANA titers
D. Elevated serum ferritin
E. Areas of relative sparing of fat on imaging

141. A 52-year old man is seen in the emergency department with elevated LFTs noted by his primary care physician when they were checked for malaise.

AST	3200 U/L
ALT	6000 U/L
Total bilirubin	2.3 mg/dL,
INR	0.9

He takes hydrochlorothiazide, rosuvastatin, metformin, phenytoin for a seizure history, and occasional ibuprofen. He admits that for the past 2 weeks he has been taking 4 to 5 gm of acetaminophen daily for right knee pain. He denies any alcohol use. Which of the following would be least helpful in the initial management of this patient?
A. Trending the INR
B. Oral N-acetylcysteine
C. Activated charcoal
D. Monitoring of his mental status
E. Checking blood pH

142. A 52-year-old man is seen in the emergency department with elevated liver function tests noted by his primary care physician when they were checked for the patient's complaints of malaise.

AST	3200 U/L
ALT	6000 U/L
Total bilirubin	2.3 mg/dL
INR	0.9

He takes hydrochlorothiazide, rosuvastatin, metformin, phenytoin for a seizure history, and occasional ibuprofen. He admits that for the past 2 weeks he has been taking 4-5 gm of acetaminophen daily for right knee pain. He denies any alcohol use. The simultaneous use of which of other drugs he is taking could increase his sensitivity to acetaminophen-induced liver injury?
A. Hydrochlorothiazide
B. Rosuvastatin
C. Metformin
D. Phenytoin
E. Ibuprofen

143. By what mechanism does phenytoin lower the threshold for acetaminophen-induced hepatotoxicity?
A. Competition for phase 2 pathways
B. Enzyme induction increasing the toxic metabolite
C. Constitutive expression of inhibitory gene products
D. Direct binding to N-acetyl-p-benzoquinone
E. Disruption of mitochondrial electron transport

144. Which of the following is true about phase 2 metabolic pathways?
A. They facilitate secretion of toxin into bile
B. They are energy dependent
C. Polymorphisms in genes responsible for their activity can be associated with cholestatic liver disease
D. They involve ABC proteins
E. They involve formation of ester links to the parent compound

145. A new compound is being studied for its ability to treat depression and has reached phase III clinical trials. In a phase III clinical trial including 600 patients, six cases of jaundice with ALT levels greater three times the upper limit normal (ULN) and bilirubin greater than two times the ULN but without alkaline phosphatase greater than two times the ULN were observed. What rate of liver failure might be expected during the marketing phase of the drug?
A. Three patients in 3000
B. One patient in 100
C. Four patients in 2500
D. Ten patients in 3000
E. One patient in 200

146. A new compound is being studied for its ability to treat depression and has reached phase III clinical trials. In a phase III clinical trial including 600 patients, six cases of jaundice with ALT levels greater three times the upper limit normal (ULN) and bilirubin greater than two times the ULN but without alkaline phosphatase greater than two times the ULN were observed. Which of the following would suggest the reaction is idiosyncratic rather than dose dependent?
A. Short latent period (hours)
B. Zonal necrosis on liver biopsy
C. Microvesicular steatosis on liver biopsy
D. Presence of a wide range of histologic changes on liver biopsy
E. Reproduction of the effect in other species

147. Which of the following patients might be at highest risk for an idiosyncratic reaction to experimental study drug?
A. A 10-year-old boy
B. A 40-year-old man with hypertension
C. A healthy 40-year-old woman
D. A 60-year-old woman with hepatitis C cirrhosis and diabetes
E. A 60-year-old man with diabetes

148. A 58-year-old female is started on a pioglitazone for a hemoglobin A1c of 7.4%, metoprolol for mildly elevated systolic blood pressure, and ciprofloxacin for dysuria and

a positive urinalysis during a new patient visit with her new primary care physician. Prior to that, she was taking an over-the-counter formulation of ginko biloba for 2 years as well as intermittent ibuprofen for chronic back pain. She reports giving blood twice in the last year without any call suggesting her blood could not be accepted. Two weeks after her appointment, her liver function tests are checked when she complains of fatigue. Laboratory values are as follows:

AST	450 U/L
ALT	660 U/L
Total bilirubin	1.1 mg/dL
Alkaline phosphatase	100 mg/dL
INR	1.1

She has no encephalopathy and otherwise feels well. Which of the following is the most appropriate next step in her management?

A. Admit to the hospital for monitoring
B. Liver biopsy
C. Stop all of her medications and monitor her liver function tests
D. Start steroids immediately
E. Order a contrasted cross-sectional abdomen imaging

149. A 58-year-old female is started on a pioglitazone for a hemoglobin A1c of 7.4%, metoprolol for mildly elevated systolic blood pressure, and ciprofloxacin for dysuria and a positive urinalysis during a new patient visit with her new primary care physician. Prior to that, she was taking an over-the-counter formulation of ginko biloba for two years as well as intermittent ibuprofen for chronic back pain. She reports giving blood twice in the last year without any call suggesting her blood could not be accepted. Two weeks after her appointment, her liver function tests are checked when she complains of fatigue, and they are as follows:

AST	450 U/L
ALT	660 U/L
Total bilirubin	1.1 mg/dL
Alkaline phosphatase	100 mg/dL
INR	1.1

She has no encephalopathy and otherwise feels well. Which of the following is a key component in proving the etiologic role of one of her medications?

A. Liver biopsy
B. History of alcohol use
C. Cross-sectional imaging
D. AST and ALT greater than 300 U/L
E. Improvement with cessation of the medication

150. A 27-year-old man is started on lamotrigine for a newly diagnosed seizure disorder. About 3 weeks later, he called about symptoms consistent with upper respiratory infection and treated himself with over-the-counter symptomatic agents with improvement in his symptoms and cessation of the over-the-counter medications after about 4 days. Another 3 weeks later, he is admitted to the hospital with headache, malaise, and a severe erythematous rash on his trunk and extremities. His liver enzymes are in the thousands with only mild elevations of total bilirubin and alkaline phosphatase. He has an eosinophilia on peripheral blood. He is not confused and his INR is normal. Which of the following is most likely to be found in this patient?

A. Mucositis
B. Cerebral edema
C. Elevated acetaminophen level
D. Neutropenia
E. Normal erythrocyte sedimentation rate

151. An 8-year-old child with systemic lupus erythematosis was given aspirin by his mother for fever and myalgia over several days. After an initial improvement, he developed worsening fatigue and malaise, so she brought him to the local emergency department. Initial vital signs showed the following:

Temperature	37.2° C
Heart rate	93 bpm
Blood pressure	104/68 mm Hg

He was alert and oriented. Laboratory tests showed AST and ALT above 3000 U/L and normal ammonia level. A liver biopsy was performed. Which of the following pathology features would be most likely to be seen on the biopsy?

A. Steatosis
B. Fibrosis
C. Hepatocellular degeneration with hydropic changes
D. Inclusion bodies
E. Hepatocyte ballooning

152. A 78-year-old woman is undergoing an urgent surgical procedure. She is obese, has type 2 diabetes, and atrial fibrillation. She has a remote history of hepatitis associated with halothane 50 years ago. What is the most reasonable way to reduce her risk of halothane hepatitis during this procedure?

A. Strict control of blood glucose
B. Perioperative zinc infusion
C. Do not use halothane
D. Give disulfiram prior to the procedure
E. Continue preoperative beta blocker

153. In a patient with history of halothane hepatotoxicity, the anesthesia team is deciding upon which agent to use to give him the lowest risk of hepatotoxicity. Which of the following is associated with the least incidence of hepatotoxicity in this patient?

A. Methoxyflurane
B. Enflurane
C. Isoflurane
D. Desflurane
E. Treichloroethylene

154. A 62-year-old immigrant man presents with right upper quadrant pain and jaundice for 2 months. Abdominal MRI and ultimately a biopsy are performed and he is diagnosed with a hepatic angiosarcoma. Upon further questioning, he reports having a wild youth and working in an industrial factory to make his ends meet in his mid to upper 20s. Which of the following was he most likely to have been exposed in his 20s that led to the development of angiosarcoma?

A. Benzene
B. Halothane
C. Dichlorodiphenyl-trichloroethane
D. Cocaine
E. Vinyl chloride monomer

155. A 54-year-old Asian immigrant woman with a history of chronic hepatitis B and her two adult daughters present to the local emergency department with abdominal pain, nausea, vomiting, diarrhea, and jaundice, which has gotten progressive over the past 36 hours. Their laboratory values showed elevation of liver enzymes: AST and ALT are >3000 IU/ML , bilirubin levels are also elevated with a range of 8 to 17 mg/dL. Liver biopsies are performed in all three and they all demonstrate nuclear inclusion bodies on electron microscopy in addition to zone 3 hepatic necrosis. Which management strategy is most likely to improve their condition?

A. Tenofovir
B. Lamivudine
C. Silibinin
D. Methylprednisolone
E. Penicillin G

156. You are visiting a newly industrializing country on a volunteer international medical program. Over the course of 2 months, you see over 20 patients with hepatotoxicity. All of them work in a local factory manufacturing industrial solvents. After you report your concern to local authorities, you see that the factory is temporarily shut down 2 weeks later for lack of compliance with safety equipment protocols. What is likely the most common route(s) of exposure to the effected patients?

A. Gastrointestinal and transdermal absorption
B. Inhalation and transdermal absorption
C. Gastrointestinal absorption via mucous membranes
D. Inhalation and ingestion
E. Accidental ingestion

157. For a patient with autoimmune hepatitis (AIH), which of the following is true regarding serologic markers?

A. The diagnostic accuracy is best achieved when ANA and SMA are both present
B. Patients with soluble liver antigen antibody (anti-SLA) have a higher likelihood of maintaining disease remission after treatment withdrawal
C. Liver-kidney microsome type 1antibodies (anti-LKM1) are most commonly found in adults
D. Atypical perinuclear antineutrophil cytoplasmic antibody (atypical pANCA) is useful in the diagnosis of type 2 AIH
E. Antibody to liver cytosol type 1 (anti-LC1) is associated with mild disease

158. A 60-year-old woman without significant past medical history is admitted after presenting to the emergency department with painless jaundice and fatigue for 2 weeks. She drinks one to two glasses of wine each night with dinner. On exam her vital signs are as follows:

Blood pressure	105/60 mm Hg
Temperature	36.9 °C
Heart rate	60 bpm

She is arousable but lethargic, has asterixis, but no stigmata of chronic liver disease. Her laboratory values are as follows:

ALT	1103 U/L
AST	957 U/L
Alkaline phosphatase	242 U/L
Total bilirubin	5.9 mg/dL
INR	2.5
Hepatitis A virus antibody	negative
HBsAg	negative
HBcAb	positive
HBsAb	positive
Hepatitis C virus antibody	negative
ANA	1:80
SMA	1:20
IgG	1700 mg/dL

Ultrasound reveals hepatomegaly. Liver biopsy is planned. Which of the following interventions is the most important next step?

A. Initiate norepinephrine
B. Initiate immediate workup for liver transplantation
C. Initiate prednisone 60 mg daily by mouth
D. ERCP
E. Initiate methylprednisolone 120 mg intravenously daily

159. Which of the following is true in patients with AIH?

A. Hyperpigmentation is a common clinical presentation
B. Asymptomatic patients usually have less severe disease and do not warrant treatment
C. In patients presenting with fulminant liver failure, it is very uncommon to find normal IgG levels
D. Anti-SLA and atypical pANCA may be helpful in diagnosing autoantibody-negative patients
E. White American patients have cirrhosis at presentation more commonly than African Americans

160. A 34-year-old woman who had fatigue and arthralgia for 3 months was found to have elevated liver enzymes as follows:

ALT	356 U/L
AST	298 U/L
Alkaline phosphatase	165 U/L
Bilirubin	1 mg/dL
INR	1.2
Creatinine	1.2 mg/dL
ANA	1:160
IgG	3200 mg/dL

Liver biopsy revealed lymphoplasmacytic portal infiltrate with moderate interface hepatitis in a background of cirrhosis. She did not have ascites, GI bleeding, or any evidence of hepatic encephalopathy. She was diagnosed with AIH and was started on combination therapy with azathioprine 50 mg daily and a tapering regimen of prednisone 30 mg daily orally. After 6 months of treatment, repeat labs today shows

ALT	401 U/L
AST	377 U/L
Alkaline phosphatase	184 U/L
Bilirubin	1.2 mg/dL
Creatinine	1.1 mg/dL
INR	1.2
IgG	3180 mg/dL

She is currently on azathioprine 50 mg daily and prednisone 10 mg daily, and she is tolerating therapy without any complication. Which of the following is the most appropriate next step in her management?

A. Discontinue prednisone and start budesonide 3 mg three times daily by mouth
B. Evaluate for liver transplantation
C. Discontinue azathioprine and start mycophenolate mofetil 1000 mg twice daily by mouth
D. Increase azathioprine to 150 mg daily and prednisone to 30 mg daily by mouth
E. Continue with current treatment regimen

161. Based on the Revised Original Scoring System for the Diagnosis of Autoimmune Hepatitis, which of the following variables increases the probability of the diagnosis?

A. Positive AMA
B. Male gender
C. Alkaline phosphatase/AST ratio >3
D. HLA DR4
E. Elevated IgM

162. An 18-year-old healthy Asian woman with no significant past medical history presents with scleral icterus, nausea, and abdominal discomfort for 1 week. She is on her second course of sulfamethoxazole-trimethoprim for a persistent urinary tract infection. On exam her vital signs are as follows:

Blood pressure	110/50 mm Hg
Heart rate	65 bpm
Temperature	36.7° C

She is alert, and oriented, well-developed. Head and neck exam is significant for scleral icterus. The rest of the exam including abdomen is unremarkable. Laboratory studies are as follows:

ALT	1585 U/L
AST	910 U/L
Total Bilirubin	3.5 mg/dL
INR	1.1
Hb	11 g/dL
Platelet count	250,000/μL
Creatinine	0.8 mg/dL

Liver ultrasound is unremarkable. ANA and ASMA are negative. IgG level 2500 mg/dL, anti-LKM1 1:320. Which of the following statements is most accurate in this patient?

A. This patient tends to have an excellent sustained response to steroids
B. There is a high chance of progression to cirrhosis and need for liver transplantation in this patient
C. Discontinuation of sulfamethoxazole-trimethoprim should lead to normalization of her liver function tests
D. Liver biopsy will show viral inclusion bodies and portal inflammation
E. There is 50% chance that atypical pANCA is found in this patient

163. A 56-year-old woman with history of Wilson Disease, status post orthotopic liver transplant in 2006, presents with elevated liver enzymes on routine testing:

ALT	375 U/L
AST	324 U/L
Alkaline phosphatase	178 U/L
Bilirubin	1.7 mg/dL
Total protein	8.2 mg/dL
Albumin	3.0 mg/dL

She denies alcohol use or new medications. Her immunosuppressive therapy consists of tacrolimus 1 mg every 12 hours; 12-hour trough level is 5.1 ng/mL. Further workup includes cytomegalovirus and hepatitis A, B and C testing, which are negative. Her ANA, ASMA, and anti- LKM1 are all negative. A liver biopsy is performed (see figure). What is the most appropriate next step in the management of this patient?

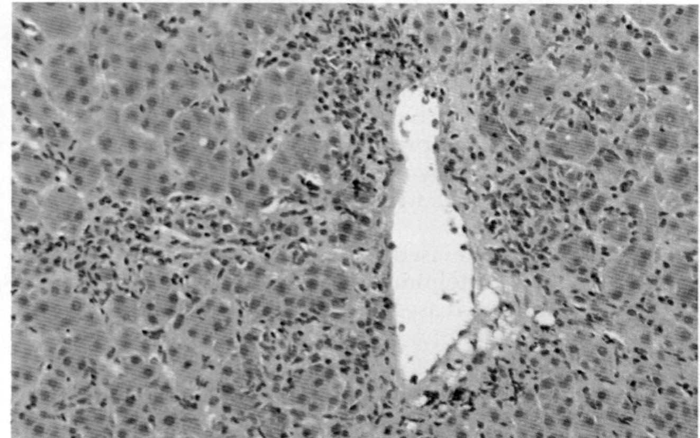

Figure for question 163.

A. Start prednisone 60 mg daily by mouth
B. ERCP
C. High-dose intravenous pulse corticosteroids
D. Increase the dose of tacrolimus
E. Start ursodeoxycholic acid

164. A 60-year-old woman presents to the office with fatigue and joint pains for 4 weeks. Her past medical history includes type 2 diabetes, hypertension, and osteoporosis. Her BMI is 41 mg/kg^2. Physical exam is significant for hepatomegaly but otherwise unremarkable. Laboratory studies reveal the following:

AST	230 U/L
ALT	294 U/L
Alkaline phosphatase	178 U/L
Bilirubin	1.1 mg/dL
INR	1.1
Albumin	4.0 mg/dL
ANA	1:160
IgG	2033 mg/dL

Viral hepatitis studies are negative. Liver biopsy reveals lymphoplasmacytic inflammation with moderate interface activity and bridging fibrosis. Which one of the following treatment regimens would you start for her?

A. Azathioprine 50 mg daily
B. Prednisone 20 mg daily
C. Prednisone 10mg daily and azathioprine 50 mg daily
D. Budesonide 3mg three times daily and azathioprine 50 mg daily
E. Tacrolimus 1mg twice daily

165. A 43-year-old woman without any significant past medical history has been seen in hepatology clinic with fatigue and mild pruritus for 6 months. Her only medication was birth control pills, which she has been taking for 8 years. Physical examination was unremarkable on presentation. Her weight was 67 kg. Initial laboratory values are as follows:

Alkaline phosphatase	213 U/L
ALT	143 U/L
AST	110 U/L
Total bilirubin	0.8 mg/dL
Total protein	8.0 mg/dL
Albumin	3.1 mg/dL
Viral hepatitis panel	negative
ANA	1:160
ASMA	negative
Anti-LKM1	negative
AMA	1:1280
IgG	3560 mg/dL

Liver biopsy was performed demonstrating portal/septal inflammatory cell infiltration consisting of an admixture of lymphocytes and plasma cells associated with foci of bile duct injury and mild interface activity. There was evidence of portal/periportal fibrosis with early bridging. She was started on ursodeoxycholic acid 500 mg twice daily. Six months later, she clinically appears the same. Laboratory values today are significant for the following:

Alkaline phosphatase	220 U/L
ALT	162 U/L
AST	128 U/L
Total bilirubin	0.8 mg/dL

What is the most appropriate next step for this patient?

A. Increase ursodeoxycholic acid to 1000 mg twice daily
B. ERCP

C. Stop ursodeoxycholic acid and start prednisone 60 mg daily
D. Continue ursodeoxycholic acid and start azathioprine 50 mg daily and prednisone 30 mg daily
E. Stop birth control pills

166. Which of the following is true regarding the prognosis of AIH?
A. A MELD score of 12 or more at presentation is associated with corticosteroid treatment failure and need for liver transplantation
B. Older patients (>40 years) are more likely to fail treatment than younger patients
C. HLA-DRB1*0301 is associated with better treatment response than HLA-DRB1*0401
D. Anti-SLA is associated with less severe disease
E. Patients who maintain normalization of liver enzymes for one year while on treatment have a low likelihood (<20%) of relapse with discontinuation of treatment

167. Which of the following statements is true about the AMA in primary biliary cirrhosis (PBC)?
A. The persistence of AMA after liver transplantation is indicative of PBC disease recurrence
B. Disease severity correlates with antibody titer
C. AMA appears to have direct cytotoxic effects in PBC
D. 60% of patients with PBC are AMA positive
E. The most frequent antigen against which AMAs are directed is pyruvate dehydrogenase complex E2 (PDC-E2)

168. A 55-year-old man presents with a 1-month history of fatigue and pruritus. He does not drink alcohol. His family history includes a sister with rheumatoid arthritis. His physical exam is normal except for nontender hepatomegaly. His laboratory studies are as follows:

Alkaline phosphatase of	278 U/L
ALT	54 U/L
AST	49 U/L
Bilirubin	0.9 mg/dL

A right upper quadrant ultrasound confirms hepatomegaly but is otherwise normal. Further testing reveals a positive AMA. Which of the following is an uncommon feature of this disease in this patient?
A. Symptoms
B. Gender
C. Age
D. Family history
E. Hepatomegaly

169. Which of the following is true regarding the pathogenesis of primary biliary cirrhosis?
A. There have been no indentified HLA class II genes linked to the disease
B. Smoking marijuana has been associated with the development of the disease
C. Patients with this disease are more likely to have a history of urinary tract infections
D. The disease has a higher concordance rate among dizygotic than monozygotic twin pairs
E. Use of minocycline has been associated with the development of the disease

170. Which of the following is true regarding symptoms related to primary biliary cirrhosis?
A. Higher fatigue levels are associated with increased risk of death and need for liver transplantation
B. A reduction in pruritus is a reliable marker for improved clinical outcomes
C. A minority of patients are asymptomatic at presentation
D. Asymptomatic patients rarely develop symptoms during long-term follow-up
E. Dry eyes and mouth are infrequent symptoms

171. A 49-year-old woman was referred to gastroenterology for evaluation of abnormal liver enzymes. She feels well outside of fatigue. She has a history of hypothyroidism and her only medication is levothyroxine. Her surgical history includes cholecystectomy at age 36. Her physical exam is normal. Laboratory values are as follows:

ALT	102 U/L
AST	94 U/L
Alkaline phosphatase	233 U/L
Bilirubin	1.1 mg/dL
Her ANA is	1:80
Anti-smooth muscle antibody (ASMA)	negative
AMA	negative
Hepatitis B surface antigen	negative
Hepatitis B surface antibody	negative
Hepatitis B core IgG	positive

MRCP reveals mild dilatation of common bile duct. A liver biopsy is performed (see figure). Which of the following is the next most appropriate step?

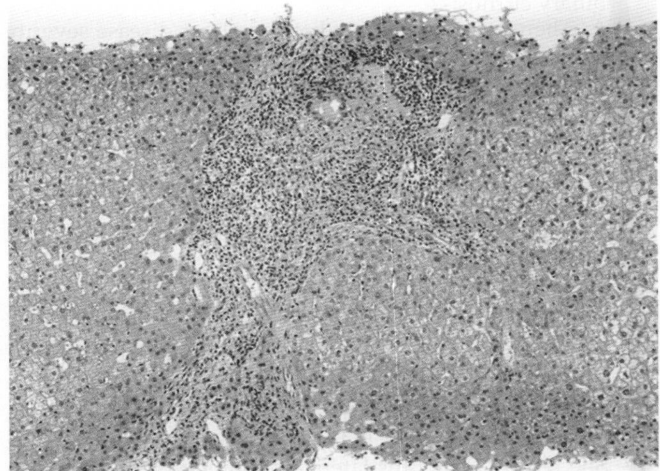

Figure for question 171.

A. ERCP
B. Colonoscopy to rule out ulcerative colitis
C. Start prednisone and azathioprine
D. Start ursodeoxycholic acid
E. Check hepatitis B e antigen

172. Which of the following is true regarding treatment of primary biliary cirrhosis with ursodeoxycholic acid (UDCA)?
A. The most effective dose of UDCA is 20-25 mg/kg/day
B. A lower rate of response is observed in women and patients diagnosed at a later age
C. Biochemical response is not a reliable predictor of long-term clinic outcomes

D. UDCA may improve liver biochemistries, but there is no evidence of improved transplant-free survival
E. One potential mechanism of action for UDCA is suppression of apoptosis

173. A 62-year-old woman presents with 3-month history of pruritus. She weighs 65 kg. Her physical exam is unremarkable. Her liver enzymes at the time of presentation include the following:

ALT	56 U/L
AST of	49 U/L
Alkaline phosphatase	434 U/L
Bilirubin	0.9 mg/dL

Further workup includes a positive AMA. Based on this, she was diagnosed with primary biliary cirrhosis and started on ursodeoxycholic acid (UDCA) 250 mg by mouth twice daily. She returns to see you for 6-month follow up. She reports good compliance with her UDCA. Repeat labs include the following:

ALT	50 U/L
AST	44 U/L
Alkaline phosphatase	430 U/L

Which of the following do you recommend?
A. Increase UDCA to 500 mg by mouth twice daily
B. Add budesonide 6 mg by mouth once daily
C. Add methotrexate 7.5 mg by mouth once weekly
D. Add azathioprine 50 mg by mouth once daily
E. Switch UDCA to cyclosporine 100 mg by mouth twice daily

174. Which of the following is true for patients with primary biliary cirrhosis?
A. There is no correlation between liver disease severity and bone loss
B. Treatment of osteoporosis with bisphosphonates is contraindicated
C. Lipid abnormalities are common; however, there is no increase in cardiovascular disease risk
D. Treatment of dyslipidemia with statins is contraindicated
E. Reduced night vision may be a sign of vitamin E deficiency

175. A 47-year-old woman with history of primary biliary cirrhosis (PBC) presents to your clinic with fatigue and an elevated alkaline phosphatase of 269 U/L. Her AMA is positive. A liver biopsy is compatible with a diagnosis of PBC and established cirrhosis. She weighs 65 kg and is started on ursodeoxycholic acid (UDCA) 900 mg per day. She returns 3 months later complaining of severe pruritus. Her liver disease remains compensated. Her laboratory values at that time include the following:

Alkaline phosphatase	170 U/L
ALT	51 U/L
AST	41 U/L
Bilirubin	0.9 mg/dL

She is started on rifampin 300 mg bid. She returns one month later and her pruritus has improved. Repeat laboratory values are as follows:

Alkaline phosphatase	195 U/L
ALT	88 U/L
AST	61 U/L
Bilirubin	3.2 mg/dL
INR	1.1
Creatinine	1.0 mg/d

What is the most appropriate next step in her management?
A. Increase UDCA to 1500 mg per day
B. Discontinue rifampin
C. Start colchicine
D. Obtain a repeat liver biopsy
E. Refer for liver transplant evaluation

176. Which of the following is true regarding primary biliary cirrhosis (PBC) and liver transplantation?
A. Overall, the number of liver transplants performed each year for PBC is on the rise
B. Compared to other etiologies, PBC patients have lower 1-year and 5-year survival rates after transplantation
C. PBC recurs after transplantation in a majority of patients
D. The presence of AMA after liver transplantation is indicative of disease recurrence
E. In patients with PBC, poor quality of life due to fatigue and refractory pruritus is an indication for liver transplantation

177. A 67-year-old woman with end-stage liver disease from hepatitis C virus develops massive hematemesis while hospitalized for spontaneous bacterial peritonitis and recently has been listed for liver transplantation. She is transferred to the intensive care unit after emergent endotracheal intubation, and is administered vasopressin, antibiotics, octreotide, and transfused 5 units of packed red blood cells. An emergent esophagogastroduodenoscopy (EGD) is performed in the intensive care unit that reveals large esophageal varices without bleeding stigmata and large amount of bright red blood in the stomach. On retroflexed view, large fundal varices extending to the gastroesophageal junction are visualized with a fibrin platelet plug. A recent MRI shows a cirrhotic liver with large amounts of ascites, patent portal vein system with a large splenorenal shunt, and associated gastroesophageal varices. Which of the following treatment options would have the highest potential to worsen the patient's ascites and esophageal varices?
A. Balloon-occluded retrograde transvenous obliteration (BRTO)
B. Transjugular intrahepatic portosystemic shunt
C. Balloon tamponade
D. Endoscopic injection of cyanoacrylate
E. Surgical portacaval shunt

178. A 52-year-old man with a history of hypertension, chronic alcohol use, tobacco use, and bouts of recurrent abdominal pain presents to the emergency department with massive hematemesis. He has a heart rate of 115 beats per minute and blood pressure is 90/40 mm Hg. Once he is resuscitated, an urgent upper endoscopy reveals the source of hemorrhage as a large isolated gastric varix with bleeding stigmata in the fundus (IGV-1) without significant esophageal varices. Which of the following findings would be most likely to be found on an abdominal MRI in this patent?
A. Nodular regenerative hyperplasia (NRH)
B. Hepatocellular carcinoma
C. Thromboses in the middle and left hepatic veins
D. Splenic vein thrombosis
E. Portal vein thrombosis

179. A 64-year-old woman is being evaluated for placement of a transjugular intrahepatic portosystemic

shunt. Portal pressure measurements are obtained. free hepatic pressure is 6 mm Hg. Wedge hepatic venous pressure is 13 mm Hg. Which of the following etiologies of portal hypertension would best explain these measurements?
A. Portal vein thrombosis
B. Constrictive pericarditis
C. Sarcoidosis
D. Alcoholic cirrhosis
E. Schistosomiasis

180. Which of the following agents is recommended for primary prophylaxis of large esophageal varices and acts to decrease both portal flow and intrahepatic resistance?
A. Prazosin
B. Isosorbide mononitrate
C. Carvedilol
D. Propranolol
E. Simvastatin

181. A 46-year-old man with known Child-Pugh class C cirrhosis due to chronic hepatitis C virus without prior variceal hemorrhage presents to the outpatient endoscopy suite for an upper endoscopy. On upper endoscopy he is found to have three channels of large esophageal varices in the distal esophagus with "red wale" stigmata. Which of the following features correlates the *least* with the patient's risk of variceal hemorrhage over the next two years?
A. Number of varices
B. Size of varices
C. Presence of bleeding stigmata
D. Elevated hepatic venous pressure gradient > 12 mm Hg
E. Child-Pugh class C cirrhosis

182. A 50-year-old man with hepatitis C virus–associated cirrhosis is transferred from the emergency department to the Intensive care unit for hematemesis. Upon arrival to the intensive care unit, he again experiences massive hematemesis and undergoes emergent endotracheal intubation. His heart rate is 115 beats per minute and blood pressure is 85/45 mm Hg. His labsoratory values are as follows:

Hemoglobin	6.5 g/dL
Platelet count	90,000/μL
INR	2.3
ALT	51 U/L
AST	68 U/L
Alkaline phosphatase	150 U/L
Total bilirubin	6.5 mg/dL
Sodium	134 mEq/L
Creatinine	1.5 mg/dL
Albumin	2.7 mg/dL

A liver ultrasound with Doppler imaging reveals a cirrhotic liver, moderate ascites, and a patent portal vein. An emergent upper endoscopy is performed which reveals large esophageal varices with a platelet-fibrin plug, and the patient undergoes successful band ligation. There was a large amount of fresh blood in the stomach obscuring the view of the stomach. Although the patient's hemodynamics stabilized, 12 hours later the patient's blood pressure decreased to 70/45 mm Hg and the heart rate increased to 120 beats per minute. Placement of a transjugular intrahepatic portosystemic shunt (TIPS) is considered in order to achieve hemostasis. Which of the following factors most strongly predicts the risk of progressive liver failure and death after placement of TIPS in this patient?
A. The patient's age
B. Etiology of liver disease
C. The total bilirubin, INR, and creatinine levels
D. Platelet count level
E. Use of a polytetrafluoroethylene-covered stent

183. A 79-year-old man with history of cirrhosis secondary to hepatitis C is seen in your clinic for evaluation. His past medical history is otherwise unremarkable. He denies any history of GI bleeding, ascites or hepatic encephalopathy. Vital signs show Heart rate is 64 bpm and blood pressure is 120/70 mm Hg. Physical exam is only significant for several spider nevi. You perform an upper endoscopy for him to screen for esophageal varices. It shows two columns of small varices in the distal esophagus. What will you recommend next?
A. Nadolol
B. Endoscopic variceal ligation (EVL)
C. Transjugular intrahepatic portosystemic shunt
D. Repeat endoscopy in 1 year
E. Repeat endoscopy in 3 years

184. A 42-year-old man with a history of alcoholism undergoes urgent upper endoscopy for massive hematemesis. On endoscopy, moderate-sized esophageal varices, which flattened with insufflation, were noted without stigmata of bleeding. The stomach had a large amount of old blood in the cardia and fundus, and large type 2 (GOV-2) varices were noted with a fibrin-platelet plug noted. Which of the following statements is correct about gastric varices?
A. The size of gastric varices is not an important risk factor for bleeding
B. Primary prophylaxis of hemorrhage with transjugular intrahepatic portosystemic shunt (TIPS) placement is strongly recommended
C. Placement of TIPS to control recent bleeding with reduction of the hepatic venous pressure gradient (HVPG) below 12 mm Hg is sufficient to prevent rebleeding from gastric varices
D. Bleeding is less likely from fundal varices compared to varices at the gastroesophageal junction
E. Risk of bleeding from gastric varices is related to severity of underlying liver disease

185. A 64-year-old woman with a history of insulin-dependent diabetes has been found to have Child-Pugh class B cirrhosis due to hepatitis C virus and a prior longstanding history of alcohol use. She has never been treated for her hepatitis C virus previously due to concerns for medical noncompliance. She states that she has had several episodes of hypoglycemia in the past on her insulin therapy and due to chronic nausea she occasionally skips meals. Her blood pressure in clinic is 105/69 mm Hg and her resting heart rate is 60 beats per minute. She undergoes a screening upper endoscopy that reveals several large esophageal varices without bleeding stigmata. Which of the following options for primary prophylaxis would be best for this patient?
A. Isosorbide mononitrate
B. Endoscopic variceal ligation
C. Nadolol
D. Transjugular intrahepatic portosystemic shunt
E. Metoprolol

186. A 61-year-old woman with history of Child-Pugh class B cirrhosis due to alcohol is transferred to the intensive care unit for massive hematemesis. She is in hemodynamic shock and has central lines placed. She is receiving intravenous fluids and undergoes endotracheal intubation in the setting of ongoing hematemesis. Which of the following interventions may result in a worse outcome for her?

A. Early administration of vasoactive drug such as octreotide
B. Broad-spectrum antibiotics such as an oral quinolone or intravenous ceftriaxone
C. Transfusion of packed red blood cells (PRBC) to at least 10 g/dL
D. EVL if esophageal varices are identified as source of hemorrhage
E. Early use of transjugular intrahepatic portosystemic shunt within 72 hours of control of bleeding if active esophageal variceal bleeding is identified

187. A 63-year-old woman with a history of diabetes, hypertension, and chronic hepatitis C virus is admitted to the hospital for 2 to 3 days of melena. She never had GI bleeding in the past. She has a blood pressure 103/63 mm Hg and her heart rate is 88 bpm. Her hemoglobin is 10.8 g/dL. It was 11.4 g/dL about 3 months ago. She undergoes upper endoscopy, which reveals small esophageal varices without bleeding stigmata. In the gastric fundus, there is diffuse mucosal oozing with a small amount of old blood and no evidence of gastric varices. The proximal gastric mucosa has a mosaic, snakeskin appearance with punctuate erythematous markings. Which of the following is recommended as the first line of treatment for her condition?

A. Nadolol and iron supplement
B. Endoscopic variceal ligation
C. Liver transplantation
D. Argon plasma coagulation (APC)
E. Transjugular intrahepatic portosystemic shunt

188. A 49-year-old woman with history of HCV cirrhosis is found to have microcytic anemia with hemoglobin of 7.3 g/dL. She undergoes upper endoscopy, which reveals in the antrum several flat erythematous stripes radiating from the pylorus with a scant amount of active oozing. Colonoscopy was unremarkable. Which of the following would be the least effective treatment for the cause of her anemia?

A. Endoscopic coagulation with a heater probe
B. Antrectomy
C. Argon plasma coagulation
D. Endoscopic radiofrequency ablation
E. Transjugular intrahepatic portosystemic shunt

189. Which of the following patients would benefit most from the successful placement of transjugular intrahepatic portosystemic shunt?

A. A 61-year-old woman found to have large GOV-2 gastric varices on upper endoscopy without history of variceal bleeding
B. A 74-year-old woman with history of congestive heart failure, NASH cirrhosis and active bleeding from esophageal varices seen on endoscopy
C. A 52-year-old man with a history of Caroli syndrome and progressive ascites
D. A 62-year-old man with alcoholic cirrhosis complicated by portopulmonary hypertension with an active esophageal variceal hemorrhage
E. A 36-year-old man with 2 weeks of ascites and right upper quadrant abdominal pain found on MRI to have a thrombus in a hepatic vein and caudate lobe hypertrophy

190. Which of the following conditions can be the cause of "pre-sinusoidal" portal hypertension?

A. Right-sided heart failure
B. Budd-Chiari syndrome
C. Constrictive pericarditis
D. Schistosomiasis
E. Inferior vena cava syndrome

191. Which of the following patterns of measurements would be expected in sinusoidal portal hypertension?
WHVP, wedged hepatic venous pressure
FHVP, free hepatic vein pressure
HVPG, hepatic venous pressure gradient

A. WHVP = Increased, FHVP = Normal, HVPG = Increased
B. WHVP = Increased, FHVP = Increased, HVPG = Normal
C. WHVP = Normal, FHVP = Normal, HVPG = Normal
D. WHVP = Increased, FHVP = Normal, HVPG = Decreased
E. WHVP = Normal, FHVP = Decreased, HVPG = Increased

192. Which of the following patterns of measurements would be expected in "post-hepatic" portal hypertension?
WHVP, wedged hepatic venous pressure
FHVP, free hepatic vein pressure
HVPG, hepatic venous pressure gradient

A. WHVP = Increased, FHVP = Normal, HVPG = Increased
B. WHVP = Increased, FHVP = Increased, HVPG = Normal
C. WHVP = Normal, FHVP = Normal, HVPG = Normal
D. WHVP = Increased, FHVP = Normal, HVPG = Decreased
E. WHVP = Normal, FHVP = Decreased, HVPG = Increased

193. A 55-year-old man with cirrhosis due to hepatitis C liver disease presents with 3 months of abdominal distention and weight gain. On physical exam, he has bulging flanks and shifting dullness on percussion. Laboratories studies include the following:

Sodium	130 mEq/L
BUN	12 mg/dL
Creatinine	0.4 mg/dL
Total bilirubin	1.3 mg/dL
Albumin	2.9 g/dL
Prothrombin time	13.4 seconds

Which of the following medical therapies is most likely to control his ascites?

A. Fluid restriction
B. Dietary sodium restriction and diuretics
C. Fluid restriction and dietary sodium restriction
D. Dietary sodium restriction
E. Single large-volume paracentesis

194. A 45-year-old man with NASH cirrhosis presents with chronic ascites requiring several paracentesis procedures over the last year. Ascitic fluid analysis is consistent with portal hypertension. He has been stable on a regimen of spironolactone 200 mg/day with furosemide 80 mg/day. When seen today, he is without complaints. On exam, he has mild ascites. Laboratory values are as follows:

Sodium	125 mEq/L
Potassium	4.3 mEq/L
Creatinine	1 mg/dL

Which of the following is the best recommendation for his management now?

A. Increase consumption of sports drinks
B. Paracentesis
C. Ensure compliance with low sodium diet
D. Transjugular intrahepatic portosystemic shunt
E. Increase diuretic doses

195. A 48-year-old man presents to the emergency department complaining of weight gain, abdominal swelling, and poor exercise tolerance. He states that over the past few months he has noticed progressive swelling in his abdomen along with shortness of breath after walking two blocks. He has a long history of alcohol abuse with multiple admissions for withdrawal. During his last admission, a right upper quadrant ultrasound revealed fatty infiltration of the liver with no signs of cirrhosis. Echocardiography revealed a normal heart size with early diastolic dysfunction. On physical exam, his respirations are normal. Cardiac exam reveals a laterally displaced PMI with regular rate and rhythm. He has bulging flanks and shifting dullness on abdominal exam. Laboratory values are as follows:

Sodium	134 mEq/L
Potassium	4.3 mEq/L
Creatinine	1.2 mg/dL
Total bilirubin	1.3 mg/dL
Albumin	3.8 g/dL
Prothrombin time	11 seconds

A diagnostic paracentesis is performed in the emergency department with the following findings:

Color Transparent yellow	
Albumin	1.0 g/dL
WBC	200,000/µL
Total Protein	1 g/dL

What is the best way to prevent recurrent episodes of ascites?

A. Evaluation and treatment of heart failure
B. Dietary sodium restriction and diuretics
C. Fluid restriction and dietary sodium restriction
D. Intensive alcohol treatment program
E. Evaluation for infectious etiology

196. A 53-year-old man presents to the emergency department for evaluation of increasing abdominal girth over the past year. He reports that his only significant past medical is hypertension that has been difficult to control. He sleeps on one pillow comfortably. His social history includes drinking 0.5 pints of vodka daily. The patient has also noticed mild swelling of his ankles and a decrease in his exercise tolerance. His physical exam includes blood pressure 175/92 mm Hg, heart rate 82 beats per minute. Lungs are clear to auscultation. On cardiac exam he has a regular rate and rhythm, prominent PMI and sternal heave. Abdominal exam reveals a protuberant abdomen with flank fullness and shifting dullness. Laboratory values are as follows:

Sodium	134 mEq/L
Potassium	4.3 mEq/L
Creatinine	1.0 mg/dL
Total bilirubin	1.2 mg/dL
Albumin	3.5 g/dL
Prothrombin time	11 seconds

A diagnostic paracentesis is performed with the following findings:

Color Transparent yellow	
Albumin	0.8 g/dL
WBC	200,000/µL
Total Protein	3.5 g/dL

What is the best next step in evaluating this patient's ascites?

A. Transthoracic echocardiogram
B. Serology for viral hepatitis
C. Gram stain of ascitic fluid
D. Right upper quadrant ultrasound
E. Liver biopsy

197. A 70-year-old woman who was recently diagnosed with ovarian cancer is being seen in your office prior to starting chemotherapy. The patient reports a 10-pound weight gain over the past year prior to her diagnosis. She recently read about how some patients develop fluid in their abdomen with progression of the disease, and she asks you if her weight gain is related to this process. She is alert and well appearing. Lung and cardiac exams are normal. Her abdomen is soft and nontender. Bowel sounds are normal. There is no dullness to percussion of her flanks. An exam for shifting dullness is equivocal. What are the chances that this patient has ascites?

A. <10%
B. 11% to 20%
C. 21% to 30%
D. 50%
E. 80%

198. A 50-year-old man with history of HCV cirrhosis presents to clinic for a follow-up visit. He was admitted to the hospital 1 month ago for tense ascites that improved with large volume paracentesis. Prior to this episode he had stable cirrhosis for 2 years. Since discharge he has felt well. He reports compliance with low sodium diet and diuretic therapy. His weight is stable since discharge. His only complaint is recent disturbance in his sleep. He finds that he no longer sleeps through the night and does not feel rested in the morning. On physical exam, he demonstrates spider angiomata and palmar erythema. Mild asterixis is observed. He has bulging flanks on evaluation of his abdomen, but he states this is no different than his baseline. Which of the following is the most appropriate next step in management?

A. Measure urine sodium to potassium ratio
B. Recommend fluid restriction
C. Hepatocellular carcinoma screening and diagnostic paracentesis
D. Measure serum ammonia level
E. Increase diuretic dose

199. Which of the following laboratory scenarios represents a contraindication to paracentesis?

A.

Platelet count	40,000/µL
INR	1.5

Fibriongen	200 mg/dL (150-350 mg/dL)
D-Dimer	150 ug/L (<300 ug/L)

B.

Platelet count	90,000/μL
INR	4.8
Fibriongen	300 mg/dL
D-Dimer	310 ug/L

C.

Platelet count	40,000/μL
INR	4.7
Fibriongen	300 mg/dL
D-Dimer	310 ug/L

D.

Platelet count	90,000/μL
INR	3
Fibriongen	100 mg/dL
D-Dimer	1000 ug/L

E.

Platelet count	80,000/μL
INR	1
Fibriongen	50 mg/dL (150-350 mg/dL)
D-dimer	290 ug/L (<300 ug/L)

200. A 60-year-old woman with a history of hepatitis C cirrhosis presents to the emergency department (ED) for evaluation of fever and abdominal pain for 3 days. She was diagnosed with cirrhosis 2 years ago with an episode of decompensation 1 year ago. She states she has been stable on diuretic therapy since that time. Three days prior to arrival, she began to notice abdominal swelling and a low-grade fever. In the ED she is alert and oriented. She has bulging flanks with shifting dullness on abdominal examination. Testing for asterixis reveals a mild flap. Laboratory values are as follows:

Sodium	134 mEq/L
Potassium	4.3 mEq/L
Creatinine	1.0 mg/dL
Total bilirubin	3.5 mg/dL
Albumin	2.6 g/dL
Prothrombin time	11 seconds

A diagnostic paracentesis is performed with the following findings:

Color	Transparent yellow
Albumin	0.8 g/dL
WBC	600,000/uL, 60% neutrophils
Total Protein	2.0 g/dL
Gram stain	Negative

Which of the following is the most appropriate next step in management?

A. Repeat paracentesis in 48 hours
B. Culture ascitic fluid at bedside
C. Send ascitic fluid to the lab for culture
D. Start oral norfloxacin
E. Start intravenous cefotaxime

201. A 48-year-old man with a history of alcohol-induced liver disease and Crohn disease is brought to the emergency department for altered mental status. The patient was staying at a homeless shelter where staff found him difficult to arouse in the morning. He does not respond to verbal commands, but does respond to noxious stimuli. A head CT is negative. His temperature is 39° C. On abdominal exam, he winces with deep palpation. Flank fullness is evident with shifting dullness. A diagnostic paracentesis is performed that demonstrates a predominance of neutrophils (PMN) count >250 cells/mm^3, and cefotaxime is started. A Gram stain of ascitic fluid finds gram positive and gram negative organisms. Which of the following is the most appropriate next step in management?

A. Check ascitic fluid lactate dehydrogenase (LDH)
B. Abdominal imaging
C. Start metronidazole
D. Await culture results
E. Repeat paracentesis in 48 hours

202. Which of the following is the first line regimen for secondary prevention of spontaneous bacterial peritonitis?

A. Doxycycline 100 mg twice daily
B. Amoxicillin 500 mg twice daily
C. Trimethoprim-sulfamethoxazole daily
D. Norfloxacin 400 mg daily
E. Ciprofloxacin 500 mg daily

203. A 55-year-old man with HCV cirrhosis and esophageal varices presents for surveillance endoscopy. His last endoscopy 1 year ago demonstrated a small column of varices that flattened with insufflation. He now has a large column of varices on endoscopy. During banding, a small amount of oozing is observed that resolves with further band placement. What is the next step in treating this patient?

A. Start norfloxacin for spontaneous bacterial peritonitis (SBP) prevention
B. Overnight observation for further bleeding
C. Endoscopy in 2 weeks
D. Endoscopy in 3 months
E. Start ceftriaxone for SBP prevention

204. A 60-year-old woman with cirrhosis due to nonalcoholic steatohepatitis presents to the emergency department complaining of shortness of breath. She was diagnosed with cirrhosis 1 year prior to presentation after developing tense ascites. She was started on sodium restriction and diuretics. She experienced an episode of hepatic hydrothorax 2 months ago that was treated with thoracentesis. Despite reported compliance with diet and medications, dyspnea slowly returned over the past month. A chest x-ray reveals right-sided pleural effusion. A thoracentesis is performed in the emergency department, and the patient is discharged with follow-up in her gastroenterologist's office. What treatment should be considered for this patient if she experiences another episode of hepatic hydrothorax?

A. Chest tube insertion
B. Pleurodesis
C. Peritoneovenous shunt
D. Video-assisted thoracoscopic surgery (VATS) to suture diaphragmatic defect
E. Transjugular intrahepatic portosystemic shunt

205. A 55-year-old man was admitted for treatment of spontaneous bacterial peritonitis (SBP). At admission he was given a dose of albumin 1.5 g/kg body weight and started on intravenous cefotaxime 2 mg every 8 hours.

On hospital day 3, he feels well. His WBC count and renal function are normal. Cultures have returned an *E. coli* species with no significant resistance to antibiotics. Which of the following is the most appropriate next step in management?

A. Administer albumin 1.5 g/kg body weight and continue cefotaxime for a total of 10 days
B. Discharge the patient on ampicillin to complete 10 days of antibiotics
C. Administer albumin 1.0 g/kg
D. Continue cefotaxime for a total of 10 days
E. Discharge the patient on daily norfloxacin to complete treatment and prevent recurrent SBP

206. A 65-year-old woman with hepatitis C virus cirrhosis returns to clinic for a 1 month follow-up. She was hospitalized 3 months ago for tense ascites, and has been seen every month since discharge. A therapeutic paracentesis during hospitalization withdrew 12 L of fluid. She was discharged on lasix 40 mg daily and spironolactone 100 mg daily. The patient reports compliance with her medications and diet. In spite of therapy, she has gained weight with re-accumulation of fluid in her abdomen. On exam, her abdomen demonstrates flank fullness and shifting dullness that has worsened since her last visit 1 month ago. Laboratory values are as follows:

Sodium	134 mEq/L
Potassium	3.8 mEq/L
Creatinine	1.1 mg/dL
Total bilirubin	2.5 mg/dL
Albumin	2.6 g/dL

A random urine sodium-to-potassium ratio is 1.5. Which of the following is the most appropriate next step in management?

A. Increase dose of lasix
B. Increase dose of spironolactone
C. Increase doses of lasix and spironolactone
D. Counsel on sodium restriction
E. Counsel on fluid restriction

207. A 54-year-old man with history of alcohol-induced cirrhosis is admitted to the hospital for treatment of cellulitis. He has a history of ascites and edema that has been relatively well controlled with a low sodium diet and diuretic therapy. At admission his abdomen is soft with flank fullness and shifting dullness. He has 2+ pitting edema in his lower extremities. Twice daily intravenous furosemide is started for diuresis. Vancomycin is started for cellulitis, and the patient improves. On hospital day 5, his creatinine is found to double to 2.6 mg/dL. Renal and GI consults are requested. What is the most likely etiology for his kidney injury?

A. Hepatorenal syndrome type 1
B. Hepatorenal syndrome type 2
C. Acute tubular necrosis
D. Diuretic-induced azotemia
E. Acute interstitial nephritis

208. A 64-year-old woman with alcoholic cirrhosis presents for follow-up in clinic. She was recently placed on the transplant list after completing an alcohol rehabilitation program. A recent MRI of the abdomen demonstrated a liver with cirrhotic morphology without any evidence of hepatocellular carcinoma. She has been on a regimen of 200 mg of spironolactone and 80 mg of furosemide daily for ascites, but she has recently noticed increasing abdominal girth. On exam, her vital signs are as follows:

Blood pressure	90/65 mm Hg
Heart rate	82 bpm
Respiration rate	18 breaths/min
Temperature	37° C

Lungs are clear to auscultation. Cardiac exam shows regular rate and rhythm. Abdomen is soft and nontender. Flank fullness and shifting dullness are present. Which of the following is the most appropriate next step in management for this patient's ascites?

A. Discontinue diuretics to improve blood pressure
B. Increase diuretic doses to improve ascites
C. Start midodrine
D. Refer for transjugular intrahepatic portosystemic shunt (TIPS)
E. Apply for MELD exception

209. A 45-year-old immigrant from Southeast Asia with a history of chronic HBV presents to the emergency department complaining of shortness of breath, abdominal pain, and increasing abdominal girth. She has intermittently followed up in an outpatient clinic, and has never been treated for HBV. Her abdomen has expanded over the past 2 weeks with worsening abdominal pain. This morning, she began to experience shortness of breath. A chest x-ray in the emergency department revealed small, bilateral pleural effusions. Her temperature is 38.5 °C. Abdominal exam reveals flank fullness, shifting dullness, and tenderness to palpation. Laboratory studies include the following:

Sodium	134 mEq/L
Potassium	4.3 mEq/L
Creatinine	1.2 mg/dL
Total bilirubin	1.3 mg/dL
Albumin	3.0 g/dL
Prrothrombin time	11 seconds

A diagnostic paracentesis is performed in the emergency department with the following findings:

Color Transparent yellow	
Albumin	2.0 g/dL
WBC	1000/μL
PMN count	40%
Total Protein	1 g/dL
Amylase	50 U/L

Antibiotics are started in the emergency department, and the patient is admitted for observation. Which of the following tests should be ordered immediately?

A. Cytology for malignancy
B. Hepatocellular carcinoma screening
C. No further diagnostic testing
D. Tuberculosis testing
E. Check serum lipase

210. In which one of the following settings is the measurement of serum ammonia most useful?

A. A 45-year-old patient with known alcoholic cirrhosis who presents to the emergency department with overt confusion
B. An 18-year-old man with carbamoyl phosphate synthetase deficiency and no other systemic conditions, who is brought to emergency department unresponsive with tonic-clonic movements

C. A 60-year-old woman with hepatitis C–related cirrhosis who presents to the hospital disoriented and with 3-week history of melena
D. A 75-year-old man with nonalcoholic steatohepatitis–related cirrhosis who developed septic shock requiring mechanical ventilation after being diagnosed with a community acquired pneumonia
E. A 60-year-old woman with autoimmune hepatitis and cirrhosis, who was diagnosed with cryptococcal meningitis 1 month ago and was started on posaconazole, and who came to the emergency department unresponsive and with active seizures

211. A 57-year-old man with known chronic hepatitis C is brought by his wife to the emergency department. He is obtunded and unable to provide any history. The wife reports that he started to experience a marked increase in his abdominal girth in the last 3 weeks and yesterday complained of abdominal pain and tremors. He was having one to two daily loose bowel movements that were brown and nonbloody. He underwent an upper endoscopy 3 months ago, which was remarkable for mild portal hypertensive gastropathy, with no gastroesophageal varices. He never suffered any episode of confusion before. He is naïve to hepatitis C therapy and his only current medication was furosemide 20 mg daily and spironolactone 100 mg daily. No recent use of alcohol or any toxic habits were reported. His vital signs are as follows:

Temperature	37.8° C
Blood pressure	90/70 mm Hg
Heart rate	105 bpm
Respiratory rate	22 breaths/min

The patient is clearly obtunded, with decrease of breath sounds on bases, and a distended abdomen with a fluid wave and shifting dullness consistent with tense ascites. Rectal exam is remarkable for a boggy prostate gland and brown stool on the rectal vault. The patient is intubated and placed on mechanical ventilation and started on intravenous fluids Laboratory studies are obtained and the patient transferred to the intensive care unit. A head CT performed earlier revealed involutional changes consistent with mild chronic encephalomalacia but no acute pathology. Which of the following is the most appropriate next step in management?

A. Start lactulose by nasogastric tube and reassess neurological status once the patient achieves more that three bowel movements daily
B. Decrease calorie protein intake to less than 1 gm/kg daily
C. Start rifaximin 550 mg orally twice daily
D. Perform a diagnostic and therapeutic paracentesis, order blood culture and ascitic fluid cultures, and start empiric broad-spectrum antibiotics
E. Place the patient on an extracorporeal albumin dialysis using a molecular absorbent recirculation system (MARS)

212. A 45-year-old woman with alcohol-related cirrhosis is transferred to your institution for consideration for liver transplant. The patient has no previous history of diabetes mellitus or renal disease. She was admitted 2 weeks ago at another hospital for the treatment of spontaneous bacterial peritonitis. Despite documented resolution of the spontaneous peritonitis with a second diagnostic paracentesis after 1 week of intravenous antibiotics, her creatinine levels increased from 0.8 mg/dL to 2.7 mg/dL with an increase in her bilirubin levels (today 4.5 mg/dL). Most recent calculated MELD score is 28. She was treated with aggressive volume expansion, with albumin 100 grams daily for the last 5 days and her diuretic therapy was discontinued on admission. A renal ultrasound demonstrated normal size kidneys with normal cortical size. No proteinuria or hematuria was identified on urine analysis and a fractional excretion of sodium of 0.7% was measured. What will be the most expected findings on renal histology if a renal biopsy is performed?

A. Normal histology
B. Proximal tubular cell necrosis and apoptosis with desquamation of cells in the lumen
C. Large glomeruli with irregular thickening of glomerular basement membrane and mesangial cell proliferation
D. Glomerular membrane thickening with capillary lumen narrowing and mesangial sclerosis and glomerulosclerosis
E. Slight mesangial hypercellularity with podocyte hypertrophy best observed on electronic microscopy

213. A 64-year-old man with alcohol-related cirrhosis is admitted to the hospital with decompensated liver disease. He was diagnosed with spontaneous bacterial peritonitis and started on antibiotics. The patient has no previous history of renal disease. After two weeks his creatinine levels increased from 0.8 mg/dL to 3.0 mg/dL with an increase on his bilirubin levels (today 4.5 mg/dL). Most recent calculated MELD score is 28. No previous episodes of significant hypotension have been documented during hospitalization. He received aggressive volume expansion, with albumin 100 gm daily for 7 days. His diuretic therapy was discontinued on admission. A renal ultrasound is unrevealing. No proteinuria or hematuria was identified on urine analysis and a fractional excretion of sodium of 0.8% was measured. What will be the most expected physiologic findings?

A. Decreased systemic vascular resistance with increased cardiac output and increased glomerular filtration rate
B. Increased systemic vascular resistance with decreased cardiac output and decreased glomerular filtration rate
C. Decreased systemic vascular resistance with decreased cardiac output and decreased glomerular filtration rate
D. Increased systemic vascular resistance with increased cardiac output and increased glomerular filtration rate
E. Increased systemic vascular resistance with increased cardiac output and decreased glomerular filtration rate

214. A 45-year-old woman with primary biliary cirrhosis and ulcerative colitis presents to the emergency department with complaints of abdominal distention, dyspnea on exertion, and fever for the last 3 days. The patient has not had recent exposure to any antibiotics. On presentation her vital signs are as follows:

Temperature	38.0° C
Blood pressure	95/76 mm Hg
Heart rate	105 bpm

The patient was admitted and started on intravenous fluid. Laboratory values are as follows:

Sodium	144 mEq/L
Potassium	3.7 mEq/L
Chloride	109 mEq/L
CO2	27 mEq/L
BUN	30 mg/dL
Creatinine	1.2 mg/dL
Ascitic Fluid	
WBC	300 polymorphonuclear cells/μL
Gram stain	gram-negative rod

What is the most appropriate next step in the management?

A. Start piperacillin/tazobactam 3.375 gm intravenously every 6 hours
B. Start cefotaxime 2 gm intravenously every 8 hours and repeat a diagnostic paracentesis routinely in 2 days
C. Start cefotaxime 2 gm intravenously every 8 hours, administer a bolus of intravenous albumin at 1.5 gm/kg, and repeat a diagnostic paracentesis routinely in 2 days
D. Start cefotaxime 2 gm intravenously every 8 hours and administer a bolus of intravenous albumin at 1.5 gm/kg now and 1.0 gm/kg on day 3
E. Start cefotaxime 2 gm intravenously every 8 hours, administer a bolus of intravenous albumin at 1.5 gm/kg now and 1.0 gm/kg on day 3, and repeat a diagnostic paracentesis routinely in 2 days

215. A 62-year-old man with alcohol-related cirrhosis is admitted to the hospital after developing a distended abdomen with abdominal discomfort. He has no previous history of diabetes mellitus or renal disease. He was diagnosed with spontaneous bacterial peritonitis and treated with cefotaxime 2 gm intravenously every 8 hours for 5 days. Three weeks after admission he developed worsening lower extremity edema, tense ascites, and lethargy. Despite documented resolution of the spontaneous bacterial peritonitis on a second diagnostic paracentesis, his creatinine level increased from 0.8 mg/dL to 2.8 mg/dL, his total bilirubin is 5.5 mg/dL and INR is 1.9. Calculated MELD score is 30. He was treated with aggressive volume expansion, albumin 100 gm daily for the last 5 days, and all diuretic therapy was discontinued on admission. A renal ultrasound showed no abnormalities. No proteinuria or hematuria was identified on urine analysis. Fractional excretion of sodium of 0.7% was measured. Which of the following is the best therapeutic management for this patient?

A. Intravenous dopamine and octreotide in combination with albumin
B. Transjugular intrahepatic portosystemic shunt placement
C. Continuous renal replacement therapy
D. Orthotropic liver transplant
E. Start tezosentan (non-selective endothelin receptor antagonist)

216. A 47-year-old man with nonalcoholic steatohepatitis–related cirrhosis presents to the clinic for follow-up visit. His liver disease has been complicated with esophageal varices with no previous history of bleeding (currently on propanolol 20 mg twice daily) and previous ascites, now well controlled with furosemide 40 mg orally once daily and spironolactone 150 mg once daily. He also has controlled hypertension and dyslipidemia. He complaints of progressive shortness of breath in the last 3 months associated with marked fatigue. He has never smoked, and has no history of toxic habits. He reports no chest pain, lower extremity swelling, or increase in abdominal girth. He reports that lying in bed improves breathing symptoms. Today at the clinic his vital signs are as follows:

Temperature	36.9° C
Blood pressure	110/76 mm Hg
Heart rate	56 beats per minute
Pulse oximetry saturation	90% on room air

Physical exam reveals clear lungs to auscultation bilaterally, a soft and depressive abdomen with no shifting dullness and no fluid wave, and no lower extremity edema. A bubble 2D echocardiogram is performed and is remarkable for an ejection fraction at 65%, no evidence of diastolic dysfunction, an estimated right ventricular systolic pressure of 28 mm Hg, and no pericardial effusions. Air bubbles are observed on the left ventricle at the fifth cardiac cycle after intravenous infusion of agitated saline. Which of the following physiologic changes might explain his current symptoms?

A. Intrinsic decrease in cardiac muscle contractility with increase in preload and increase in systemic vascular resistance causing pulmonary congestion
B. Pulmonary inflammation causing airway obstruction, mucosal edema, eosinophil infiltration causing ventilation-perfusion mismatch
C. Microvascular dilatation in the precapillary and capillary pulmonary arterial circulation mediated by nitric oxide
D. Vascular medial proliferation and hypertrophy, plexiform arteriopathy and in situ vascular thrombosis of pulmonary microvasculature
E. Extracellular matrix deposition and scar formation in pulmonary interstitium

217. A 66-year-old man is referred to your clinic for liver transplant evaluation. He was diagnosed with chronic hepatitis C–related cirrhosis 10 years ago. He also has controlled hypertension and high cholesterol. He had presented with severe volume overload requiring therapeutic paracentesis on several occasions. His volume overload has been better controlled in the last 3 months after his diuretic therapy was optimized; however, he complaints today of marked fatigue and dyspnea on exertion. Today at the clinic his vital signs are as follows:

Temperature	36.7° C
Blood pressure	145/89 mm Hg
Heart rate	76 beats per minute
Pulse oximetry saturation is	97% on room air

Physical exam reveals clear lungs to auscultation bilaterally, positive jugular venous distention, soft and depressive abdomen with no shifting dullness, fluid wave, or lower extremity pitting edema. A bubble 2D echocardiogram is performed and is remarkable for an ejection fraction of 60%, moderate diastolic dysfunction, moderate tricuspid regurgitation, and an estimated right ventricular systolic pressure of 56 mm Hg. No air bubbles are observed on the left ventricle after intravenous infusion of agitated saline. Right heart catheterization reveals a mean pulmonary arterial pressure of 34 mm Hg, a pulmonary capillary wedge pressure of 13 mm Hg and a pulmonary vascular resistance of 300 dynes-sec-cm^{-5}. Which of the following might explain the etiology of this patient's symptoms?

A. Intrinsic decrease in cardiac muscle contractility with increase in preload and increase in systemic vascular resistance causing pulmonary congestion
B. Pulmonary inflammation causing airway obstruction, mucosal edema, eosinophil infiltration causing ventilation-perfusion mismatch
C. Microvascular dilatation in the pre-capillary and capillary pulmonary arterial circulation mediated by nitric oxide
D. Vascular medial proliferation and hypertrophy, plexiform arteriopathy and in situ vascular thrombosis on pulmonary microvasculature
E. Extracellular matrix deposition and scar formation in pulmonary interstitium

218. A 47-year-old man with hepatitis C–related cirrhosis presents for a follow-up visit. His liver disease has been complicated with ascites in the past requiring paracentesis on two previous occasions. He is currently using furosemide 40 mg orally once daily and spironolactone 150 mg once daily. Last paracentesis was 1 year ago. He also has well-controlled diabetes mellitus type II. Today, he complains of worsening shortness of breath in the last 3 months associated with moderate to severe dyspnea on exertion. He denies chest pain, lower extremity swelling, or increase in abdominal girth. He reports that lying in bed improves his respiratory symptoms. Vital signs are as follows:

Temperature	36.5° C
Blood pressure	109/66 mm Hg
Heart rate	56 beats per minute
Pulse oximetry saturation at rest	88%

Physical exam reveals clear lungs to auscultation bilaterally, a soft and depressive abdomen with no shifting dullness and no fluid wave, and no lower extremity edema. Chest CT without contrast revealed no abnormalities on the lung parenchyma. A bubble 2D echocardiogram is performed and is remarkable for an ejection fraction of 68%, no diastolic dysfunction, an estimated right ventricular systolic pressure of 25 mm Hg, and no pericardial effusions. Air bubbles are observed on the left ventricle at the fourth cardiac cycle after intravenous infusion of agitated saline. Laboratory values are as follows:

Sodium	143 mEq/L
Potassium	3.8 mEq/L
Chloride	103 mEq/L
CO2	24 mEq/L
BUN	15 mg/dL
Creatinine	0.7 mg/dL
Total Bilirubin	1.6 mg/dL
INR	1.4
WBC	2600/µL
Hemoglobin	12.0 g/dL
Platelet count	100,000/µL
Arterial blood gas	
pH	7.37
pO2	48 mm Hg
pCO2	60 mm Hg
Calculated MELD score	12

Which of the following is the best therapeutic management for this patient?

A. Start on home oxygen
B. Start inhaled epoprostenol
C. Start intravenous epoprostenol
D. Start sildenafil 20 mg three times daily
E. Refer for liver transplant

219. A 53-year-old woman with primary biliary cirrhosis, diagnosed 3 years ago after suffering from severe pruritus, presents to your clinic for follow-up evaluation. She is currently using ursodeoxycholic acid at 15mg/kg/day and multivitamins. Three years ago she had elevated antimitochondrial antibodies, elevated liver enzymes with an alkaline phosphatase of 405 U/L and GGT levels of 102 U/L. At that time she had an abdominal MRI, which was remarkable for a nodular appearing liver with mild splenomegaly and no ascites. A colonoscopy 3 years ago was remarkable for a 0.5 cm sessile polyp with tubular histology, which was completely removed with no complications. An upper endoscopy 1 year ago was remarkable for a column of small varices completely obliterated on air insufflation. The patient had an abdominal sonogram performed 3 months ago showing liver with nodular contour, no ascites, and portal vein with hepatopetal flow. She also has hypothyroidism and hypercholesterolemia. She denies family history of GI malignancies. She reports feeling well, following a healthy diet, and is compliant with a regular exercise program. Physical exam today reveal no stigmata of chronic liver disease. Laboratory values are as follows:

Sodium	138 mEq/L
Potassium	4.0 mEq/L
Chloride	98 mEq/L
BUN	9 mg/dL
Creatinine	0.7 mg/dL
Albumin	3.6 g/dL
Total Bilirubin	1.0 mg/dL
INR	1.3
Alkaline phosphatase	150 U/L
GGT	23 IU/L
WBC	4600/µL
Hemoglobin	13.5 g/dL
Platelet count	145,000/µL
Calculated MELD score	9

What is the most appropriate next step in the management of this patient?

A. Surveillance colonoscopy
B. Abdominopelvic CT with intravenous contrast with triphasic protocol
C. Liver biopsy
D. Bone densitometry scan
E. Upper endoscopy for esophageal varices surveillance

220. A 66-year-old man is referred to your clinic for liver transplant evaluation. He was diagnosed with nonalcoholic steatohepatitis–related cirrhosis 15 years ago. He also has controlled hypertension, diabetes mellitus type II, and hypertriglyceridemia. He complains today of worsening exertional dyspnea, orthopnea, chest pressure, and lightheadedness. His current medications include propranolol 20 mg twice daily, furosemide 40 mg orally twice daily, spironolactone 200 mg once daily, sliding scale insulin, and atorvastatin 40 mg once daily. Today at the clinic his vital signs are as follows:

Temperature	36.7° C
Blood pressure	122/74 mm Hg
Heart rate	76 bpm
Pulse oximetry saturation	97% on room air

Physical exam reveals clear lungs to auscultation bilaterally, positive jugular venous distention, soft and depressive abdomen with no shifting dullness and no fluid wave, and lower extremity pitting edema. EKG revealed no ischemic changes, unspecific T wave changes on precordial leads and mild QTc prolongation. You refer the patient for dobutamine stress test where he reaches maximum expected heart rate, with ejection fraction of 68% and no ischemic changes. A bubble 2D echocardiogram is performed and is remarkable for moderate diastolic dysfunction, moderate to severe tricuspid regurgitation, and an estimated right ventricular systolic pressure of 52 mm Hg, and no bubbles on left ventricle after 7 cardiac cycles. Which of the following is the most appropriate next step?

A. Left heart catheterization
B. Right heart catheterization
C. Increase furosemide to 80 mg twice daily
D. Technetium ventilation/perfusion scan
E. Liver Transplant

221. A 67-year-old woman comes to your clinic for liver transplant evaluation. She was diagnosed with autoimmune hepatitis–related cirrhosis 20 years ago after presenting with esophageal variceal bleeding. She also has controlled hypertension and dyslipidemia. Today, she complains of marked exertional dyspnea, orthopnea, and chest pressure. Her current medications include propranolol 20 mg twice daily, furosemide 40 mg orally once daily, spironolactone 150 mg once daily, and atorvastatin 40 mg once daily. Today her vital signs are as follows:

Temperature	37.7° C
Blood pressure	100/70 mm H
Heart rate	56 beats per minute
Pulse oximetry saturation	96% on room air

Physical exam reveals clear lungs to auscultation bilaterally, positive jugular venous distention, soft and depressive abdomen with no shifting dullness and no fluid wave, and no lower extremity pitting edema. EKG revealed no ischemic changes. A dobutamine stress test, where patient reach maximum expected heart rate, had no ischemic changes. A bubble 2D echocardiogram is performed and is remarkable for an ejection fraction at 60%, moderate diastolic dysfunction, severe tricuspid regurgitation, and an estimated right ventricular systolic pressure of 55 mm Hg. Right heart catheterization reveals a mean pulmonary arterial pressure of 53 mm Hg, a pulmonary capillary wedge pressure of 12 mm Hg ,and a pulmonary vascular resistance of 330 dynes-s-cm^{-5}. What is the most appropriate next steps in this patient?

A. Discontinue propranolol and perform upper endoscopy
B. Discontinue furosemide
C. Liver transplant
D. Left heart catheterization
E. Chest CT with intravenous contrast

222. A 67-year-old woman with primary biliary cirrhosis (PBC) presents to the emergency department with complaints of marked fatigue, tense ascites, and jaundice. She was diagnosed with PBC after presenting with ascites and pruritus. She was started at that time on ursodeoxycholic acid 15mg/kg/day, furosemide 40 mg once daily, spironolactone 150 mg once daily, vitamin D, and calcium supplementation. Her clinical course has been stable until 3 months ago when she started experiencing worsening of the abdominal distention. She reports being compliant with current medications; however, she admits occasional indulgences with high sodium intake. Her last upper endoscopy was 3 years ago when one column of small esophageal varices was identified with mild portal hypertensive gastropathy. At that time nonselective beta-blockers were prescribed; however, the patient discontinued therapy after she developed lightheadedness and dizziness. The patient reports no recent episode of fever, chills, chest pain, abdominal pain, bloody vomits, black stools, or hematochezia. Her vital signs are as follows:

Temperature	37.5° C
Blood pressure	100/70 mm Hg
Heart rate	96 bpm
Pulse oximetry saturation	96% on room air

Physical exam is remarkable for a holosystolic murmur, soft and depressive distended abdomen with shifting dullness consistent with tense ascites and lower extremity pitting edema. Laboratory tests reveal the following:

Sodium	132 mEq/L
Potassium	3.6 mEq/L
Chloride	98 mEq/L
CO2	20 mEq/L
BUN	19 mg/dL
Creatinine	0.9 mg/dL
Albumin	2.9 g/dL
Total Bilirubin	3.5 mg/dL
INR	1.9
Alkaline phosphatase	230 U/L
GGT	89 U/L
WBC	2600/µL
Hemoglobin	8.0 g/dL
Platelet count	100,000/µL
Blood culture	negative
Calculated MELD score	18

The patient is admitted and ultrasound-guided diagnostic and therapeutic paracentesis is performed, which revealed no evidence of spontaneous bacterial peritonitis. Abdominal MRI with contrast revealed a shrunken, cirrhotic liver with no parenchymal lesions, significant collateral circulation with canalization of the umbilical vein, esophageal varices, and ascites. 2D echocardiogram is remarkable for a hyperdynamic left ventricle with ejection fraction of 65% to 70%, mild tricuspid regurgitation, and an estimated right ventricular systolic pressure of 28 mm Hg. What is the most appropriate next step?

A. Upper endoscopy
B. Transfuse 4 units of fresh frozen plasma (FFP) and proceed with upper endoscopy
C. Transfuse one unit of packed red blood cells (PRBCs) and proceed with upper endoscopy
D. Transfuse 4 units of FFP and proceed with transjugular intrahepatic portosystemic shunt (TIPS)
E. Transfuse one unit of PRBCs and proceed with TIPS

223. In which of the following patients is liver transplantation absolutely contraindicated?

A. A 45-year-old woman with transfusion-related hepatitis C and end-stage liver disease, with a history of breast cancer diagnosed at age 35 who underwent bilateral modified radical mastectomy and chemotherapy, and is currently in remission
B. A 52-year-old man with chronic hepatitis B who was recently diagnosed with a 5 cm liver mass consistent with hepatocellular carcinoma
C. A 62-year-old woman with primary biliary cirrhosis with a MELD score of 22, with recent right heart catheterization consistent with portopulmonary hypertension (POPH) and a mean pulmonary artery pressure of 52 mm Hg.
D. A 65-year-old man with alcoholic cirrhosis, who has been abstinent from alcohol for 8 months, and presents with a MELD score of 20 and partial portal vein thrombosis.
E. A 45-year-old woman with nonalcoholic steatohepatitis–related cirrhosis with a BMI of 50 mg/kg^2, who presents with acute kidney injury, volume overload, and a MELD score of 30.

224. A 56-year-old man with hepatitis C–related cirrhosis presents to the emergency department with a complaint of worsening abdominal distention and abdominal pain.

Abdominal sonogram revealed ascites with hepatofugal flow at the portal vein consistent with portal vein thrombosis. Which of the following abnormalities could contribute to the formation of an acute portal vein thrombus?

A. Factor VII deficiency
B. Factor IX deficiency
C. Factor II deficiency
D. Thrombomodulin deficiency
E. Factor X deficiency

225. A 64-year-old man with known chronic hepatitis C was brought by his wife to the emergency department. He was lethargic and unable to provide a reliable medical history. The wife reported that he had several episodes of chills and fever associated with dysuria 3 weeks ago. He was having one to two daily loose bowel movements that were brown and nonbloody. A urinalysis was ordered and confirmed urinary tract infection. The patient was treated with intravenous antibiotics and started on lactulose with resolution of the hepatic encephalopathy. He was discharged home and returned to your clinic in 2 weeks. The patient's relative reports he continued with sporadic episodes of confusion and flapping tremors of distal upper extremities. He has been using lactulose as prescribed, and is having three to four loose bowel movements daily. You prescribe rifaximin 550 mg daily and schedule a follow-up appointment in 3 weeks. On the follow-up visit patient's relative reports no major improvement of clinical symptoms. The patient has no signs or symptoms of infection, has not started any new medication (except for the one prescribed), and has no electrolytes disorders or signs suggestive of dehydration. Which of the following is the most probable effective therapy in this patient?

A. Start probiotics
B. Start intravenous albumin
C. Flumazenil
D. Intravenous L-ornithine-L-aspartate (LOLA)
E. Daily protein intake of less than 1g/kg/day

226. A 25-year-old woman is brought to the emergency department by her family for confusion over the past 12 hours and is found to be in acute liver failure (ALF). According to discussion with her family, the patient was started on a medication for latent tuberculosis 2 weeks ago but they cannot remember the name of the medication. They estimate that she drinks approximately three glasses of wine each night. She has a history of ulcerative colitis and thyroiditis. The patient's family denies any obvious depression and states that they cannot imagine her willingly overdosing on any medication in an attempt to hurt herself. Which of the following is the least likely cause of her acute liver failure?

A. Autoimmune hepatitis
B. Wilson disease
C. Alcohol resulting in alcoholic hepatitis
D. Drug-induced liver injury secondary to isoniazid
E. Acetaminophen overdose

227. A 26-year-old woman is transferred to the intensive care unit with a 24-hour history of somnolence and required endotracheal intubation. Her family states that she has never been hospitalized before and they are unaware of any prior liver problems. The family states she drinks one to two beers per week and denies knowledge of any illicit drug use. Laboratory studies are as follows:

ALT	742 U/L
AST	1904 U/L
Alkaline phosphatase	28 IU/L
Total bilirubin	8 mg/dL
Hemoglobin	6.8 gm/dL
INR	2.9

Which of the following tests would be best help to establish the diagnosis of this patient in this clinical scenario?

A. Genetic testing for *ATP7B*
B. Urinary copper excretion level
C. Serum ceruloplasmin level
D. Liver biopsy with hepatic copper quantification
E. Penicillamine challenge

228. A 64-year-old man presents to the emergency department with lethargy and confusion. His family states that he drinks up to a bottle of wine daily and has a remote history of illicit drug use. According to the family, he strained his back 2 weeks ago and since then has been taking a pain medication but they are unsure of the name. They are unaware of any other medications. On exam, he is lethargic, slow to respond to questions, and is unable to name the year. He has asterixis. His laboratory tests reveal the following:

ALT	2493 U/L
AST	3984 U/L
Alkaline phosphatase	194 U/L
Total bilirubin	4.2 mg/dL
Creatinine	2.3 mg/dL
INR	3.5
Acetaminophen serum concentration	15 mcg/mL
HBsAg	negative
HBcAb	positive
HBsAb	positive

Which of the following would you recommend?

A. Corticosteroids
B. Activated charcoal
C. Intravenous acyclovir
D. Entecavir
E. N-acetylcysteine

229. A 23-year-old woman in her third trimester of her first pregnancy develops abdominal pain, nausea and vomiting, fever, and confusion. On exam she has mild scleral icterus, somnolence, asterixis, and no rashes. Her laboratory values are significant for the following:

ALT	4239 U/L
AST	5203 U/L
Total bilirubin	4.3 mg/dL
Platelet count	142,000/μL
INR	3.2
Creatinine	2.1 mg/dL
LDH	223 U/L
IgG level	1293 mg/dL

Urinalysis does not reveal proteinuria. She undergoes a transjugular liver biopsy, which reveals extensive hepatocyte necrosis and intranuclear inclusion bodies. Which of the following is the most likely diagnosis?

A. Hemolysis, elevated liver enzymes, and low platelet count syndrome (HELLP syndrome)
B. Herpes simplex virus (HSV)
C. Acute fatty liver of pregnancy
D. Cholestasis of pregnancy
E. Autoimmune hepatitis

230. A 25-year-old woman with a history of depression, substance abuse, and prior admissions to a psychiatric hospital is admitted to the intensive care unit with mental status changes. She was obtunded and not responsive to stimuli on arrival to the emergency department and underwent endotracheal intubation. Her family member states that they found her at home in her room unconscious with an empty acetaminophen bottle. She is started on N-acetylcysteine, given fluid resuscitation, broad-spectrum antibiotics, and sedation. She is found to have the following labsoratory values:

ALT	6,435 U/L
AST	8678 U/L
Alkaline phosphatase	168 U/L
Total bilirubin	3.3 mg/dL
Platelet count	179,000/μL
INR	3.5
Creatinine	1.6 mg/dL
Arterial Blood Gas (ABG) pH	7.32
Acetaminophen serum concentration	264 mcg/mL

Which of the following factors portends a poor prognosis for this patient according to the King's College Criteria?
A. Grade of encephalopathy
B. ALT
C. Arterial blood gas
D. Bilirubin
E. Acetaminophen level

231. A 42-year-old woman with a history of rheumatoid arthritis and diabetes is admitted to the intensive care unit with mental status changes. The family is present and state that she drinks one to two glasses of wine after dinner each night, does not smoke, and has no known use of illicit drugs. They deny a history of depression and she is employed as a secretary. For her worsening arthritic symptoms, her rheumatologist placed the patient on prednisone and then rituximab a few weeks ago. On exam, she is somnolent and able to provider her name but not the place or year. She has no stigmata of chronic liver disease and her right upper quadrant is mildly tender without guarding. She has asterixis present. Laboratory values are as follows:

ALT	2493 U/L
AST	3984 U/L
Alkaline phosphatase	226 IU/L
Total bilirubin	5.2 mg/dL
Creatinine	1.6 mg/dL
INR	2.5
Acetaminophen serum concentration undetectable	
Hepatitis A IgM	negative
HBsAg	positive
HBcAb	positive
HBsAb	negative
Hepatitis C virus antibody	positive
Hepatitis C virus RNA level	9.3 million U/mL
Antinuclear antibody (ANA)	negative
Anti-smooth muscle antibody (ASMA)	negative
Serum IgG level	1863 mg/dL

Which of the following agents is the most appropriate to treat the cause of her acute liver failure?
A. N-Acetylcysteine
B. High-dose glucocorticoids
C. Direct-acting antiviral regimen for hepatitis C virus
D. Tenofovir
E. Intravenous acyclovir

232. Which of the following statements regarding HEV is correct?
A. It is commonly acquired by using the contaminated needle
B. Acute liver failure due to HEV has a worse prognosis in pregnant patients
C. Among patients that become infected with HEV, pregnant women are more likely to develop acute liver failure
D. Although HEV infection is common in India, it is a very rare cause of acute liver failure in that country
E. HEV infection is the second cause of acute liver failure in the United States

233. A 42-year-old man with a history of intravenous drug use is admitted to the hospital with two weeks of progressive jaundice, malaise, polyarticular arthritis, and right upper quadrant discomfort. He is coherent on exam and his vital signs are stable. Laboratory values are as follows:

ALT	2,642 U/L
AST	1984 U/L
Alkaline phosphatase	103 U/L
Total bilirubin	8.1 mg/dL
Creatinine	0.8 mg/dL
INR	1.8
Acetaminophen serum concentration	undetectable
HAV antibody	positive (IgM negative)
HBsAg	positive
HBcAb	positive (IgM positive)
HBsAb is	negative
HCV antibody is	negative

The patient never develops mental status changes and is provided supportive care. Over the next few days, his ALT and AST decrease to below 300 U/L, his INR improves to 1.4, and the patient is discharged from the hospital. He returns 12 days later to the hospital with confusion. At that time his laboratory values are as follows:

ALT	2,930 U/L
AST	2,783 U/L
INR	3.8
Total bilirubin	12.9 mg/dL

Which of the following statements describes the most likely cause of the patient's worsening course?
A. The patient has acute liver failure from acute hepatitis C virus
B. The patient has acute liver failure due to coinfection with HBV and hepatitis D virus (HDV)
C. The patient has a relapsing form of HAV
D. The patient has acute liver failure due to HEV
E. The patient likely has drug-induced liver injury (DILI)

234. A 55-year-old man with acute liver failure (ALF) from hepatitis B virus is placed on a ventilator due to progressive encephalopathy, and is administered propofol. He is sedated and the nurse notes posturing of his upper extremities bilaterally. His heart rate is 48 bpm and his blood pressure is 183/97 mm Hg. What is the first-line therapy for elevated intracranial pressure (ICP) in this patient?

A. Barbiturates
B. Glucocorticoids
C. Hyperosmotic agents
D. Induction of hypothermia
E. Hyperventilation

235. What is the most common cause of acute liver failure in the United States?
A. Alcohol hepatitis
B. Acetaminophen overdose
C. NSAIDs use
D. Hepatitis B infection
E. Hepatitis E infection

236. A 40-year-old woman with a history of chronic hepatitis B virus infection is found on routine ultrasound to have a 2.2 cm mass in the right lobe of her liver. She has been taking oral contraceptive pills (OCP) for a total of 8 years of her life. She denies any abdominal pain. A triphasic CT scan finds a 2.5 cm lesion in the right lobe of her liver with arterial enhancement in the arterial phase, followed by central washout and capsular enhancement in the portal-venous and delayed phases. The spleen size is normal. A CT scan of her lungs shows no suspicious lesions. Her platelet count, liver enzymes, and INR are normal. Her serum alpha-fetoprotein (AFP) level is 10.1 ng/mL. An upper endoscopy revealed no masses or evidence of portal hypertension. Which of the following options would be the best treatment for the described lesion?
A. Surgical resection
B. Repeat CT scan in 6 months to assess for interval changes
C. Discontinuation of oral contraceptive therapy and surgical resection if becomes symptomatic
D. Targeted CT-guided biopsy of the lesion
E. No further treatment necessary

237. A 58-year-old man with chronic hepatitis C virus and known cirrhosis is found on surveillance imaging to have a 3.3 cm lesion in the right lobe of his liver. The MRI shows enhancement of the lesion during the arterial phase with late central washout and capsular enhancement. His spleen is 15.1 cm and he has a small volume of ascites. Laboratory studies are as follows:

Platelet count	85,000/μL
Alpha-fetoprotein	34.5 ng/mL
INR	1.9
Bilirubin level	2.4 mg/dL

A chest CT scan does not reveal any abnormalities. Which of the following treatments would be associated with the lowest risk of recurrence?
A. Radiofrequency ablation (RFA)
B. Transarterial chemoembolization (TACE)
C. Orthotopic liver transplantation
D. Surgical resection
E. Sorafenib therapy

238. A 52-year-old man with history of alcohol-induced cirrhosis is found to have hepatic lesions on imaging consistent with hepatocellular carcinoma and is referred to clinic at a liver transplant center for evaluation. His MRI is reviewed and reveals three lesions measuring 1.3 x 1.9 cm, 2.7 x 2.0 cm, and 1.4 x 1.0 cm. The MRI reveals large volume ascites, a 16.7 cm spleen, and a tumor thrombus in the right hepatic portal vein associated with one of the lesions. Prior to his referral to the transplant center, he had the largest lesion treated with transarterial chemoembolization. The radiologist comments that this lesion has had "partial response" to the locoregional therapy. The patient's calculated MELD score is 12 and his alpha-fetoprotein (AFP) level is 62.4 ng/mL. CT scan of his chest reveals no abnormalities. Which of the following features would prevent this patient from being considered a suitable liver transplant candidate?
A. Elevated AFP level
B. Size and number of lesions
C. Prior locoregional therapy
D. Tumor thrombus
E. Partial response to locoregional therapy

239. A 52-year-old woman presents to gastroenterology clinic for evaluation of painless jaundice. MRI reveals a 2.2 cm lesion located at the hepatic duct bifurcation with associated left-sided intrahepatic biliary ductal dilation. The lesion is hypo-intense on T1 images and has progressive enhancement on portal venous and delayed phases. There is a 1.3 cm lymph node in the porta hepatis. There is no radiographic evidence of portal hypertension or underlying cirrhosis. The surgeons are considering the patient for surgical resection or liver transplantation but request your opinion on the best means to make a diagnosis prior to surgery?
A. Upper endoscopic ultrasound (EUS) with fine needle aspiration (FNA) of the lesion
B. Positron emission tomography-computed tomography (PET-CT)
C. Endoscopic retrograde cholangiopancreatography (ERCP) with brushings and intraductal forceps biopsies and possible stent placement
D. Triphasic CT scan
E. Perform upper endoscopy and colonoscopy to assess for primary source

240. A 62-year-old man with a history of diabetes, chronic obstructive pulmonary disease (COPD), and hypertension presents to his primary care physician with 5 months of progressive fatigue, abdominal pain, sclera icterus, abdominal distension, and an unintentional 15-pound weight loss. He is barely able to lift himself out of a chair to a standing position. The patient occasionally drinks alcohol, smokes a pack of cigarettes a day, and has spent most of his life in an industrial factory working with chemical production of vinyl chloride. A CT scan of the abdomen reveals hepatosplenomegaly, large amount of ascites, and a vague mass in the right lobe of the liver. A targeted biopsy of the mass reveals dilated cavernous vascular spaces lined by markedly pleomorphic neoplastic cells. Which would be the best course of action?
A. Transarterial chemoembolization to downstage the tumor to qualify for liver transplantation
B. Sorafenib therapy
C. Discuss goals of life and consider transfer to hospice
D. Provide reassurance
E. Surgical resection

241. Which of the following is the most common benign tumor of the liver?
A. Focal nodular hyperplasia (FNH)
B. Hepatic adenoma

C. Hemangioma
D. Mesenchymal hamartoma
E. Von Myenberg complex

242. A 52-year-old obese woman undergoes an abdominal CT scan for episodic right upper quadrant pain that occurs after eating fatty meals. She is found to have a 3.7 cm lesion in the right hepatic lobe without evidence of underlying liver disease/fibrosis. It is well demarcated; hypodense on precontrast images, and shows early peripheral enhancement followed by late "filling in" of contrast consistent with a hemangioma. Which of the following is the most appropriate step in management?
A. Right hepatectomy
B. MRI with gadoxetate contrast
C. Hepatic artery angiography with embolization of the lesion
D. No further intervention
E. Targeted biopsy of the lesion

243. A 33-year-old Caucasian woman presents to her primary care doctor for dull, constant, right upper quadrant pain for the past 4 months. She is otherwise doing well and denies weight loss, jaundice, or pruritus. She denies any known prior problems with her liver. She takes minocycline for acne and an oral contraceptive (OCP). A CT scan reveals a well-demarcated 6 cm lesion in the right hepatic lobe that is initially isodense but with contrast shows peripheral enhancement with heterogeneous appearance and subsequent centripetal flow during the portal venous phase. During the late phase the lesion becomes hypodense. A percutaneous targeted liver biopsy was interpreted by the pathologist as "normal hepatic parenchyma with normal hepatocytes." Which of the following is most likely?
A. Focal nodular hyperplasia (FNH)
B. Regenerative nodule
C. Hepatic adenoma
D. Nodular regenerative hyperplasia (NRH)
E. Von Myenberg complex

244. A 33-year-old Caucasian woman presents to her primary care doctor for dull, constant, right upper quadrant pain for the past 4 months. She is otherwise doing well and denies weight loss, jaundice, or pruritus. She denies any known prior problems with her liver. She takes minocycline for acne and an OCP. A CT scan reveals a well-demarcated 6 cm lesion in the right hepatic lobe that is initially isodense but with contrast shows peripheral enhancement with heterogeneous appearance and subsequent centripetal flow during the portal venous phase. During the late phase the lesion becomes hypodense. A percutaneous targeted liver biopsy was interpreted by the pathologist as "normal hepatic parenchyma with normal hepatocytes." Which of the following would you recommend?
A. Discontinuation of OCP and referral for surgical resection
B. ERCP
C. Reassurance
D. Repeat imaging in 6 months
E. Repeat biopsy of the lesion since likely missed

245. A 43-year-old woman with a history of hypertension, tobacco history, and prior appendectomy is found on a contrast-enhanced CT scan of the abdomen to have a 4.5 cm hepatic lesion (see figure). Which of the following statements is true about this lesion?

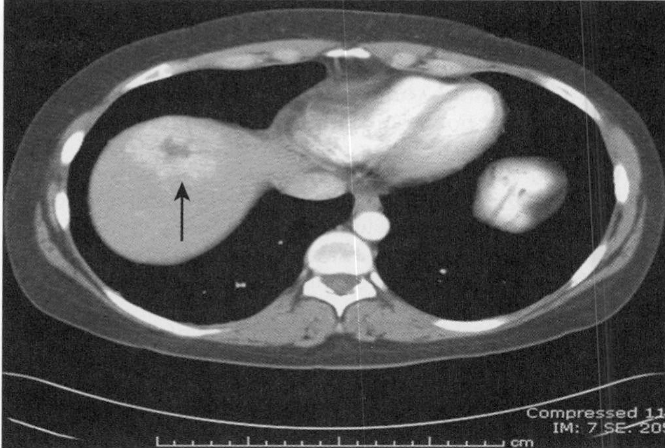

Figure for question 245.

A. It is a benign lesion but can undergo malignant transformation
B. It is at increased risk of rupture in pregnancy
C. It would expect a "cold spot," representing no active uptake on a technetium sulfur colloid scan
D. The natural history of this lesion predicts stability or may regress over time
E. Locoregional therapy with embolization or surgical resection is indicated

246. A 61-year-old man presents with fatigue, abdominal distension, and lower extremity edema for the past 3 months. He has a remote history of polysubstance abuse, and quit alcohol use one year ago. He states that his mobility is limited and can no longer walk to his mailbox. On exam, he appears chronically ill, has mild sclera icterus, temporal wasting, a moderately distended abdomen, 1+ pitting edema to his shins bilaterally, and telangiectasias on his upper chest and nose. His laboratory tests reveal the following:

Total bilirubin	5.2 mg/dL
INR of	1.7
Creatinine	1.1 mg/dL

An MRI of his abdomen reveals a lesion in segment 7 measuring 3.2 cm with arterial enhancement, venous-phase washout, as well as moderate ascites with a 16 cm spleen. A chest CT does not show any abnormalities. Which of the following would be the best management for this patient?
A. Sorafenib
B. Refer for surgical resection
C. Refer to liver transplant center
D. Refer to interventional radiology for transarterial chemoembolization
E. Hospice consultation

247. Which of the following statements is correct regarding fibrolamellar hepatocellular carcinoma?
A. It occurs in patients older than 60 years old
B. Alpha-fetoprotein (AFP) level is usually above 100 ng/mL
C. It almost always arises in a noncirrhotic liver
D. It carries a worse prognosis than conventional hepatocellular carcinoma (HCC)
E. Its response to chemotherapy is significantly better than conventional HCC

248. In which of the following scenarios would the patient benefit most from surgical resection?
- **A.** A 42-year-old man with an extrahepatic 2.7 cm cholangiocarcinoma involving the common bile duct with hepatic artery encasement but no evidence of metastasis
- **B.** A 42-year-old asymptomatic woman with autosomal dominant polycystic kidney disease and innumerable hepatic cysts ranging from 1 to 3 cm
- **C.** A 30-year-old asymptomatic woman with a 5 cm hepatic adenoma who is considering getting pregnant
- **D.** A 52-year-old man with HCV, cirrhosis, and a 3.4 cm hepatocellular carcinoma without metastasis, total bilirubin of 6.2 mg/dL, large volume ascites, platelet count of 100,000/μL
- **E.** A 59-year-old woman with a history of ulcerative colitis and hepatic nodules found to have nodular regenerative hyperplasia on liver biopsy

249. A 19-year-old man is transferred from a community hospital after a suicidal attempt. Per his family, the patient ingested more than 75 tablets of acetaminophen 500 mg approximately 19 hours ago. He was promptly treated with N-acetylcysteine (NAC) at the local hospital but was found to have renal failure. He is transferred for the initiation of hemodialysis. On admission the patient is alert and nontoxic. He states the overdose was an impulsive action and expresses regret. There is no prior history of suicidal attempts. Past history is unremarkable. Vital signs are as follows:

Temperature	37.3° C
Blood pressure	120/67 mm Hg
Heart rate	105 bpm
Respiratory rate	21 breaths/min

On exam, the patient is alert and oriented to time, place, and person. His sclera is icteric but exam is otherwise unremarkable. Laboratory values are as follows:

ALP	221 U/L
ALT	6772 U/L
AST	5961 U/L
Total bilirubin	3.8 mg/dL
INR	3.7
Creatinine	4.6 mg/dL
Platelet count	167,000/μL
WBC	7600/μL

In addition to continuing NAC, what is the most appropriate next step?
- **A.** Await psychiatric consultation
- **B.** List for a liver transplant
- **C.** List for combined liver and kidney transplant
- **D.** Liver biopsy
- **E.** Renal biopsy

250. A 41-year-old woman with end-stage liver disease (ESLD) from autoimmune hepatitis is awaiting liver transplant. Her main symptom is fatigue. A suitable donor becomes available and the patient comes in for liver transplant. A Swan-Ganz catheter is placed for intraoperative monitoring and reveals the following:

Mean pulmonary artery pressure	80 mm Hg
Pulmonary capillary wedge pressure	10 mm Hg
Pulmonary vascular resistance	500 dynes/cm^2

Which of the following is the most appropriate next step in management?
- **A.** Proceed with liver transplant as planned
- **B.** Begin intravenous epoprostenol
- **C.** Begin intravenous heparin
- **D.** Abort liver transplant
- **E.** Obtain an emergent echocardiogram and proceed with a transplant if normal

251. Which of these patient scenarios qualifies for a MELD exception?
- **A.** A patient with chronic HCV, 2 lesions consistent with hepatocellular carcinoma (3.3 cm and 1.6 cm)
- **B.** A patient with portopulmonary hypertension (POPH) and mean pulmonary artery pressure (MPAP) of 45 mm Hg on treatment
- **C.** A patient with hepatopulmonary syndrome (HPS) and Pa02 of 65 mm Hg on room air
- **D.** A patient with primary hyperoxaluria and end-stage renal disease requiring hemodialysis
- **E.** A patient with refractory ascites unresponsive to diuretics

252. A 62-year-old man is 7 years post–orthotopic liver transplant (OLT) for alcoholic liver disease and HCV cirrhosis with multifocal hepatocellular carcinoma (2 lesions 3 cm and 2.2 cm in diameter). Post-transplant history is notable for chronic renal insufficiency and recurrent HCV. He smokes 1 pack per day for 30 years. He presents with 2 months of a "sore tongue." No improvement with antifungal/steroid rinses. He denies fevers, night sweats, or weight loss. His medication includes sirolimus 4 mg daily, metoprolol 25 mg twice daily, and aspirin 81mg daily. Physical exam is significant for oral thrush, 1 cm ulcer on the right side of the tongue and firm cervical lymphadenopathy. Laboratory values are as follows:

WBC	4500/μL
Hematocrit	36%
Platelet count	135,000/μL
ALT	23 U/L
AST	43 U/L
Bilirubin	1.2 mg/dL

An abdominal CT scan does not reveal any significant lymphadenopathy. The liver graft appears normal with no suspicious lesions. What is the most likely diagnosis?
- **A.** Mucormycosis
- **B.** Posttransplant lymphoproliferative disorder (PTLD)
- **C.** Recurrent hepatocellular carcinoma
- **D.** Oropharyngeal squamous cell carcinoma (SCC)
- **E.** Sirolimus toxicity

253. A 67-year-old man is 5 days post–living donor liver transplantation with a choledocho-choledochostomy for HCV cirrhosis complicated by hepatocellular carcinoma. You note that his right abdominal drain is now draining bile. On exam he has low grade fever and mild abdominal tenderness. Laboratory studies are as follows:

Bilirubin	3.5 mg/dL
AST	100 U/L
ALT	121 U/L
ALP	211 U/L
WBC	10,500/μL
Hematocrit	32%

A hepatobiliary (HIDA) scan shows evidence of a bile leak from the site of anastomosis. Which of the following is the most appropriate next step in the management of this patient?
- **A.** Reassurance
- **B.** Start 14-day course of broad-spectrum antibiotics
- **C.** ERCP
- **D.** Laparoscopic bile duct repair
- **E.** Surgical bile duct revision with Roux-en-Y anastomosis

254. A 45-year-old man with history of liver transplant for primary sclerosing cholangitis 4 years ago presents with abnormal liver function tests. He has been on a stable dose of tacrolimus for the past 3 years. He was admitted to the hospital 1 month ago with fever and seizures, and was discharged 2 weeks later on multiple new medications. His tacrolimus trough level now is less than 2 ng/mL, whereas it usually ranges between 6 ng/mL to 8 ng/mL (normal range 5-20 ng/mL). Which of the following medications has likely caused this?
   A. Phenytoin
   B. Itraconazole
   C. Diltiazem
   D. Fluconazole
   E. Levetiracetam

255. A 64-year-old woman is 2 years post–liver transplant for cryptogenic cirrhosis complicated by hepatocellular carcinoma (HCC). She has had elevated liver function tests for the past 2 months. Her past medical history is significant for diabetes, hypertension, and dyslipidemia. She is obese with a BMI of 35 mg/kg^2. Laboratory studies are as follows:

ALT	74 U/L
AST	63 U/L
ALP	90 U/L
Bilirubin	0.8 mg/dL
Tacrolimus trough level	6.7 ng/mL (5-20 ng/mL)

Abdominal ultrasound shows diffuse steatosis with no bile duct dilatation. Liver biopsy shows 50% steatosis with a mixed inflammatory infiltrate and perivenular fibrosis; bile ducts appear normal; no significant plasma cell infiltrate noted. What is the most likely diagnosis?
   A. Acute cellular rejection
   B. Autoimmune hepatitis
   C. Recurrent nonalcoholic fatty liver disease (NAFLD)
   D. Anastomotic biliary stricture
   E. Chronic rejection

256. A 52-year-old man is 3 months post–living donor liver transplant for primary sclerosing cholangitis. His posttransplant course was complicated by an episode of steroid resistant rejection, which was treated with thymoglobulin 1 week posttransplant. He now presents with diarrhea, fever, nausea, and vomiting. Current medications include tacrolimus, prednisone, and mycophenolate mofetil. On exam he is toxic appearing, with dry mucous membranes and diffuse abdominal tenderness. Laboratory studies are as follows:

ALT	132 U/L
AST	113 U/L
ALP	120 U/L
Bilirubin	0.9 mg/dL
WBC	1900/μL
Creatinine	3 mg/dL

What is the most likely diagnosis?
   A. Acute rejection
   B. Graft-versus-host-disease (GVHD)
   C. Bile leak
   D. Ascending cholangitis
   E. CMV gastroenteritis

257. You see a 67-year-old woman who is post–liver transplant 1 week ago for primary biliary cirrhosis. She had a prolonged hospitalization pretransplant with variceal bleeding, encephalopathy, acute kidney injury, and catheter-related sepsis. The patient was improving posttransplant; however, over the past few days she has become progressively more obtunded. Medications include tacrolimus, prednisone, mycophenolate mofetil, acyclovir, sulfamethoxazole/trimethoprim, metoclopramide, and fluconazole. Laboratory studies are as follows:

WBC	6500/μL
Hematocrit	36%
Platelet count	120,000/μL
ALT	65 U/L
AST	57 U/L
Bilirubin	0.9 mg/dL
BUN	43 mg/dL
Creatinine	1.4 mg/dL

Head CT scan is normal. EEG shows seizure activity. Cerebral spinal fluid analysis is negative. What is the most likely cause of her altered mental status?
   A. Steroid-induced psychosis
   B. CNS toxoplasmosis
   C. HSV encephalitis
   D. Tacrolimus neurotoxicity
   E. Uremic encephalopathy

258. A 65-year-old man post–liver transplant 2 years ago for hepatocellular carcinoma (HCC) presents with 6 weeks of dyspnea. Three months ago he was switched from tacrolimus to sirolimus due to renal insufficiency. He otherwise feels well and denies any fever or cough. Physical exam is unremarkable except for fine crackles on lung exam. Chest x-ray shows bilateral pulmonary infiltrates. Chest CT is suggestive of an interstitial process. Echocardiogram is normal. What is the most likely cause of these pulmonary infiltrates?
   A. Pneumocystis carinii pneumonia
   B. Posttransplant lymphoproliferative disorder (PTLD)
   C. Sirolimus-induced toxicity
   D. Congestive heart failure (CHF)
   E. Pulmonary metastasis from HCC

ANSWERS

1. **C** (S&F ch71)
   The liver forms as an outgrowing diverticulum of proliferating endodermal cells present in the ventral floor of the foregut during the third week of gestation.

2. **D** (S&F ch71)
   Riedel lobe is an anatomic variation that indicates a prominent right liver lobe extending below the level of the umbilicus. It is diagnosed by ultrasound but may be mistaken for an abdominal mass. It is more commonly seen in females. It is not associated with abnormal liver enzymes or increased risk of malignancy.

3. **B** (S&F ch71)
   Abernethy malformation is a congenital extrahepatic portocaval shunt. There are two known types of this anomaly. In type 1, the portal vein is absent and the portal blood is diverted into the inferior vena cava. Type 1 malformation is more common in girls and is associated with hepatic tumors such as focal nodular hyperplasia in addition to congenital

extrahepatic anomalies, including biliary atresia and cardiac defects. In type 2 Abernethy malformation, a side-to-side anastomosis of the portal vein with the inferior vena cava leads to shunting, so the portal vein is technically present. It is not associated with extrahepatic malformations.

4. B (S&F ch71)
Although rare variants may arise from the SMA, the hepatic artery typically arises from the celiac trunk.

5. C (S&F ch71)
Hepatoblasts are dipotent cells that arise from hepatic stem cells and give rise to hepatocytes and cholangiocytes. They are present throughout the parenchyma in the fetal liver but only in the canal of Herring in adult patients. Numbers typically decline with age and wax and wane when there is any parenchymal injury.

6. C (S&F ch71)
Kupffer cells and hepatic NK cells are the main resident cells of immune surveillance. Kupffer cells are categorized as tissue macrophages and have the ability to phagocytose large particles.

7. A (S&F ch71)
Extrahepatic biliary development depends upon the expression of sex-determining region Y-box 17 *(SOX17)*. The expression of *SOX17* is controlled by homolog of hairy/enhancer-of-split 1 (*HES1*). Insufficient *SOX17* expression has been linked to the development of congenital biliary atresia.

8. B (S&F ch62 and 71)
Alagille syndrome is the most common type of familial intrahepatic cholestasis. The hallmark of this syndrome is paucity of interlobular bile ducts. It is an autosomal dominant disease with incomplete penetrance and variable expressions. Mutations in jagged1 (*JAG1*) gene have been found in 94% of all the cases. A mutation in *NOTCH2* receptor gene has been shown in patients with Alagille syndrome who did not manifest *JAG1* mutations. Mild to moderate mental retardation has been noted in only 15% to 20% of patients with this syndrome. On the basis of some retrospective studies, 20-year predicted life expectancy is 75% for all patients and 80% for those who did not require liver transplantation.

9. B (S&F ch72)
Stellate cell activation is the central event in hepatic fibrosis. Kupffer cells or tissue macrophages are responsible for removing toxic or foreign substances. Pit cells are natural killer cells of the liver. Cholangiocytes are bile duct epithelial cells. Sinusoidal cells have a specialized endothelial lining, which serves as a selective barrier between the blood and the hepatocytes.

10. A (S&F ch72)
Adult hepatocytes contribute to liver regeneration after partial hepatectomy. Only when the proliferation of adult hepatocytes is inhibited because of toxic or physical injuries do progenitor cells or (also called oval cells) proliferate. Stellate cells play a role in fibrosis progression. Pit cells are natural killer cells of the liver.

11. D (S&F ch72)
α-1 antitrypsin inhibits elastin, and a missense mutation can lead to α1-antitrypsin deficiency and associated liver disease. α1-acid glycoprotein inhibits proliferating response of peripheral lymphocytes to mitogens. α1-antichymotrypsin inhibits chymotripsin-like serine proteinase. Serum amyloid A is produced in the liver but its function is unknown. Transferrin is an iron-binding protein and is increased in iron deficiency.

12. B (S&F ch72)
ApoB-100 is synthesized in the liver and is one of the major apolipoproteins associated with triglyceride transport and is the predominant transport carrier in VLDL. ApoB-48 is similar to ApoB-100 except it is synthesized in the small intestine and is part of the chylomicron remnant. Apo-E is synthesized in the liver and is important for removal of lipoprotein remnants in the serum. Absence of Apo-E leads to reduced clearance of chylomicron and VLDL remnants and increases risk of atherosclerosis. ApoA-1 is the major component of HDL lipoproteins. ApoC is also synthesized in the liver and is composed of three different genes that may inhibit the uptake of chylomicron remnants by the liver.

13. D (S&F ch72)
Tangier disease or familial alpha-lipoprotein deficiency is an autosomal recessive disorder characterized by the accumulation of cholesteryl esters in reticuloendothelial cells in combination with near absence of serum HDL cholesterol. It is caused by mutations in the gene encoding ATP-binding cassette transporter A1 (ABCA1) and increases the risk of atherosclerotic heart disease by four- to sixfold. Lecithin-cholesterol acyltransferase (LCAT) enhances cholesterol esterification in the plasma. Hepatic TG lipase (HTGL) is involved in lipolysis of VLDL or IDL and plays a role in LDL formation. Cholesteryl ester transfer protein (CETP) mediates the exchange of cholesteryl esters from HDL and TGs from chylomicrons or VLDL. HMG-CoA reductase is the rate-limiting enzyme in hepatic cholesterol synthesis.

14. D (S&F ch73)
Dubin Johnson syndrome is a rare genetic syndrome characterized by an isolated direct hyperbilirubinemia, and is due to a defect in the gene that encodes multidrug-resistance protein 2 (MRP2) and does not lead to adverse clinical outcomes. Biopsy often reveals black tissue due to pigment accumulation. Rotor syndrome also causes benign direct hyperbilirubinemia but the liver is normal in appearance. Gilbert disease and Crigler-Najjar syndrome types 1 & 2 are due to indirect hyperbilirubinemia.

15. B (S&F ch73, ch76, ch86, ch87, ch90)
Patients with nonalcoholic fatty liver disease often have other coexisting metabolic risk factors including central obesity, diabetes, hypertension, and dyslipidemia. ALT is greater than AST and biopsy reveals macrovesicular steatosis. Alcoholic hepatitis presents with AST greater than ALT (usually 2:1 or 3:1) and AST is rarely greater than 300. Autoimmune hepatitis is more predominant in women and classic biopsy findings consist of interface hepatitis and a lymphoplasmacytic infiltrate. Wilson disease is largely diagnosed in younger patients and the alkaline phosphatase is disproportionately low. Ischemic hepatitis presents with an AST/ALT greater than 20 to 25 times normal and is usually precipitated by some type of hemodynamic instability.

16. C (S&F ch73)
The increased AST seen in alcoholic liver disease is due to deficiency of pyridoxal 5'phosphate which is a cofactor in ALT production, thus leading to decreased levels of ALT

(rather than an increased production of AST). 5'nucleotidase is associated with canalicular and sinusoidal plasma membranes and is primarily increased in hepatobiliary disease. Antibodies to tissue transglutaminase are found in celiac disease.

17. C (S&F ch73, ch91)
This patient fits the demographics for primary biliary cirrhosis (PBC) that is often seen in middle-aged women and characterized by cholestatic liver disease (elevation in alkaline phosphatase) and pruritus. A positive AMA is diagnostic for PBC. An ACE level can be useful in identifying patients with sarcoidosis. An ASMA is often positive in patients with autoimmune hepatitis and presents with a hepatocellular pattern of injury (elevated AST and ALT). Ferritin can be elevated in hemochromatosis, but is also an acute phase reactant and can be seen in many chronic liver disease conditions. Copper overload is seen in patients with Wilson disease but a low ceruloplasmin level aids in diagnosis.

18. E (S&F ch73)
Vascular endothelial cells produce Factor VIII; all other clotting factors are produced in the liver.

19. E (S&F ch74)
Certain patients with chronic HBV are at an increased risk for hepatocellular carcinoma (HCC). The American Association for the Study of Liver Diseases (AASLD) recommends routine HCC screening for patients with HBV who have a positive family history of HCC, Asian males age > 40 and Asian females age >50, African patients age > 20, and patients with cirrhosis. Treatment with antivirals including tenofovir or PegIFN is not indicated in this patient since he is in the inactive carrier stage. A liver biopsy is not going to impact management since his liver function tests are within normal range and his viral load is low, making treatment with antivirals unnecessary at this point. Screening should include at least an ultrasound every 6 months.

20. C (S&F ch74)
20% to 40% of patients with cirrhosis have osteopenia or osteoporosis, therefore, all patients waiting for liver transplantation should have bone densitometry. Calcium, phosphorus, vitamin D, and testosterone levels (in males) should be checked and all patients should receive calcium 1000 to 1200 mg/d and vitamin D 400 to 800 IU/d. Patients with documented osteoporosis may be treated with bisphosphonates. A liver biopsy is not warranted in this patient with established cirrhosis. An MRI is also not necessary in this scenario since the patient has already had abdominal imaging (ultrasound) for hepatocellular carcinoma screening. A macroaggregated albumin scan is helpful to confirm the presence of intrapulmonary shunting in patients with suspected hepatopulmonary syndrome (HPS) and is not relevant in this patient in view of his normal PaO2.

21. A (S&F ch74)
Spontaneous bacterial peritonitis (SBP) is an ominous complication of end-stage liver disease. A diagnosis is based on ascitic fluid cell count analysis demonstrating a neutrophil count of more than 250/mm^3. Patients with a positive gram stain can also be treated as SBP even if their neutrophil count is less than 250. All patients should be placed on long-term antibiotics for secondary prophylaxis following an episode of SBP. The patient is not a candidate for a liver transplant given his ongoing alcohol abuse. He already had an ultrasound so an MRI is not necessary at this point. An EGD is warranted for variceal screening, and outpatient paracentesis is also useful for symptom relief; however the most important step in this patient's management is to initiate secondary prophylaxis with norfloxacin. Other options include trimethoprim/sulfamethoxazole as well as ciprofloxacin (dosed once weekly).

22. C (S&F ch74)
Patients with HBV and cirrhosis should receive antiviral treatment if they have any detectable level of virus. A liver biopsy to document grade of inflammation is not necessary. Treatment with interferon is contraindicated in cirrhosis given the significant side effects associated with interferon, which are usually poorly tolerated by cirrhotic patients. An MRI is not necessary since the patient already had an ultrasound to screen for hepatocellular carcinoma.

23. A (S&F ch74)
The patient's tumor is within Milan criteria (1 lesion <5 cm or 2 to 3 lesions with none of the lesions exceeding 3 cm, and no vascular invasion or metastasis). He does not appear to have any contraindications for liver transplant (no medical comorbidities and good psychosocial support) and he should therefore be referred for an evaluation. Surgical resection is a potential option in patients with compensated cirrhosis (Child-Pugh class A) who have good synthetic function (normal bilirubin) and a normal platelet count. This patient has decompensated liver disease and portal hypertension and therefore is not a candidate for surgical resection. Antiviral therapy may be useful prior to transplant but will not impact his prognosis in the setting of his hepatocellular carcinoma. Observation alone is not enough at this time since his tumor is large enough to earn a MELD exception.

24. E (S&F ch74)
This patient has type 1 hepatorenal syndrome (HRS) and her 3-month mortality without a liver transplant is very high. Renal function typically returns to normal following a liver transplant and a kidney transplant is therefore not necessary at this point. Dialysis may be necessary as a bridge to transplantation; however, the patient at this time does not appear to have any life threatening electrolyte disturbance or volume overload and dialysis is not necessary at this time. She has already received intravenous fluids without any improvement and additional fluid may result in volume overload, and is not likely to provide any benefit.

25. D (S&F ch74)
This is a typical presentation of hepatopulmonary syndrome (HPS) that can develop in 10% of patients with cirrhosis and portal hypertension. Diagnostic criteria include evidence of intrapulmonary shunting, an elevated alveolar-arterial gradient and arterial hypoxemia in the absence of lung parenchymal disease. An echocardiogram with a bubble study is the diagnostic modality of choice to screen for this condition. Patients with PaO2 <60 mm Hg qualify for a MELD exception and should be referred for a transplant. Hypoxemia typically resolves posttransplant. A chest CT and bronchoscopy are not likely to add any additional useful information. The patient is young and not likely to have underlying coronary artery disease or chronic obstructive pulmonary disease (COPD), particularly since she is non-smoker.

26. D (S&F ch74)
Patients with PSC who develop jaundice should undergo an MRCP to evaluate for any new or dominant

strictures and the presence of a liver mass. If a dominant stricture is found, then ERCP is indicated to obtain brush cytology or biopsy, and attempt to stent the stricture. A liver biopsy is not likely to add any useful information. His symptoms do not suggest acute cholangitis and antibiotics are therefore not necessary. The patient may be a candidate for a liver transplant; however, he should be evaluated for a possible cholangiocarcinoma first.

27. A (S&F ch74)
In patients with compensated cirrhosis, cardiovascular disease is the most common cause of death. Stroke, malignancy (hepatocellular carcinoma [HCC] and non-HCC malignancies), and renal disease are the other common causes of death. In patients with decompensated cirrhosis, complications of portal hypertension, HCC, and sepsis are the most common causes of death.

28. E (S&F ch75)
This patient presents with a history and exam supporting a diagnosis of type IV hemochromatosis. Type IV hemochromatosis, also known as ferroportin disease, results from a mutation in ferroportin, reducing its ability to export iron. Iron is sequestered in the reticuloendothelial system, and a liver biopsy will reveal excess iron in Kuppfer cells. It is the only form of hemochromatosis resulting in anemia. Other clues in the question stem include the autosomal dominant inheritance pattern, normal serum iron, and normal total iron binding capacity. The other options represent forms of hemochromatosis inherited in an autosomal recessive pattern, and will be much less likely to present with anemia.

29. E (S&F ch75)
Hemochromatosis is a disease of incomplete penetrance. Not all patients develop symptoms, even if they inherit the autosomal recessive *C282Y/C282Y* genotype associated with the disease. Women have a much lower penetrance than men. This is likely a result of menses, childbirth, and genetic modifiers. This patient has a 1/4 chance of inheriting the *C282Y/C282Y* genotype. Further, women who are *C282Y* homozygotes have ~1% chance of developing iron overload–related disease. Therefore, without knowing her genotype, she has a 1/400 chance of developing iron overload–related disease. Option A is her risk of inheriting the genotype. Option B is the risk of a man inheriting the homozygous genotype and developing symptomatic disease with the given a penetrance of 28% in males. Options C and D are incorrect.

30. A (S&F ch75)
Phlebotomy is the treatment of choice for hemochromatosis. In the age of genetic testing, many patients are identified prior to the development of symptomatic iron overload. The initial goal of therapy is to remove 1 to 2 units of blood per week until the patient achieves mild anemia with normalization of ferritin. This patient, therefore, has reached the goal for the initial treatment and should be transitioned to maintenance phlebotomy. Low iron diet has no role in the treatment of hemochromatosis. Phlebotomy to hemoglobin of 10.0 g/dL will not benefit this patient. Liver biopsy would not benefit this patient and, in fact, is rarely used with the advent of less invasive testing. Serum iron levels are not used for monitoring the effect of phlebotomy.

31. E (S&F ch75)
An asymptomatic male with no laboratory findings suggesting elevated iron levels should not receive any further testing for hemochromatosis. Transferrin saturation and ferritin are the two best tests for screening a patient for risk of iron overload. He can continue to be screened with these tests given the risk of inheriting the *C282Y* mutation. Other tests are not merited at this time. HLA typing is not used for diagnosis of hemochromatosis. Testing for *C282Y* genotype would be the test of choice for diagnosing hereditary hemochromatosis if his screening labs were abnormal. MRI and biopsy of the liver can be used to assess the extent of hepatic damage from symptomatic iron overload.

32. B (S&F ch75)
This patient presents with multiple symptoms of iron overload due to hereditary hemochromatosis. This patient has the classic symptoms of skin bronzing and diabetes. Other symptoms related to iron overload include cardiomyopathy/arrhythmia, hypogonadism, arthropathy, joint space changes, liver injury/cirrhosis, and fatigue. Most patients now present prior to the onset of symptoms. If a patient does present with symptoms related to iron overload, phlebotomy could lead to improvement in many of these symptoms. The physical changes to joint spaces are the only manifestation of iron overload listed that does not improve with phlebotomy. Hypogonadism is another symptom that does not improve with phlebotomy. Other symptoms usually improve with phlebotomy.

33. A (S&F ch75)
This patient's presentation is highly suggestive of hereditary hemochromatosis. Approximately 75% of patients present without symptoms of iron overload. Routine laboratory studies and family history offer clues to diagnosis. This patient's family history and elevated iron saturation increase the likelihood of hereditary hemochromatosis, and as such, confirmatory testing should be pursued. The test of choice for confirming hereditary hemochromatosis is genetic testing. *C282Y* is the most common genotype leading to hereditary hemochromatosis. Serum ferritin can support the diagnosis of iron overload, but cannot confirm the diagnosis of hereditary hemochromatosis. Hereditary hemochromatosis was initially associated with specific HLA types, but the advent of genetic testing for specific mutations responsible for the disease limits the utility of HLA typing. MRI cannot be used to diagnose hereditary hemochromatosis, however, T2-weighted MRI is used to follow the level of iron deposition in patients diagnosed with the disease. Phlebotomy should not be initiated until a diagnosis of hereditary hemochromatosis is confirmed.

34. B (S&F ch75)
This patient presents with a normocytic anemia in the setting of longstanding rheumatoid arthritis. Her laboratory values and history are consistent with a diagnosis of anemia of chronic disease. This results from chronic inflammation, which leads to IL-6–mediated hepatic expression of hepcidin (see figure). Hepcidin acts as a master regulator of iron stores in the body. It binds to ferroportin on the basolateral surface of enterocytes and prevents the passage of iron from the digestive tract to the circulation, thus lowering iron absorption without leading to iron deficiency. The others are genes associated with iron homeostasis. Mutations in the *HFE* gene are the most common etiology for hereditary hemochromatosis.

Mutations in the the *ferroportin*, *BMP*, and *HAMP* genes are associated with less common forms of hereditary hemochromatosis.

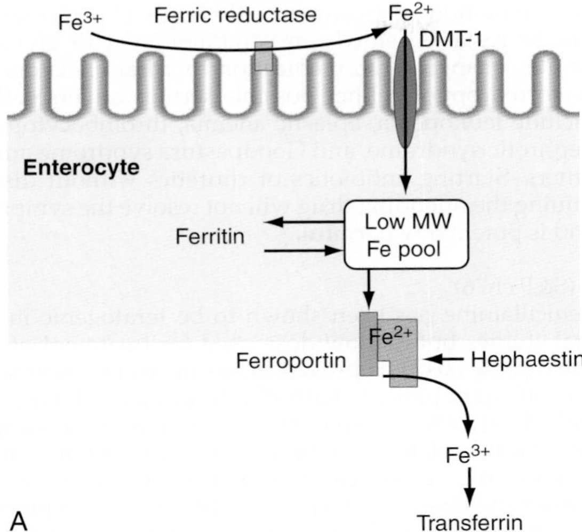

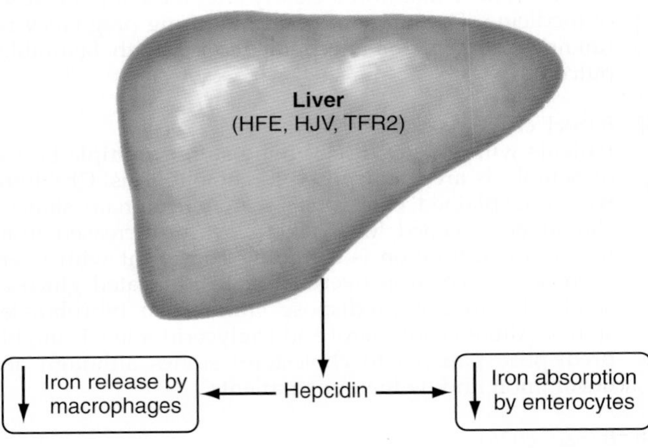

Figure for answer 34.

35. C (S&F ch75)
Elevated transferrin saturation is the most sensitive and specific test for iron overload. While genetic testing would tell if the patient has a risk of developing hemochromatosis, the disease has a penetrance of only 28%. Thus a positive genetic test would still have to be followed for iron overload. ALT elevation is not specific for iron overload. Serum ferritin elevation can result from multiple inflammatory processes, and therefore is not specific enough for symptomatic iron overload. Iron binding capacity is not specific for iron overload.

36. E (S&F ch75)
Testing the wife for the *HFE* mutation would be the best way to screen the children for their risk of developing hereditary hemochromatosis (HH). If the wife is negative, the children do not need to be tested. If the wife is positive for a mutation associated with (HH), then the children should be screened for the *HFE* mutation. As the disease only has a penetrance of ~28% in males, measuring serum ferritin and TIBC can be used for predicting the development of symptomatic iron overload if the children test positive for mutations associated with HH.

37. D (S&F ch75)
Oral iron chelation therapy is a common therapy for patients with transfusion-associated iron overload. These patients by definition cannot tolerate phlebotomy. Deferasirox is the only currently available oral iron chelation therapy available for this patient. This medication, however, carries several black box warnings including renal failure, hepatic failure, and gastrointestinal hemorrhage. Other options have not been found to be side effects of therapy with deferasirox.

38. B (S&F ch76)
This patient has a family history and liver biochemical test (elevated liver enzymes and low alkaline phosphatase) consistent with Wilson disease. The described histology is consistent with early histologic findings of Wilson disease. Also, changes in hepatocellular mitochondria are an important feature of Wilson disease. Insulin resistance has been associated with nonalcoholic fatty liver disease (NAFLD). Although steatosis is a feature of NAFLD, the patient is young with no metabolic risk factors that might increase his risk of NAFLD. Elevated ferritin levels are a common feature of hemochromatosis and other inflammatory conditions. None of the histological findings favors a diagnosis of hemochromatosis in this patient. Elevated anti–smooth muscle antibodies are more characteristic of autoimmune hepatitis (AIH). Interface hepatitis with plasmacytic infiltrates is a more characteristic histological finding in AIH. A low alpha1-antitrypsin level in serum is a finding consistent with alpha1-antitrypsisn deficiency. Alpha1-antitrypsisn deficiency is a common liver condition diagnosed in neonates and children and can present with asymptomatic elevation of liver enzymes. The most classic histological finding of alpha1-antitrypsisn deficiency is intracellular globules accumulation on the endoplasmic reticulum that stain positive with periodic Acid-Shiff (PAS).

39. C (S&F ch76)
This young patient has clinical and biochemical findings suggestive of Wilson disease. These include findings suggestive of portal hypertension (ascites), mild elevation of liver enzymes, and low to normal alkaline phosphatase levels and indirect hyperbilirubinemia (which might be a finding consistent with hemolysis). A 24-hour urine collection for copper, preferably three separate collections, is a useful diagnostic approach. The basal 24-hour urine copper excretion is elevated two to three times that of normal in the vast majority of patients with Wilson disease. The urine collection should be complete; volume and creatinine levels should be measured and special caution should be taken to avoid other sources of copper contamination. Although performing a slit-lamp exam looking for Kayser-Fleischer rings might be easy and cost-effective, approximately 40% to 60% of patients with exclusively hepatic involvement will have absent Kayser-Fleischer rings. Also this patient does not have neurological manifestations that might suggest brain involvement. Serum ceruloplasmin alone is an unreliable diagnostic method for Wilson disease. Immunological methods, which measure both apoceruloplasmin and holoceruloplasmin, overestimate the true amount of functional ceruloplasmin. Serum ceruloplasmin might be elevated with hepatic inflammation and, on the other hand, low ceruloplasmin level is not specific for Wilson disease,

and might occur in malabsorption, nephrotic syndrome and other chronic liver diseases. More than 500 mutations have been identified in the ATP7B gene in different populations. Gene mutation analysis is particularly challenging in Japanese and Mediterranean populations, in which no mutation is present in high frequency. Percutaneous liver biopsy might be diagnostic in a patient with Wilson disease; however, the risk of complication should be expected in a patient with ascites and coagulopathy, and biopsy should not be the next diagnostic approach.

40. D (S&F ch76)
Genetic screening of first-degree relatives, when the patient's DNA is available for mutation analysis, is the most reliable test to identify affected individuals. All first-degree relatives should be screened for Wilson disease and not just the siblings. In the absence of genetic analysis, screening should include physical exam, liver biochemical tests, serum copper and ceruloplasmin measurements, 24-hour urinary copper collection, and slit-lamp examination.

41. C (S&F ch76)
This patient is presenting with acute liver failure secondary to Wilson disease. Mortality of acute liver failure secondary to Wilson disease (which is characterized by acute hemolytic anemia, altered mental status, deterioration of liver function, renal dysfunction, and coagulopathy) is high and the patient should be referred for liver transplant emergently. This patient might present some laboratories findings suggestive of autoimmune disease, such as positive ANA and inclusive autoimmune markers. It is very important to differentiate these two diagnoses because treatment might be different and time sensitive. The combination of the ratio of alkaline phosphatase to bilirubin levels of less than 4 and the AST to ALT ratio greater than 2.2 is specific for the diagnosis of acute Wilson disease with liver failure. Options A and B might be recommended treatments for mild and severe flare of autoimmune hepatitis. In this case, the clinical history and the low alkaline phosphatase, with laboratories consistent with hemolytic anemia (elevated LDH levels, indirect hyperbilirubinemia) favor the diagnosis of Wilson disease. Choice D is the recommended therapy for acetaminophen intoxication that more commonly presents with marked elevation (usually above 1000 IU/L) of liver enzymes. The serology tests are not consistent with active hepatitis B infection in this patient.

42. D (S&F ch76)
Wilson disease might be complicated by extrahepatic complications. Renal disease, mainly Fanconi syndrome might be prominent. This is secondary to the toxicity of copper on renal tubules. Findings might include microscopic hematuria, aminoaciduria, phosphaturia, and defective acidification of the urine. Penicillamine, an effective medication for Wilson disease might cause several adverse effects. Among the severe side effects include rashes (elastosis perforans serpiginosa), hypothyroidism, severe proteinuria, leucopenia, thrombocytopenia, and aplastic anemia. It is unlikely that this patient's renal signs and symptoms are caused by this medication. Hepatorenal syndrome is a severe renal dysfunction in patients with end-stage liver disease caused by splanchnic vasodilation, renal vasoconstriction and cardiac dysfunction. It is unlikely that interstitial nephritis is causing all the findings on the urinalysis in this patient. The patient does not have biochemical findings consistent with a severe prerenal state.

43. D (S&F ch76)
This patient is presenting a severe adverse reaction to D-penicillamine. A febrile reaction with rash and proteinuria might develop in some patient 7 to 10 days after initiation of treatment. Although D-penicillamine can be restarted slowly in combination with glucocorticoids, changing the medication to other chelators is a preferred option. Other possible serious adverse effects include leukopenia, aplastic anemia, thrombocytopenia, nephrotic syndrome, and Goodpasture syndrome among others. Starting antibiotics or diuretics without discontinuing the offending drug will not resolve the symptoms and is potentially harmful.

44. B (S&F ch76)
Penicillamine has been shown to be teratogenic in animal studies but the low dose used for treatment of Wilson disease has been proved to be safe in clinical practice. For pregnant patients with Wilson disease who are controlled on penicillamine, treatment must be continued because complete discontinuation may result in postpartum hepatic decompensation. However, it is advised to reduce the dose of penicillamine by 25% of the prepregnancy dose especially if cesarean delivery is anticipated in view of the concern of wound healing. Liver function tests need to be monitored closely after reducing the dose of medicine. The safety of trientine during pregnancy is unknown, except for anecdotal reports with favorable outcomes.

45. B (S&F ch76)
Patients with Wilson disease who suffer multiple bouts of hemolysis are predisposed to cholelithiasis. Children with unexplained cholelithiasis, of bilirubinate stones, should be screened for Wilson disease. Increased iron transferrin saturation is a finding consistent with liver cirrhosis and/or iron overload states. Elevated glucose levels should not predispose children to bilirubinate stones. Altered cholesterol and triglycerides levels might predispose patients to cholesterol stones although an uncommon finding in young patients.

46. B (S&F ch76)
Ceruloplasmin is an acute-phase reactant and might be elevated in pregnancy, inflammatory states (including hepatic inflammation), and with the use of exogenous estrogen. The rest of the above conditions are commonly associated with low ceruloplasmin levels.

47. C (S&F ch76)
Neurologic manifestations in Wilson disease follow two main patterns that include movement disorders and spastic dystonia. Movement disorders, such as loss of fine motor control and tremors, usually occur earlier in the course of the disease. Spastic dystonic presentations, such as dysarthria, rigidity, or drooling tend to develop later. Intellectual function is not impaired in Wilson disease and seizures are uncommon.

48. C (S&F ch77)
This infant is presenting with typical signs and symptoms of a urea cycle disorder (UCD). Patients with UCDs have elevated blood ammonia levels as a consequence of the disruption of their urea cycle, and the elevated ammonia results in the signs and symptoms of the disease. Presentation is often confused for sepsis, and bacterial blood cultures will not make the diagnosis in these patients. Quantitative urine ALA and PBG can be used

to diagnose porphyrias. Arterial blood gas in this patient may show a respiratory alkalosis from hyperventilation secondary to hyperammonemia; however, this is not specific to UCDs. Serum phenylalanine can help diagnose tyrosinemia.

49. D (S&F ch77)
Of all the congenital disorders of glycosylation, only type Ib responds clinically to dietary mannose, however, hepatic fibrosis can occur despite clinical improvement. Patients with this type of disease have a defect in phosphomannose isomerase, which converts fructose-6-phosphate to mannose 6-phosphate. These patients develop diarrhea, hepatic fibrosis, hypoglycemia, and recurrent vomiting.

50. B (S&F ch77)
This patient has alpha1-antitrypsin deficiency leading to cirrhosis and decompensation with ascites. He may also have pulmonary disease based on his history of asthma. The mechanism of hepatocyte injury is buildup of the abnormal Z protein in hepatocytes and subsequent activation of caspase pathways, endoplasmic reticulum stress responses, and autophagic responses. Increased fatty acid influx into the liver is a mechanism of liver injury in glycogen storage disease type 1. Uninhibited neutrophil elastase activity is the mechanism of pulmonary injury in patients in alpha1-antitrypsin deficiency, but does not play a role in hepatic injury. Accumulation of fumarylacetoacetate and maleylacetoacetate occurs in tyrosinemia. Obstruction of small bile ducts can occur in many types of liver disease, including cystic fibrosis related liver disease, but is not a primary mechanism of liver injury in alpha1-antitrypsin deficiency.

51. E (S&F ch77)
Typical histological findings in hepatic tissue of alpha1-antitrypsin deficiency, which lead to liver injury, are described in E. While not always present, the PAS-positive, diastase-resistant globules are the histological hallmark of the disease. Myelosomes on electron microscopy are seen in congenital disorders of glycosylation. Micronodular cirrhosis, bile duct plugging, steatosis, and giant cell transformation are microscopic findings of tyrosinemia. Steatosis and iron deposition are found in porphyrias and many other liver injuries. Hepatocyte pallor and minimal fatty infiltration are associated with urea cycle disorders.

52. A (S&F ch77)
The short vignette describes an infant with Zellweger syndrome, a peroxisomal disorder and one of the bile acid synthesis defects. In addition to the characteristics described in the question stem, these infants frequently have large anterior fontanelles, impaired hearing, retinopathy, cataracts, skeletal changes, and hepatomegaly with progressive liver disease. Mutation of the *CFTR* gene causes cystic fibrosis. Strict protein avoidance is necessary for patients presenting acutely with urea cycle disorders. Cutaneous vesicles and bullae in light exposed areas are typical of cutaneous porphyrias. Continuous nighttime tube feeding is often necessary in patients with glycogen storage diseases.

53. B (S&F ch78)
A 2010 publication of 1158 cases of HAV infection reported principal risk factors as follows: international travel (45.8%), contact with someone infected with HAV (14.8%), children in daycare center or employee (7.6%), exposure during food or waterborne outbreak (7.2%), history of illicit drug use (4.3%), and history of men having sex with men (3.9%).

54. C (S&F ch78 and www.cdc.gov)
For healthy persons aged 12 months to 40 years, single-antigen hepatitis A vaccine at the age-appropriate dose is preferred to IG because of vaccine advantages that include long-term protection and ease of administration. Hepatitis A vaccine or IG should be administered to all previously unvaccinated household and sexual contacts of persons with serologically confirmed hepatitis A virus.

55. E (S&F ch78)
This patient has hepatitis A infection with prolonged cholestasis, which is a rare variant and resolves spontaneously usually in 10 to 12 weeks. The treatment is conservative with reassurance of the patient. It is acceptable to consider abdominal ultrasound to exclude extrahepatic biliary obstruction, but no other invasive or expensive test including ERCP, liver biopsy, or abdominal MRI is indicated in this patient. There is no increased mortality rate and liver transplant evaluation is not necessary.

56. C (S&F ch78)
In addition to age, the most important risk factors for fulminant hepatic failure (FHF) and mortality include underlying liver disease and chronic viral hepatitis. Mode of transmission of the virus does not increase the risk of FHF. The highest mortality rates occur in persons older than 75 years. The risk is mildly higher in blacks and non-whites than in whites, and in men greater than women. Creatinine level greater than 2 has been also shown to be a clinical predictor of FHF-associated mortality.

57. D (S&F ch78)
Fecal-oral contact is the primary route of transmission by either person-to-person contact or ingestion of contaminated food or water. In rare cases, transmission of HAV by parenteral route has been documented, and cyclical outbreaks have been seen in injection and noninjection drug users and men who have sex with men.

58. B (S&F ch78)
This is an example of relapsing form of hepatitis A virus (HAV) infection. It is seen in 10% to 15% of cases with acute hepatitis A infection within a 6-month period after full recovery of the initial illness. The relapsing phase is usually milder than the first acute period. Hepatitis A virus shedding in the stool is common during the relapsing phase and these patients may remain infectious. It is not associated with chronic hepatitis A infection or increased mortality and the prognosis is excellent. Anti-HAV IgM and IgG are usually detectable during relapsing phase. Appropriate recognition of this condition is essential to avoid any invasive unnecessary tests like ERCP or liver biopsy.

59. D (S&F ch79)
Hepatitis B is acquired via direct contact with infected blood or body fluids. It is primarily spread via heterosexual contact (40%), injection drug use (15% to 20%), or homosexual contact (12%) in low prevalence areas such as the United States and West Europe. In high prevalence areas like China, vertical transmission from mother to child is the most common cause of infection. Hepatitis B is not spread by fecal-oral contamination. Although hemodialysis and unsterile tattoo practices can certainly increase the risk of acquiring hepatitis B, they are not the most common modes of viral infection.

60. B (S&F ch79)
In high prevalence areas like China, vertical transmission from mother to child is the most common cause of infection. Hepatitis B is acquired via direct contact with infected blood or body fluids. It is primarily spread via heterosexual contact (40%), injection drug use (15% to 20%) or homosexual contact (12%) in low prevalence areas such as the United States and West Europe. Although unsterile tattoo practices can certainly spread the virus, it is not the most common cause of viral infection.

61. E (S&F ch79)
Hepatocellular carcinoma (HCC) surveillance is recommended for: Asian male HBV carriers over age 40 and female carriers over age 50, HBV carriers with a family history of HCC, HBV carriers born in Africa and over age 20 and HBV carriers with cirrhosis.

62. E (S&F ch79)
The age at which a person becomes infected with HBV is a principal determinant of the clinical outcome. Perinatal exposure leads to chronic HBV carrier state in 95% of people. Children who are exposed to the virus during the first 5 years of life have a 30% chance of chronic hepatitis B. Only 2% to 5% of adults who are exposed to the virus become chronically infected.

63. A (S&F ch79)
Acute hepatitis B resolves in over 95% of adults infected with the virus. However, acute liver failure can occur in 1% of patients who present with acute hepatitis B. The rate of spontaneous survival in acute liver failure caused by hepatitis B virus is only ~20%.

64. B (S&F ch79)
In patients who develop immunity due to hepatitis B virus vaccination, all markers are negative except for hepatitis B surface antibody. Choice A represents a person with past infection (anti-HBc positive) who now has immunity (anti-HBs positive). Choice C is a person who has active infection. Choice D is a person who has never been exposed to hepatitis B but can be susceptible to the virus. Choice E represents a patient who is chronically infected.

65. E (S&F ch79)
This patient is in the immune tolerant phase of HBV infection characterized by normal liver enzymes and high viral load. She needs to start hepatocellular carcinoma (HCC) surveillance due to family history of HCC. She does not require treatment and can be monitored closely. A liver biopsy is not recommended; however, if performed it would show minimal necroinflammatory activity and no significant fibrosis.

66. D (S&F ch79)
Patients in need of immunosuppressive drug therapy and who are positive for HBsAg and anti-HBc benefit from prophylactic antiviral therapy to prevent reactivation of hepatitis B. Antiviral therapy is generally recommended to start at least 1 week prior to initiation of the immunosuppressive drug and to be continued for 6 to 12 months after discontinuation of treatment.

67. B (S&F ch79)
Entecavir and tenofovir are highly efficacious and have a high genetic barrier to resistance. They are the preferred first-line agents for antiviral therapy. Lamivudine, adefovir, and telbivudine have high rates of resistance and are no longer preferred as first-line agents. In the era of these new effective antivirals, interferon-based treatment is not recommended due to its frequent side effects and the potential risk of decompensation of liver disease with advanced fibrosis.

68. A (S&F ch79)
Administering antiviral therapy during the third trimester of pregnancy and continuing it for a brief period of time after delivery (e.g., 4 weeks postpartum) greatly diminishes both the risk of infection to the newborn and prevents postpregnancy flares of disease caused by recovery of immunologic function in the mother, respectively. Although none of the current antiviral agents are licensed for use in pregnancy, lamivudine has the greatest amount of safety data from HIV-positive mothers. It is pregnancy class B in HIV-infected pregnant women but category C in HBV-infected women. Because it has an excellent safety record and the most extensive use during pregnancy, its use has been recommended for highly viremic mothers. The risk of developing drug-resistant HBV can be anticipated to be small because of the need for short-term treatment. There is no role for the combination of lamivudine and adefovir in this population and pegIFN is contraindicated for use in pregnant women.

69. D (S&F ch79)
The patient in choice D is presenting with acute hepatitis B and rate of spontaneous recovery is greater than 95%. All HIV-HBV coinfected patients, regardless of CD4 count, should be treated for hepatitis B infection due to increased risk of death from liver disease in that population. All patients with active viremia and cirrhosis should be treated with antiviral therapy to prevent decompensation of liver disease and reactivation of hepatitis B. The patient in choice E likely has long-standing hepatitis B from vertical transmission and now has evidence of active viremia and fibrosis (stage 2), and should be treated.

70. C (S&F ch80)
NS3 is a serine protease responsible for cleavage of the HCV polyprotein. The other proteins serve different functions in HCV replication.

71. D (S&F ch80)
In Egypt, 15% of the population has hepatitis C and more than 90% have genotype 4 infection. Genotypes 1, 2, and 3 are most common in the United States and Europe. Genotype 6 is found predominantly in Asia.

72. C (S&F ch80)
The worldwide prevalence of hepatitis C is increasing while the incidence of acute hepatitis C is declining. The age group with the highest prevalence of hepatitis C has shifted from 35-44 years to 55-64 years. The prevalence of hepatitis C is higher in males and African Americans.

73. A (S&F ch80)
It is recommended that all persons born between 1945-1965 be tested for anti-HCV antibody. Receiving a blood transfusion prior to 1992, when HCV blood testing was implemented, and illicit intravenous drug use are risk factors for hepatitis C. There are no specific recommendations for HCV testing based on alcohol consumption. The source of transmission is unknown in one third of cases with HCV infection, and as many as half of patients with hepatitis C may have a normal ALT at any given time.

74. B (S&F ch80)
Younger and female patients have the lowest rates for HCV chronicity. The rate of spontaneous clearance is higher in symptomatic patients in whom jaundice develops and with CC IL28 polymorphism. There is no known influence of genotype in the development of HCV chronicity. African Americans may have a higher rate of viral persistence than whites or Hispanics. Chronicity may be less common in cases of infection acquired by injection than in those who acquire HCV infection by blood transfusion.

75. E (S&F ch80)
This patient has hepatitis C–related cyroglobulinemia. All of the above treatments have been used to treat cryoglobulinemia with variable success, however, the best long-term treatment is directed at HCV. Achieving a sustained viral response leads to resolution of cryoglobulinemia.

76. C (S&F ch80)
Patients who are immunocompromised or on hemodialysis may have negative hepatitis C virus antibody testing and require virologic assays to diagnose hepatitis C. Hepatitis B surface antigen is negative, indicating the patient does not have hepatitis B; hepatitis A IgG indicates previous infection or vaccination. ANA is positive in 9% of patients with hepatitis C. Ordering a tissue transglutaminase in an African-American, asymptomatic patient to rule out celiac disease has a low yield.

77. D (S&F ch80)
Male gender, substantial alcohol consumption, and type 2 diabetes are all risk factors of hepatocellular carcinoma (HCC). Patients with hepatitis C and cirrhosis have a 1% to 4% per year risk of hepatocellular carcinoma. Coffee consumption has been reported to have a beneficial effect on overall mortality in patients with hepatitis C, not an increased risk of HCC.

78. E (S&F ch80)
Obesity is associated with progression of hepatic fibrosis in patients with hepatitis C. Age greater than 40 years, male gender, and white race are also associated with progression of fibrosis. While accelerated disease progression has been described with genotype 3, this is not the case for genotype 1. Viral load is not associated with progression of fibrosis.

79. C (S&F ch80)
Nucleos(t)ide polymerase inhibitors are potent, pangenotypic, and have a high barrier to resistance (see table at the end of the chapter). The other drugs do not meet these characteristics. Sofosbuvir is an example of a nucleotide polymerase inhibitor.

80. E (S&F ch80)
Sustained viral response is associated with regression of fibrosis and reduction in hepatic inflammation. Long-term follow-up studies confirm sustained responses in more than 98% of cases if the patient is HCV RNA negative in serum 24 weeks after completion of antiviral therapy (definition of sustained viral response). Quality of life improves with SVR. SVR reduces, but does not eliminate, the risk for hepatocellular carcinoma.

81. B (S&F ch80)
High hepatitis C viral loads after transplant are associated with an increased severity of HCV recurrence and graft loss. Older donor age is associated with an increased risk of graft loss. Use of high dose corticosteroids may lead to an increase in fibrosis progression and poor long-term outcome. Patients have a 25% chance of developing cirrhosis 5 years after liver transplantation. Low dose corticosteroids may be used in patients with HCV infection after liver transplant.

82. E (S&F ch81)
This patient most likely has hepatitis B with hepatitis D superinfection secondary to intravenous drug use. Antihepatitis D IgM is the best test to diagnosis acute hepatitis D, and is confirmed by HDV RNA. Hepatitis D antigen can be detected in hepatocytes by immunohistochemical staining, however, its reliability decreases as the hepatitis D infection becomes chronic. Measurement of serum hepatitis D antigen is not reliable secondary to the presence of high titers of neutralizing antibodies, which may interfere with detection of the antigen. CMV infection is possible, but less likely in an immunocompetent patient. Hepatitis A IgM and hepatitis C PCR would be the best tests to diagnosis acute hepatitis A and C, respectively (see table at the end of the chapter).

83. A (S&F ch81)
HBV and HDV coinfection usually leads to resolution of both infections, while superinfection leads to chronic HBV and HDV in 70% of cases. Coinfection most often presents with positive hepatitis B core IgM confirming acute hepatitis B virus infection. Superinfection more often leads to rapid disease progression and higher risk for hepatocellular carcinoma. Double peak in ALT is seen in coinfection as HDV infection is established after HBV infection in these cases (see figure).

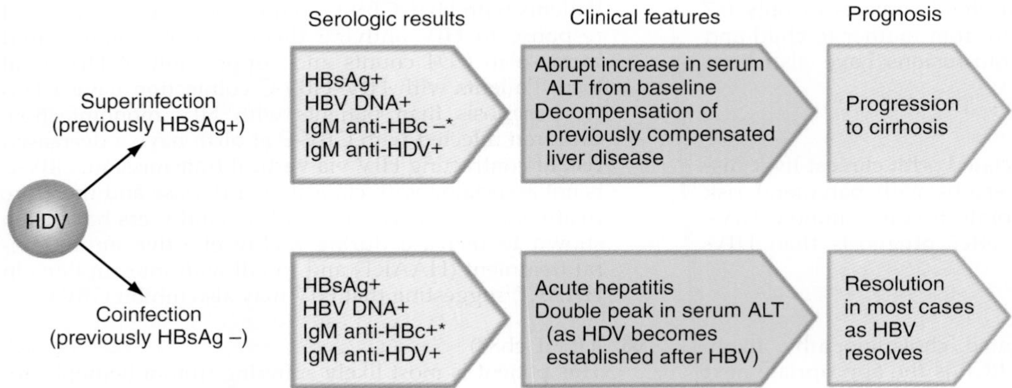

Figure for answer 83.

84. C (S&F ch81)
The only therapeutic option for treatment of hepatitis D is interferon-α (IFN-α), which has side effects that include flu-like symptoms, cytopenias, and depression. The sustained virologic response (SVR) rates with pegylated IFN-α for at least 48 weeks have been reported to be between 17% and 47%, with relapse rates of 2% to 14%. The shorter the duration of disease, the more likely you are to achieve a sustained viral response. While tenofovir is efficacious in the treatment of hepatitis B, it lacks efficacy against hepatitis D. The addition of lamivudine to interferon therapy does not improve response rates compared to interferon alone.

85. B (S&F ch82)
There is no documented animal-to-human transmission for genotype 1 infection but genotype 3 infection is likely via consumption of undercooked meat. Genotype 1 does not have an animal reservoir while genotype 3 does (pigs, wild boars, and deer). Genotype 1 infection occurs in large epidemics, small outbreaks, and frequent sporadic cases while genotype 3 occurs as cases of sporadic acute hepatitis. Genotype 1 does not lead to chronic infection while genotype 3 can lead to chronic infection in immunosuppressed patients. Genotype 1 occurs in young, otherwise healthy persons while genotype 3 occurs in elderly patient with comorbid conditions.

86. C (S&F ch82)
Pregnant women with hepatitis E infection, in their second or third trimester, have mortality rates of 5% to 25%. Fulminant hepatic failure developed in ~22% of affected pregnant women. In nonpregnant women, mortality rates are low: 0.07% to 0.6%.

87. D (S&F ch82)
In patients with chronic HEV infection, withdrawal or reduction in dose of immunosuppressive medication can lead to the disappearance of HEV viremia in one third of patients. Termination of pregnancy has not been proven to be beneficial in pregnant patients with acute or chronic HEV. Choices B and C, although viable treatment options, are contraindicated in pregnant women. Supportive therapy and close monitoring is not the *best* option in this patient.

88. B (S&F ch82)
The predominant route of transmission is fecal-oral and most occur due to consumption of fecally contaminated drinking water. Person-to-person transmission is uncommon with rates among household contacts of only 0.7 to 2.2%. Vertical transmission from mother to child and transmission from blood transfusions have also been documented.

89. B (S&F ch83)
GBV-C infection is not associated with clinical liver disease. GBV-C is found in persons with parenteral risk factors, and HCV–GBV-C coinfection is common. HIV–GBV-C coinfection has a better prognosis than HIV-monoinfected patients.

90. A (S&F ch83)
This patient has AIDS-related cholangiopathy, likely related to CMV infection. ERCP is the appropriate next step and papillotomy with or without biliary stent placement may improve cholestasis. Antiviral therapy has no effect on this syndrome. Cholelithiasis does not cause irregular intrahepatic ducts and therefore cholecystectomy is not indicated. Fluconazole will be effective in treatment of the patient's thrush but will have no effect on cholangiopathy. In the setting of AIDS, the patient is not a liver transplant candidate.

91. C (S&F ch83)
The liver biopsy shows multinucleated hepatocytes and eosinophilic viral inclusions (Cowdry type A) consistent with HSV hepatitis. Mucocutaneous lesions are seen in only half of the cases. High-dose intravenous acyclovir is effective treatment for HSV hepatitis and appears to be safe in pregnancy. There is no evidence of autoimmune hepatitis or hepatitis C and therefore prednisone and sofosbuvir/ribavirin are not indicated. The patient does not need a liver transplant at this time as she does not meet criteria for acute liver failure. Emergent delivery provides no benefit in the treatment of HSV hepatitis.

92. C (S&F ch83)
TTV is also called *transfusion transmitted virus* and was described in 1997. TTV can be spread by both parenteral and fecal-oral routes. It is a nonenveloped, single-stranded DNA virus. TTV is commonly found worldwide. The reported prevalence among blood donors has been reported approaching 100% in some studies. Most infected persons have no biochemical or histologic evidence of liver disease.

93. E (S&F ch83)
This patient likely has EBV mononucleosis. Nine out of ten of patients with acute mononucleosis have serum transaminitis up to two to three times the upper limit of normal. Elevated levels of alkaline phosphatase are common, and mild hyperbilirubinemia is observed in about half of the cases. Liver biopsy is rarely necessary for diagnosis but, if done, shows portal and sinusoidal mononuclear cell infiltration with no disruption of hepatic architecture. CMV can present with mononucleosis-like illness, however, the diagnosis would be confirmed by CMV IgM, not IgG. The other options are not consistent with the described clinical presentation.

94. B (S&F ch83)
This infant has congenital CMV syndrome characterized by jaundice, hepatosplenomegaly, thrombocytopenic purpura, and severe neurologic impairment. Histopathologic findings in CMV hepatitis include hepatocyte nuclei containing large "owl's eye" viral inclusions.

95. C (S&F ch83)
Patients with HIV–GBV-C coinfection have an improved response to HIV antiviral therapy with a more rapid increase in CD4 counts and suppression of HIV viral load. Patients with HIV–GBV-C coinfection have a better prognosis than patients with HIV monoinfection. Children infected with GBV-C at birth have a decreased risk of contracting HIV via vertical transmission. GBV-C is not associated with clinical liver disease and therefore treatment is not necessary. GBV-C viral titers have been shown to increase during highly effective antiretroviral treatment (HAART) and to fall with interruptions in HAART, suggesting that HIV may also inhibit GBV-C.

96. A (S&F ch83)
This patient is most likely suffering from a hemophagocytic syndrome, also known as hemophagocytic lymphohistiocytosis (HLH), which is characterized by fever, hepatosplenomegaly, cytopenia, abnormal liver function

tests, and very high serum ferritin level (usually above 10,000 mcg/L). It is caused by natural killer T-cell dysregulation resulting in lymphocyte proliferation and activation with uninhibited hemophagocytosis as well as cytokine production. It is associated with primary or reactivated EBV infection. The other viruses are not associated with this condition. This syndrome may also be seen with hematologic malignancies or collagen vascular diseases.

97. D (S&F ch84)
Fifty percent of patients with disseminated gonococcal infection have elevated serum alkaline phosphatase and 30% to 40% have elevated AST levels with normal total bilirubin. The patient above has Fitz-Hugh-Curtis syndrome, a perihepatitis due to direct spread of the infection from the pelvis, which can be seen with gonococcal infection or Chlamydia infection. Most patients have a history of pelvic inflammatory disease and on exam, a characteristic friction rub can be heard over the liver. There is no evidence of gallbladder wall thickening, pericholecystic fluid, or stranding to suggest acute cholecystitis. Yersinia can cause an ileocolitis in children and terminal ileitis or mesenteric adenitis in adults and is often associated with arthritis, cellulitis, and erythema nodosum. Legionella infection is often manifested by pneumonia. *Salmonella typhi* infection or typhoid fever is a systemic infection that can cause fever, tender hepatomegaly, elevations in serum aminotransferases, and in some cases jaundice.

98. B (S&F ch84)
Bacillary angiomatosis (*Bartonella henselae* or *Bartonella quintana*) is primarily seen in patients with AIDS or other immunodeficiency states and is frequently associated with exposure to cats. Patients present with blood-red papular skin lesions, persistent fever, bacteremia, and sepsis. The bacilli can infect the liver, lymph nodes, pleura, bronchi, bones, brain, bone marrow, and spleen. In hepatic infection, serum aminotransferases are elevated and peliosis hepatitis is seen on biopsy. *Coxiella burnetti* or Q fevers is typically acquired by inhalation of animal dusts and is characterized by relapsing fevers, headaches, myalgias, pneumonitis, and culture-negative endocarditis. Liver involvement is common and is manifested predominantly by elevated alkaline phosphatase levels. Liver biopsy shows fibrin ring granulomas. Fitz-Hugh-Curtis Syndrome is a perihepatitis caused by infection with gonococcus or *Chlamydia* and associated with pelvic inflammatory disease. Brucellosis is acquired from infected pigs, cattle, goats, and sheep and manifests as an acute febrile illness. Liver biopsy shows noncaseating hepatic granulomas. Bartonella infection is endemic to Colombia, Ecuador, and Peru and causes an acute febrile illness accompanied by jaundice, hemolysis, hepatosplenomegaly, and lymphadenopathy.

99. C (S&F ch84)
The patient has Weil syndrome from leptospirosis, which is characterized by jaundice in the first phase and fevers, hepatitis, marked jaundice, and renal injury from acute tubular necrosis in the second phase. Hemorrhagic complications are frequent and are the result of capillary injury caused by immune complexes. The diagnosis is made on clinical grounds in conjunction with a positive blood or urine culture in the first and second phase, respectively, and confirmed by serologic testing. Doxycycline is effective if given within the first several days of the illness.

100. A (S&F ch84)
Acute malaria is made by clinical history, physical exam, and identification of parasites on peripheral thin and thick blood smears. Because the number of parasites in the blood may be small, repeated smear examinations should be performed when the index of suspicion is high.

101. B (S&F ch84)
This patient has visceral leishmaniasis, which is transmitted by the sandfly bite. It usually begins with a papular or ulcerative skin lesion at the site of the sandfly bite and, after an incubation period of months to years, symptoms of fevers, weight loss, diarrhea, and progressive painful hepatosplenomegaly develop. Cutaneous gray hyperpgimented spots (kala-azar) are characteristically seen in patients from the Indian subcontinent. *Plasmodium falciparum* infection causes malaria, which typically manifests with cyclic fevers, malaise, anorexia, nausea, and diarrhea. Tender hepatomegaly with splenomegaly is common. Babesiosis is a malaria-like illness, which causes fever, anemia, mild hepatosplenomegaly, and abnormalities on liver biochemical tests. Amebiasis (caused by *Entamoeba histolytica*) can cause fever, right upper quadrant pain, and peritonitis. Elevated right hemidiaphragm and hepatic cysts are seen on imaging. *Toxoplasma gondii* can cause a mononucleosis-like illness with fever, chills, headache, lymphadenopathy, and occasional hepatosplenomegaly.

102. E (S&F ch84)
Visceral larva migrans is a nematodal infection (toxicariasis). Examples of causative parasites are *Toxicara canis* and *Toxicara cati.* Infection occurs worldwide, and is common in children. It is acquired when embryonated eggs in soil or food are ingested. Pica is a risk factor. ELISA is the most commonly used serologic test for accurate diagnosis with a very high sensitivity and specificity. Stool studies are not useful because these organisms do not produce eggs in humans nor do they remain in the GI tract. Blood cultures and urine cultures are not helpful. Liver biopsy is not routinely recommended especially if done blindly, however, it can help differentiate between visceral larva migrans from hepatic capillariasis.

103. B (S&F ch84)
Choice B correctly depicts the accurate life cycle of *Schistosoma* species (see figure).

104. E (S&F ch84)
Chronic schistosomal infection can lead to hepatic complications, including periportal fibrosis, presinusoidal occlusion, and ultimately portal hypertension due to the inflammatory reaction to eggs deposited in the liver. The lungs can also be affected when eggs or adult worms pass through the liver into the systemic circulation, causing pulmonary hypertension. Treatment is praziquantel. Echinococcal infection leads to hydatid cysts in the liver and are largely asymptomatic. If they grow large enough they can cause low-grade fever, pain, tender hepatomegaly, and if they rupture can cause trauma into the lungs, leading to dyspnea and hemoptysis. Treatment is either surgical removal of the cyst or PAIR (puncture, aspiration, injection of a scolicidal agent and re-aspiration). Albenadoze can also be used if surgical options are not available. Histoplasmosis infection is acquired through the respiratory tract and in most cases confined to the lungs; in chronic progressive disseminated histoplasmosis, hepatomegaly and splenomegaly may be seen. Treatment includes amphotericin B, fluconazole, or itraconazole.

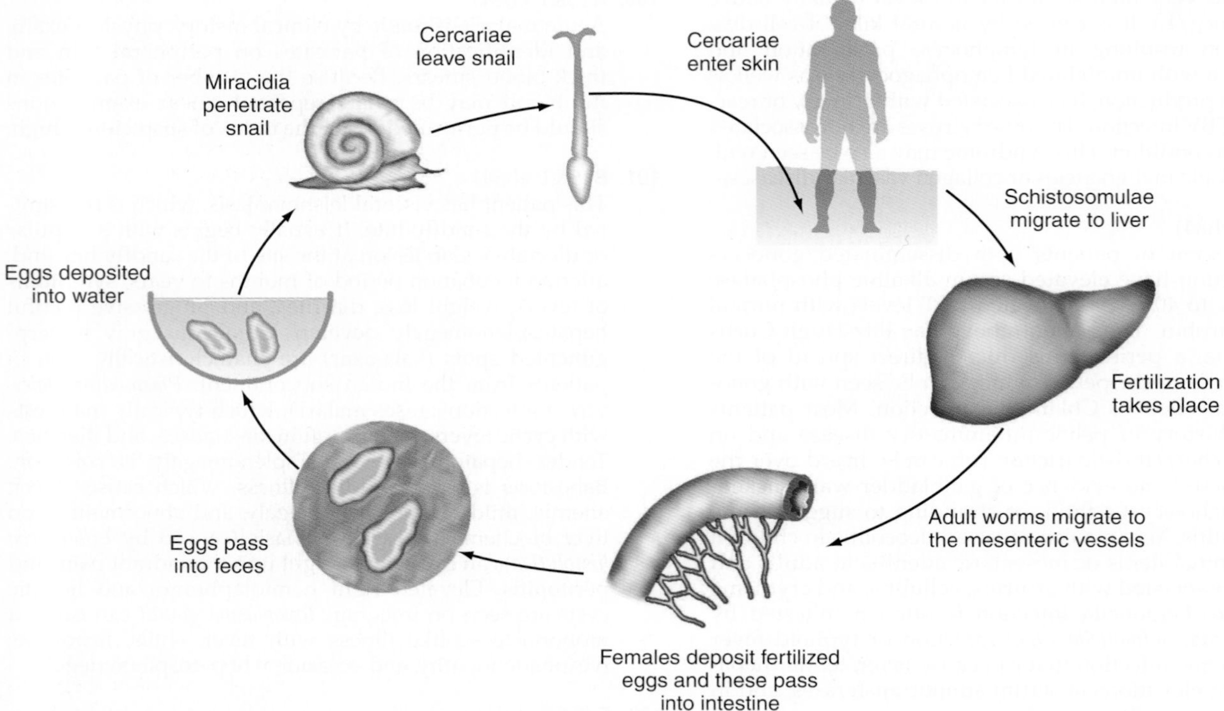

Figure for answer 103.

Acute strongyloides infection can lead to a pruritic eruption, fever, cough, wheezing, abdominal pain, diarrhea, and eosinophilia. In immunocompromised patients, hyperinfection can cause involvement of liver, lung, and brain. Treatment is ivermectin or albendazole. Trichinella infection can cause diarrhea, fever, myalgias, periorbital edema, and marked eosinophilia; jaundice may result from biliary obstruction. Treatment consists of steroids to relieve allergic symptoms, followed by treatment with albendazole or mebendazole.

105. C (S&F ch84)
Choice C describes the accurate life cycle of the *Echinococcus* species. Choice D depicts the accurate life cycle of the *Schistosoma* species.

106. C (S&F ch84)
Amebiasis is treated by oral or intravenous metronidazole and then the addition of an oral luminal amebicide such as iodoquinol, paromomycin, or diloxanide furoate. Histoplasmosis treatment includes amphotericin B, fluconazole, or itraconazole. Trichinella treatment consists of steroids to relieve allergic symptoms, followed by treatment with albendazole or mebendazole. Treatment of strongyloides is ivermectin or albendazole. *S. typhi* is usually treated with a third-generation cephalosporin or a fluoroquinolone.

107. C (S&F ch85)
A Doppler ultrasound showing absent flow in the hepatic veins has a high sensitivity and specificity for BCS. Ten percent of cases occur in patients taking OCP. The pattern of liver function tests is not suggestive of alcoholic hepatitis where you would expect an AST/ALT ratio >2. Similarly, imaging and presentation are not suggestive of a hepatic adenoma or cholecystitis. The patient's CBD is not dilated on imaging and no stones are noted, making a diagnosis of choledocholithiasis unlikely.

108. D (S&F ch85)
Hepatic artery aneurysm (HAA) can be iatrogenic from hepatobiliary surgery, but may also be due to atherosclerotic disease or underlying connective tissue diseases such as Ehler-Danlos and SLE. Patients with multiple HAA or nonatherosclerotic HAA are at a high risk for rupture, which carries a high risk of mortality and treatment is warranted. The treatment of choice is embolization by interventional radiology. A biopsy is not warranted. HAA is not an indication for a liver transplant. Oral contraceptives are not involved in the pathogenesis of hepatic artery aneurysms, therefore there is no need to discontinue these medications.

109. E (S&F ch85)
This is a typical presentation for sinusoidal obstruction syndrome, which almost always occurs in patients receiving high-dose myeloablative chemotherapy in preparation for a bone marrow transplant. Treatment is symptomatic and symptoms typically resolve within a few weeks. Some patients may develop fulminant liver failure and this has high mortality. Patients who develop this condition are usually not candidates for a liver transplant in view of their cancer diagnosis. Transjugular intrahepatic portosystemic shunt may be helpful to ameliorate symptoms but is not the initial treatment of choice. There is no role for anticoagulation in this setting.

110. D (S&F ch85)
Peilosis hepatis is a relatively rare condition associated with the presence of large blood-filled cavities on histological examination of the liver. Associated conditions include infection with HIV, Bartonella, renal transplantation, and use of anabolic steroids. The histopathology

slide shows the typical enlarged blood-filled cyst surrounded by interrupted hepatocyte plates and sinusoid walls, which is typical of this condition.

111. B (S&F ch85)
Congenital porto-systemic shunts typically present at an early age but may occasionally present in an elderly patient. Recurrent episodes of encephalopathy associated with elevated ammonia levels in the absence of cirrhosis or portal hypertension is typical. In addition to medical treatment, the optimal intervention is to embolize the shunt. This usually resolves symptoms. A liver transplantation is rarely warranted. Urea cycle defects may cause a similar presentation, however, this patient has a clear shunt on imaging and this must be addressed first. Symptomatic treatment with lactulose and rifaximin is helpful; however, a more definitive approach would be to embolize any visible shunt. The patient is already on an adequate dose of lactulose and therefore increasing this dose is not warranted. Rifaximin may be added if embolizing the shunt is impossible or unsuccessful.

112. D (S&F ch85)
Patients with Budd-Chiari syndrome typically have a sub-acute presentation and often present with established cirrhosis. A fulminant presentation is very rare and most often seen amongst pregnant females usually in the setting of another underlying hypercoagulable condition. This condition carries very high mortality without a liver transplant. Anticoagulation is not likely to benefit this patient and may increase her risk of bleeding. Surgical shunting carries a very high mortality rate in this scenario and transjugular intrahepatic portosystemic shunt is also not likely to provide much benefit. The patient must be urgently evaluated for a liver transplant.

113. A (S&F ch85)
Patients with sinusoidal obstruction syndrome (SOS) typically present with new onset ascites, hyperbilirubinemia, and hepatomegaly. Many medications have been associated with SOS including azathioprine. While patients with ulcerative colitis are at higher risk for primary sclerosing cholangitis, the absence of any significant abnormality on MRCP makes this less likely. Similarly, there is no mention of occluded hepatic veins to suggest Budd-Chiari syndrome and no symptoms suggestive of underlying congestive heart failure or an allergic reaction.

114. C (S&F ch85)
Patients with established cirrhosis who present with new onset ascites should have abdominal imaging to evaluate for a portal vein thrombosis. This patient has an acute portal vein thrombus. In addition to evaluating for underlying hypercoagulable conditions, the patient should receive anticoagulation. Recanalization occurs in about 80% to 90% of patients who receive anticoagulation. Prior to starting treatment it is recommended to screen these patients for varices and initiate appropriate prophylaxis if these are present to reduce the risk of bleeding. Thrombolysis is associated with high risk of bleeding and is not indicated. Surgical thrombectomy and transjugular intrahepatic portosystemic shunt are more invasive procedures and not warranted particularly given the high response rate to anticoagulation. A transplant evaluation is not indicated at this time particularly since the patient's MELD score is low.

115. D (S&F ch85)
Patients with cirrhosis should be periodically screened for varices. Cavernous transformation indicates that this portal vein thrombus is chronic rather than acute. Long-term oral anticoagulation is not indicated in patients with chronic portal vein thrombosis as it will not lead to resolution of the thrombus and will increase the patient's risk for bleeding. An exception to this is if the patient has an underlying hypercoagulable condition. Surgical thrombectomy is associated with increased morbidity and mortality and is unlikely to provide any benefit in this setting since the patient has established portal hypertension. The patient does not have any symptoms such as ascites or refractory variceal bleeding to warrant referral for transjugular intrahepatic portosystemic shunt.

116. D (S&F ch86)
Hepatomegaly is found in approximately 75% of patient with fatty liver and alcoholic hepatitis and is the most common physical finding in these patients. Jaundice and ascites can be found in approximately 60% of patients, and is more frequent in patients with severe disease. Splenomegaly was found in approximately 26% of patients admitted with alcoholic liver disease. Displaced PMI is a finding consistent with cardiomegaly. Spider telangiectasias and lower extremity edema are other findings that can present in a patient with cirrhosis.

117. B (S&F ch86)
This patient's findings are consistent with severe alcoholic hepatitis. Patients with severe alcoholic hepatitis can present with modest elevation of serum aminotransferases, usually with an AST/ALT ratio greater than 2, in combination with elevated bilirubin levels, alkaline phosphatase levels, coagulopathy, fever in the absence of infection, and occasionally leukocytosis, with levels consistent with a leukemoid state. The use of prednisolone in patients with a Maddrey's discriminative function more than 32 have been demonstrated to reduce the mortality on several clinical trials. The combination of prednisolone and pentoxifylline has not proved to be superior to monotherapy with prednisolone. N-acetylcysteine is indicated for acetaminophen toxicity and has not demonstrated any role in management of alcoholic hepatitis. Tenofovir is an antiviral drug indicated for the treatment of chronic hepatitis B. This drug may also have some role in the treatment of acute liver failure secondary to acute hepatitis B, however, this patient serology is consistent with hepatitis B exposure, not active infection. He does not have a confirmed chronic hepatitis C and therapy with sofosbuvir and simeprevir is not indicated at this moment.

118. D (S&F ch86)
This patient's findings are consistent with severe alcoholic hepatitis. Patients with severe alcoholic hepatitis can present with modest elevation of serum aminotransferases, usually with an AST/ALT ratio greater than 2, in combination with elevated bilirubin levels, alkaline phosphatase levels, and coagulopathy, fever in the absence of infection and occasional leukocytosis with levels consistent with a leukemoid state. This patient does not have a serology consistent with acute hepatitis B. Acute hepatitis B might present with jaundice; however, it is characterized for marked elevation on aminotransferases. Acute hepatitis C is a rare cause of acute hepatitis and usually presents with marked elevation on serum aminotransferases (above 1000 U/L). Acetaminophen intoxication can also cause acute hepatitis and acute liver failure, particularly in alcoholics; however, it is more characterized with marked elevation of serum aminotransferases usually

around 1000 U/L. This patient, despite elevated serum ferritin and iron saturation, does not have diagnostic criteria for hereditary hemochromatosis.

119. B (S&F ch86)
Heavy alcohol consumption is one of the most important risk factors for the development of liver cirrhosis. Twenty ounces of wine is equal to approximately to 56 gm of alcohol daily, which is above the threshold to develop alcohol liver disease for a woman. The relative risk of liver cirrhosis is tenfold to thirtyfold higher for a heavy alcohol user with chronic hepatitis C. High cholesterol levels and insulin resistance are metabolic risk factors that have been associated with liver inflammation and disease, however, they are not as important as alcohol use for the development of liver cirrhosis. Moderate coffee consumption has been identified as a protective factor in patients with hepatitis C in some studies. A positive serology for hepatitis B core antibody does not increase the risk of cirrhosis.

120. A (S&F ch86)
This patient has histopathological findings consistent with alcoholic cirrhosis. Obesity, smoking, continuous alcohol use, and hepatitis C are well-recognized risk factors for the development of hepatocellular carcinoma. Previous exposure to hepatitis B with a positive hepatitis B core antibody is not a risk factor for hepatocellular carcinoma. Hypercholesterolemia, diabetes mellitus type II and age are not considered strong risk factors for the development of hepatocellular carcinoma.

121. D (S&F ch86)
The findings in this patient are consistent with alcoholic hepatitis. Several clinical features have been associated with severe disease in alcoholic hepatitis. Among them are hepatic encephalopathy, prolongation of the prothrombin time, bilirubin, renal insufficiency, leukocytosis, and age. These clinical features have been incorporated in different score models (Maddrey discriminative function, Lille score, Glasgow alcoholic hepatitis score, ABIC score) to calculate mortality risk and decide therapy on patients with alcoholic hepatitis. Hemoglobin level, hypokalemia, platelet count and AST/ALT ratio have not been associated with severe disease in patients with alcoholic hepatitis.

122. B (S&F ch86)
Prognosis of patients with alcoholic cirrhosis depends on the development of various liver-related complications. A Danish population-based study described the 1-year mortality of patients who presented with no complications, patients who presented with ascites, patients who presented with esophageal varices, patients who presented with esophageal varices and ascites, and patients who presented with hepatic encephalopathy. One-year mortality was 15% to 20% for patients with no complications, 20% for patients with esophageal varices, 30% after the development of ascites, 50% for those with esophageal varices and ascites, and 65% for patients with hepatic encephalopathy. Several score models have been used to stratify the mortality risk in patients with alcoholic cirrhosis. Among them are the Child-Pugh-Turcotte score, MELD score, and the Beclere model.

123. D (S&F ch86)
Patients with alcoholic disease can develop clinical deterioration after the ingestion of hepatotoxic drugs and herbal remedies. One of the most well known is the use of acetaminophen in patients with chronic alcohol use. Heavy alcohol use (and smoking) induces the CYP2E1, making them susceptible to acetaminophen intoxication secondary to glutathione depletion and rapid production of n-acetyl-p-benzoquinone (NAPQI). These patients might develop acetaminophen intoxication, even using acetaminophen at therapeutic levels for days to weeks. Despite the fact that clinical findings of alcoholic hepatitis and acetaminophen intoxication might be indistinguishable, in patients with acetaminophen toxicity the serum aminotransferases are usually elevated more than 1000 U/L. Acetaminophen levels are not helpful, especially if the time of last ingestion is not known. This patient has a serology of previous exposure to hepatitis B, and is not at risk of hepatitis B reactivation or acute hepatitis B. Liver failure secondary to hepatitis C is a very rare presentation. This patient does not have risk factors for acute exposure to hepatitis C and her positive serology might be secondary to chronic hepatitis C for needle sticks in the past. Elevated ferritin levels and iron saturation is commonly seen in patients with alcoholic liver disease. This patient does not fit the diagnostic criteria for hereditary hemochromatosis.

124. A (S&F ch86)
Obesity and smoking are two major risk factors associated with alcoholic liver disease progression and risk of hepatocellular carcinoma. Although this patient might have vitamin deficiencies, vitamin supplementation has not been demonstrated to decrease risk of hepatocellular carcinoma. Silymarin has been studied on patients with alcoholic liver disease, but it has not demonstrated to decrease the risk of hepatocellular carcinoma or disease progression. Pentoxifylline improves survival in patients with severe alcoholic hepatitis who are not candidates for prednisolone, but does not reduce the risk of hepatocellular carcinoma or disease progression.

125. E (S&F ch86)
Accurate assessment of nutritional status on a patient with alcoholic liver disease can be difficult. Many of the typical tests used as surrogate markers for nutrition can be altered secondary to the liver disease. Visceral proteins such as albumin and pre-albumin are produced in the liver and can be altered secondary to the liver disease. BMI is a poor marker of nutrition in a patient with fluid retention and creatinine-height index is not reliable in a patient with altered renal function. SGA is a simple bedside tool, which can be used to assess malnutrition, particularly in patients with ascites and muscle wasting.

126. D (S&F ch86)
This patient is presenting with clinical findings consistent with zinc deficiency that might complicate alcoholic liver disease. Zinc deficiency can cause skin lesions, night blindness, mental irritability, confusion, hepatic encephalopathy, anorexia, altered taste and smell, hypogonadism, and altered wound healing in patients with alcoholic liver disease. Lactulose is indicated for the treatment of hepatic encephalopathy; however, it is not a good alternative on patients with active diarrheas and will not help to resolve the rest of patient symptoms. Rifaximin is indicated in combination with lactulose for the treatment of hepatic encephalopathy. Patients with alcohol abuse can present with vitamin B_{12} deficiency, which is characterized for macrocytic anemia, and in severe cases impaired proprioception and subacute combined degeneration of the spinal cord. Patients with liver disease might be at

risk of vitamin A deficiency, which is characterized for impaired night vision, xerophthalmia, and xerosis.

127. D (S&F ch86)
The findings in this patient are consistent with severe alcoholic hepatitis. The use of prednisolone in patients with a Maddrey's discriminative function more than 32 has been demonstrated to reduce the mortality on several clinical trials. However, a dramatic reduction in survival has been shown in patients treated with glucocorticoids who had severe renal disease. Pentoxifylline is an alternative to therapy with steroids in patients with severe alcoholic hepatitis, who are not candidates for glucocorticoid therapy (active gastrointestinal bleeding, systemic infection, or renal insufficiency). The combination of prednisolone and pentoxifylline has not been proved to be superior to monotherapy with prednisolone. N-acetylcysteine is indicated for acetaminophen toxicity and has no demonstrated role in alcoholic hepatitis. Tenofovir is an antiviral drug for the treatment of chronic hepatitis B. This drug may have some role in acute liver failure secondary to acute hepatitis B, however, this patient's serology is consistent with previous hepatitis B exposure.

128. D (S&F ch86)
The clinical findings are consistent with severe alcoholic hepatitis. The 90-day mortality of patients who require intensive care unit management of 3 or more failing organ systems exceeds 90%. Patients with severe alcoholic hepatitis admitted with multiorgan failure have an extremely poor prognosis, and will benefit from palliative care team evaluation within the first days of admission to provide appropriate support to patients and relatives. A dramatic reduction in survival has been demonstrated in glucocorticoid-treated patients with severe renal disease, active infection, and/or GI bleeding. The combination of prednisolone and pentoxifylline has not proved to be superior to monotherapy with prednisolone. MARS is FDA approved for the treatment of severe drug-induced liver injury and refractory hepatic encephalopathy; its role in severe alcoholic hepatitis with multiorgan failure is not well defined. Patients with severe alcoholic hepatitis, who are actively using alcohol, are not considered suitable candidates for liver transplant. In addition, this patient has other findings that can be considered contraindications for liver transplant (e.g., active systemic infection, multiorgan failure, dependence on vasopressors).

129. D (S&F ch86)
Several pathophysiologic mechanisms have been identified in the development of alcoholic liver disease. Alcohol-induced intestinal dysfunction and endotoxemia has been identified as a mechanism promoting liver injury. High alcohol intake causes increased hepatic superoxide generation in the liver mitochondria with increasing generation of electrons along the respiratory system transport chain and increased NADH/NAD+ ratio. Deficiency of SAMe in alcoholic patients was first noted in the 1980s. SAMe is the primary biologic methyl donor through a transmethylation pathway that is a precursor of glutathione. Elevated levels of S-adenosylhomocyteine (SAH) and homocysteine have been identified in patients with alcoholic liver disease. Elevated SAH has been shown to sensitize hepatocytes to TNF-mediated destruction. Elevated biliary production of endothelin-1 with increased nitric oxide production and subsequent pulmonary vasodilation is a proposed mechanism for the development of hepatopulmonary syndrome (see S&F ch94).

130. E (S&F ch86)
The clinical presentations of this patient are consistent with alcoholic hepatitis. Patients with alcoholic hepatitis, with a Maddrey's discriminant function (DF) below 32, have a good prognosis and are well-treated with nutritional and supportive care. Occasionally, patients with alcoholic hepatitis can be misdiagnosed for Budd-Chiari syndrome on the basis of failure to visualize the hepatic veins on Doppler ultrasound, rapid deterioration, hepatomegaly, or caudate lobe hypertrophy. Careful evaluation of clinical presentations and biochemical features typical of alcoholic hepatitis (e.g., modest AST/ALT elevation with a 2:1 ratio vs. marked elevation of aminotransferases on Budd-Chiari syndrome) is required to distinguish between these two conditions. Failure to identify the correct diagnosis before initiating treatment with anticoagulation therapy or vascular shunts can increase mortality in patients with alcoholic hepatitis.Patients with mild alcoholic hepatitis (DF less than 32) will not benefit from glucocorticoid therapy.

131. B (S&F ch87)
This patient has some classic features for nonalcoholic steatohepatitis including obesity, recent weight gain, possible pre-diabetes, and mild liver enzymes elevation with ALT greater than AST. In addition to evaluation for other common causes of elevated liver tests (e.g., chronic viral etiologies, not listed as a choice), an ultrasound is the next best step because it is noninvasive, relatively inexpensive, and sensitive for steatosis. FibroSURE is relatively expensive and more appropriate for determining degree of steatohepatitis or fibrosis than it is for diagnostic purposes. While this patient may eventually be considered for bariatric surgery, nothing in the question stem suggests simple lifestyle modifications have been tried. A liver biopsy may also eventually be necessary to confirm the suspected diagnosis and stage the degree of fibrosis; however, it is premature in this patient. A CT of the abdomen is a reasonable alternative to ultrasound; however, it is more expensive and includes ionizing radiation without significant advantages for diagnosis of fatty liver disease.

132. A (S&F ch87)
Distinguishing between alcoholic steatohepatitis and nonalcoholic steatohepatitis is not reliably possible by histopathology. Options B to D are all evidence of fatty deposition in hepatocytes. Acidophil bodies mark hepatocyte death and are nonspecific.

133. E (S&F ch87)
The best first step in a patient with steatohepatitis who has not made an effort at diet, exercise, and lifestyle modification is to pursue lifestyle changes that promote weight loss and insulin sensitization. There is significant debate over the use of pharmacologic therapy for NASH with lack of clear guidelines and concerns based upon subpopulation and other comorbid risks.

134. A (S&F ch87)
NAFLD has been associated with colonic adenomas, metabolic syndrome, diabetes, vitamin D deficiency, cardiovascular disease, obstructive sleep apnea, hypothyroidism, polycystic ovary syndrome, pancreatic steatosis, and elevated serum uric acid levels. The other choices are not known to be associated with NAFLD.

135. B (S&F ch87)
Patients with NAFLD are clearly at high risk for cardiovascular, which is the primary cause of death in this population. choices, A, C, and D are certainly concerns, especially if she is cirrhotic, evidence of which is lacking based on this question stem. While she is female, ovarian cancer is not a relatively high risk for her epidemiologically.

136. D (S&F ch87)
Vitamin E has not been studied as a treatment for NASH in patients with diabetes and there are concerns about potential risks that could be exacerbated in diabetic patients (including cardiovascular risks). The guidelines recommend caution in using vitamin E in diabetic patients with NASH. Age, gender, atorvastatin, or hydrochlorothiazide use are not specific concerns or contraindications for vitamin E use.

137. B (S&F ch87)
The image shows the appearance of focal fatty liver on CT scan. The lesion is nonspherical shape, does not show mass effect, and has CT attenuation values consistent with soft tissue. Altered venous flow to the liver, tissue hypoxia, and intestinal malabsorption of lipoprotein are hypothesized pathogenesis mechanisms, though the exact cause is unknown. Dysplastic growth of hepatocytes could be seen in a dysplastic nodule or hepatocellular carcinoma. Hepatitis B virus is a possibility in a patient from an endemic country such as China, but it is not a known cause of focal fatty liver, nor is trauma.

138. A (S&F ch87)
This is the radiographic description of focal fatty liver. Focal fatty liver is a benign lesion. It isn't unreasonable to confirm the diagnosis with a different imaging modality, but the patient can be very reasonably reassured about its benign nature and likelihood of resolution. Biopsy would not be necessary with typical imaging findings of focal fatty liver and without arterial enhancement, mass effect, irregular shape, history of malignancy, mixed hypoechogenicity or hyperechogenicity on ultrasound. TACE, liver transplantation, and referral to an oncologist might all be things to do if a diagnosis of hepatocellular carcinoma was made.

139. C (S&F ch87)
Donor liver grafts with steatosis are associated with an increased risk of primary graft nonfunction and poorer overall outcomes. This is especially true if the liver graft has more than 60% steatosis. There is no known association with steatotic liver grafts and posttransplant malignancies. A patient who receives a steatosis liver graft would not be at increased risk of weight gain. Conversely, if they have trouble with primary nonfunction or other outcomes, the patient might have trouble gaining weight. Pretransplant hepatitis C recurs after transplant almost universally, regardless of the fat content of the liver graft. Posttransplant alcohol use is unrelated to the fat content of the donor liver.

140. B (S&F ch87)
AST and ALT levels greater than 10 times the upper limit of normal would be very unusual for NASH and should prompt looking for other causes of liver injury. Many patients with NASH have mild elevation of liver function tests with ALT greater than AST, which is often helpful in distinguishing it from alcoholic hepatitis. They also frequently have low positive ANA titers. Elevated serum ferritin is often seen, as is Kupffer cell accumulation of iron on liver biopsy (secondary to iron overload). Imaging often shows steatosis but with focal areas of sparing.

141. C (S&F ch88)
Based on his history and presenting laboratory values, you should be suspicious about acetaminophen overdose. Osmotic cathartics or binding agents have little to no role in the management of acetaminophen overdose. Trending his INR, oral N-acetylcysteine, and monitoring his mental status are standards in managing acetaminophen overdose. Checking his blood pH is an important aspect of the King's College Criteria, a prognostic scoring system.

142. D (S&F ch88)
Drugs like phenytoin and zidovudine can lower the dose threshold for acetaminophen-induced hepatotoxicity. While the other drugs present could be involved in idiosynchratic drug reactions, they do not lower the threshold for acetaminophen-induced hepatotoxicity.

143. A (S&F ch88)
Phenytoin reducing the dose threshold for acetaminophen-induced hepatotoxicity is a classic example of inhibition of drug metabolism. In this case, competition for phase 2 pathways, such as glucuronidation and sulfation, facilitates the presentation of unconjugated drug to the cytochrome P450 (CYP) system. The other choices have no relevance to phenytoin's role in acetaminophen-induced hepatotoxicity.

144. E (S&F ch88)
Formation of ester links to make a compound or metabolite more water soluble is a mechanism employed by phase 2 (conjugation) reactions. Phase 3 reactions involve secretion of drugs, drug metabolites, or their conjugates into bile. Several transporters participate and adenosine triphosphate-binding cassette (ABC) proteins are involved and require energy from ATP hydrolysis. Polymorphisms involving the genes responsible for Phase 3 reactions have been associated with human cholestatic liver diseases.

145. A (S&F ch88)
This is Hy's rule, which states that elevations of serum ALT levels to threefold or more above the ULN with an associated increase in the serum bilirubin concentration (at least two times the ULN), without an elevation of serum alkaline phosphatase elevation greater than two times the ULN, indicate the potential for the drug to cause acute liver failure at a rate of about 10% of the number of cases of jaundice. One percent of the patients in the trial met criteria; therefore, 0.1% could be expected during the marketing phase to have acute liver failure, or three in 3000.

146. D (S&F ch88)
Idiosyncrasy refers to the susceptibility of rare persons to hepatotoxicity from a drug that in conventional doses is usually safe. It is frequently characterized by a variable duration of latency, a wide range of histologic changes on biopsy, and lack of reliable injury in nonhuman species. Dose-dependent hepatotoxicity usually occurs after a short latent period (hours), is characterized by zonal necrosis or microvesicular steatosis on biopsy, and can be reproduced in nonhuman species. The prototypical drug for dose-dependent hepatotoxicity is acetaminophen.

147. D (S&F ch88)
For dose-dependent hepatotoxins, drug dose, drug serum levels, and duration of intake increase the risk of

hepatotoxicity. For idiosyncratic reactions, several factors other than genetic predisposition have been linked to higher risks. The most important factors are age, gender (frequently higher in females), exposure to other substances, a family history of previous drug reactions, other risk factors for liver disease/concomitant liver disease, and other medical disorders. Choice D has the most of these risk factors, so it is the best answer for highest risk of idiosyncratic hepatotoxicity.

148. C (S&F ch88)
In addition to checking for other common causes of mild to moderate liver enzymes elevation, all of her medications should be stopped if it is safe to do so, as it is in this case. This includes her chronic other-the-counter medications as well. Then her LFTs and INR should be monitored for resolution of the hepatitis. Provided they return to normal, her essential medications can be reintroduced while carefully monitoring her LFTs. At this point, with only mild to moderate elevatation of her liver enzymes without evidence of synthetic dysfunction, hospitalization would be unnecessary. Likewise, it is premature for a liver biopsy, though it can be considered if there is no improvement with medication withdrawal and the remainder of the workup is unrevealing. Contrasted cross-sectional imaging is unnecessary at this point, but could be a part of an evaluation for liver disease or advanced fibrosis depending on the course of her follow-up. There is no role for steroids in drug-induced liver injury (DILI).

149. E (S&F ch88)
In most cases of DILI, there should be discernible and progressive improvement after cessation of the offending medication, termed dechallenge. Clinical recovery from some medications, like amiodarone, may take months and can confound diagnosis and management. In carefully selected situations, rechallenge can be undertaken to confirm DILI or prove/disprove a particular drug as the offending agent. An example of a situation where rechallenge may be reasonable is when a particular drug is felt to be medically necessary and without adequate alternative. Regardless, rechallenge, if undertaken, should be done carefully and with informed consent of the patient. Liver biopsy during DILI can sometimes help, but most often is not specific for implicating an individual drug. A history of alcohol use can increase the risk of drug injury to some drugs, but is not specific in its own right. Cross sectional imaging will not implicate a specific drug. DILI is often accompanied for high liver enzymes elevation in the thousands, but this can occur with several drugs, both idiosyncratic and dose-dependent reactions, as well as liver injuries other than DILI.

150. A (S&F ch88)
His history and presentation are concerning for drug reaction with eosinophilia and systemic symptoms (DRESS) Syndrome. Patients with DRESS syndrome can develop Stevens-Johnson syndrome with mucositis. Cerebral edema is a risk of patients with fulminant hepatic failure with encephalopathy and coagulopathy, neither of which he has. While he was taking over-the-counter medications, which could have included acetaminophen, he has not taken them in weeks and thus would not have an elevated acetaminophen level. Furthermore, acetaminophen toxicity would not explain the rash or eosinophilia. Patients with DRESS syndrome usually have neutrophilia, not neutropenia. They also usually have elevations of acute phase reactants like the erythrocyte sedimentation rate.

151. C (S&F ch88)
The purpose of this question is to differentiate salicylate hepatotoxicity from Reye's syndrome. Among the features typical of Reye's syndrome, this child does not have encephalopathy, or elevated ammonia. Reye's syndrome is characterized by steatosis on biopsy, and the absence of steatosis differentiates Reye's syndrome from salicylate hepatotoxicity, which typically shows a nonspecific focal hepatitis with hepatocellular degeneration and hydropic changes. One would not expect significant fibrosis in the acute drug hepatotoxicity period. Inclusion bodies and hepatocyte ballooning are not typical of salicylate hepatotoxicity.

152. C (S&F ch89)
The best method to prevent halothane hepatotoxicity is avoidance of halothane, and there are many better options for anesthesia available in countries with modern medical capabilities. Both zinc and disulfiram have been studied but not proven effective in humans for preventing halothane toxicity. Control of her blood sugar and continuation of her chronic beta blocker therapy may be reasonable perioperative strategies, but they are unlikely to play any role in reducing her risk of halothane hepatotoxicity should she be given halothane.

153. D (S&F ch89)
The extent to which haloalkane anesthetics are metabolized by CYP enzymes predicts the likelihood of liver injury. Halothane is metabolized 20% to 30%, methoxyflurane 30%, enflurane 2%, sevoflurane 1%, isoflurane 0.2%, and desflurane less than 0.2% (see table at the end of the chapter).

154. E (S&F ch89)
Exposure to vinyl chloride is associated with a risk of angiosarcoma development with a mean latency of 25 years after exposure. Dichlorodiphenyl-trichloroethane is associated with hepatocellular carcinoma. Benzene, halothane, and cocaine are not known to be directly associated with hepatic malignancy.

155. C (S&F ch89)
This presentation and clinical findings are consistent with mushroom toxicity from *Amanita phylloides* or *Amanita verna*. Ingestion of these mushrooms has a high mortality from acute liver failure. The best data supports the use of silibinin (isolated from milk thistle) over other agents including penicillin G. There is no known role for steroid therapy. While hepatitis B virus is mentioned in the question, the simultaneous acute presentation of liver injury in all three patients suggest a form of poisoning rather than a flare up of hepatitis B. Therefore, treatment with antiviral medications such as tenofovir or lamivudine is unlikely to be useful.

156. B (S&F ch89)
The most common routes of industrial chemicals causing exposure, especially in an industrial setting, are through inhalation and transdermal absorption. Safety equipment, such as protective gloves/suites and respirators, may be required to reduce risks. Gastrointestinal absorption would require ingestion, accidental or intentional, which would be less likely given the apparent safety equipment protocol noncompliance.

157. A (S&F ch90)
The diagnostic accuracy for AIH is best when ANA and SMA are both present (74%). Patients with anti-SLA have a higher likelihood of disease relapse after treatment withdrawal. Anti-LKM1 is most commonly found in children. Atypical pANCA is common in type 1 AIH and may be useful in evaluating patients who lack ANA and SMA. Anti-LC1 is associated with severe liver inflammation and rapid progression to cirrhosis.

158. B (S&F ch90)
This patient is presenting with fulminant liver failure from autoimmune hepatitis. While corticosteroid therapy should be considered, the most appropriate next step is liver transplant evaluation. Her presentation is not suggestive of biliary obstruction or ischemic hepatitis.

159. D (S&F ch90)
Thirteen percent of patients with AIH are negative for ANA, SMA and anti-LKM1. Atypical pANCA and anti-SLA may be helpful to reclassify these patients as classic AIH. Hyperpigmentation is very uncommon in patients with AIH and would be more suggestive of primary biliary cirrhosis. Asymptomatic patients have a similar frequency of cirrhosis as symptomatic cases. Untreated asymptomatic patients have a reduced survival and therefore warrant treatment consideration. Serum IgG levels are normal in 25% to 39% of patients presenting with fulminant liver failure due to AIH.

160. D (S&F ch90)
This patient has had a suboptimal response to initial standard therapy for AIH as evidenced by worsening of transaminitis after 6 months of treatment. The most appropriate next step, according to the AASLD guidelines, is increasing the dosage of immunosuppression with prednisone and azathioprine. There is no indication for budesonide in patients not responding to prednisone, and it is not recommended to use this therapy in patients with cirrhosis. The patient remains compensated with a low MELD score, and therefore, transplant is not necessary at this point. Finally, the use of mycophenolate mofetil in the treatment of AIH has been studied in small single-center experiences as first-line or salvage therapy. It is not part of the standard treatment and its use in AIH must be highly individualized and carefully monitored.

161. D (S&F ch90)
HLA DR3 or DR4 support the diagnosis of autoimmune hepatitis (AIH). Elevated IgM is found in patients with primary biliary cirrhosis, while elevated IgG supports a diagnosis of AIH. Alkaline phosphatase/AST<1.5 also supports the diagnosis of AIH, while alkaline phosphatase/AST >3 and positive AMA levels are more suggestive of primary biliary cirrhosis. Female gender is a risk factor for AIH (see table at the end of the chapter).

162. B (S&F ch90)
This patient has type 2 autoimmune disease, which is more common in women and is associated with LKM1 antibody. Liver biopsy classically shows lymphoplasmacytic infiltrate with interface activity. The clinical course is often aggressive resulting in cirrhosis within a 3-year period. These patients, especially young adults with autoimmune hepatitis (AIH) (between 18 to 40 years of age) have a high rate of treatment failure (exceeding 20%) to steroids. Elevated IgG level and anti-LKM1 antibody are strongly suggestive of autoimmune hepatitis in this patient, not viral (CMV or HSV) or drug-induced hepatitis. Atypical pANCA is present in 50% to 92% of type 1 AIH. It is absent in type 2 AIH.

163. A (S&F ch90)
The biopsy demonstrates centrilobular zone 3 necrosis with hepatocyte rosettes. This clinical scenario is consistent with posttransplant de novo autoimmune hepatitis which is seen in up to 4% of liver transplant patients. Treatment is similar to that of autoimmune hepatitis and consists of initiation of oral prednisone; intravenous pulse corticosteroids is not necessary. Tacrolimus trough level is in therapeutic range (5-20 ng/mL) for liver transplant, and there is no role for increasing the dosage. Ursodeoxycholic acid or ERCP are not indicated in de novo AIH.

164. D (S&F ch90)
Budesonide in addition to azathioprine is an efficacious option for treatment of autoimmune hepatitis (AIH) that results in less corticosteroid-related side effects. Azathioprine monotherapy is not recommended as initial therapy. Higher doses of prednisone are recommended for initial monotherapy (60 mg daily) or in combination with azathioprine (30 mg daily). Tacrolimus is usually reserved for AIH refractory to conventional treatment.

165. D (S&F ch90)
Based on serology studies and liver biopsy findings, this patient has evidence of autoimmune hepatitis and primary biliary cirrhosis overlap syndrome. In these patients it is reasonable to start the most benign treatment, ursodeoxycholic acid, and follow clinical response. Despite the correct dose of ursodeoxycholic acid (13-15 mg/kg daily), this patient demonstrated a worsening of transaminitis, which is best treated with the addition of azathioprine and prednisone. The patient is already on appropriate weight-based ursodeoxycholic acid and increasing the dose will be of no benefit. There is nothing to suggest PSC or need for ERCP in this patient. The pathogenesis of this patient's illness appears autoimmune in nature and not a drug hepatotoxicity.

166. A (S&F ch90)
A MELD score of 12 or more at the time of presentation identifies 97% of persons who will fail conventional glucocorticoid therapy, die of liver failure, or require liver transplantation. Older patients and those with HLA-DRB1*0401 are more likely to respond to conventional treatment. Anti-SLA is associated with more severe disease and long-term treatment dependence. Relapse occurs in half of patients within 6 months of treatment discontinuation even in the patients who maintained normal liver enzymes on treatment.

167. E (S&F ch91)
The most frequent antigen against which AMAs are directed is PDC-E2. AMA does not appear to have direct cytotoxic effects in primary biliary cirrhosis (PBC). This is evidenced by (1) persistence of AMA after liver transplantation without evidence of disease recurrence, and (2) disease severity does not correlate to antibody titer. 90% to 95% of patients with PBC are AMA positive.

168. B (S&F ch91)
Primary biliary cirrhosis (PBC) is predominantly found in women, with a female-to-male ratio of 9:1. The most common symptoms include fatigue and pruritus. It is commonly seen that relatives of patients with PBC have other autoimmune conditions. Approximately 25% of patients with PBC have hepatomegaly.

169. C (S&F ch91)
Patients with primary biliary cirrhosis (PBC) are more likely to have had a urinary tract infection within the 5 years preceding the diagnosis of PBC compared to matched controls. Several HLA class II genes have been linked to PBC. While the disease is associated with tobacco smoking, no association exists with marijuana smoking. Minocycline has been associated with the development of autoimmune hepatitis, not PBC.

170. A (S&F ch91)
Higher fatigue levels are associated with increased risk of death and need for liver transplantation. Pruritus may occur at any point in the course of the disease and often resolves as the disease progresses. Sixty percent of patients are asymptomatic at the time of diagnosis; however, it is not uncommon to develop symptoms during the course of the disease. Dry eyes and dry mouth are common complaints among patients with primary biliary cirrhosis.

171. D (S&F ch91)
The biopsy shows mononuclear inflammatory cells of the portal tract with some disruption of the limiting plates. The bile ducts are surrounded by inflammatory cells. This patient has AMA-negative primary biliary cirrhosis and should be started on ursodeoxycholic acid. A majority of these patients will be ANA positive; however, the biopsy does not suggest autoimmune hepatitis. Therefore, there is no indication for prednisone and azathioprine. Her MRCP reveals a mild dilated common bile duct that is common in the setting of previous cholecystectomy. There is no indication of primary sclerosing cholangitis (PSC), and therefore, ERCP and colonoscopy are not indicated.

172. E (S&F ch91)
An important role of apoptosis in the pathogenesis of primary biliary cirrhosis (PBC) is emerging and these findings could explain in part the mechanism of UDCA, an agent shown to suppress apoptosis. The most effective dose of UDCA is 13-15 mg/kg/day. A lower rate of response is observed in men and patients diagnosed at an earlier age (before age 30). Biochemical response to UDCA is predictive of better long-term clinical outcomes. Several studies have shown UDCA improves transplant free survival in PBC.

173. A (S&F ch91)
The appropriate dose of UDCA for primary biliary cirrhosis (PBC) treatment is 13-15 mg/kg/day. Based on this, the patient's UDCA dosing is suboptimal and should be increased to 500 mg by mouth twice daily. Although budesonide may benefit patients with PBC, the data is too limited to currently support its use. Methotrexate, azathioprine, and cyclosporine have no benefit in PBC.

174. C (S&F ch91)
Lipid abnormalities are found in up to 85% of patients with primary biliary cirrhosis (PBC); however, the risk of myocardial infarction and stroke does not appear to be increased. The use of statins is safe among PBC patients who would benefit from lipid-lowering therapy. In patients with PBC, the severity of osteoporosis increases as liver disease advances, and treatment with bisphosphonates appears safe. Reduced night vision may be an indication of vitamin A deficiency.

175. B (S&F ch91)
The most appropriate next step is discontinuation of rifampin. Rifampin is effective in the treatment of pruritus; however, it is associated with reversible liver injury in 15% of patients. Currently the patient is on the appropriate weight-based dose of UDCA (13-15 mg/kg/day) and increasing the dose provides no benefit. Colchicine has no proven benefit in the treatment of primary biliary cirrhosis. A repeat liver biopsy is of little utility and unnecessary. The patient's MELD score is only 12 and therefore liver transplant evaluation is unnecessary at this time.

176. E (S&F ch91)
The development of complications from chronic cholestasis, including fatigue, refractory pruritus, or persistent hyperbilirubinemia in the absence of cirrhosis or malignancy should prompt physicians to consider referral for liver transplantation. From 1995 to 2006, the absolute number of liver transplants performed for primary biliary cirrhosis (PBC) each year decreased. Liver transplant survival outcomes for PBC are similar or exceed transplantation for other etiologies. PBC can recur after transplantation, but not in a majority of patients (0 to 35%). AMA levels may persist after liver transplantation and do not correlate with recurrent PBC.

177. A (S&F ch92)
BRTO may be associated with increase in portal pressure to the liver and can worsen ascites and esophageal varices. TIPS is effective in decreasing portal pressures and is an effective treatment for gastroesophageal varices and refractory ascites. Balloon tamponade and cyanoacrylate injections would not affect portal pressures. Surgical creation of a portacaval shunt is very effective at decompressing gastroesophageal varices and treating ascites. This is in contrast to selective and partial portosystemic shunts, which may increase the risk of ascites because hepatic sinusoidal pressure is not reduced.

178. D (S&F ch92)
Given the patient's history with risk factors for pancreatitis, the patient's bleeding isolated fundal varix is most likely related to splenic vein thrombosis caused by chronic pancreatitis. The splenic vein courses along the posterior surface of the pancreas, and inflammation can lead to thrombosis. Since the short gastric veins drain the fundus, splenic vein thrombosis can lead to the development of isolated gastric fundal varices. NRH is a cause of noncirrhotic portal hypertension that is usually diagnosed by liver biopsy and is not particularly associated with the formation of fundal varices. The risk of variceal hemorrhage may be increased in patients with hepatocellular carcinoma but would not have a predisposition for fundal varices. Budd-Chiari syndrome (thrombosis in the hepatic veins) is a cause of posthepatic portal hypertension and can present with variceal hemorrhage, but would not be an expected cause of isolated fundal varices. Portal vein thrombosis is a cause of prehepatic portal hypertension but would not be expected to cause isolated fundal varices.

179. D (S&F ch92)
The measurements show a normal free hepatic venous pressure and elevated wedge pressure, with an elevated hepatic vein pressure gradient (HVPG) of 7 mm Hg (which is the difference between the wedge hepatic pressure and free hepatic vein pressure). This is consistent with sinusoidal causes of portal hypertension, such as alcoholic cirrhosis. Portal vein thrombosis leads to prehepatic portal hypertension, while sarcoidosis and schstosomiasis lead to presinusoidal portal hypertension. In

these two types of portal hypertension, measurements should show a normal free hepatic venous pressure and a normal HVPG. Constrictive pericarditis leads to posthepatic portal hypertension, which results in elevation of both free and wedge hepatic pressures and a normal HVPG. Refer to the table at the end of the chapter.

180. C (S&F ch92)
Carvedilol has both nonselective B-adrenergic blockade as well as weak alpha-receptor blockade activity, which is thought to decrease portal flow and intrahepatic vascular resistance, respectively. Propranolol, on the other hand, is a nonselective beta-blocker that blocks β1-adrenergic and β2-adrenergic receptors to decrease cardiac output and portal flow. It is not thought to have any effect on intrahepatic resistance. Prazosin (an α-1 adrenergic blocker), isosorbide mononitrate (a nitrate), and simvastatin have all been show to decrease intrahepatic vascular resistance but are clinically rarely used for this purpose.

181. A (S&F ch92)
The number of varices is the least important variable for predicting the patient's risk of future hemorrhage. The size of the varices, presence of bleeding stigmata, elevated HVPG, and Child-Pugh class have been shown to be the most important predictors of bleeding.

182. C (S&F ch92)
The MELD formula was originally derived to predict survival in patients undergoing transjugular intrahepatic portosystemic shunt (TIPS) placement and has been widely validated and uses the bilirubin, INR, and creatinine. This patient's calculated MELD score of 27 predicts a high (76%) 3-month mortality. Studies have shown that older patients have higher post-TIPS mortality and incidence of hepatic encephalopathy (Casadaban et al., Dig Dis Sci 2014 and Parvinian et al J Vasc Interv Radiol 2013) and this patient is relatively young. Although the etiology of liver disease was originally a factor in calculating the MELD score, it has been removed. The platelet level may be related to bleeding-related complications associated with the procedure but is not a powerful predictor of outcomes. Recent widespread use of polytetrafluoroethylene-covered stents has significantly reduced the rate of shunt stenosis but has not been associated with worsening trend of liver failure.

183. D (S&F ch92)
Primary prophylaxis of esophageal variceal hemorrhage in patients with cirrhosis who only have small varices includes repeat endoscopy in 1 to 2 years. If there are no varices seen, the endoscopy needs to be repeated in 2 to 3 years. Nadolol or EVL are both acceptable measures if large varices are found during screening endoscopy. There is no role for transjugular intrahepatic portosystemic shunt as the primary prophylaxis of esophageal variceal hemorrhage in cirrhotic patients.

184. E (S&F ch92)
Studies have suggested that the risk of bleeding is more likely in patients with more severe cirrhosis as measured by MELD score or Child-Pugh score. In contrast to esophageal varices, reduction of HVPG < 12 mm Hg itself may be ineffective to control or prevent bleeding from gastric varices. Therefore, if large gastric varices are still visualized on portogram, obliteration embolization should strongly be considered. In general, small varices are less likely to bleed than similar-sized esophageal varices due to overlying gastric mucosa and decreased transmural pressure gradient in the abdomen. Due to complications related to transjugular intrahepatic portosystemic shunt, especially in decompensated cirrhotics and unclear rate of hemorrhage, primary prophylaxis with TIPS placement is not recommended. Gastric varices are only to bleed when they are large (>20 mm in diameter). Bleeding is more likely in patients with IGV1 and GOV2 (fundal varices) compared to other types of gastric varices that involve gastroesophageal junction.

185. B (S&F ch92)
Guidelines recommend either EVL or nonselective beta-blockers (NSBB) like nadolol for primary prophylaxis of patients with moderate or large-sized varices. Choice of treatment between these modalities may be determined by treating provider and patient preferences. In this patient EVL, would be preferred since use of NSBB requires compliance by patients and should not be used in insulin-dependent diabetes with episodes of hypoglycemia. Nitrates can decrease portal pressure by decreasing portal venous blood flow and possibly by a reduction in intrahepatic resistance; however, its use is no longer recommended for primary prophylaxis and is associated with limiting side effects. Transjugular intrahepatic portosystemic shunt is not recommended for primary prophylaxis of bleeding from esophageal varices. Metoprolol is not an NSBB and should not be used for primary prophylaxis.

186. C (S&F ch92)
A growing body of evidence suggests that there is risk of increasing portal pressures and rebleeding by over-transfusing PRBC to levels of 10 g/dL. A restrictive transfusion strategy with a threshold of 7 g/dL may produce better outcomes. Early administration of vasoactive drugs such as octreotide in the United States or terlipressin around the world decrease portal blood flow and is associated with improved hemostasis and shorter hospitalization length. Use of an oral quinolone like norfloxacin or intravenous cetriaxone is recommended because antibiotics have been shown to decrease mortality and reduce risk of recurrent bleeding. Endoscopic therapy such as EVL is recommended to achieve hemostasis, if possible. Recent data shows that patients considered at high risk of treatment (Child-Pugh class C or Child-Pugh class B with active bleeding) have a reduced rate of treatment failure and mortality from early use of transjugular intrahepatic portosystemic shunt.

187. A (S&F ch92)
This is a presentation of chronic, slow bleeding from portal hypertensive gastropathy (PHG). Beta-blockers and iron supplements are recommended for patients with severe PHG and anemia. EVL is ineffective for controlling diffuse bleeding from portal hypertensive gastropathy. APC is used for treatment of gastric antral vascular ectasia (GAVE), which is most common in the antrum rather than fundus. Transjugular intrahepatic portosystemic shunt or liver transplant are not the first-line treatment for slow bleeding from PHG; however, patients who are transfusion dependent from PHG despite beta blockade and iron supplement may be considered for TIPS.

188. E (S&F ch92)
Gastric antral vascular ectasia (GAVE) is an uncommon cause of upper gastrointestinal bleeding seen both in patients with cirrhosis and connective tissue diseases. Since GAVE does not seem to be a direct result of portal hypertension, reduction of the portal pressure gradient with measures such as transjugular intrahepatic portosystemic shunt or beta blockade is ineffective. A variety of endoscopic treatments, such as thermal coagulation,

argon plasma coagulation, and radiofrequency ablation may be used in addition to supportive measures. Antrectomy is effective if patients are suitable surgical candidates and have failed endoscopic therapy.

189. E (S&F ch92)
Although it may be technically difficult, transjugular intrahepatic portosystemic shunt (TIPS) placement in Budd-Chiari syndrome can decompress congested hepatic segments with good outcomes. TIPS placement is not recommended for primary prophylaxis of gastric varices. Advanced age and congestive heart failure are contraindications to TIPS. Patients with Caroli syndrome have multiple cystic dilations of intrahepatic biliary ducts and TIPS placement may involve transversal of a cyst resulting in hemorrhage with poor outcomes, and is a contraindication. Placement of TIPS immediately increases venous return to the heart and decreases systemic vascular resistance, and patients with pulmonary hypertension may not be able to handle the increased volume.

190. D (S&F ch92)
Schistosomiasis is one of the most common causes of noncirrhotic portal hypertension worldwide. As part of the life cycle, eggs inhabit the mesenteric veins and may get trapped in terminal portal venules, which results in chronic inflammation and later fibrosis. In early stages, the site of portal resistance is presinusoidal and later sinusoidal. The remainders of the listed conditions are examples of "post-hepatic" portal hypertension.

191. A (S&F ch92)
When the site of increased resistance is located at the sinusoidal level, the WHVP will be increased and the FHVP will be normal, resulting in an increased hepatic venous pressure gradient (HVPG) (see table at the end of the chapter).

192. B (S&F ch92)
Causes of posthepatic portal hypertension result in increased FHVP and thus increased WHVP. However the difference between the two (HVPG) will be normal since the site of resistance is not at the sinusoidal level. See table at the end of the chapter.

193. B (S&F ch93)
Dietary sodium restriction and diuretics are the treatment of choice for end-stage liver disease (ESLD) patients with ascites. Patients who are adherent to a low sodium diet should lose weight while on diuretic therapy. Diuretic doses can be titrated as needed. Fluid restriction is not recommended for treatment of ascites, and should be avoided in all cases where the patient's sodium is >120 mEq/L. Dietary sodium restriction alone is not the treatment of choice for ascites. Single large-volume paracentesis will have no effect on preventing future episodes of ascites.

194. C (S&F ch93)
The treatment of choice for ascites is diuretics and sodium restriction. This patient has been on diuretics, but compliance with the low sodium diet should be confirmed prior to initiating any changes to his therapy. Sports drinks are not an effective source of electrolytes. Transjugular intrahepatic portosystemic shunt (TIPS) is an appropriate second-line therapy for patients with truly diuretic-resistant ascites. If this patient is compliant with a low sodium diet, then a trial of increased diuretic doses should be initiated prior to considering TIPS.

195. D (S&F ch93)
Alcohol abuse is one of the few reversible causes of ascites. In the absence of cirrhosis, this patient could avoid further episodes of ascites if he can abstain from alcohol. In the setting of chronic alcoholism, cardiac dysfunction can certainly lead to ascites. While this patient's displaced PMI on exam provides evidence of cardiomegaly, cardiac ascites typically presents with an ascitic fluid protein level >2.5g/dL. Dietary sodium restriction and diuretics are the mainstay of ascites treatment in the setting of portal hypertension, especially when the patient has cirrhosis. This patient, who does not have evidence of cirrhosis on recent imaging, could benefit with intense alcohol rehabilitation. There is no reported fever or elevated WBC count to suggest an infectious etiology. There are not enough WBCs in the ascitic fluid to suggest spontaneous bacterial peritonitis.

196. A (S&F ch93)
This patient's history and exam are suggestive of a cardiac abnormality. While liver disease and heart disease can both lead to ascites, an ascitic fluid protein level >2.5 g/dL points to heart failure as the etiology of ascites. His elevated blood pressure, prominent PMI, and sternal heave also suggest heart failure as the etiology of ascites. The normal bilirubin, albumin, and prothrombin time lower the likelihood of liver disease as the etiology for his ascites. There are no signs to suggest an infection.

197. A (S&F ch93)
Flank fullness with shifting dullness is the most specific physical exam finding for ascites. In the absence of these findings, a patient has a ≤10% chance of having fluid in their abdomen. Shifting dullness does not offer much insight into the presence of absence of ascites.

198. C (S&F ch93)
Any chronic liver disease patient with an acute disruption of their baseline should be screened for hepatocellular carcinoma. The patient should also have a diagnostic paracentesis given at the onset of symptoms consistent with hepatic encephalopathy. Random urine sodium-to-potassium ratios can be used to help identify patients that are not adhering to a low sodium diet. Patients with a ratio >1 who are not losing weight are not likely adherent to a low sodium diet. Fluid restriction is not recommended for controlling ascites. This patient has clinical signs of hepatic encephalopathy, and will not benefit from having ammonia levels measured. As the patient's weight remains stable, without evidence of worsening ascites, he does not need to have his dose of diuretics increased.

199. D (S&F ch93)
Patients with cirrhosis tend to have multiple laboratory indicators of coagulopathy. These patients, however, tend to have a balance of abnormalities of pro- and anti-coagulants with relatively preserved coagulation. As such, there are few contraindications to paracentesis. The procedure can be safely performed in patients with an INR up to ~8, and with platelet levels >20,000/μL. The only true contraindication to paracentesis is disseminated intravascular coagulation (DIC). The elevated D-dimer, low fibrinogen, and elevated INR seen in (D) suggest DIC, and therefore, would preclude paracentesis in a patient with these values.

200. E (S&F ch93)
Any patient with cirrhosis and ascites presenting with fever and abdominal pain should be evaluated

immediately for spontaneous bacterial peritonitis (SBP). The elevated WBC count with a predominance of neutrophils (count >250 cells/uL) suggests SBP. Ascitic fluid cultures should be sent at the time of the diagnostic paracentesis, The lab results obtained from this patient require immediate antibiotic treatment. Studies have shown that intravenous third generation cephalosporins, such as cefotaxime, provide broad antibiotic coverage for the majority of organisms that cause SBP. Oral norfloxacin can provide antibiotic coverage for SBP, however, studies have shown lower efficacy when compared to intravenous cefotaxime. norfloxacin can be used to prevent recurrent episodes of SBP. A repeat paracentesis will offer no new information. Any delay in antibiotic initiation can lead to significant morbidity and mortality.

201. B (S&F ch93)
Infection of ascitic fluid is usually the result of spontaneous bacterial peritonitis (SBP). A single organism typically causes SBP. The bacterial load is usually so low that a gram stain does not stain positive for any organisms. The patient in this case presents with signs of a severe infection. The ascitic fluid confirms a suspected infection, however, the presence of multiple organisms on gram stain suggests a secondary bacterial peritonitis. Given the patient's history of Crohn disease, intestinal perforation should be suspected. Abdominal imaging to confirm perforation should be obtained immediately. Testing ascitic fluid LDH can support secondary bacterial peritonitis if the value is >225 U/L, however, the polymicrobial gram stain obviates the need for LDH testing. Metronidazole should be started for anaerobic coverage; however, finding and repairing intestinal perforation should be the top priority. Awaiting culture results or repeating paracentesis would delay treatment, leading to a significant increase in mortality.

202. D (S&F ch93)
Oral Norfloxacin 400 mg daily is the treatment of choice for secondary prevention of spontaneous bacterial peritonitis (SBP). Ciprofloxacin and rimethoprim-sulfamethoxazole can both be used for secondary prevention, but are usually considered second-line agents. Amoxicillin and doxycycline are not used for prophylaxis.

203. C (S&F ch93)
This use of antibiotics to prevent SBP in patients with actively bleeding varices has been confirmed in multiple tries. The increased risk of SBP with active variceal bleeding appears to be associated more with shock than bleeding. This patient has minor oozing during a routine banding procedure and should not be managed as a case of overt gastrointestinal bleeding.

204. E (S&F ch93)
Hepatic hydrothorax can occur in patients with end-stage liver disease. These patients typically have a small defect in the diaphragm allowing for the passage of fluid between the peritoneum and thoracic cavity. Sodium restriction, diuresis, and intermittent thoracentesis are the first-line therapy for hepatic hydrothorax. Transjugular intrahepatic portosystemic shunt can be considered in patients with uncontrollable symptoms who do not respond to first-line therapy. Chest tube insertion can be difficult to remove, and should not be placed in patients with hepatic hydrothorax. VATS with pleurodesis can be considered in these patients, but they tend to be poor surgical candidates. Peritoneovenous shunts should not be pursued in these patients.

205. C (S&F ch93)
Patients diagnosed with SBP should receive albumin 1.5 g/kg on admission and then 1.0 g/kg on day 3 after admission. There is no need to give intravenous cefotaxime for 10 days. Discharging the patient on oral antibiotics without giving a second dose of albumin would not be recommended. After the second dose of albumin, this patient could likely be discharged on oral antibiotics.

206. D (S&F ch93)
Patients who truly adhere to a low sodium diet should lose weight if their random urine sodium-to-potassium ratio is greater than 1. As this patient's ratio is 1.5, she should not be gaining weight. Counseling this patient to ensure she is truly complying with a low sodium diet could help avoid an unnecessary alteration of her medications. If she is truly adhering to a 2 g/day sodium diet, then increasing the dose of her diuretics can be considered. Many patients are incorrectly labeled as diuretic resistant. The sodium-to-potassium ratio should be checked prior to making alterations of a patient's medications. Fluid restriction should not be recommended for ascites prevention.

207. D (S&F ch93)
This patient, who was given multiple doses of intravenous furosemide, should be evaluated for diuretic-induced azotemia.. Intravenous furosemide should be avoided in patients with cirrhosis. While effective for diuresis in heart failure, intravenous furosemide can rapidly lead to azotemia that can be confused with hepatorenal syndrome type 1. Hepatorenal syndrome type 2 does not present this acutely. Acute tubular necrosis and acute interstitial nephritis are less likely in this clinical scenario. This patient's renal dysfunction may be reversed with intravenous fluids and discontinuation of diuretics.

208. C (S&F ch93)
Midodrine is an alpha-adrenergic receptor agonist used as an antihypotensive. Its hemodynamic effects improve renal blood flow and creatinine clearance. In patients with a systolic blood pressure less than 100 mm Hg, midodrine can be started at 5 mg by mouth three times daily, and titrated to achieve a 10 mm Hg increase in blood pressure or a systolic blood pressure greater than 100 mmHg. This increase in blood pressure can improve the efficacy of diuretics in a hypotensive cirrhotic patient. In the absence of azotemia, there is no need to stop diuretics in a cirrhotic patient. Diuretic dose should not be increased without addressing the patient's hypotension. Transjugular intrahepatic portosystemic shunt can be pursued for patients with refractory ascites, however, this patient cannot yet be labeled as refractory. There is no MELD exception for this patient at this time.

209. D (S&F ch93)
This patient has signs and symptoms of tuberculous peritonitis. Any immigrant presenting with abdominal pain, fever, and ascites should be evaluated for tuberculosis. Further evidence supporting tuberculosis in this patient include left-sided pleural effusion, serum-ascites albumin gradient (SAAG) <1.1, and elevated peritoneal WBC count without a predominance of neutrophils. Malignancy related effusion would be unlikely to present with a left-sided pleural effusion. The patient's age also lowers the likelihood of malignant ascites. Hepatocellular carcinoma (HCC) should be suspected in any patient with chronic liver disease who presents with new onset ascites; however, this patient's laboratory studies and presentation are unlikely to support HCC. Pancreatic ascites can present with neutrophilic

ascites and a SAAG <1.1; However, the low ascitic fluid amylase lowers the likelihood of pancreatic ascites.

210. B (S&F ch94)
No specific marker is reliable for the diagnosis of hepatic encephalopathy. However blood ammonia levels might be a useful indicator of hepatic encephalopathy in a patient with urea cycle syndromes with no cirrhosis or portal hypertension. Serum ammonia blood level is commonly measured on patients with cirrhosis and portal hypertension, but it is not sensitive or specific for hepatic encephalopathy. Several factors might raise the ammonia levels on sample (GI bleeding, ingestion of certain medications, the use of tourniquet when sample is drawn), and make this laboratory test of poor value for hepatic encephalopathy diagnosis.

211. D (S&F ch94)
The most important step in the management of acute hepatic encephalopathy (HE) is to identify precipitating factors and start treatment directed toward eliminating or correcting those factors, in this case suspected infection. The use of nonabsorbable disacharides has been an effective treatment for acute and chronic hepatic encephalopathy, producing catharsis and colonic acidification. However, is inappropriate to start lactulose therapeutically without addressing precipitating events of HE. In the past, restricting protein intake was recommended on the treatment of HE; however, recent studies have suggested that limiting protein-calorie intake is not beneficial in patients with HE. Rifaximin is a poorly absorbed antibiotic that was approved by the FDA in 2010, in combination with lactulose, for the treatment of chronic HE and for the reduction of overt HE in patients with advanced chronic liver disease. However, as discussed above it is inappropriate to start monotherapy with this drug without addressing precipitating events of HE. MARS demonstrated reduction in blood ammonia levels and improvement in severe HE in patients with acute-on-chronic liver failure. MARS was recently approved by the FDA for treatment of refractory encephalopathy. Its role on the treatment of acute encephalopathy is not defined.

212. A (S&F ch94)
This patient is most probably presenting with hepatorenal syndrome (HRS). Pathophysiology of HRS is complex and incompletely understood. Three components contribute to the initiation and perpetuation of the disorder: (1) arterial vasodilation on the splanchnic and systemic circulation, (2) renal arterial vasoconstriction and (3) cardiac dysfunction. HRS is a functional disorder and no laboratory or imaging studies alone are enough to establish the diagnosis. In HRS, the kidneys are histologically intact. Another possible renal disorder that can complicate advanced cirrhosis is acute tubular necrosis. Option C is characteristic of membrano-proliferative glomerulonephritis. Option D is histological findings of membranous glomerulonephritis. Findings on option E are consistent with minimal change disease.

213. C (S&F ch94)
This patient meet the diagnostic criteria for hepatorenal syndrome (HRS) defined by the International Ascites Club Consensus Workshop in 2007 that include: cirrhosis with ascites, serum creatinine greater than 1.5 m/dL, lack of improvement in creatinine levels after diuretic withdrawal and significant volume expansion, absence of shock, no evidence of recent use of nephrotoxic drugs, and lack of renal parenchymal disease. HRS physiology is not completely understood; however, three major components of its pathophysiology include arterial vasodilation in the splanchnic and systemic circulation with reduction of the effective circulatory volume, renal arterial vasoconstriction, and cardiac dysfunction. When patients with cirrhosis develop portal hypertension in the early stages, increase in cardiac output compensates for the decrease in effective circulatory volume and causes a hyperdynamic circulation. However, recent data demonstrate that cardiac output is impaired in patients with cirrhosis that develop HRS compared with patient with no HRS, suggesting that cardiac dysfunction is an important factor in the development of HRS, thus options D and E are incorrect.

214. D (S&F ch94)
Patients with hepatorenal syndrome (HRS) have a high mortality rate compared with other cirrhotic patients. This underscores the importance of prevention of HRS addressing intravascular depletion, avoiding nephrotoxic drugs, and using antibiotics in cirrhotic patients when indicated. The use of cefotaxime in combination with intravenous albumin, within 6 hours after diagnosis of spontaneous bacterial peritonitis (SBP) and then on day 3 has demonstrated to decrease the mortality rate in cirrhotic patients. Routine follow-up diagnostic paracentesis is not generally indicated after the diagnosis of SBP, unless the patient presents symptoms of active infections or there is a concern of an atypical or nosocomial infection. Piperacillin/tazobactan is not the recommended first-line agent for the treatment of SBP.

215. D (S&F ch94)
Liver transplantation is the only modality that has the potential to reverse the renal dysfunction and the liver disease, and should be considered in all patients with hepatorenal syndrome (HRS) who are candidates for transplant. The uses of dopamine in combination with octeotride and albumin have not improved the outcome of HRS. Transjugular intrahepatic portosytemic shunt (TIPS) placement is an effective treatment for refractory ascites, which is a precursor of HRS; however, TIPS can seriously complicate liver function, especially in patient with decompensated liver disease and high MELD score. Continuous renal replacement therapy is a treatment for acute on chronic renal dysfunction, but it not effective in HRS. One trial demonstrated that the use of nonselective endothelin receptor antagonist (to reduce intrarenal vasoconstriction) in patients with HRS type 2 was deleterious.

216. C (S&F ch94)
This patient has diagnostic criteria for hepatopulmonary syndrome, which is characterized by microvascular dilatation in the precapillary and capillary pulmonary arterial circulation mediated by nitric oxide overproduction. Option A is the classic presentation of congestive heart failure, which is characterized by volume overload, pulmonary edema, extremity swelling, orthopnea, and no platypnea. Option B is more characteristic of chronic obstructive pulmonary disease. Opion D shows the expected findings of pulmonary artery hypertension. Option E is expected in pulmonary fibrosis.

217. D (S&F ch94)
The findings in this patient are consistent with portopulmonary hypertension (POPH). The mechanisms of development of POPH are poorly understood. Histologically POPH shares the same findings as seen in pulmonary artery hypertension. Choise A is the classic presentation

of congestive heart failure. Choice B is characteristic for chronic obstructive pulmonary disease. Choice C shows the expected findings of hepatopulmonary syndrome. Choice E is expected in pulmonary fibrosis.

218. **E** (S&F ch94)
This patient meets the diagnostic criteria of hepatopulmonary syndrome (HPS). The patient has evidence of severe disease. Patients with severe HPS (resting pO2 less than 60 mm Hg) have a high mortality and poor outcome if not transplanted and should be considered for exception point for MELD score. Phosphodiesterase inhibitors and prostacyclin analogs have no role in the treatment of HPS, and are used for some patients with portopulmonary syndrome. Although oxygen therapy has been used for HPS, no study has demonstrated clinical benefits of this approach.

219. **D** (S&F ch94)
This patient has a diagnosis of primary biliary cirrhosis (PBC) with findings consistent with cirrhosis, and no recent hepatic decompensation. The prevalence of osteoporosis is high in patients with liver cirrhosis (12% to 55%) and is considerably high in patient with cholestasis, as in a patient with PBC or PSC. Bone mineral density screening for osteoporosis is appropriate in patients with PBC and PSC. The use of calcium and vitamin D and therapeutic bisphosphonates seems to improve bone mineral density and appears to have no significant side effects in this population. This patient has an average risk for colorectal cancer with a recent colonoscopy (3 years ago) and has no indication for a colonoscopy at this moment. The Patient has a recent acceptable negative study for surveillance of hepatocellular carcinoma, with no signs or symptoms suggestive of malignancy, so an abdominal CT with contrast is not indicated at this moment. She will not benefit from a liver biopsy at this moment, especially with evidence of PBC in remission with current ursodeoxycholic acid therapy. Of note, mild elevations of alkaline phosphatase can be observed in patients with osteoporosis. The patient has a recent upper endoscopy with evidence of small esophageal varices with low risk of bleeding, a Child-Pugh score of 5 (class A), and no recent liver decompensation. Current clinical guidelines endorse surveillance endoscopy every 2 years in patients with small varices, with no previous bleeding, on no primary prophylaxis, and no recent liver decompensation.

220. **B** (S&F ch94)
This patient has clinical findings and studies worrisome for portopulmonary hypertension (POPH). Right heart catheterization with measurement of pulmonary artery hemodynamics should be performed in all patients with suspected POPH to confirm diagnosis and assess severity of the condition. Findings on pulmonary artery catheterization are useful to distinguish between volume overload and hyperdynamic circulation in POPH and help the clinician to tailor therapy. Left catheterization alone will not help to establish POPH diagnosis, and is more useful to rule out coronary artery disease. This patient had a negative noninvasive cardiac stress test, and the benefit of a left heart catheterization at this moment is questionable. Although increase of diuretics might help with symptoms of overload, this alone will not be appropriate. A ventilation/perfusion scan can help to assess pulmonary shunting as the etiology of pulmonary symptoms; however, this patient has a negative bubble echocardiogram. POPH should be completely characterized before referring a patient for liver transplant. The outcome of liver transplant in patients with severe POPH is poor, and this is not a suitable therapeutic option for this patients.

221. **A** (S&F ch94)
This patient meets diagnostic criteria for severe POPH, based on the results of right heart catheterization. Withdrawal of beta-adrenergic blocker therapy has been shown to improve right-side cardiac function in patients with POPH and is an acceptable therapy. Patients with POPH who have severe disease are not suitable candidates for liver transplant in view of dismal prognosis. Treatment of this patient consists of diuretic to reduce volume overload and oxygen therapy, if hypoxemic. Studies have demonstrated benefits with the use of prostacyclin analogs, endothelin receptor antagonists, and phophodiesterase-5 inhibitors. These therapies are used with more frequency by clinicians. This patient had as negative noninvasive cardiac stress test, and the benefit of a left heart catheterization at this moment is questionable. The patient has an identified etiology for his respiratory symptoms, so a chest CT with intravenous contrast is of no benefit at this moment.

222. **A** (S&F ch94)
The patient is presenting with acute liver decompensation manifested by tense ascites, symptomatic anemia, and jaundice. The patient has a previous endoscopy with evidence of varices. Surveillance of esophageal varices is indicated in any patient who presents with acute liver decompensation, particularly in a patient with symptomatic anemia and previous intolerance to nonselective beta-blockers. Elevated INR is not considered a risk factor for spontaneous bleeding in patients with cirrhosis. Although it is common practice to administer vitamin K, FFP, and occasionally Factor VIIa in patients with chronic liver disease (especially in the setting of invasive procedure) there is no clinical evidence that this approach reduces the chance of bleeding. Moreover, the volume of FFP (>6 units) required to achieve a significant reduction of INR is associated with other complications (e.g., acute lung injury, volume overload). There is no indication for PRBC transfusion in this patient who has no signs of active bleeding and is hemodynamically stable. Recent studies have shown increased mortality in stable patients with hemoglobin levels above 7g/dl that receive PRBC transfusion in the setting of GI bleeding. Although transjugular intrahepatic portosystemic shunt (TIPS) is an indicated therapy for esophageal varices and ascites, this patient has a high risk of 3-month mortality after TIPS placement with her current MELD score. Optimization of diuretic therapy and low sodium intake is a more appropriate approach at this moment.

223. **C** (S&F ch94)
The patient in vignette C has a diagnosis of severe POPH. The outcome of liver transplant in a patient with severe POPH is poor, and these patients are not suitable candidates for liver transplant. Patients with history of solid tumors and prolonged documented remission are acceptable candidates for liver transplant. Hepatocellular carcinoma that meets the Milan Criteria is an indication for liver transplant; this patient might qualify for exception MELD points. Partial vein thrombosis is not an absolute contraindication for liver transplant; vascular problems on potential transplant candidates should be evaluated on an individual bases. Although patients with morbid obesity have a higher morbidity and mortality in some series compared with nonobese patients, improvement in surgical techniques and perioperative and postoperative

care has improved the outcomes of these patients significantly. Morbid obesity is not an absolute contraindication for liver transplantation.

224. D (S&F ch94)
The reason that patients with cirrhosis are at increased risk of thrombotic events (portal vein thrombosis, pulmonary embolism and deep vein thrombosis) is deficiency of endogenous anticoagulants including protein C, protein S, tissue plasminogen activator, and thrombomodulin. The progressive loss of hepatocytes in patients with cirrhosis leads to progressive loss of procoagulant factors, in particular those dependent of vitamin K (II, VII, IX, X). Deficiency of procoagulant factors predispose cirrhotic patient to bleeding, not thrombosis.

225. D (S&F ch94)
Intravenous LOLA, a salt of the aminoacids ornithine and aspartic acids, has been demonstrated to improve hepatic encephalopathy (HE) in cirrhotic patients compared with lactulose. This medication activates the urea cycle and stimulates ammonia clearance. Intravenous LOLA is an acceptable alternative therapy or adjunct therapy for patients with HE, which is unresponsive to conventional therapies. Probiotics have been used to modulate intestinal flora and decrease ammonia production. Unfortunately, a recent Cochrane Database review was unable to conclude their benefit and this therapy is generally not indicated for treatment of HE. Intravenous albumin is not an effective therapy for HE. Flumazenil is a benzodiazepine receptor inhibitor, which might transiently improves mental status in overt HE with no improvement on recovery or survival, thus it is not indicated for long-term treatment. Limiting protein intake is not beneficial in patients with HE.

226. C (S&F ch95)
This young patient drinks 3 glasses of wine each night, which can cause alcoholic hepatitis and even alcoholic cirrhosis in the long-term; however, it is unlikely to be the cause of acute liver failure. Patients with alcoholic hepatitis usually have underlying advanced fibrosis or cirrhosis from chronic alcohol consumption. Autoimmune hepatitis can present as ALF and is commonly seen in patients with other autoimmune conditions such as ulcerative colitis; it is identified in both genders and at any age but is more common in females in their 40's and 50's. Wilson disease can present with acute liver failure; it can first present with either hepatic or neuropsychiatric manifestations. Isoniazid is one of the most common causes of serious idiosyncratic liver injury. Acetaminophen overdose remains the most common cause of ALF in the United States and in the United Kingdom, and approximately half of cases are thought to be unintentional or "therapeutic misadventures." The risk may be increased by preceding chronic alcohol consumption and malnutrition.

227. B (S&F ch95)
This patient's presentation is highly suggestive of fulminant liver failure due to Wilson disease, which typically presents with a markedly subnormal alkaline phosphatase level, AST:ALT ratio >2.2, alkaline phosphatase:total bilirubin ratio <4, and hemolytic anemia. Urinary copper excretion is useful to make the diagnosis, and 24-hour excretion >100 mcg is very suggestive. Presence of mutations in *ATP7B* is very suggestive of Wilson disease and is useful for family screening; however, processing this laboratory study is slow and should not be used in a critically ill patient as described. The serum ceruloplasmin level may be normal or even elevated (especially in acute hepatitis) in patients with Wilson disease and thus a normal level is not sufficient to rule out Wilson disease. Histologic findings in Wilson disease are nonspecific and hepatic copper quantification is a slow process that can lead to false negatives; in this coagulopathic, critically ill patient with other noninvasive means of making the diagnosis, a liver biopsy should be used as a measure of last resort. Penicillamine should not be used in patients with fulminant liver failure and encephalopathy with hemolytic crisis; rather, consideration for rapid copper removal such as plasma exchange and urgent liver transplantation should be considered.

228. E (S&F ch95)
This is a typical presentation for acetaminophen overdose. Many cases of unintentional acetaminophen overdose are result of excessive ingestion of medications that contain acetaminophen over a period of days, which renders use of the Rumack-Matthew nomogram inappropriate for treatment with N-acetylcysteine. N-acetylcysteine is most effective when administered soon after ingestion but is still beneficial in later stages. Corticosteroid use is not routinely recommended in acetaminophen overdose. Gastrointestinal decontamination with activated charcoal may be useful in patients that present within 4 hours of a single ingestion of acetaminophen, but likely has limited utility after that. Intravenous acyclovir may be empirically started in any patient in which herpes simplex virus hepatitis is clinically considered, but would less likely be the case in this scenario. This patient's viral panel is consistent with prior exposure and clearance of hepatitis B virus, not active infection, and thus entecavir would not be indicated.

229. B (S&F ch95)
While several of these conditions can have similar presentations in the third trimester of pregnancy, a liver biopsy with viral inclusion bodies is very suggestive for HSV hepatitis. The characteristic rash is present in less than half of affected patients. HSV hepatitis needs to be identified promptly because intravenous acyclovir improves mortality. HELLP syndrome can present similarly but often with components of preeclampsia and proteinuria in almost all patients. Acute fatty liver of pregnancy also presents in the third trimester of pregnancy with similar symptoms although typically does not have such a high aminotransferase levels. A liver biopsy is diagnostic with characteristic microvesicular fatty infiltration of hepatocytes. Cholestasis of pregnancy occurs in the second and third trimester and is characterized by pruritus and elevated bile acid concentrations; it is not a cause of fulminant liver failure. Autoimmune hepatitis can initially present during pregnancy and is characterized by autoimmune serologies and elevated IgG level with a characteristic liver biopsy, which is not seen in this case.

230. A (S&F ch95)
For cases of acetaminophen overdose, the King's College criteria predict a poor prognosis in patients with an arterial pH <7.25 or INR > 6.5, creatinine >3.4 mg/dL, or grade 3 to 4 hepatic encephalopathy.

231. D (S&F ch95)
This patient likely has reactivation of hepatitis B virus from the recent addition of rituximab. Reactivation can be associated with a range of manifestations from asymptomatic patients to acute liver failure, such as this patient. Prompt

recognition is essential and initiation of antiviral therapy with agents such as tenofovir or entecavir is essential. The risk of reactivation can be eliminated by recognition of risk and initiation of antiviral prophylaxis in appropriate patients prior to initiation of immunosuppressive agents, such as rituximab. This case of acute liver failure (ALF) is unlikely to be due to acetaminophen overdose. High-dose steroids can be used if autoimmune hepatitis is suspected; although this patient has hyperglobulinemia, this is nonspecific and could be elevated in conditions such as rheumatoid arthritis. Although this patient may have chronic hepatitis C virus, it is not a cause of acute liver failure. Intravenous acyclovir may be empirically started whenever herpes hepatitis is considered until the PCR returns, but it is unlikely in this scenario to be the cause.

232. C (S&F ch95)
Although pregnant women with HEV are at higher risk of developing ALF than those that are not pregnant, the outcomes of patients with ALF from HEV are not affected by pregnancy status. HEV is a waterborne virus similar to hepatitis A. HEV is the most common cause of ALF in India but has not commonly been identified as the cause of ALF in the United States or United Kingdom.

233. B (S&F ch95)
The patient initially had acute liver injury secondary to acute infection with HBV as indicated by the positive IgM HBcAb. Patients with coinfection with HBV and HDV can have a bimodal pattern to their presentation; the second peak is consistent with significant acute liver failure as replication of HDV increases and may have a poor prognosis. While acute infection with HCV can cause acute liver injury and initially have a negative HCV antibody, HCV is an exceedingly rare cause of acute liver failure. The patient has previously been exposed to HAV but the negative IgM indicates lack of acute infection. This is unlikely to be caused by HEV or DILI.

234. C (S&F ch95)
Hyperosmotic agents such as mannitol are the first-line means of treatment in patients with acute liver failure and elevated ICP. Glucocorticoids have not been shown to be of benefit in patients with ALF and ICP; additionally there is concern for infection. Barbiturates, indomethacin, induction of hypothermia, and hyperventilation are considered the second line of treatment. Induction of hypothermia has been used at many centers with promising results but needs further research. Hyperventilation also helps at least transiently, and may delay the onset of cerebral herniation.

235. B (S&F ch95)
Acetaminophen overdose is the cause of acute liver failure (ALF) in 46% of the cases. In India, hepatitis E is the leading cause of ALF (more than 35% of the cases). The risk of developing ALF with NSAIDs is very low at 0.001%. Alcohol hepatitis is the leading cause of chronic liver failure, not acute liver failure.

236. A (S&F ch96)
The radiographic findings are classic for hepatocellular carcinoma and surgical resection would be most appropriate. Although direct measurement of hepatic venous pressure gradient (HVPG) to further assess may be considered prior to surgical resection, the normal platelet levels, normal spleen size, as well as lack of endoscopic evidence of varices speak against the presence of portal hypertension. Watchful waiting or no further treatment of hepatocellular carcinoma in this situation would not be appropriate. Discontinuation of OCP's would be appropriate for a hepatic adenoma. For lesions greater than 2 cm with classic radiographic features of hepatocellular carcinoma as above, a liver biopsy is not usually considered necessary and may carry some risk of seeding the tumor.

237. C (S&F ch96)
While all of the listed options have a potential role in the management of hepatocellular carcinoma, liver transplantation in appropriate candidates without extrahepatic disease within the Milan criteria carries the lowest 5-year tumor-free survival and overall survival rates. Given this patient's evidence of portal hypertension with cirrhosis he would not be a suitable surgical resection candidate. RFA and TACE would be possible options but have a higher recurrence rate and are occasionally used while patients await liver transplantation. Systemic therapy with sorafenib has been shown to have modest survival benefit in patients with advanced hepatocellular carcinoma but preserved hepatic function.

238. D (S&F ch96)
The presence of a tumor thrombus is considered extrahepatic disease and would represent tumor progression outside of Milan criteria, portending a poor prognosis. His described lesions are within the Milan criteria by size but not by the tumor thrombus. Prior treatment with locoregional therapy is not considered a contraindication to transplantation and is often used in patients on the waiting list in effort to decrease the risk of hepatocellular carcinoma progression and recurrence after transplantation. Although studies have demonstrated that very elevated AFP levels (such as above 400 ng/mL) are associated with higher risk of recurrence after liver transplantation, this patient's AFP is not as significantly elevated. Partial response to locoregional therapy (a greater than 50% decrease in enhanced areas) may prompt repeat attempt at therapy but is not generally considered a contraindication to transplantation.

239. C (S&F ch96)
ERCP will potentially provide both diagnostic and therapeutic utility in the setting of this suspected peri-hilar cholangiocarcinoma. There are a variety of tools that can be used to maximize the yield of obtaining a tissue diagnosis such as brushings, intraductal forceps biopsies, cholangiography, and Fluorescence in situ hybridization (FISH) depending on local expertise. Placement of a biliary stent can decompress the biliary system. If stent placement is unsuccessful by ERCP, a percutaneous approach as percutaneous transhepatic cholangiography (PTC) can be considered. Upper EUS with FNA may be useful to get a diagnosis as well but has the potential for causing peritoneal seeding and should be avoided if surgical resection or liver transplant is being considered. A PET-CT may show an enhancing lesion and could be useful to screen for obvious metastatic disease but may not make a diagnosis. A triphasic CT may be suggestive of the diagnosis but would be unlikely to add further information than the MRI above. An upper endoscopy and colonoscopy may be appropriate to eliminate the upper GI tract and colon as source of a primary malignancy with hepatic metastasis but would not otherwise be the best means to make the diagnosis.

240. C (S&F ch96)
This is a typical presentation for angiosarcoma, which bears a very poor prognosis and has little meaningful

potential therapies. Exposure to vinyl chloride is a risk factor for development for hepatic angiosarcoma. Unfortunately, the patient has poor functional status and would likely not be a suitable candidate for any therapy, and comfort-based goals of care should be discussed with the patient and the family. The patient would not be considered for liver transplantation and sorafenib therapy would not be appropriate. Reassurance is not appropriate and the patient would likely not benefit from surgical resection given the poor outcomes and his poor functional status.

241. C (S&F ch96)
Hepatic hemangiomas are the most common benign tumor of the liver and are found in about 7% of autopsies.

242. D (S&F ch96)
Hepatic hemangiomas are often found incidentally on imaging. It is a benign lesion and does not need any intervention, such as a surgical resection or locoregional therapy. An MRI could also be used to confirm the diagnosis if in question; however, the findings of the CT scan in this case are classic. In general biopsy should be avoided since it would be of limited value and is associated with serious bleeding complications.

243. C (S&F ch96)
This is a typical presentation of a hepatic adenoma in a female on longstanding OCP therapy; when large they may present symptomatically with chronic pain. The CT scan findings are characteristic and may have a heterogenous appearance due to hemorrhage or necrosis. Liver biopsy or FNA may prove useless since histology mimics normal hepatic parenchyma.

244. A (S&F ch96)
This is a typical presentation of a hepatic adenoma in a female on longstanding OCP therapy. In general, hepatic adenomas that are larger than 5 cm or lesions causing symptoms should be surgically resected since these lesions are thought to be at risk for rupture and malignant transformation to hepatocellular carcinoma. Discontinuation of OCPs should be recommended given the association with estrogen. ERCP would not be diagnostic or therapeutic. Reassurance in large, symptomatic lesions as described would be inappropriate in most cases. Radiographic surveillance would be appropriate for small asymptomatic lesions. There would likely be no utility in repeat biopsy. Hepatic adenoma can mimic normal hepatic parenchyma on biopsy; on larger tissue the absence of bile ducts and central veins may be appreciated.

245. D (S&F ch96)
The CT shows arterial enhancement of a lesion with lack of enhancement of a central stellate scar, which is a classic finding seen in focal nodular hyperplasia (FNH). These lesions are benign and characterized by a stable course that may even disappear over prolonged observation. There is not thought to be any risk of malignant transformation or rupture in pregnancy as seen in hepatic adenomas. Prior to the availability of high-quality MRI scans with liver-specific gadolinium-based contrast agents, the technetium sulfur colloid scan was frequently used to differentiate FNH from hepatic adenomas but has limited specificity. Most FNH lesions showed active uptake since they contain Kupffer cells in contrast to hepatic adenomas. No specific treatment such as chemoembolization or resection is indicated.

246. C (S&F ch96)
This fits the radiographic description of a hepatocellular carcinoma in a decompensated cirrhotic patient. The lesion is within Milan criteria and the patient should be worked up for liver transplantation. Given his hyperbilirubinemia and poor functional status, sorafenib would not be indicated in this circumstance. Surgical resection in a decompensated cirrhotic patient with hyperbilirubinemia would have very poor outcome and would likely result in catastrophic complications and further hepatic decompensation. While locoregional therapy is often well tolerated in patients with compensated cirrhosis, this patient's poor performance status and hyperbilirubinemia would likely deem him not a candidate. Consideration for hospice could be appropriate if the patient did not wish to undergo transplantation or was found not to be a suitable candidate.

247. C (S&F ch96)
The fibrolamellar variant of hepatocellular carcinoma almost always is found in noncirrhotic liver. It typically occurs in young patients, does not produce AFP and is seen equally in both genders. Patients with fibrolamellar hepatocellular carcinoma are more often a candidate for surgical treatment and therefore it carries a better prognosis than conventional hepatocellular carcinoma (HCC). However, the response of fibrolamellar variant of hepatocellular carcinoma to chemotherapy is not any better than conventional HCC.

248. C (S&F ch96)
A large hepatic adenoma in a female considering pregnancy should strongly be considered for surgical resection prior to pregnancy given the risk of rupture and associated high mortality. Hepatic artery encasement is considered a contraindication for surgical resection in patients with cholangiocarcinoma. In a patient with polycystic liver disease and no dominant cyst with few symptoms, surgical intervention may be fraught with complications and provide little benefit at this point. A patient with hepatocellular carcinoma within Milan criteria but with decompensated cirrhosis and evidence of portal hypertension should be considered for liver transplantation rather than resection. Nodular regenerative hyperplasia is a form of noncirrhotic portal hypertension that can be caused by a variety of medications and predisposing conditions and is not an indication for surgical resection.

249. B (S&F ch97)
This patient presents with fulminant liver failure secondary to acetaminophen ingestion. Drug- induced liver injury accounts for the majority of cases of liver failure with acetaminophen being the most often implicated drug. In the absence of any obvious contraindications for a transplant, all patients with acute liver failure should be referred to a transplant center promptly. Acute kidney injury is common in this scenario and typically is reversible with supportive care, so a kidney transplant is not warranted. A liver biopsy is not needed to establish the diagnosis. A psychiatric evaluation is warranted, however, should not delay a transplant evaluation.

250. D (S&F ch97)
Portopulmonary hypertension occurs in about 5% to 10% of patients referred for a liver transplant. Mean pulmonary artery pressures >50 mm Hg are associated with very high perioperative mortality and are a contraindication to surgery. Patients with a MPAP >35 mm Hg typically require treatment first, and can only be listed for a

transplant if treatment successfully reduces the MPAP to <35 mm Hg. An echocardiogram is helpful to assess for any valvular pathology or any evidence of right ventricular dysfunction; however, even a normal echocardiogram does not change the fact that this patient has a high perioperative mortality. Epoprostenol (Flolan), a prostacyclin, is one of the medications used to treat portopulmonary hypertension; however, treatment is typically needed for weeks to months in order to effectively lower pulmonary pressures to within target range. Intravenous heparin may be useful in patients where pulmonary hypertension is the result of a pulmonary embolus, but is not indicated in this particular case.

251. D (S&F ch97)
Patients with primary hyperoxaluria and renal failure qualify for a MELD exception of 28. The patient with hepatocellular carcinoma has disease outside Milan criteria and therefore does not qualify for a MELD exception. Patients with POPH need to have an MPAP <35 mm Hg on treatment to qualify for a MELD exception. Patients with HPS need to have a PaO2 <60 mm Hg on room air to qualify for exception points. Refractory ascites alone does not qualify a patient for a MELD exception.

252. D (S&F ch97)
New or recurrent malignancy is a common cause of morbidity and mortality in solid organ transplant recipients. The most common malignancy is posttransplant lymphoproliferative disorder (PTLD) followed by skin cancer. Recurrent hepatocellular carcinoma (HCC) occurs in up to 10% of patients with disease that was originally within Milan criteria; however, this is not a typical presentation. Patients with a history of alcohol abuse are at an increased risk for oropharyngeal SCC and esophageal carcinoma. Recurrent HCC is unlikely in this case since CT scan does not show any abnormal lesions. Metastatic HCC is typically seen in lungs and bone but is not likely to present with an oral ulcer. PTLD is possible, however, not likely to present with an oral ulcer. Sirolimus can cause oral ulcers; however, the presence of significant lymphadenopathy is more consistent with a diagnosis of cancer.

253. C (S&F ch97)
The initial treatment for a bile leak is an ERCP with biliary stenting. Surgical revision is required if an ERCP is unsuccessful. A laparoscopic approach is not recommended in this setting. Percutaneous drainage of a biloma and/or antibiotics is helpful, particularly if an infection is suspected.

254. A (S&F ch97)
Phenytoin can induce cytochrome p450 and increase metabolism of tacrolimus, leading to lower levels. The patient's tacrolimus dose should be increased to maintain adequate drug levels. The remaining medications listed are negative inducers of cytochrome p450 and will actually result in increased levels of tacrolimus for the same dose; therefore, patients started on any of these medications should have their tacrolimus doses reduced.

255. C (S&F ch97)
Recurrence of disease is a common cause of morbidity in patients post–liver transplant. This patient has several risk factors for the metabolic syndrome as well as evidence of steatosis on imaging. This is suggestive of underlying NAFLD. Her tacrolimus dose has been stable and her levels being adequate makes rejection unlikely. Her ultrasound also does not show any evidence of biliary dilation to suggest a stricture. Autoimmune hepatitis recurs in up to 40% of patients posttransplant; however, this scenario and presentation is more consistent with recurrent NAFLD. The lack of a plasma cell infiltrate on pathology also makes autoimmune hepatitis unlikely.

256. E (S&F ch97)
Opportunistic infections are most common in the first 6 months post–liver transplantation. Patients with CMV viremia can have various presentations. Typical symptoms associated with CMV gastroenteritis include diarrhea, which may be bloody, fever, and abdominal pain; and patients may appear quite toxic. Rejection is not typically associated with fever or significant GI symptoms. The patient's bilirubin is normal, which makes cholangitis less likely. The symptoms are also not suggestive of a bile leak. GVHD is common amongst bone marrow transplant recipients but does not usually occur in liver transplant patients.

257. D (S&F ch97)
Altered mental status in the perioperative period is often multifactorial. An infection should always be ruled out. The patient's CSF analysis is bland which rules out HSV and toxoplasmosis. The patient's BUN is not significantly elevated and this makes uremic encephalopathy unlikely. Steroids can cause psychosis, however, the most likely cause of altered mental status in this scenario is tacrolimus-induced neurotoxicity. This will resolve once tacrolimus is discontinued. This patient should be switched to an alternative immunosuppressant such as sirolimus or everolimus. Other common side effects of tacrolimus include nephrotoxicity, hypertension, and myelosuppression.

258. C (S&F ch97)
This is a typical presentation of sirolimus-induced lung toxicity. Pneumocystis pneumonia typically occurs in the first 6 months posttransplant and is not likely to occur several years posttransplant. The patient's echocardiogram is normal making CHF an unlikely cause in this scenario. PTLD is a common malignancy posttransplant but the chest CT findings are not suggestive of this diagnosis. Similarly, the chest CT does not show any evidence of metastatic disease. Discontinuation of sirolimus leads to improvement of symptoms.

TABLE FOR ANSWER 79 Relative Properties of Classes of Direct-Acting Antiviral Agents in Clinical Development

	Properties		
Drug Class	**Potency**	**Pan-Genotypic Efficacy**	**Barrier to Resistance**
Protease inhibitors (second generation)	++ - +++	+ - ++	+ - ++
Non-nucleos(t)ide polymerase inhibitors	+ - ++	±	±
Nucleos(t)ide polymerase inhibitors	+ - +++	+++	++ - +++
NS5A inhibitors	+++	+ - ++	+ - ++

+, Lowest; +++, highest.

TABLE FOR ANSWER 82 Diagnostic Markers for HDV Infection, Their Importance, and Potential Weaknesses

Diagnostic Markers and their Importance	Potential Weaknesses
IgG Anti-HDV	
Positive in all persons exposed to HDV; persists long term, even after viral clearance May indicate active or past infection; not a neutralizing antibody	May not be elevated in immunocompromised persons
IgM Anti-HDV	
Positive in acute infection; negative in past infection May be used as a surrogate marker for HDV replication Decrease in titers and subsequent clearance in chronic HDV infection is a predictor of spontaneous or therapy-induced remission	Often persists in chronic infection, particularly with active liver disease Neither 100% sensitive nor specific for HDV replication
HDAg	
Can be demonstrated in hepatocytes by immunohistochemical staining	The reliability of immunochemistry decreases as the disease becomes chronic The presence of high titers of neutralizing antibodies (anti-HDV) interferes with detection of HDAg Less sensitive than molecular assays
HDV RNA (Qualitative)	
Marker of HDV replication Positive in all patients with chronic HDV infection Negative in spontaneous or treatment-induced viral clearance	Variability in the HDV genome and assay primers influences the sensitivity of HDV RNA detection No WHO standardized assay
HDV RNA (Quantitative)	
Used to measure the level of HDV RNA in serum Useful method for predicting and monitoring treatment response	HDV RNA may be present at a lower titer than the limit of detection (as low as 10 copies/mL) Levels do not reflect the grade or stage of liver disease May be useful for monitoring patients during therapy with interferon, but there is no WHO-standardized assay Results may differ significantly among laboratories
HBsAg (Quantitative)	
May be useful for predicting or monitoring treatment response during therapy with interferon, because a falling titer heralds HBsAg loss and hence HDV RNA clearance	Confined to research laboratories in the United States but commercially licensed in Asia and Europe

HBsAg, Hepatitis B surface antigen; HDAg, hepatitis D antigen; IgG, immunoglobulin G; IgM, immunoglobulin M.

TABLE FOR ANSWER 153 Hepatotoxic Anesthetics Other Than Halothane

Anesthetic	Percent Metabolized	Incidence of Hepatotoxicity	Cross-reactivity with Other Haloalkanes	Other Clinical Features
Methoxyflurane	>30	Low	Yes	Nephrotoxicity
Enflurane	2	1 in 800,000	Yes	Similar to halothane
Isoflurane	0.2	Rare	Yes	Similar to halothane
Desflurane	<0.2	Few reports	Yes	Cardiac toxicity, malignant hyperthermia
Sevoflurane	Minimal	Rare	Uncertain	None reported

TABLE FOR ANSWER 161 Revised Original Scoring System for the Diagnosis of Autoimmune Hepatitis

Category	Variable	Score
Gender	Female	+2
AP/AST	>3 <1.5	−2 +2
Gamma globulin or IgG level	>2.0 times ULN 1.5-2.0 times ULN 1.0-1.5 times ULN <1.0 times ULN	+3 +2 +1 0
ANA, SMA, or anti-LKM1 titer	>1:80 1:80 1:40 <1:40	+3 +2 +1 0
AMA	Positive	−4
Viral markers	Positive Negative	−3 +3
Drug history	Yes No	−4 +1
Alcohol consumption	<25 g/day >60 g/day	+2 −2
HLA	DR3 or DR4	+1
Concurrent immune disease	Thyroiditis, UC, synovitis, others	+2
Other liver-defined autoantibodies	Anti-SLA, anti-actin, anti-LC1, atypical pANCA	+2
Histologic features	Interface hepatitis Plasmacytic infiltrate Rosettes None of above Biliary changes Other features	+3 +1 +1 −5 −3 −3
Treatment response	Complete Relapse	+2 +3
Pretreatment Score		
Definite diagnosis		>15
Probable diagnosis		10-15
Post-treatment Score		
Definite diagnosis		>17
Probable diagnosis		12-17

AMA, Antimitochondrial antibodies; ANA, antinuclear antibodies; anti-LC1, antibodies to liver cytosol type 1; anti-LKM1, antibodies to liver-kidney microsome type 1; anti-SLA, antibodies to soluble liver antigen; AP/AST (or AP/ALT), ratio of serum alkaline phosphatase level to serum AST (or serum ALT) level; IgG, immunoglobulin G; pANCA, perinuclear antineutrophil cytoplasmic antibodies; SMA, smooth muscle antibodies; ULN, upper limit of normal.

TABLE FOR ANSWERS 179, 191, and 192 Use of Hepatic Vein Pressure Gradient in the Differential Diagnosis of Portal Hypertension

Type of Portal Hypertension	WHVP	FHVP	HVPG
Prehepatic	Normal	Normal	Normal
Presinusoidal	Normal	Normal	Normal
Sinusoidal	Increased	Normal	Increased
Postsinusoidal	Increased	Normal	Increased
Posthepatic			
Heart failure	Increased	Increased	Normal
Budd-Chiari syndrome	—	Hepatic vein cannot be cannulated	—

FHVP, Free hepatic vein pressure; HVPG, hepatic vein pressure gradient; WHVP, wedged hepatic venous pressure.

CHAPTER

10

Small and Large Intestine

Julia Massaad, Khaled Abdeljawad, Kavya M. Sebastian, Nikrad Shahnavaz, Sagar Shroff, Joshua Novak, Tanvi Dhere, Sonali Sakaria, Rahul Maheshwari, Jennifer Christie, Muhammad Fuad Azrak, and Emad Qayed

QUESTIONS

1. A 71-year-old man presents to the emergency department with acute abdominal pain that started 2 hours prior to presentation. He is tachycardic, sweaty, and in severe discomfort. His abdomen is diffusely tender with decreased bowel sounds. Computed tomography scan (CT) scan of the abdomen reveals free air in the peritoneal space. Which of the following is the least likely location of the bowel perforation?
   A. Transverse colon
   B. Cecum
   C. Proximal jejunum
   D. Hepatic flexure
   E. Ascending colon

2. You are doing a small bowel enteroscopy on a 56-year-old man as part of workup for chronic diarrhea and malabsorption. You took biopsies from the duodenum and jejunum, but your technician forgot to label the jars in which the samples were placed. Which histologic finding is characteristic of duodenal tissue?
   A. Presence of finger-shaped villi
   B. Brunner glands
   C. Presence of enteroendocrine cells
   D. Presence of enterochromaffin cells
   E. Absence of goblet cells

3. Which of the following is true about the abdominal wall anomalies omphalocele and gastroschisis?
   A. In omphalocele, there is no sac covering the extruded intestine
   B. The umbilical cord should be clamped 2 cm from the abdominal wall after delivery
   C. Increased maternal alpha-fetoprotein (AFP) is expected in the prenatal period in both conditions
   D. Extraintestinal anomalies are more common in gastroschisis than in omphalocele
   E. Gastroschisis is most commonly located to the right of the umbilical cord

4. A 1-day-old male neonate is having bilious vomiting and poor feeding. Physical exam reveals an irritable baby with a distended abdomen and a normal perineal exam. Plain abdominal films show a double-bubble sign. The diagnosis of duodenal atresia is made. Which of the following is true in this condition?
   A. It is a result of an ischemic insult
   B. It is more common than duodenal stenosis
   C. Typically, it is located proximal to the ampulla of Vater
   D. On plain films, the small air bubble corresponds to the gastric bubble
   E. A small percentage of patients born with duodenal atresia have associated anomalies

5. A 2-day-old male newborn is about to be discharged from the nursery unit, but his mother notices that he has not passed stool yet. Exam reveals a distended abdomen. Rectal examination results in expulsion of retained fecal material. Plain film shows distended proximal loops of bowel. What is the next step in management?
   A. Reassure the mother and tell her that treatment is indicated after 3 months
   B. Perform a contrasted enema on a prepared colon
   C. Perform anal manometry as it has a low false-positive rate
   D. Perform suction biopsy of the rectal mucosa 2 cm above the mucocutaneous junction
   E. Perform a flexible sigmoidoscopy, since the presence of a normal full rectum and dilated proximal bowel on sigmoidoscopy is diagnostic

6. A 26-year-old Puerto Rican woman presents to your office for evaluation of 6 months of mild crampy diffuse abdominal pain, which occurs on most weekday mornings. She usually has complete resolution of her symptoms as the day progresses and never has symptoms at night. She has tried modifying her diet to exclude gluten and dairy products, but she noted no change in symptoms. She also has not seen variation of the symptoms depending upon whether she skips breakfast or eats before work. Two or three times a week, she will experience small-volume loose-quality stools after the cramping begins, which often results in alleviation of the abdominal pain. Her weight is stable, and she denies any nausea or vomiting. She has not seen any blood in her stool. She has no past medical history and does not take medications on a regular basis. She notes a family history of an uncle with colon cancer at 62 years of age and a first-degree cousin with a history of Crohn's disease. She takes ibuprofen 800 mg twice daily for 2 to 3 days a month during her menstrual cycle. She drinks 2 to 4 beers or glasses of wine a week, but she does not smoke or use recreational drugs. She started her first job after completing graduate studies 3 months ago, and she is working 12 to 14 hours daily on weekdays. On physical exam, she is a well-developed, anxious-appearing female in no acute distress. Vital signs are stable, and her exam is otherwise unremarkable. Which of the following is the most likely underlying mechanism to explain her presentation?

A. Nerve loss of the intestinal wall with feeble contractions and slow transit
B. Altered function of the interstitial cells of Cajal (ICC) with abnormal patterning of contractions
C. Muscular hypertrophy with high-amplitude forceful contractions
D. Altered afferent function with increased visceral sensitivity and disordered motility
E. Myocyte and mitochondrial abnormalities with inadequate force for transit and mixing

7. Which of the following is correct regarding normal small intestinal motor and sensory function?
A. Deep plexus is present within the circular muscle, and its ganglia are connected to those of the submucosa by interganglionic fascicles
B. Intrinsic sensory neurons synapse in the intramural plexuses where they induce excitation via release of dopamine
C. The myenteric interstitial cells of Cajal are distributed within the muscle layers where they are innervated preferentially by intrinsic enteric motor neurons
D. Intestinofugal neurons have peripheral terminals within the intestinal wall, which sense and receive information regarding intestinal distention
E. Myocytes communicate electrically via gap junctions, physically specialized areas of cell-to-cell contact

8. An 84-year-old Haitian man is brought to the emergency department with new onset confusion and agitation of 6-hour duration. The nursing home noticed that he was behaving in an agitated fashion, speaking to his empty room as if someone were present, and becoming combative with the nursing staff. The patient had previously been known to be oriented to self and place, and calm with no history of violent behavior. The staff also reports that he has had decreased urination and significant constipation, which is different from his baseline. His son is concerned due to the patient's lack of bowel movements for 4 days when typically the patient has 1 to 2 bowel movements on a daily basis. No changes have been made recently to his diet or medications. He has a notable history of Parkinson's dementia, hypertension, hyperlipidemia, allergic rhinitis, mild depression, and diabetes mellitus type 2. His medications include a daily low-dose aspirin, diphenhydramine, simvastatin, metformin, benztropine, nortriptyline, and hydrochlorothiazide.

On exam, vital signs are as follows:

Temperature	38° C
Heart rate	127 bpm
Blood pressure	163/95 mm Hg
Respiratory rate	16/min
Oxygen saturation	97% on room air

He is notably agitated and speaking to the walls. He continually reaches out to touch the air in front of him. He does not speak in a coherent fashion, and he is continually trying to rise from his stretcher, requiring restraining by the emergency department staff. He is flushed appearing without evidence of diaphoresis. His pupils are widely dilated and minimally reactive to light. The exam is limited by the patient's lack of cooperation, but it is only otherwise notable for a mildly distended soft abdomen with decreased bowel sounds. The patient appears to have mild tenderness over all quadrants as noted by his grimacing and pushing your hand away. Laboratory values demonstrate the following:

WBC	13,400 cells/μL
Hemoglobin	13.7 g/dL
Platelet count	217,000/μL
Lactate	1.46 mg/dL
Lipase	49 U/L
BUN	69 mg/dL
Creatinine	1.93 mg/dL
Glucose	93 mg/dL
Urinalysis	>20 leukocytes/high power field (HPF) present, + nitrite, 3 + blood

Which of the following is the immediate next best step?
A. Administer physostigmine
B. Draw blood for aerobic and anaerobic cultures
C. Obtain a 12-lead electrocardiogram (ECG)
D. Electively intubate for airway protection
E. Obtain a PO contrast CT of the abdomen and pelvis

9. A 49-year-old African-American woman with a history of diabetes mellitus for 10 years, hypertension, and dyslipidemia presents to your office with a reported history of abdominal bloating and discomfort approximately 2 to 3 hours after meals in the last 6 months. She is on an insulin regimen and has maintained a hemoglobin A1c of 9.7% over the last year. She also takes hydrochlorothiazide and simvastatin. She denies any nausea or vomiting. Her chart reveals that her primary care provider obtained a 4-hour gastric emptying study 2 months ago, which was normal with no evidence of gastroparesis. The patient has had no changes in bowel habits, and her weight is stable. She does not smoke, drink, or use recreational drugs. She has a history of a normal upper endoscopy and colonoscopy performed last year. On exam, she is well appearing with stable vital signs, and she has no notable findings aside from mildly hypoactive bowel sounds. Which of the following is the next best step in her diagnostic workup?
A. Small bowel follow-through study
B. Obtain a 6-hour gastric emptying study
C. Lactulose breath test
D. Small bowel manometry
E. MRI of the abdomen

10. Which of the following is correct regarding small intestinal motor activity?
A. Small intestinal contractions arise when an electrical action potential is superimposed on the slow wave
B. Slow waves lead to small intestinal contractions in a one-to-one fashion
C. Pattern of small intestine motility is generally consistent
D. Various input of stimuli, such as distention of the small intestine, are perceived by receptors within the mucosa
E. Small bowel transit time is determined by the rate of gastric emptying, as determined by the gastric pacemaker

11. A 20-year-old Caucasian woman is referred to your office for evaluation of poor oral intake and recurrent abdominal pain in the last 12 months. She has a history of stage IV ovarian rhabdomyosarcoma diagnosed at age 17 for which she was treated with chemotherapy and radiation with complete remission achieved last year. At this time, her oncologist notes that she remains disease free on her most recent staging studies. However, she has had at least ten lengthy hospitalizations over the last year for recurrent nausea, vomiting, and abdominal pain. Multiple CTs

and MRIs of her abdomen have been obtained during these episodes with findings of thickened, edematous diffusely dilated loops of small bowel, but no obstruction or transition points were noted. She has typically been managed with bowel rest, resuscitation, and after eventual resolution of her symptoms, discharge from the hospital. However, her mother, who accompanies her today, remains very concerned due to her daughter's 33-pound weight loss over the last year. She reports that regardless of how bland or soft a meal she cooks for her daughter, the patient continues to have nausea and occasional vomiting, although this is improved by use of antiemetics. The patient also notes chronic abdominal pain with bloating that is worsened by food intake. When she does keep food down, she experiences foul-smelling, greasy diarrhea several hours later. She denies any blood in her stool. On exam, her vital signs are as follows:

Temperature	36.9° C
Heart rate	103 bpm
Blood pressure	91/57 mm Hg
Oxygen saturation	100% on room air
Height	65 inches
Weight	83 lb

She is a cachectic female in no acute distress but fatigued-appearing. She is noted to have temporal wasting with a scaphoid abdomen that is mildly distended but otherwise nontender with no rigidity, rebound, or guarding. She has hyperactive bowel sounds throughout all quadrants. What is the next best step of management?

A. Inpatient hospitalization with initiation of central parenteral nutrition (CPN)
B. Outpatient MR enterography
C. Clinic visit for surgical consultation
D. Inpatient hospitalization with trial of slow administration of postpyloric enteral feeds
E. Proceeding with an upper endoscopy and colonoscopy with random duodenal and colonic biopsies

12. A 55-year-old Caucasian man with a history of myotonic dystrophy is admitted to the medical floor due to complaints of abdominal bloating, nausea, and intermittent explosive liquid bowel movements of watery, nonbloody consistency occurring every 3 to 4 days for the last 2 weeks. His last bowel movement was this morning. The patient denies any recent travel or changes in his dietary habits. His neurologist saw him 4 weeks ago, and his neurologic exam was found to be stable with no changes required in management. He has a history of a ventriculoperitoneal shunt, which was placed 1 year ago for normal pressure hydrocephalus. This has been complicated by one occasion 2 months ago when the patient presented to the emergency department for severe headaches and was found to have malpositioning of the catheter, requiring repositioning with a hospitalization that lasted 1 week in duration. Today, he only has a mild headache that has been present for the last 2 hours. He denies fevers, but he has mild chills and sweats at home. On exam, vital signs are as follows:

Temperature	36.8° C
Heart rate	76 bpm
Blood pressure	124/73 mm Hg
Oxygen saturation	96% on room air

He appears to be in mild distress and uncomfortable. Cardiac and pulmonary exams are benign. His abdomen is noted to be tense and distended with hypoactive bowel sounds. Tenderness is present throughout all quadrants. There is no rigidity, rebounding, or guarding. The abdomen is tympanitic to percussion. In addition to initial laboratory studies, which of the following would be the next best step?

A. CT scan of the abdomen with PO contrast
B. *Clostridium difficile* toxin polymerase chain reaction (PCR) study
C. Plain upright film of the abdomen
D. Surgical consultation
E. Flexible sigmoidoscopy

13. You are called to see a 42-year-old Caucasian woman in the rehabilitation unit for constipation in the last 6 months. She sustained an injury at the level of T4 7 years ago with resultant complete paraplegia of the lower extremities. Her providing team is requesting further diagnostic evaluation for a chronic history of constipation with infrequent small amounts of pellets or liquid stool occurring once every 7 to 10 days. She has bloating and abdominal discomfort secondary to this, but otherwise she denies any severe abdominal pain, nausea, vomiting, or blood in her stool. Her weight is stable, and her appetite is good. She has a history of chronic pain secondary to complications from the car accident that led to her spinal cord injury and is on hydrocodone daily. She has a family history notable for a mother who was diagnosed with colorectal cancer (CRC) at age 62 years. On exam, her vital signs are as follows:

Temperature	37.6° C
Heart rate	84 bpm
Blood pressure	109/72 mm Hg
Oxygen saturation	95% on room air

Exam is otherwise only notable for a soft, mildly distended abdomen with normal bowel sounds with mild tenderness on deep palpation throughout all quadrants. There is dullness to percussion. An abdominal x-ray done at bedside that is only significant for fecal load throughout the colon. Which of the following is the next best step in management?

A. Colonoscopy
B. Breath testing for small intestinal bacterial overgrowth
C. MR enterography
D. Decreasing opioid dosing and initiating an aggressive bowel regimen
E. Surgical consultation

14. A 38-year-old African-American woman presents to your clinic with a 4-month history of epigastric discomfort, bloating, and diarrhea. Her symptoms are worsened by food intake. She reports a 5-pound weight loss in the last 6 months. The stools are malodorous and greasy at times, but she has never seen melena or blood in them. She traveled to Paris, France, on a business trip 2 weeks ago, but otherwise, she has not left the area. She has a history of recurrent ear infections, and occasionally requires courses of antibiotics. She recalls that her last infection was a little over a year ago. She is also undergoing a workup with her dermatologist for gradual development of tight and shiny skin over both of her hands over the last year. She has been noticing a thickened and puffy texture to the skin with the same tight quality over her face, particularly around the orbits of her eyes. She denies taking any chronic or over-the-counter medications. She has a family history notable for Crohn's disease of both her mother and her sister. She denies any history of surgical procedures. On exam, she is well-appearing with stable vital signs and findings of mildly hyperactive bowel sounds. Laboratory values demonstrate the following:

WBC	10,700/µL
Hemoglobin	11.3 g/dL

HCT	33.9%
MCV	98 fL/cell
Platelet count	253,000/μL
Lipase	34 U/L
Vitamin B_{12}	142 pg/mL
Folate	20 ng/mL
Lactate	1.6 mg/dL
ESR	49 mm/hr
C-reactive protein	8.3 mg/mL

Which of the following is the next best diagnostic management for this patient?

A. *C. difficile* toxin PCR study
B. MR enterography
C. Upper endoscopy and colonoscopy with random biopsies
D. Stool cultures
E. Glucose breath testing

15. A 57-year-old Caucasian man previously in good health presents to you for a second opinion regarding chronic diarrhea of 6 months duration. He has 10 to 15 watery, nonbloody bowel movements a day. He has lost 25 pounds to date. He has diffuse abdominal pain of a bloated nature. He has undergone evaluation with a previous gastroenterologist with negative stool studies for *Salmonella*, *Shigella*, *Campylobacter*, and *Escherichia coli*. A *C. difficile* toxin PCR study was negative. He also has records of an unremarkable upper endoscopy and colonoscopy. Pathology reports demonstrate no histologic abnormalities of the duodenal, ileal, or colonic biopsies. The patient has normal levels of gastrin, chomogranin A, urine 5-hydroxyindoleacetic acid (5-HIAA), and serum vasoactive intestinal peptide (VIP). He has a CT of the abdomen and pelvis from last month with no abnormal findings. His symptoms have been severe enough to require 3 hospitalizations in the last 2 months for volume depletion. Use of antidiarrheals decreases the frequency and volume of his stools, but the patient continues to have mild symptoms and is still losing weight. He also reports episodes of feeling faint upon standing. On exam, vital signs are as follows:

Temperature	37.1° C
Heart rate	113 bpm
Blood pressure	62/49 mm Hg
Oxygen saturation	88% on room air

He appears to be a thin, ill-appearing male. Cardiovascular exam is notable for elevated jugular vein pressure (JVP) and a pericardial rub, and auscultation of lungs reveals clear breath sounds bilaterally. Abdomen is soft, diffusely tender throughout all quadrants, and moderately distended. Bowel sounds are normal, and the abdomen is dull to percussion. Bilateral lower extremities are noted to have 2+ pitting edema. The patient is admitted to the intensive care unit for further workup and resuscitation. Which of the following studies would provide the best information for further management?

A. Video capsule enteroscopy
B. Octreotide scan
C. Fecal elastase
D. Myocardial biopsy
E. MR enterography

16. A 34-year-old Caucasian woman who is 29 weeks into her first pregnancy is referred to your office by her obstetrician due to a history of constipation in the last 3 months. She was in good health prior to the onset of pregnancy and takes no medications either prescribed or over-the-counter aside from prenatal vitamins, which she began taking 6 months prior to conception. She has had a change from a daily soft bowel movement to 2 to 3 hard consistency bowel movements a week, which often required straining to pass. She has had no melena, hematochezia, or bright red blood per rectum. However, she is experiencing some discomfort due to the presence of hemorrhoids, which are painful during straining upon defecation. She is otherwise well with her pregnancy, progressing as expected and with a healthy fetus. She is concerned about this change in her bowel habits due to a family history notable for a maternal grandmother with colon cancer at age 62 years. Which of the following is the next best step?

A. Evaluation with colonoscopy
B. Thyroid function studies
C. CT scan of the abdomen and pelvis
D. Fecal occult blood testing
E. Reassurance and establishment of a daily bowel regimen

17. Which of the following is true regarding interstitial cells of Cajal (ICC)?

A. ICC are neuronal in origin
B. Increased numbers or volume of ICC has been associated with normal aging
C. ICC play an important role in water and electrolyte secretion
D. ICC are major targets of neurotransmitters such as acetylcholine and nitric oxide
E. ICC are recognized by their immunoreactivity for platelet-derived growth factor receptor α (PDGFRα)

18. A 21-year-old man presents to your clinic for follow-up of gastroesophageal reflux disease (GERD). His symptoms are well controlled with lifestyle changes. He is an avid runner and wonders how his GI system adapts to his activity during sports. Which of the following can you tell him regarding the mechanisms that modify his bowel activity during exercise?

A. The parasympathetic nervous system is responsible for modified bowel activity during exercise
B. The mechanisms responsible for regulation of the GI tract during exercise are driven by a powerful cholinergic drive from preganglionic nerve cell bodies from the spinal cord
C. Branches of the vagus nerve reach the prevertebral ganglia, from where they innervate the colon, assisting in modifying bowel activity during exercise
D. In response to exercise, nerve fibers from prevertebral ganglia cause vasodilation of the mucosal and submucosal blood vessels
E. Reflexive to exercise, axons act on the circuitry of the submucosal plexus to promote epithelial secretion

19. Which of the following is true regarding colonic motility?

A. Phase III of the interdigestive migrating myoelectric-motor complex does not contribute to ileocecal transit
B. Solids and liquids spend the same amount of time in each region of the colon
C. The ileocecal junction is not an actual sphincter
D. Retrograde movement of colonic contents is considered pathologic
E. Proximal colonic emptying occurs independent of wall tone

20. Which of the following medications works by activating chloride channels on the intestine?

A. Ondansetron
B. Lubiprostone
C. Alosetron

D. Prucalopride
E. Bisacodyl

21. What is the principal driving force behind fluid secretion in the intestines?
A. Apical sodium channels
B. Nutrient-coupled sodium transport
C. Transcellular movement of chloride
D. Transport of bicarbonate
E. Osmotic pressure

22. A 23-year-old female medical student presents to the emergency department with diarrhea and dehydration. While taking her medical history, it is revealed that she returned from Africa 2 days ago, where she was performing missionary work. She denies any fevers or chills but states that she is having 15 to 20 watery bowel movements daily. She had been in another emergency department 1 day ago, but was discharged home. Her stool studies reveal fecal electrolytes (Na^+ 104, K^+ 30), and her fecal calprotectin and fecal leukocytes are both negative. What is the most likely mechanism for her underlying diarrhea?
A. Endotoxic damage by bacteria to the intestinal villi
B. Consumption of hyperosmotic solutions
C. Inhibition of the *CFTR* gene expression
D. Cyclic adenosine monophosphate (cAMP) inhibiting reabsorption of intestinal secretion
E. cAMP increasing chloride channel activity

23. A 46-year-old man with Crohn's disease underwent an end-colostomy with closure of the distal colonic segment (Hartmann's procedure) around 6 months ago. He has been experiencing tenesmus and bloody/mucus discharge from the rectal pouch. An endoscopic examination of the rectum shows erythema and edema without ulcerations. Biopsy reveals acute prominent lymphoid hyperplasia and chronic inflammatory cell infiltration. Deficiency of which of the following substances in the diverted colon can be the cause of this condition?
A. Bile acids
B. Long-chain fatty acids
C. Short-chain fatty acids (SCFA)
D. Bicarbonate
E. Chloride

24. Which of the following is correct regarding potassium transport in the small intestine and colon?
A. Passive absorption in the small intestines, and active transport in the colon
B. Active transport in the small intestines, and passive absorption in the colon
C. Passive absorption in both small intestine and colon
D. Active transport in both small intestine and colon
E. Active transport in the small bowel and no absorption the colon

25. Which of the following is true regarding butyrate and propionate?
A. They are absorbed in the jejunum and aid in reabsorption of fluids in the small intestines
B. They are generated by bacterial fermentation from indigestible carbohydrates and are a major source of metabolic fuel for colonocytes
C. They are readily utilized by enterocytes as a source of metabolic fuel
D. They must be digested by colonic flora or can result in an osmotic diarrhea
E. They are 10- to 12-carbon fatty acids

26. Which of the following statements is correct regarding glucagon-like peptide 1 (GLP-1) and GLP-2 and their role in digestion?
A. GLP-1 and GLP-2 are secreted by the pancreas in response to luminal protein
B. GLP-1 decreases appetite and increases gastric emptying
C. GLP-1 and GLP-2 are high in the fasting state and decrease rapidly after nutrient digestion
D. GLP-1 and GLP-2 are co-secreted by enteroendocrine cells in the small and large intestine in response to fat and carbohydrate
E. GLP-1 and GLP-2 are co-secreted by enteroendocrine cells in the small intestines in response to protein

27. A 45-year-old African-American woman is referred to you by her primary care physician with complaints of bloating, occasional diarrhea, and gastroesophageal reflux disease. She denies any weight loss, blood in her stool, fevers, or chills. She has no history of abdominal surgery, and denies any recent travel or antibiotic use. Stool cultures, anti–tissue transglutaminase (tTG) and anti-endomysial antibodies are negative with a normal total serum IgA. She recently had a CT scan of the abdomen and pelvis that was unremarkable. She denies any changes in her diet and cooks at home. She does drink three lattes from her local coffee shop daily. The patient states that her diarrhea improved when she recently went camping for 2 weeks. What is the etiology of her abdominal bloating?
A. An allergy to a protein in wheat
B. Small intestinal bacterial overgrowth (SIBO)
C. A deficiency in a brush border membrane hydrolase
D. Chronic pancreatitis
E. Ulcerative colitis (UC)

28. Which of the following conditions can cause steatorrhea as the result of deactivation of pancreatic lipase?
A. Zollinger-Ellison syndrome (ZES)
B. High-dose proton-pump inhibitors (PPI)
C. Post–Billroth I surgery
D. Small intestinal bacterial overgrowth
E. Atrophic gastritis

29. Which of the following enzymes plays the key role in conversion of trypsinogen to its active form, trypsin?
A. Enterokinase
B. Elastase
C. Chymotrypsin
D. Carboxypeptidase A
E. Carboxypeptidase B

30. A 35-year-old woman presents to clinic with symptoms of dyspepsia and increasing lower extremity paresthesia. She denies any weight loss, melena, or rectal bleeding. Upon further questioning, the patient has a history of Crohn's disease and had some type of surgery in the past. Her hemoglobin is 9 g/dL, and her platelet count is 250,000/μL. Deficiency of which of the following micronutrients is the most likely etiology of this patient's symptoms?
A. Iron
B. Cobalamin
C. Vitamin C
D. Folic acid
E. Niacin

31. A 45-year-old homeless man presents to the emergency department with fatigue. He denies any rectal bleeding or melena and eats regularly at a local shelter. He was admitted last month to the hospital with alcohol withdrawal. Physical examination is significant for a thin male, nail pitting, and BMI of 18 kg/m^2. Initial laboratory values are as follows:

Hemoglobin	9.5 g/dL
WBC	4000/μL
Platelet count	300,000/μL
MCV	105 fL

What is the most likely etiology of this patient's anemia?

A. Iron deficiency
B. Hypothyroidism
C. Copper deficiency
D. Folate deficiency
E. Peptic ulcer disease

32. A 45-year-old woman with a history of diabetes mellitus type 2 presents to clinic with complaints of fatigue and dyspnea on exertion in the last 3 months. On further questioning she admits to drink 1 to 2 pints of beer daily in the last year. Physical examination is significant for bilateral 1+ pitting edema. Basic laboratory values are as follows:

Hemoglobin	12.0 g/dL
WBC	5000/μL
Platelet count	350,000/μL
MCV	95 fL
INR	1.0
AST	130 U/L
ALT	61 U/L
Total bilirubin	1.0 mg/dL

What is the most likely etiology of the patient's fatigue?

A. Iron deficiency
B. Cobalamin deficiency
C. Thiamine deficiency
D. Copper deficiency
E. Folate deficiency

33. A 37-year-old woman presents to clinic with complaints of acid reflux for the last year. She has a history of a Roux-en-Y gastric bypass 3 years ago. Routine blood tests are as follows:

Hemoglobin	10 g/dL
WBC	2500/μL
Platelet count	300,000/μL
MCV	77 fL
Iron	60 μL/dL
Ferritin	120 μL/L

What is the etiology of the patient's anemia?

A. Iron
B. Cobalamin
C. Thiamine
D. Copper
E. Folate

34. A 46-year-old man presents to clinic with a history of chronic hypokalemia and diarrhea. You discover that the etiology of patient's diarrhea is steatorrhea secondary to chronic pancreatitis. You add pancreatic enzyme supplementation, which helps to improve the diarrhea. You also discover that he has profound hypomagnesemia, and you decide to add oral supplements. Which of the following is correct regarding magnesium absorption in the small intestine?

A. At basal state, magnesium absorption is greater in the jejunum compared to other parts of small bowel
B. Duodenum is the main site for magnesium absorption
C. Jejunal absorption of magnesium is increased by vitamin D
D. Ileal absorption of magnesium is increased by vitamin D
E. On normal dietary intake, overall efficiency of magnesium absorption is more than 50%

35. A 45-year-old woman presents to the emergency department with complaints of diarrhea, fatigue, and weight loss of 6 months duration. She also reports worsening shortness of breath and cough. Social history is significant for drinking one glass of wine twice a week with dinner for the last 20 years. On physical exam, vital signs are as follows:

Temperature	97° F
Heart rate	95 bpm
Respiratory rate	18 breaths/min
Blood pressure	105/65 mm Hg
BMI	18 kg/m^2

She appears undernourished. Neck exam reveals a jugular venous pressure of 15 cm H_2O. Abdominal examination reveals moderate ascites. The liver edge is palpable 4 cm below the right costal margin, with a liver span of 14 cm on percussion. She has pitting lower extremity edema up to her midcalves. Echocardiogram reveals a mildly dilated right ventricle, normal left ventricle, and thickened ventricular walls. Fecal fat was measured at 20 g/day. What is the likely diagnosis?

A. Exocrine pancreatic insufficiency
B. Systemic amyloidosis
C. Celiac disease
D. Small bowel bacterial overgrowth
E. Anorexia nervosa

36. A 45-year-old African-American woman presents with complaints of abdominal bloating, diarrhea, and intermittent nausea and vomiting of 6 months duration. Her symptoms are exacerbated with food. She reports passing foul smelling stools without blood. She notes that she has to frequently wear gloves while inside or outside during the winter. She also reports severe heartburn, for which she takes omeprazole twice daily. Social history is significant for drinking one glass of wine twice a week with dinner for the last 20 years. On physical exam, vital signs are as follows:

Temperature	98° F
Heart rate	75 bpm
Respiratory rate	16 breaths/min
Blood pressure	115/65 mm Hg
BMI	20 kg/m^2

She has no scleral icterus. She has a small ulcer on the tip of the left index finger. Her abdomen is tender to palpation in the epigastrium. She has a nonitchy macular rash on both elbows. Laboratory values are as follows:

WBC	6000/μL
Hemoglobin	10.5 g/dL
Creatinine	1 mg/dL
Bilirubin	1.5 mg/dL
Alkaline phosphatase	118 IU/L
ALT	25 IU/L
AST	22 IU/L

Fecal occult blood is negative. There are no fecal leukocytes. Which of the following is likely to be found on further evaluation of this patient?

A. Multiple peptic and duodenal ulcerations on upper endoscopy
B. Significantly delayed intestinal transit seen on barium small bowel follow-through
C. Greater than 20 intraepithelial lymphocytes per 100 epithelial cells on colonic biopsies

D. Architectural distortion and chronic inflammation on colonic biopsy
E. Villous atrophy and increased intraepithelial lymphocytes on duodenal biopsy

37. Which of the following can be seen in folate deficiency?
A. High serum homocysteine level
B. Low serum homocysteine level
C. High serum methylmalonic acid level
D. Low serum methylmalonic acid level
E. High serum citruline level

38. A 52-year-old woman presents to your clinic with 6 months history of bloating, nonbloody diarrhea, and excessive gas. She has a history of multiple abdominal surgeries for adhesions and small bowel obstruction in the past as a result of severe endometriosis. A small bowel follow-through study last month did not show any evidence of obstruction but was significant for several jejunal diverticula. Elevation of which of the following lab parameters is most likely in this patient?
A. Vitamin B_{12} level
B. Folate level
C. INR
D. Thiamin level
E. Nicotinamide level

39. A 26-year-old African-American woman presents to your clinic with 1-year history of nonbloody diarrhea and bloating. She denies any history of surgery in the past but has experienced at least 6 episodes of pharyngitis and sinusitis in the last 3 years. On physical exam, vital signs are as follows:

Temperature	97° F
Heart rate	86 bpm
Respiratory rate	16 breaths/min
Blood pressure	110/65 mm Hg
BMI	19 kg/m^2

The rest of the exam is unremarkable except mild pallor. Laboratory values are as follows:

WBC	5000/μL
Hemoglobin	10.1 g/dL
MCV	108 fL
Ferritin	100 μL/L
Folate	2 ng/mL
Vitamin B_{12}	80 pg/mL (normal range 150-750 pg/mL)
Creatinine	1 mg/dL
Bilirubin	1.1 mg/dL
Alkaline phosphatase	118 IU/L
ALT	48 IU/L
AST	47 IU/L

Upper endoscopy is performed, which is unremarkable, but small bowel biopsies show villous shortening, an increased number of lymphocytes in the epithelium, and absence of plasma cells. What is the most likely diagnosis in this patient?
A. Celiac disease
B. Small intestinal bacterial overgrowth
C. Common variable immunodeficiency (CVID)
D. Zollinger-Ellison syndrome (ZES)
E. Lactose malabsorption

40. Which of the following statements is correct regarding lactose intolerance?
A. It is more common in Northern Europeans compared to Middle Easterners
B. Consuming whole milk rather than skim milk can reduce the symptoms
C. Persistence of symptoms while patient is on lactose-free diet rules out the diagnosis of lactose intolerance
D. Lactase deficiency usually produces more severe symptoms in children compared to adults
E. There is a clear relation found between the amount of lactose ingestion and the severity of the symptoms

41. Which of the following statements is correct regarding the pathophysiology of small intestinal bacterial overgrowth?
A. Mucosal injury by the bacteria will lead to increase in brush-border enzymes, hence the carbohydrate maldigestion
B. Luminal competition with the host for nutrients can lead to consumption of thiamine, B_{12}, and other vitamins
C. Diarrhea is caused by the synthesis of acetaldehyde
D. Injury to the epithelial barrier will decrease intestinal permeability and as a result will lead to malabsorption
E. Diarrhea usually occurs as a result of the effect of deconjugated bile salts on the small bowel

42. Which of the following can be found in patients with small intestinal bacterial overgrowth?
A. High vitamin B_{12} level
B. High folate levels
C. High thiamine level
D. High nicotinamide level
E. High INR level

43. A 33-year-old woman with a long-standing history of diabetes presents to you for evaluation of nausea and bloating. She has a history of hysterectomy and a small ileal diverticulum incidentally noted on prior abdominal imaging. Which of the following factors puts her at highest risk for small intestinal bacterial overgrowth?
A. Younger age
B. History of ileal diverticula
C. History of hysterectomy
D. History of diabetes
E. Antacids consumption

44. Which of the following statements is true regarding the hydrogen breath testing used in the diagnosis of small intestinal bacterial overgrowth?
A. Exercise and smoking can lead to false positive results
B. Gastroparesis can lead to false negative results
C. Oral flora does not have any effect in the interpretation of the study
D. Patients are advised to fast for 12 hours prior to the test
E. Methanogenic bacteria can give false positive results

45. Which of the following is correct regarding the diagnosis of small intestinal bacterial overgrowth (SIBO)?
A. Most small intestinal biopsies from patients with SIBO have villus atrophy
B. When performing jejunal aspirates, greater than 10^5 colony-forming units (CFU)/mL is diagnostic in all geographic regions
C. During the lactulose hydrogen breath test (LHBT), the first peak is related to hydrogen production by the oral flora
D. Breath tests are cheaper than jejunal aspirates
E. Fecal calprotectin is usually high in patients with SIBO

46. Which of the following contributes to the mechanism of liver injury in patients with small intestinal bacterial overgrowth?
A. Deconjugation of primary bile acids
B. Consumption of dietary proteins
C. Fermentation of unabsorbed carbohydrates
D. Synthesis of acetaldehyde
E. Loss of brush-border enzymes

47. Which of the following conditions is linked to small intestinal bacterial overgrowth?
A. Hysterectomy
B. Hyperthyroidism
C. Colonic diverticulosis.
D. Ileocecal valve resection
E. Ulcerative colitis

48. A 19-year-old man with a history of partial enterectomy due to intestinal ischemia with resultant 130 cm of small intestine with an ileal colonic anastomosis presents to the emergency department with right flank pain. Abdominal CT demonstrates parenchymal inflammation of the right kidney with dilation of the right ureter. What is the likely treatment that would have prevented this patient's symptoms?
A. Low fat diet
B. Low oxalate diet
C. Limit simple sugars in diet
D. Low calcium diet
E. Cholestyramine

49. A 40-year-old woman with a history of short bowel syndrome is brought to the emergency department by her husband with symptoms of confusion and inappropriate behavior of 1-day duration. The husband says that she has had extensive small intestinal surgery. She has been depressed lately due to the death of family pet and has been eating excessive sweets to cope. She takes diphenoxylate/atropine for her diarrhea and a multivitamin. She is used to drinking one glass of wine with dinner three times a week for the past 10 years. On physical examination, the patient is disoriented with an ataxic gait. Eye examination reveals bilateral nystagmus. Laboratory values are as follows:

Sodium	145 mEq/L
Chloride	98 mmol/L
Bicarbonate	15 mmol/l
Potassium	4.0 mEq/L
Lactic acid	0.6 mmol/L
Creatinine	2.2 mg/dL

Which of the following is the most likely etiology of the patient's presentation?
A. Alcohol intoxication
B. Salicylate overdose
C. Fermentation of unabsorbed carbohydrates
D. Dehydration precipitating renal failure
E. Thiamine deficiency

50. A 33-year-old woman with short bowel syndrome who is dependent on total parenteral nutrition (TPN) is admitted to the hospital with severe shortness of breath. She has not been administering her TPN for some time because she is tired of hooking up the bag every night. Physical examination reveals a jugular venous pressure of 15 cm H_2O and bilateral inspiratory and expiratory crackles. Heart auscultation reveals an S3 gallop. There is bilateral lower extremity edema to the midcalves. Which of the following explains the patient's presentation?
A. Copper deficiency
B. Vitamin D deficiency
C. Chromium deficiency
D. Selenium deficiency
E. Manganese deficiency

51. A 45-year-old man with a history of short bowel syndrome who is dependent on TPN is seen in clinic for follow-up. His wife noticed that his eyes turned yellow several weeks ago. She also reports that his arms and body sometimes twist into abnormal postures. On physical exam, the patient has scleral icterus. He is noted to have a resting tremor, has an unstable gait, and is slightly confused. Laboratory values are as follows:

Total bilirubin	6.0 mg/dL
Alkaline phosphatase	305 U/L
AST	100 U/L
ALT	120 U/L
Creatinine	0.8 mg/dL

You order a right upper quadrant ultrasound, which demonstrates no gallbladder wall thickening, with a common bile duct diameter of 6 mm. What is the likely etiology of this patient's symptoms?
A. Thiamine deficiency
B. Copper deficiency
C. Cobalamin deficiency
D. Selenium toxicity
E. Manganese toxicity

52. A 47-year-old man with short bowel syndrome who has been on TPN for 3 years presents to your clinic for follow-up visit. He denies any complaint except mild tenderness at the site of tunneled catheter. On physical exam his vital signs are as follows:

Temperature	36.8° C
Heart rate	66 bpm
Blood pressure	110/75 mm Hg

Exam of the catheter site shows some tenderness and erythema at the exit site. Also, some discharged pus is noted on the dressing. The rest of the exam is unremarkable. What is the most appropriate next step in this patient?
A. Stop using the catheter and continue with oral nutrition for 2 weeks before restarting TPN
B. Remove the catheter and replace with a new one at a different site
C. Send blood culture and start antibiotics based on culture results
D. Send culture of the pus, start piperacillin/tazobactam while awaiting results
E. Send culture of the pus, start vancomycin while awaiting results

53. A 50-year-old man presented for a resection of large cecal adenoma. During the surgery the distal ileum is injured, and the patient undergoes a partial enterectomy with ileocolonic anastomosis. He now presents to you with complaints of diarrhea. Fecal leukocytes are negative, as is *C. difficile* toxin PCR. Fecal fat is 6 g/24 hours. His diarrhea is not responding well to loperamide. Which of the following is the most likely etiology of his diarrhea?
A. Fat malabsorption
B. Bile acid deficiency
C. Osmotic diarrhea from unabsorbed bile acids
D. Secretory diarrhea from unabsorbed bile acids
E. Osmotic diarrhea from unabsorbed simple carbohydrates

54. A 54-year-old woman with short bowel syndrome who has been on TPN for 2 years presents to your clinic with complaint of slowed rate of TPN, which is resistant to flushing of the catheter in the last 3 days. She denies any other complaint. She remembers one episode of occlusion of the catheter "by a clot" 6 months ago. On physical exam, her vital signs are as follows:

Temperature	37.1° C
Heart rate	86 bpm
Blood pressure	100/70 mm Hg

Exam of the catheter site is unremarkable. What is the most appropriate next step in this patient?
A. Empirically treat with tissue plasminogen activator (tPA)
B. Attempt aspiration through the catheter
C. Start empiric vancomycin
D. Radiologic contrast study of the catheter
E. Remove and replace the catheter

55. Which of the following is true regarding teduglutide in patients with short bowel syndrome?
A. It has been approved to be used for up to 1 year
B. It is a synthetic analog of glucagon-like peptide 2 (GLP-2)
C. Teduglutide administration is associated with decreased plasma citrulline levels
D. Nephropathy is a common side effect of this medication
E. Its use results in more significant improvement in nitrogen absorption than fluid absorption from the small bowel

56. A 41-year-old man with history of short bowel syndrome who has been on TPN for 2 years presents to GI clinic for follow-up. His wife has noticed worsening jaundice in addition to episodes of confusion in the last 3 months. He complains of increased size of his belly. The physical exam shows:

Temperature	36.7° C
Heart rate	84 bpm
Respiratory rate	16/min
Blood pressure	100/68 mm Hg

Significant jaundice, nontense ascites, and bilateral lower edema up to the knees are remarkable in the exam. Laboratory values are as follows:

Hemoglobin	10 g/dL
WBC	4000/μL
Platelet count	109,000 /μL
Total bilirubin	8.0 mg/dL
Alkaline phosphatase	155 U/L
AST	40 U/L
ALT	50 U/L
Creatinine	1.8 mg/dL
INR	1.9

What would be the best long-term treatment plan for this patient?
A. Small intestinal transplantation
B. Combined small intestine–liver transplantation
C. Teduglutide
D. Intestinal lengthening procedure
E. Optimization of TPN regimen

57. A 40-year-old man with SBS presents to clinic for follow-up. He has chronic diarrhea that has been stable. The patient states he only had small intestinal resection, and his entire colon is still intact. He denies any shortness of breath or cough. He reports difficulty with driving at night and dry eyes. He is eating well with no restrictions on his diet. Which of the following would explain the patient's symptoms?
A. Fat malabsorption
B. Vitamin B_{12} deficiency
C. Folate deficiency
D. Niacin deficiency
E. Fermentation of unabsorbed carbohydrates

58. A 32-year-old Caucasian woman with history of chronic generalized abdominal discomfort, bloating, and loose stool for the last 4 years presents to your clinic for a second opinion. She remembers that she had an upper endoscopy and colonoscopy about 2 years ago, which were both unremarkable. She mentions that in the last 3 months after reading a book about the effect of diet on health, she has been on strict gluten free diet (GFD) and has noted significant improvement in her symptoms. She would like to stay on a GFD because she is very worried to experience her symptoms again if she goes back on gluten-containing diet. However, she is curious to know if she has celiac disease or not. What test would you recommend to her at this time?
A. Upper endoscopy with small bowel biopsy (at least 6 biopsies)
B. IgA anti-tTG antibody
C. Genetic testing for human leukocyte antigen (HLA)-DQ2/DQ8
D. IgG anti–deamidated gliadin peptides (DGP)
E. No further test is necessary. Her symptoms improvement on the GFD confirms celiac disease

59. When examining a small intestinal biopsy of a patient with celiac disease, which of the following findings is expected to be seen?
A. The disease process that only affecting the mucosa
B. Eosinophilic cytoplasm of the enterocytes
C. Increased intraepithelial neutrophils
D. Shorter crypts
E. Decreased cellularity of the lamina propria

60. When counseling patients with celiac disease, which of the following would you advise them to avoid?
A. Rice
B. Corn
C. Barley
D. Sorghum
E. Millet

61. A 32-year-old woman is referred to you for evaluation of abdominal bloating. She denies any change in bowel habits or anemia. Her past medical history is remarkable for idiopathic infertility. Her laboratory values show positive IgA tTG antibody. You perform an upper endoscopy with biopsies of the small bowel, which comes back normal. What is the best next step in her management?
A. Inform her that she has celiac disease and needs to be on a strict gluten free diet for the rest of her life
B. Inform her that you are concerned she has latent celiac and will need to adhere to a strict gluten free diet as this might be contributing to her bloating and infertility
C. Order serum IgA level
D. Order genetic testing for celiac disease
E. Order IgA antigliadin antibody to confirm the diagnosis of celiac disease

62. A 23-year-old Caucasian man with history of iron deficiency anemia is referred to your clinic for second opinion. He denies any history of GI bleeding. He has never been on a gluten free diet. He had an upper endoscopy with small bowel biopsies that suggested celiac disease.

However, IgA tTG and IgA endomysial antibodies were negative. He also had a colonoscopy, which was unremarkable. You checked his serum IgA level, which was undetectable. Which of the following is the most appropriate test in this patient?

A. Genetic HLA testing
B. IgA antigliadin antibody
C. IgG antigliadin antibody
D. IgG anti-tTG antibody
E. IgG anti-DGP antibody

63. A 42-year-old woman presents to your office for diarrhea, fatigue, and weight loss for the past few years. She had tried several types of diets until she started a gluten free diet a few weeks ago and felt remarkably better. Her physical exam is unremarkable, and basic laboratory values show no abnormalities. Her IgA-tTG is positive. She underwent an esophagogastroduodenoscopy (EGD) and small bowel biopsies were obtained, and were normal. What is the best next step in her management?

A. Reassure the patient and schedule a routine follow-up
B. Check HLA-DQ2 and -DQ8; positive results confirm the diagnosis
C. Obtain barium study of the small intestine
D. Start a gluten challenge for at least 2 weeks and repeat biopsies
E. Repeat IgA-tTG to avoid false positive results

64. A 39-year-old man is referred to you from his dermatologist's office for evaluation. He was diagnosed with dermatitis herpetiformis 6 months ago and has been on dapsone with good response in skin rash. However, the rash and pruritus return each time that dapsone is discontinued. He has no gastrointestinal complaints. You ordered celiac disease serologic testing and endoscopy with small bowel biopsies, and they both came back negative. What is the best step in the management of this patient?

A. Instruct patient to continue with dapsone for the rest of his life
B. Stop dapsone and start strict gluten free diet (GFD)
C. Start GFD and continue with dapsone for 6 months and then taper off dapsone if skin lesions resolve
D. Check HLA-DQ2/DQ8
E. Add oral steroids to dapsone regimen

65. When counseling patients with celiac disease about diet, which of the following advice is correct?

A. Oats should be completely avoided
B. Dairy products should be avoided at the beginning of treatment
C. Nutritional deficiencies are not an issue after symptom improvement and weight gain on gluten free diet
D. Medications and vitamin supplements are all gluten free
E. Avoidance of all types of alcoholic beverages is essential

66. A 44-year-old woman with history of celiac disease presents to you for persistent symptoms of abdominal pain, bloating, and diarrhea. She was diagnosed with celiac 5 years ago based on an elevated tissue transglutaminase antibody level and abnormal small bowel biopsies. She has been on a strict gluten free diet for 5 years, but reports persistent symptoms. Her weight is stable. You perform a tissue transglutaminase level, and it is elevated. What is the most likely etiology for her symptoms?

A. Continued ingestion of gluten
B. False positive diagnosis of celiac disease
C. Microscopic colitis
D. Refractory celiac disease
E. Ulcerative jejunitis

67. Which of the following is true regarding malignancies related to celiac disease?

A. Intestinal lymphomas related to celiac disease are usually of B-cell origin
B. Enteropathy-associated T-cell lymphoma (EATL) usually responds to gluten free diet (GFD)
C. EATL has a poor prognosis
D. Patients with untreated celiac disease have a similar risk of nonlymphoma malignancies compared to the general population
E. Even with strict GFD, the risk of all malignancies is significantly increased compared to the general population

68. An 18-year-old woman presents for evaluation of anemia, gas, and intermittent diarrhea. She put herself on a gluten free diet for the past 3 months and reports she is feeling better. Her tTG antibody level 6 months ago was normal. She had an upper endoscopy with small bowel biopsies 6 months ago that did not show any small bowel abnormalities. Her hemoglobin is 11 g/dL with an MCV of 90 fL, and they have not changed significantly in the last 6 months despite being on a gluten free diet. The patient believes she has celiac disease and would like a repeat endoscopy to ensure that she is absorbing iron now that she has been on a gluten free diet. Which of the following is the most appropriate next step?

A. Repeat EGD
B. Reassure her that she does not need endoscopic evaluation because her celiac disease is asymptomatic now that she is on a gluten free diet
C. Recommend a colonoscopy
D. Reassure the patient that she has nonceliac gluten intolerance and that repeating the endoscopy will not be helpful
E. Prescribe B_{12} injections, as she is probably B_{12} deficient, hence, the lack of improvement in her hemoglobin

69. A 58-year-old Caucasian man with history of celiac disease diagnosed in his 20s presents to your clinic with a 4-month history of severe abdominal pain, weight loss, and diarrhea despite being on gluten free diet. A small bowel barium contrast study was perfomed (see figure). Which of the following statements is correct regarding this patient's condition?

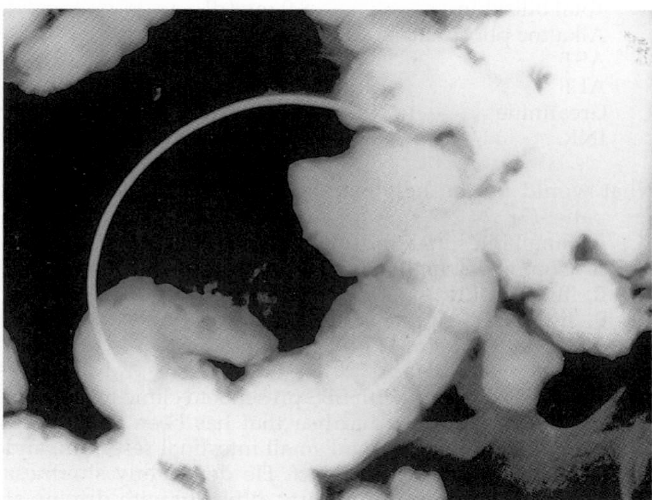

Figure for question 69.

A. The treatment is strict gluten free diet
B. The 5-year survival rate is 80%
C. It is always associated with T-cell lymphoma
D. Corticosteroids can cause worsening of this condition
E. The most effective treatment is surgery

70. A 29-year-old healthy man traveled to Mexico to visit his girlfriend. During his stay, he ate at local restaurants and drank tap water. Upon his return, he starts complaining of watery diarrhea and abdominal bloating. Which of the following pathogens is the most likely etiology to his symptoms?
A. *Vibrio cholera*
B. *Giardia lamblia*
C. *Cryptosporidium*
D. Enterotoxin-producing *Escherichia coli*
E. *Campylobacter jejuni*

71. Which of the following is correct regarding the epidemiology of tropical sprue?
A. It may occur in indigenous residents
B. Sporadic tropical sprue cases are no longer reported
C. It affects children more frequently than adults
D. Tropical sprue epidemics have been increasing in the last decade
E. Exposure to epidemic sprue is not protective against a second wave

72. A 42-year-old healthy man who recently stayed in India for 3 months on a business trip presents with diarrhea, bloating, and a 35-pound weight loss in the last 2 months. During his stay there, he had a flu-like illness with fatigue, low-grade fevers, and watery diarrhea. If the diagnosis of tropical sprue is suspected, which of the following is correct regarding histologic examination of the GI tract?
A. Villus to crypt ratio of 5:1 on a jejunal biopsy
B. Significant and complete villus atrophy
C. Infiltration of the lamina propria with intraepithelial lymphocytes is diagnostic
D. Atrophic gastritis is common
E. If scalloping of the duodenum is seen, then celiac sprue is more likely to be the cause

73. A 43-year-old man presents to your clinic for abdominal pain, diarrhea, weight loss, and anemia. His symptoms started several weeks ago. He recently moved back to the United States to receive medical attention after living in Costa Rica for 6 months. He describes steatorrhea, peripheral neuropathy, and excessive bruising. You suspect he has tropical sprue. What diet would you recommend for him?
A. High calorie, low protein, high fat diet
B. High calorie, high protein, high fat diet
C. Low calorie, high protein, low fat diet
D. Low calorie, low protein, low fat diet
E. High calorie, high protein, low fat diet

74. A 38-year-old man, with no family history of colon cancer, who has tropical sprue, is admitted for abdominal distension, decreased bowel sounds, and nausea. His last bowel movement was an hour ago. An abdominal CT scan shows a significantly dilated colon without small bowel dilation. Surgery is consulted for impending perforation. The patient is hemodynamically stable with a normal WBC count. He started tetracycline 24 hours earlier and reports his abdominal distension has been progressively getting worse. The surgical attending calls you to discuss a treatment plan. What would you recommend next?
A. Surgical colectomy
B. Colonoscopy
C. Surgical cecostomy
D. Correct electrolyte imbalance, and monitor closely with frequent abdominal exam closely
E. Switch to an intravenous antibiotic as patient is probably not absorbing the tetracycline

75. A 48-year-old Haitian woman is referred to you for intermittent dysphagia of 3 months duration. You perform an upper endoscopy, which does not show any esophageal pathology, but incidentally you notice flattening of the villi in the duodenum. You biopsy her duodenum, and the pathologist calls to inform you that she seems concerned about celiac disease based on the histologic features on the biopsies. The patient denies any symptoms of diarrhea, abdominal pain, or weight loss. Her laboratory values are as follows:

Hemoglobin	13 g/dL
WBC	8000/μL
Platelet count	185,000/μL
Total bilirubin	1.1 g/dL
Alkaline phosphatase	78 U/L
ALT	38 U/L
AST	35 U/L
INR	1.1
Folate	18 ng/mL
B_{12} level	650 pg/mL
Serum IgA level	300 mg/dL
Anti-tTG IgA	negative

Which of the following is the most likely diagnosis?
A. Serology-negative celiac disease
B. Tropical sprue
C. Whipple's disease
D. Tropical enteropathy
E. Common variable immune deficiency (CVID)

76. A 75-year-old Indian woman is admitted to the hospital for abdominal pain of 6 weeks duration. The pain became so severe that her daughter brought her to the emergency department. On your initial assessment, the patient is hemodynamically stable with diffuse abdominal tenderness on exam. Abdominal imaging shows terminal ileal and right colonic wall thickening without obstruction, but with a few enlarged mesenteric lymph nodes. The emergency department physician would like to start her on steroids for possible Crohn's disease. Her most recent colonoscopy was normal 2 years ago. What would you recommend as the next step in the management of this patient?
A. Abdominal MRI
B. Start mesalamine
C. Colonoscopy
D. Agree with intravenous steroids
E. Surgical consult

77. Which of the following is true about Whipple's disease?
A. It is caused by a gram-negative bacterium
B. It is more common in females
C. It is more common in Africans
D. It is not seen in children
E. It leads to symptomatic neurologic manifestations in the majority of patients

78. You are evaluating a 52-year-old white man who is referred for evaluation of chronic watery diarrhea of 9-month duration, as well as occasional subjective low-grade fevers. The patient reports a 22-lb weight loss and abdominal pain. Physical examination reveals inguinal lymphadenopathy. Laboratory evaluation shows a mild leukocytosis and negative blood cultures. Whipple's disease is one of the possibilities on your differential diagnosis. Which of the following findings is associated with Whipple's disease?

A. Erythrocytosis
B. Decreased serum carotene level
C. Normal C-reactive protein
D. Low stool fat content
E. High serum iron levels

79. You are consulted on a 58-year-old white man who complains of mild diarrhea for 3 months. His primary care physician suspects Whipple's disease because the patient is a farmer. He orders a stool test for *Tropheryma whipplei* PCR, and it is positive. The patient denies any other complaints, including fever, weight loss, abdominal pain, neurologic, cardiac, pulmonary, or rheumatologic symptoms. Abdominal imaging is normal. The primary care physician recommends treatment with antibiotics for 1 year. You perform an upper endoscopy with eight small bowel biopsies. The pathologist calls you to tell you that the histology on the biopsies is normal without any evidence of Whipple's disease. What is the next step in the management?

A. Antibiotics for 1 year
B. Enteroscopy and small bowel biopsy
C. Reassure the patient that he does not have Whipple's disease
D. Colonoscopy and biopsy
E. Treat with antibiotics for 1 month

80. Which of the following statements is correct regarding the pathologic findings in Whipple's disease?

A. Periodic acid–Schiff (PAS)–positive macrophages in extraintestinal organs are specific findings of Whipple's disease
B. Structurally intact bacteria are present intracellular
C. Mucosal infiltration by positive PAS cell appears patchy
D. Histologic findings disappear within 2 weeks after adequate treatment
E. Positive PAS stain reflects the glycoprotein

81. Four weeks after a 53-year-old man with Whipple's disease was started on trimethoprim/sulfamethoxazole, he starts complaining of worsening of symptoms. He now develops worsening arthralgias, fevers, and severe abdominal pain. On history taking, you realize the patient had been on steroids for 8 weeks prior to being diagnosed with Whipple's disease as his primary care physician thought his symptoms were related to an inflammatory arthritis. What would be your next course of action?

A. Switch from trimethoprim/sulfamethoxazole to tetracycline
B. Suspect that you made the wrong diagnosis and repeat the workup
C. Consult rheumatology to assist with the management of arthralgias
D. Add another antibiotic to the current regimen
E. Start prednisone

82. A 60-year-old white man with progressive dementia, weight loss, arthralgias, and diarrhea is diagnosed with Whipple's disease and treated with tetracycline for 1 year. The patient has complete resolution of all symptoms within 3 months of treatment. However, 6 months after finishing therapy, he presents with insomnia, progressive dementia, and syncope. CT scan of the head shows no focal lesions. You suspect a central nervous system (CNS) relapse. Which of the following is true regarding this condition?

A. Initial treatment with oral tetracycline lowers the likelihood of CNS relapse
B. Prognosis of CNS relapses depends on the choice of initial treatment
C. CNS relapses usually respond to treatment with tetracycline
D. Trimethoprim/sulfamethoxazole is not associated with CNS relapses
E. CNS relapses are rarely seen in patients treated with a 2-week course of intravenous penicillin plus streptomycin, followed by tetracycline for 1 year

83. When choosing an antibiotic for the management of Whipple's disease, which of the following is the most important factor to consider?

A. Parenteral route
B. Gram-negative coverage
C. Ability to cross the blood-brain barrier
D. Second-generation cephalosporin
E. Short-term therapy but high doses

84. A 37-year-old female aid worker travels to Asia following a natural disaster and develops severe diarrhea. Hundreds in the local population are afflicted with the same illness, consisting of large-volume watery stools with resultant significant fluid and electrolyte losses. Under the microscope, the causative pathogen is found to be gram-negative, short, and curved rod-appearing, like a comma. Which of the following is true regarding the above illness?

A. Most patients who come in contact with the organism develop clinical illness
B. Biopsy of the small bowel would demonstrate inflammation and ulcerations
C. The bacterial toxin increases adenylate cyclase activity, resulting in elevated levels of cAMP
D. Antimicrobial therapy is not recommended
E. The bacteria primarily affect the colon

85. A 61-year-old man with a past medical history of hepatitis C cirrhosis presents to the emergency department with a worsening, painful skin lesion that started on his foot 3 days ago. He recently returned from a trip to southern Alabama and spent several days swimming in the Gulf of Mexico and reports suffering a minor cut on the bottom of his foot. Currently his vital signs are as follows:

Heart rate	105 bpm
Blood pressure	90/60 mm Hg
Temperature	38.0° C

Physical examination is significant for the patient appearing in mild distress with hemorrhagic bullae and erythema spreading superiorly from his left foot. Which of the following is true regarding the causative pathogen?

A. The bacteria are characterized as gram-positive, short, curved rods
B. The bacteria carry a higher incidence rate but lower severity of illness in patients with underlying liver disease
C. Preventive measures include avoiding raw seafood
D. Vancomycin is recommended for severe infection
E. Septicemia due to this organism carries mortality rate for at-risk populations at around 10%

86. A 78-year-old male nursing home resident with a past medical history of hypertension and dyslipidemia presents to the emergency department with bloody diarrhea for 1 day. He reports he had watery, non-bloody diarrhea associated with abdominal cramping for 3 days preceding the bloody diarrhea. He also reports nausea, vomiting, and chills. Several other residents at his nursing home are hospitalized with similar illnesses. Physical examination is significant for the patient appearing to be in moderate distress with moderate diffuse abdominal tenderness without rebound tenderness or guarding. Laboratory studies are as follows:

WBC	17,000/μL with 85% neutrophils
Hemoglobin	8.3 g/dL
Platelet count	72,000/μL
Sodium	132 mEq/L
Potassium	3.2 mEq/L
Chloride	102 mEq/L
HCO_3^-	18 mEq/L
BUN	110 mg/dL
Creatinine	3.4 mg/dL
Glucose	85 mg/dL

The patient previously had normal laboratory values 6 months ago. What is the most likely pathogen causing this patient's illness?

A. *Shigella dysenteriae*
B. *E. coli*
C. *Yersinia enterocolitica*
D. *V. cholerae*
E. *Salmonella enterica*

87. A 33-year-old man presents to the emergency department with abdominal pain and watery diarrhea for 4 days. CT scan of the abdomen and pelvis demonstrates terminal ileal thickening without evidence of obstruction. Which of the following is known to commonly cause terminal ileitis?

A. *V. cholerae*
B. *Y. enterocolitica*
C. Enteropathogenic *E. coli* (EPEC)
D. Enteroinvasive *E. coli* (EIEC)
E. *C. jejuni*

88. A 32-year-old female immigrant from Mali presents to your clinic with abdominal pain, diarrhea, and weight loss for the last 6 weeks. She reports good appetite, but having lost 20 pounds despite this. Occasionally, she sees blood in her stool and notes fullness in the right side of her abdomen. She immigrated to the United States over 20 years ago and notes no other sick contacts. Her vital signs are as follow:

Heart rate	84 bpm
Blood pressure	134/72 mm Hg
Temperature	36.9° C

Physical examination demonstrates a palpable right lower quadrant abdominal mass with mild right lower quadrant tenderness. Laboratory studies are as follows:

WBC	8200/μL
Hemoglobin	10.1 g/dL
Platelet count	324,000/μL

Basic metabolic panel and hepatic function panel are unremarkable. CT scan of the abdomen/pelvis demonstrates thickening of the terminal ileum and cecum with surrounding lymphadenopathy. Colonoscopy demonstrates multiple superficial ulcers throughout the ascending colon, cecum, and terminal ileum with surrounding erythema. The patient develops severe abdominal pain, and a CT scan of the abdomen shows a cecal perforation. A right hemicolectomy is performed, and a colon micrograph of the surgical specimen is shown. What is the most likely diagnosis?

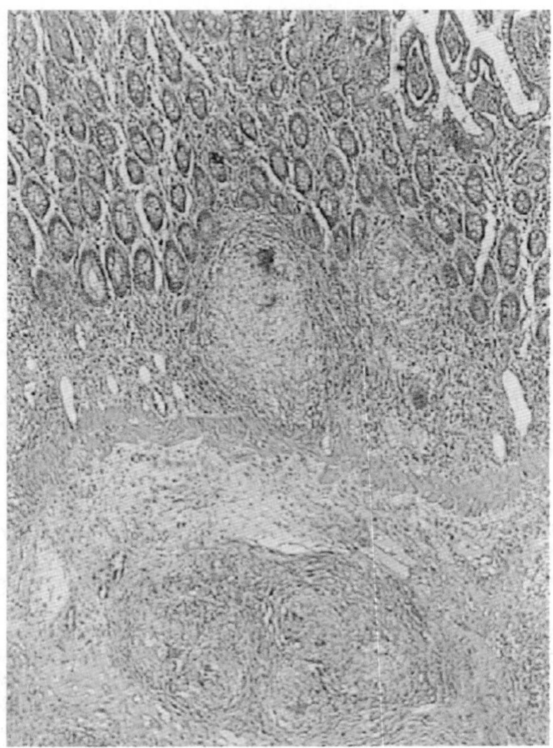

Figure for question 88.

A. *Mycobacterium tuberculosis*
B. *Yersinia enterocolitica*
C. Crohn's disease
D. Behçet's disease
E. *Entamoeba histolytica*

89. Which of the following general principles regarding oral intake is true in managing infectious diarrhea?

A. Reduced-osmolarity oral rehydration solutions (ORS) should be avoided due to the risk of hyponatremia
B. Dairy products should be avoided due to the possibility of secondary lactose deficiency
C. Oral feeding should be started only after the diarrhea resolves
D. ORS should not be given in patients who are vomiting
E. ORS generally carry glucose to increase calorie intake

90. A 41-year-old man with history of insulin-dependent diabetes mellitus sees you in clinic for watery diarrhea for the last 2 days. He also complains of nausea, low-grade fever, and malaise. His wife suffered from similar symptoms 5 days ago that have since resolved. Vital signs are as follows:

Heart rate	90 bpm
Blood pressure	124/72 mm Hg
Temperature	37.4° C

Physical examination is remarkable only for a tired-appearing man of stated age with mild diffuse abdominal tenderness. Stool cultures are negative, and a presumptive diagnosis of norovirus infection is made. Which of the following is true regarding norovirus?

A. Alcohol-based hand sanitizer is considered equivalent to soap-and-water hand hygiene in preventing norovirus infection
B. Ill individuals should be excluded from work for 48 to 72 hours after illness to prevent further spread of the disease
C. Norovirus is only symptomatic in individuals that are immunocompromised
D. The majority of patients who acquire norovirus do not exhibit symptoms
E. Antivirals are recommended to decrease disease duration and severity

91. You are called to see a 67-year-old man with past medical history of hemochromatosis and diabetes mellitus admitted to the hospital for the last 2 days with diarrhea and fevers. The patient states he has had fever, abdominal pain, diarrhea, and vomiting for the last week. The diarrhea is watery and up to 1.5 L per day. He lives on a pig farm in the rural part of the state and prepares his own sausages. He has no travel history. No other family members are sick, and he does not smoke, consume alcohol, or use any other types of drugs. Vital signs are as follows:

Heart rate	110 bpm
Blood pressure	82/56 mm Hg
Temperature	38.6° C

Physical examination demonstrates an individual of stated age in moderate distress, with chills and mild to moderate right lower quadrant abdominal tenderness without rebound tenderness or guarding. CT scan of abdomen/pelvis demonstrates mild wall thickening of the terminal ileum without evidence of intestinal obstruction. Ileocolonoscopy revealed normal ileal and colonic mucosa, and ileal and colonic biopsies were unremarkable. Routine stool culture is negative, but microscopy reveals leukocytes and red blood cells. Blood cultures are preliminarily positive for a gram-negative rod. What is the most likely pathogen causing this patient's illness?

A. *Y. enterocolitica*
B. *V. cholerae*
C. *S. enterica*
D. *Mycobacterium tuberculosis*
E. *S. dysenteriae*

92. A 48-year-old woman with history of diabetes mellitus and recent diarrheal infection is in the hospital for the second time in the last month. She presents at this admission with symmetric weakness that has progressively worsened, requiring intubation and mechanical ventilation. She had previously been hospitalized with bloody diarrhea, low-grade fevers, abdominal pain, myalgias, anorexia, and vomiting, but no stool culture had been sent. Her diarrheal illness resolved with supportive care. Currently the patient's vital signs are as follows:

Heart rate	85 bpm
Blood pressure	110/64 mm Hg
Temperature	37.4° C
Oxygen saturation	100% on 40% FiO_2
Respiratory rate	12 breaths/min on the mechanical ventilator

Physical examination is notable for a sedated female of stated age on a mechanical ventilator. Which of the following is true regarding the patient's illness?

A. Sexual partners of the patient should be empirically treated with antibiotics
B. A common extraintestinal manifestation includes cellulitis
C. Toxic megacolon is a common complication that requires close clinical monitoring
D. It is caused by a motile, comma-shaped, gram-negative rod bacterium with a polar flagellum
E. The pathogen is rarely acquired via contaminated foods

93. A 19-year-old African-American man with a past medical history of sickle cell anemia and gastroesophageal reflux disease (GERD) is admitted to the hospital with diarrhea. The patient states that over the last 48 hours he has experienced fevers, abdominal cramping, nausea, and vomiting. He characterizes the diarrhea as watery and large volume. He takes omeprazole daily for his GERD. He is a nonsmoker, nondrinker, and works as a bank teller. Vital signs are as follows:

Heart rate	110 bpm
Blood pressure	94/70 mm Hg
Temperature	38.4° C

Physical examination is remarkable for a man of stated age in mild distress and mild diffuse tenderness throughout the abdomen without rebound tenderness or guarding with hyperactive bowel sounds. Laboratory studies are as follows:

WBC	17,300/μL
Neutrophils	85%
Hemoglobin	8.4 g/dL (baseline 9-10 g/dL)
Creatinine	1.3 mg/dL

He has otherwise unremarkable basic metabolic panel and hepatic function panel. The patient is treated with supportive care but, subsequently during the hospitalization, develops persistent fevers and a new diastolic heart murmur. Which of the following is true regarding the patient's causative pathogen?

A. The patient's sickle cell anemia predisposes him to invasive infections
B. One subtype of the causative bacterium can cause hemolytic-uremic syndrome (HUS) through release of Shiga toxins
C. The colon is the typical site of invasion in the GI tract
D. The pathogen is typically acquired from human feces
E. Enteritis and diarrhea need to precede bacteremia

94. A 82-year-old male patient presents to the emergency department with fevers, abdominal pain, and diarrhea. The patient states feeling quite weak currently and initially had 3 days of fevers, abdominal pain, and watery diarrhea that has since turned bloody in the last couple days. Stool culture grows *S. dysenteriae*. Which of the following is true regarding *S. dysenteriae* infection?

A. Early administration of antibiotics can cause development of hemolytic-uremic syndrome (HUS)
B. In patients with shigellosis and meningismus, the organism can be isolated from the cerebrospinal fluid (CSF)
C. Vaccination is an important method of prevention in patients at risk
D. Chronic carriers of *Shigella* rarely become symptomatic with the strain they carry
E. Men who have sex with men are at increased risk of shigellosis

95. A 43-year-old man is admitted to the hospital with fevers, headaches, diarrhea, and abdominal pain of 3 days duration. He is a journalist and recently returned from an assignment in rural Kenya. He describes his pain as having lasted for the last week and localized to the right lower quadrant. He also notes green diarrhea over the same time period. More recently, he has noted fullness in his left abdomen with a rash on his chest. Vital signs are as follows:

Blood pressure	94/52 mm Hg
Heart rate	54 bpm
Temperature	38.9° C

Physical examination demonstrates a male of stated age in moderate distress and rose spots on the chest. Abdominal examination is significant for moderate right lower quadrant tenderness with splenomegaly. What is the most likely pathogen causing this patient's illness?

A. *Vibrio parahaemolyticus*
B. *Salmonella typhi*
C. *E. coli*
D. *C. jejuni*
E. *Y. enterocolitica*

96. A 32-year-old previously healthy woman presents to your clinic after having gone to the emergency department with diarrhea, nausea, and vomiting a few weeks ago. She had these symptoms for a day and describes the diarrhea as watery, estimating less than 1 L in stool output. She had not had any fevers. She had recently returned from a trip to the Alabama coast where she had consumed oysters and swam in the Gulf of Mexico. She had been sent home, and her symptoms had resolved within 2 days. Which of the following was the most likely causative organism?

A. *V. parahaemolyticus*
B. *S. enterica*
C. Shiga toxin–producing *E. coli*
D. *C. jejuni*
E. *Y. enterocolitica*

97. A 46-year-old man with Crohn's disease, which has been well controlled on adalimumab, is seen in your clinic for follow-up visit. In addition to adalimumab, he only takes warfarin 5 mg daily for a history of 2 episodes of deep vein thrombosis (DVT) in the past. He informs you that he is planning a 10-day trip to a rural area in India for business. He asks you about the necessity of chemoprophylaxis for traveler's diarrhea in his case. What would you recommend?

A. Azithromycin
B. Rifaximin
C. Bismuth subsalicylate
D. Loperamide
E. No chemoprophylaxis is indicated. Safe eating and drinking is what he needs

98. Which of the following statements about foodborne diseases is correct?

A. Foodborne disease from *C. jejuni* is more common in the summer
B. The most commonly confirmed pathogen in cases of foodborne illness is *Shigella*
C. The incidence of vibriosis is declining
D. The annual rate of foodborne disease with *V. vulnificus* is lower in patients with liver disease compared to the general population
E. PPI use may alter innate defense mechanisms against foodborne illness

99. A 37-year-old woman presents to the emergency department with her 11-month-old son because 2 days ago, the baby had severe vomiting and diarrhea. The mother is relieved that the diarrhea resolved after the first day with no stool output since. She is concerned that, in the last 24 hours, he has not been nursing or eating and has appeared "limp and listless." Upon further discussion, she notes that his 7-year-old brother had the flu recently, and she would like for the baby to be tested for this. Until he became ill, the baby had been in good health and had begun eating a solid diet this week with scrambled eggs in addition to soft vegetables harvested from the family farm several months prior. Upon exam, the infant is noted to be afebrile but lethargic appearing, with loss of reflexes and diminished muscle tone. The baby's skin is noted to be flushed, and his vital signs demonstrate a fluctuating heart rate and blood pressure. His breathing is slightly labored. A rapid noncontrast CT of the brain is obtained and found normal. A chest x-ray is unremarkable for an acute cardiopulmonary process. The infant is admitted to the pediatric intensive care unit for initiation of supportive care and resuscitation. What is the next best step in the management?

A. Nasopharyngeal swabs for rapid diagnostic confirmation of the influenza virus
B. Stool and serum samples for botulinum neurotoxin
C. Stool culture for *Salmonella* while initiating empiric therapy with a fluoroquinolone
D. Emergent neurology consultation for electromyography
E. Contact the state health department to obtain botulism antitoxin

100. A 45-year-old Caucasian man presents to your gastroenterology clinic because of 2 days of nausea and vomiting with copious nonbloody diarrhea and abdominal cramps. He notes severe fatigue and felt faint when he stood up after getting out of bed this morning. He reports that he was previously in good health, and last week he returned from a summer vacation visiting his brother who lives in Maryland along the Chesapeake Bay. He recalls that he enjoyed spending most of his time down by the water where he played water sports in addition to eating meals from the beach vendors. Aside from a history of hyperlipidemia, the patient denies any significant medical history. He notes no history of tobacco use. He consumes a bottle of wine and 4 to 5 glasses of scotch daily. Vital signs are as follows:

Temperature	39.3° C
Heart rate	107 bpm
Blood pressure	98/63 mm Hg

Upon standing, the patient's heart rate is 124 bpm, and his rechecked blood pressure is 79/52 mm Hg. He is noted to be an ill-appearing male on exam with a BMI of 48 kg/m^2. Erythematous bullous lesions are noted over his upper and lower extremities. The patient is directly admitted to the intensive care unit for supportive care. Which of the following initial diagnostic studies would assist with determining the prognosis of his illness?

A. Complete blood count, complete metabolic panel, and coagulation profile
B. Chest x-ray
C. A noncontrast CT of the head
D. Skin biopsy
E. Multiple sets of aerobic and anaerobic blood cultures

101. A 38-year-old African-American woman presents to the emergency department with vomiting, severe abdominal cramps, and severe watery diarrhea of 12 hours duration. She reports attending a barbecue 24 hours prior, where beef and pork were grilled in the backyard to feed up to 100 guests. She has heard from several friends also present at the barbecue that at least 13 more individuals have developed similar symptoms. On exam, the patient's vital signs are as follows:

Temperature	37.1° C
Heart rate	87 bpm
Blood pressure	132/66 mm Hg

She appears to be in no acute distress with moist mucous membranes and an unremarkable exam, aside from mild diffuse abdominal tenderness throughout all quadrants. She has no rebound, guarding, rigidity, or distention. The patient asks for more information regarding how to prevent future illness. Which of the following is correct regarding her diagnosis?

A. Most infections are the result of cutaneous exposure to or inhalation of infected spores
B. Diarrhea occurs as a consequence of toxin-stimulated intestinal secretion that is mediated by changes in intracellular calcium
C. Infection results in almost 20% of all deaths from food-borne illness with possible development of neurologic sequelae secondary to CNS involvement
D. Maximum activity takes place in the ileum with inhibition of glucose transport, resulting in damage to the intestinal epithelium with subsequent protein loss
E. Mode of transmission is usually from food handler to food product

102. A 68-year-old Chinese women presents to the emergency department with her sister because she developed an itchy sensation all over her skin accompanied by a rash and palpitations shortly after eating her lunch 4 hours ago. She reports that she consumed a tuna salad dressed with peanuts, croutons, and lemon-pepper dressing. She is concerned that she could have had an allergic reaction to the peanuts, although her sister expresses surprise as the patient just had a peanut butter and jelly sandwich the previous day with no similar reaction. On exam, the patient is noted to be afebrile with vital signs as follows:

Heart rate	112 bpm
Blood pressure	109/74 mm Hg

Oral exam reveals a normal-appearing tongue and mucous membranes with no obstruction of her airway. Her skin is diffusely erythematous, and cardiac auscultation reveals tachycardia. Exam is otherwise unremarkable. What do you advise the patient and her sister?

A. The patient should have blood cultures and stool cultures collected as she appears to be suffering from an infectious gastroenteritis and requires antibiotic therapy
B. The patient should be admitted to the intensive care unit with plans for intubation of her airway as respiratory compromise will eventually ensue
C. The patient's current symptoms are the result of a one-time reaction for which she may take antihistamines and expect for her symptoms to resolve within the day
D. The patient has developed a severe peanut allergy and should undergo allergy testing for confirmation in addition to complete avoidance of peanuts
E. The patient needs to be given an immediate dose of botulism antitoxin

103. A 34-year-old Caucasian man presents to your office with symptoms of vomiting that began 5 hours ago. He has mild abdominal cramps, but he denies diarrhea. He has no hematemesis or coffee grounds emesis. He recalls that he was coming home from his night shift job 8 hours ago and stopped by a fast food restaurant to have a meal of chicken fried rice on the way. On exam, he is a well-nourished though fatigued-appearing male. His vital signs are as follows:

Temperature	36.9° C
Heart rate	89 bpm
Blood pressure	124/69 mm Hg

Aside from dry mucous membranes, the remainder of his physical exam is unremarkable. What is the most likely cause of food poisoning in this patient?

A. *Staphylococcus aureus*
B. *Bacillus cereus*
C. *Clostridium perfringens*
D. *S. typhi*
E. *Campylobacter*

104. A 24-year-old Caucasian man presents to an emergency department in Tokyo because of shortness of breath and face numbness of 2 hours duration. He is being carried by his roommate due to difficulty walking, and most of the history is provided by his roommate due to the patient's slurred speech. His roommate notes that 3 hours prior, the patient had 5 beers and used marijuana while out with his friends at a street festival. He also ate grilled chicken, sushi, and fried oysters, which were being sold by street vendors at the event. On exam, vital signs are as follows:

Temperature	37.4° C
Heart rate	49 bpm
Blood pressure	73/55 mm Hg.
Respiratory rate	36 breaths/min
Oxygen saturation	89% on room air

The patient is in mild distress with dry heaving. His cardiac exam is notable for bradycardia, and he is noted to be tachypneic with stridor. He is noted on neurologic exam to have loss of sensation to pinprick over his face and extremities as well as diminished deep tendon reflexes. He has dysarthria but is oriented to self, place, and time. An electrocardiogram is performed and demonstrates first degree atrioventricular (AV) block. His roommate is going to contact the patient's parents and would like to speak to you for further information about his condition. Which of the following is correct?

A. The patient's presentation is most likely secondary to ingestion of contaminated oysters
B. The patient's neurologic and cardiac findings are due to effects on the potassium channels in nerve tissue that prevents depolarization and propagation of action potentials
C. The patient's expected mortality approaches 50%, but should he survive the first 24 hours, he will make a full recovery
D. The next step in management is to proceed with gut lavage and administration of activated charcoal, which is gold-standard therapy
E. The molecule that results in a presentation such as the patient's is a heat-labile enterotoxin

105. Which of the following statements about food poisoning is correct?

A. Infection with *C. perfringens* type A results in vascular thrombosis with subsequent intestinal necrosis
B. *S. aureus* has a total of 5 different enterotoxins, which may result in food poisoning

C. *B. cereus* results in infection of GI mucosa due to endospores with formation of endotoxin complexes that result in local tissue damage with edema, mucosal ulcerations, and systemic toxemia
D. Scombroid poisoning is associated with a high mortality rate
E. Ciguatera poisoning resolves within the first 24 hours of infection with no residual effects

106. A 78-year-old Caucasian woman who is a nursing home resident with a history of Alzheimer dementia is admitted to the inpatient medicine team with severe diarrhea. She is a poor historian, but her nursing aide who accompanies her states that the patient has had 10 to 12 loose, large-volume, malodorous stools both during the day and night regardless of food intake for a duration of 5 days now. She was well until 10 days prior to admission when she developed shortness of breath. She was subsequently diagnosed by the nursing home physician as having pneumonia, and she was treated with a course of levofloxacin, which has been completed successfully. She had a syncopal episode at the nursing home earlier today, and she was found to have a blood pressure of 74/49 mm Hg. She was sent to the hospital for further workup and management. Her medications from the nursing home chart include omeprazole and metformin. She is noted to have a drug allergy history to erythromycin, with reported action of nausea and vomiting. On exam, her vitals signs are as follows:

Temperature	38.8° C
Heart rate	119 bpm
Blood pressure	81/56 mm Hg
Oxygen saturation	94% on room air

In general, she is a lethargic-appearing elderly female who is minimally interactive. She is noted to have dry mucous membranes. Cardiac exam is notable for tachycardia, and her lungs are clear to auscultation bilaterally. Her abdomen is firm and distended with guarding and rebound tenderness throughout all quadrants. Bowel sounds are diminished. A KUB is obtained that shows dilation of the ascending and transverse colon with maximal dilation diameter of 8 cm. Laboratory values are notable for the following:

WBC	28,300/μL
Hemoglobin	12.7 g/dL
Hematocrit	38.1%
Platelet count	167,000/μL
Lactate	3.12 mg/dL
BUN	57 mg/dL
Creatinine	2.3 mg/dL

Which of the following is the next best step in management?
A. Colonoscopy with random biopsies
B. Fecal microbiota transplantation (FMT)
C. Surgery consultation
D. Administration of intravenous antihistamines and intramuscular epinephrine
E. Initiation of oral and rectal vancomycin

107. Which of the following is a feature characteristic of antibiotic-associated diarrhea?
A. Antiperistaltic agents are contraindicated
B. Evidence of inflammatory colitis on abdominal imaging
C. There is often previous history of symptoms of diarrhea with antibiotics
D. May result in severe illness with subsequent sepsis
E. Symptoms persist for 2 weeks or longer after withdrawal of offending antibiotic(s)

108. A 63-year-old woman with a history of mild *C. difficile* colitis twice in the last 3 months, requiring outpatient antibiotic treatment each time, presents to your clinic for follow-up. She states she was in good health until 5 days ago when she developed new onset diarrhea with watery, nonbloody bowel movements up to 5 to 6 times a day. She is otherwise well with no complaints of fevers, weight loss, or syncope. She has mild abdominal cramps with her diarrhea. She is currently taking no medications aside from hydrochlorothiazide for mild hypertension. You check a *C. difficile* toxin PCR, which returns positive. Which of the following is the most appropriate treatment?
A. Vancomycin 125 mg orally 3 times daily for 10 to 14 days
B. Metronidazole 500 mg orally 3 times daily for 10 to 14 days
C. Fecal microbiota transplantation via nasogastric tube administration
D. Vancomycin in tapered and pulsed doses
E. Teicoplanin 100 mg twice day for 10 days

109. Which of the following is correct regarding *C. difficile* infection?
A. Colonization rates of *C. difficile* in infants and children up to 2 years of age are reported to reach 25% to 80% with subsequent development of colitis
B. High concentrations of serum IgG antitoxin A antibody confers a protective benefit against *C. difficile*-associated diarrhea and colitis
C. Common antibiotics associated with *C. difficile* infection include aminoglycosides and tetracyclines
D. Use of proton-pump inhibitors results in increased incidence of *C. difficile* infection
E. Patients undergoing cytotoxic chemotherapy for malignancy are at risk for *C. difficile* infection only if treated for recurrent infections with several courses of antibiotics

110. An 83-year-old African-American female with a history of coronary artery disease, peripheral vascular disease, and chronic renal insufficiency is brought into the emergency department after being found down in her assisted living facility. During transportation to the hospital, the patient had developed pulseless electrical arrest. Resuscitative efforts were undertaken with the patient recovering normal sinus rhythm within 4 minutes of initiation of chest compressions and epinephrine administration. Upon arrival, her vital signs are as follows:

Temperature	39.9° C
Heart rate	42 bpm
Blood pressure	64/42 mm Hg

She has been intubated and is deeply sedated on a ventilator. No family or witnesses are available for further history. Exam is notable for an elderly, fragile-appearing female. Cardiac exam is notable for bradycardia but is otherwise unremarkable. Respiratory exam reveals prominent right lower rales. Abdomen is soft, nondistended, and normal bowel sounds are present. Extremities have weak peripheral pulses with cool skin, and the patient is noted to be missing several digits from her hands and feet. Upon transferring her from the stretcher to the bed, the patient is noted to pass large quantities of watery, malodorous brown stool with copious dark red blood and clots. Laboratory values are as follows:

WBC	29,300/μL
Hemoglobin	11.7 g/dL (baseline 13.1)

Hematocrit	35.1%
Platelet count	169,000/μL
INR	0.92
Lactate level	2.94 mg/dL
BUN	97 mg/dL
Creatinine	4.1 mg/dL (baseline 2.3)

The patient is admitted to the intensive care unit where she is aggressively resuscitated and stabilized. You are called for a gastroenterology consult, and 24 hours later, you perform a colonoscopy at bedside. This shows a 10 cm segment of yellow and white thick exudates in a circumferential fashion at the splenic flexure in a contiguous fashion. There are no discrete ulcerations or mucosal breakdown seen. The colonic mucosa proximal and distal to this area appear normal, and no blood is seen throughout the exam. Which of the following is the next best step in management?

A. Intravenous fluids with vasopressor support as needed
B. Urgent fecal microbiota transplant
C. CT angiography with embolization
D. Empiric initiation of oral and rectal vancomycin administration
E. Surgical evaluation for emergent left hemicolectomy

111. A 53-year-old Caucasian male presents for a follow-up office visit after completion of therapy for his second episode of *C. difficile* infection. He was first treated 7 months ago for a mild and uncomplicated episode of *C. difficile* infection with a 14-day course of metronidazole. His second episode was 2 months ago and responded well to a repeat 14-day course of metronidazole. He states that he was well until 10 days ago when he developed intermittent looser quality stools 1 to 2 times daily. He never has nocturnal symptoms. He denies any melena or bloody stools. He denies any recent antibiotic use, travel, or changes in diet. His weight is stable, and his appetite is good. He states that the days when the diarrhea occurs alternates with days with normal formed bowel movements. He notes that he has some mild bloating and diffuse abdominal cramping, which is relieved by passage of stool. His vital signs are stable, and his exam is unremarkable. You check a *C. difficile* toxin PCR study, which returns negative. Which of the following is the next best step in this patient's management?

A. Colonoscopy with random biopsies
B. Small bowel bacterial overgrowth breath testing
C. MR enterography
D. As needed use of antidiarrheals and antispasmodics
E. Initiation of a vancomycin taper

112. A 34-year-old woman is seen in your clinic for follow-up of treatment for recurrent mild *C. difficile* colitis. She is currently on oral vancomycin in tapered dose with significant improvement in her diarrhea. Her husband, who is healthy and asymptomatic, mentions that he had his stool checked by his primary care physician, which returned positive for *C. difficile* toxin by enzyme immunoassay. What would be your recommendation for the husband?

A. Check stool for *C. difficile* toxin PCR; treat with oral vancomycin if positive
B. Start oral vancomycin for 14 days
C. Start oral metronidazole for 14 days
D. Start fidaxomicin for 10 days
E. Hand hygiene

113. A 76-year-old Indian woman presents to your outpatient clinic due to the gradual onset of severe abdominal pain over the last 7 days. She notes that in the last 48 hours, she has developed profuse bloody diarrhea. She notes that she recently moved in with her daughter 2 weeks ago after leaving her village in India. She had chicken fried rice from a fast food establishment for the first time last week. She is adjusting to the diet at her daughter's house as she is used to growing her own food and drawing her water from the local well in her village. She notes a 5-pound weight loss. On exam, she is an afebrile, thin female in no acute distress, appearing mildly fatigued with dry mucous membranes. Her exam is notable for slight tachycardia and a soft but distended abdomen that is moderately tender to deep palpation throughout all quadrants. Rectal exam reveals no stool in the vault, but there are traces of old blood on the glove upon withdrawal. Stool specimen for ova and parasites with hematoxylin-eosin (H&E) stain is shown (see figure). Which of the following is the most likely infection in this patient?

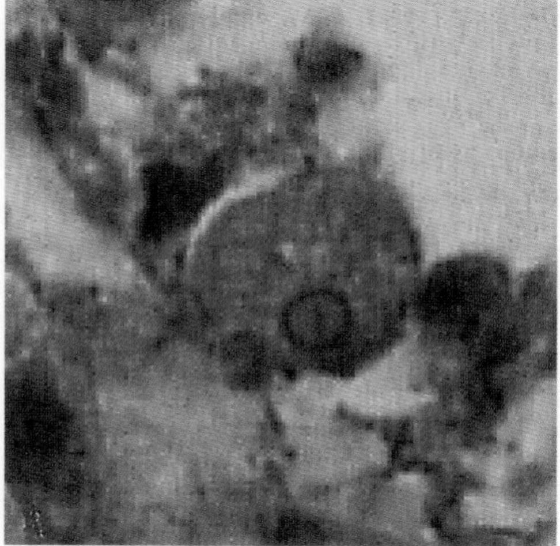

Figure for question 113.

A. *Giardia intestinalis*
B. *Isospora belli*
C. *Cryptosporidium*
D. *Cyclospora cayetanensis*
E. *Entamoeba histolytica*

114. A 24-year-old African-American woman presents to your office with diarrhea that began 2 weeks ago. She states that her symptoms initially consisted of bloating and cramps with 1 to 2 watery stools daily, but currently, her symptoms have progressed to 10 to 12 large-volume nonbloody bowel movements present regardless of food intake and including nocturnal symptoms. Otherwise, she notes a foul smell to her stools. She has had to cancel many of her plans for the last week due to fatigue. She had begun using a new creamer in her coffee a week prior to symptom onset and has noted worsening of symptoms with its use. She denies any recent travel and is largely at home as a homemaker who assists in managing her husband's business. She mainly leaves the house to take her 2-year-old to and from daycare. Both her husband and son are well with no symptoms similar to the patient's. She has been taking 1600 to 2400 mg of ibuprofen on a daily basis over the last month after straining her back during a training session at her gym. On exam, she is noted to have lost 10 pounds since her primary care provider's note 2 months prior. Her vital signs are as follows:

Temperature	37.1° C
Heart rate	94 bpm
Blood pressure	101/64 mm Hg
Oxygen saturation	98% on room air

Physical exam is notable for mild diffuse tenderness in all abdominal quadrants, but the patient otherwise appears well. What would you recommend next to confirm the diagnosis in her?

A. Enzyme-linked immunosorbent assay (ELISA) or direct immunofluorescent antibody microscopy of stool samples
B. Colonoscopy
C. Upper endoscopy with biopsy of small bowel
D. Stool exam for ova and parasite
E. Upper endoscopy with duodenal aspiration

115. A 44-year-old Caucasian man presents to your office with 9 days history of profuse watery diarrhea. He reports mild abdominal pain, but otherwise has no complaints. He denies any recent travels as he has remained in town during his summer vacation and spent time playing tennis and swimming at the public pool. He did eat take-out fried chicken 2 weeks ago, but otherwise, he has not eaten outside of the home. He has a medical history of hyperlipidemia and hypothyroidism, but otherwise, he does not follow routinely for medical care. He denies tobacco use, but he does admit to drinking 3 to 4 glasses of wine daily. He has a history of occasional intravenous drug use. His mother has a history of diverticulitis, but otherwise, he denies any significant history of gastrointestinal disorders among his relatives. On exam, the patient has vital signs as follows:

Temperature	37.3° C
Heart rate	92 bpm
Blood pressure	105/67 mm Hg
Oxygen saturation	99% on room air
BMI	17.6 kg/m^2

In general, he is a thin-appearing male in no acute distress. Oral exam is notable for a slight hyperemic and edematous appearance to the oropharyngeal mucosa with no overlying exudates. He is mildly tachycardic on exam. He also has tender subcentimeter, diffuse cervical and axillary lymphadenopathy. Examination of stool with acid-fast stains demonstrates multiple oocysts. Which of the following is the next best step in management?

A. Treatment with nitazoxanide and serologic testing for human immunodeficiency virus (HIV)
B. Evaluation with colonoscopy to obtain random biopsies
C. High resolution imaging of the abdomen and pelvis with an MR enterography
D. Duodenal aspirate for confirmation of disease followed by a course of metronidazole
E. Treatment with levofloxacin and inspection of the establishment from which he purchased fried chicken

116. You are called for an inpatient GI consultation to the bedside of a 27-year-old Venezuelan woman with abdominal pain for 7 days. She is visiting her sister, who lives in the United States. Her sister notes that the patient has appeared fatigued since arrival and has had concerning puffiness around her eyes. The patient has been short of breath at home and cannot walk up the single flight of stairs to her room despite typically being strong enough to work a 12-hour day as a field laborer at a local farm. The patient was brought to the hospital yesterday with lethargy, massive abdominal, distention, and constipation. On exam, vital signs are as follows:

Temperature	40.2° C
Heart rate	43 bpm
Blood pressure	73/59 mm Hg
Oxygen saturation	91% on 2 L nasal cannula

She is minimally responsive and somnolent. Her jugular venous pressure is 10 cm, and she is bradycardic. Auscultation of her lungs reveals bibasilar rales. Her abdomen is notably distended though soft with hypoactive bowel sounds and dullness to percussion. A barium enema is obtained (see figure). Which of the following is true regarding this patient?

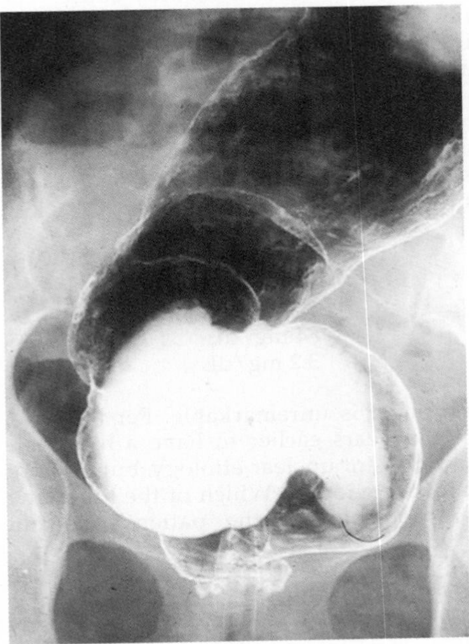

Figure for question 116.

A. Diagnosis will only be possible via demonstration of positive antibody testing through the Centers for Disease Control and Prevention (CDC)
B. The patient should be moved to a critical care setting for rapid administration of neostigmine
C. The patient will likely have an abnormal electrocardiogram
D. Disease acquirement varies by genetic predisposition and is not preventable, but she will respond to emergent reversal of her severe hypothyroidism
E. The patient has previously undiagnosed coronary artery disease

117. A 63-year-old Caucasian woman presents to your clinic with a history of now resolved 4 days of diarrhea. Her symptoms were mild with nonbloody, watery stool. She had mild abdominal cramps but no fever, nausea or vomiting. She denies any recent sick contacts, and she has not traveled outside of the country in several years. Her primary care provider checked infectious stool studies at the time and called to report that she was noted positive for *Blastocystis hominis*. She is back to baseline health at this time, but she would like an opinion regarding further management. Which of the following is correct regarding *Blastocystis* infection?

A. There is an association with inflammatory bowel disease
B. Asymptomatic patients with *B. hominis* found in stool need to be treated
C. It is only seen in the tropics
D. It is associated with other unrecognized infections in more than 50% of cases
E. Greater levels of parasitic infection correlate with increased gastrointestinal symptoms

118. A 65-year-old Vietnam War veteran is admitted to the intensive care unit with polymicrobial sepsis with blood cultures growing *E. coli* and *K. pneumoniae*. His past medical history is significant for chronic obstructive pulmonary disease (COPD) and chronic tobacco abuse. The patient was initially started on oral prednisone 40 mg daily after being diagnosed with a COPD exacerbation, and his respiratory symptoms improved significantly. However, his condition has worsened in the last 24 hours. He is currently intubated for hypoxia with interstitial pneumonitis evident on chest x-ray. His physical examination is unremarkable. His Laboratory values are remarkable for the following:

Hemoglobin	12.3 g/dL
WBC	18,400/μL
Neutrophils	80%
Eosinophils	10%
BUN	84 mg/dL
Creatinine	3.2 mg/dL

His hepatic function panel is unremarkable. Per his wife, he had been noted years earlier to have a high percentage of eosinophils of unclear etiology, but had not had GI complaints previously. Which of the following infections is responsible for the patient's current symptoms?
A. *Enterobius vermicularis*
B. *Stronglyoides stercoralis*
C. *Ancylostoma duodenale*
D. *Trichuris trichiura*
E. *Taenia saginata*

119. A 52-year-old Chinese immigrant man is admitted to the medicine ward with 2 weeks of worsening right upper quadrant pain and jaundice. He immigrated to the United States 15 years ago and states he previously underwent intervention for recurrent biliary infections in China. His vital signs are as follows:

Heart rate	100 bpm
Blood pressure	110/72 mm Hg
Temperature	37.2° C

Physical examination is significant for right upper quadrant abdominal tenderness without rebound tenderness or guarding as well as jaundice. His laboratory studies are as follows:

Bilirubin	7.2 mg/dL
Direct bilirubin	5.2 mg/dL
AST	120 U/L
ALT	140 U/L
Alkaline phosphatase	342 U/L

Abdominal ultrasound delineates moderate intrahepatic ductal dilation without evidence of choledocholithiasis. endoscopic retrograde cholangiopancreatography (ERCP) demonstrates marked dilation of the intrahepatic biliary ducts and a mass-like hilar stricture causing narrowing of the common, right, and left hepatic ducts. Which of the following is contributory to the patient's current clinical condition?
A. *Necator americanus*
B. *Diphyllobothrium latum*
C. *Clonorchis sinensis*
D. *Schistosoma mansoni*
E. *Dipylidium caninum*

120. A 27-year-old Puerto Rican man presents to the emergency department with hematemesis. Following stabilization, endoscopy reveals large esophageal varices with red wale sign that are successfully banded. Abdominal MRI demonstrates enlarged left hepatic lobe and splenomegaly, but normal liver morphology and flow through the hepatic artery without evidence of thrombosis. Which of the following is responsible for the patient's current clinical condition?
A. *Ascaris lumbricoides*
B. *T. saginata*
C. *Ancylostoma ceylonicum*
D. *S. mansoni*
E. *S. stercoralis*

121. A 53-year-old woman with a past medical history of asthma sees you in clinic for evaluation of anemia. She reports no history of GI bleeding and is currently postmenopausal. She takes a yearly fishing trip with her family to Alaska where they often consume the raw fish they catch. Physical examination is unremarkable. Laboratory studies are remarkable for the following:

Hemoglobin	10.8 g/dL
MCV	112 fL
Folate	9.8 ng/mL
Vitamin B_{12}	100 pg/mL

Which of the following is responsible for the patient's anemia?
A. *D. latum*
B. *Taenia solium*
C. *Hymenolepis nana*
D. *C. sinensis*
E. *Schistosoma japonicum*

122. A 34-year-old Indian man with a past medical history of hypertension sees you in clinic for evaluation of iron deficiency anemia. He recently immigrated to the United States. Laboratory values are as follows:

Hemoglobin	10.8 g/dL
MCV	72 fL
WBC	7200/μL
Eosinophils	11%
Ferritin	8 ng/mL
Iron	22 μL/dL
Total iron binding capacity	420 μL/dL
Iron saturation	5.2%

EGD and colonoscopy are unremarkable. Which of the following is responsible for this patient's anemia?
A. *Opisthorchis viverrini*
B. *T. solium*
C. *C. sinensis*
D. *E. vermicularis*
E. *A. duodenale*

123. A 71-year-old Caucasian man presents to your outpatient clinic for evaluation of symptoms of nausea and occasional vomiting, which have progressed in severity over the last month. He reports early satiety and has noted an unintentional weight loss of 15 pounds. He notes decreased frequency of bowel movements in the last 2 weeks although the consistently has remained soft.

He has not seen any melena, hematochezia, or bright red blood per rectum. He has no history of nonsteroidal antiinflammatory drug (NSAID) use. He notes an unremarkable EGD performed for gastroesophageal reflux disease last year at the same time as his normal screening colonoscopy. He has recently traveled to West Africa on business, but he denies any sick contacts. He reports 4 to 5 beers daily in addition to 2 packs of cigarettes daily and rare recreational marijuana use. On exam, he is noted to have the following vital signs:

Temperature	36.9° C
Heart rate	103 bpm
Blood pressure	83/69 mm Hg
Oxygen saturation	100% on room air
BMI	38.3 kg/m²

He is a well-developed male in mild distress. The remainder of his exam is pertinent for a soft but distended abdomen with rare bowel sounds, moderate tenderness to light palpation throughout all quadrants, and no rigidity or rebound tenderness. Slight guarding is present. Murphy's sign is negative. Laboratory values are drawn and return with the following values:

WBC	12,000/µL (8200/µL, 1 year ago)
Hemoglobin	9.7 g/dL (13/µL, 1 year ago)
MCV	71 fL (86/µL, 1 year ago)
Platelet count	243,000/µL
ALT	63 U/L
AST	23 U/L
Alkaline phosphatase	84 U/L
Total bilirubin	0.7 mg/dL
INR	0.93

After inpatient admission and resuscitation, which of the following is the next best step?

A. Fecal occult blood testing of the patient's stool
B. EGD and colonoscopy with random duodenal and colonic biopsies
C. Four-hour scintigraphic gastric emptying study
D. CT enterography
E. Biopsy of the liver

124. A 53-year-old Asian woman with a history of abdominal pain for 1 year undergoes workup with her primary care provider demonstrating a midjejunal mass on imaging, which is confirmed on single balloon enteroscopy to be a gastrointestinal stromal tumor (GIST). Which of the following is a characteristic of a small intestine GIST?

A. Small bowel GISTs most commonly exhibit malignant behavior
B. GISTs commonly express KIT or CD117
C. GISTs commonly are S100 positive
D. The most useful indicators of survival are the anatomic site of the tumor and the presence of cystic spaces
E. The mainstay of therapy for advanced GISTs is chemotherapy and radiation therapy

125. Which of the following is correct regarding the risk factors associated with small intestine tumors?

A. Patients carrying a diagnosis of familial adenomatous polyposis (FAP) require periodic screening for periampullary duodenal carcinoma
B. Patients who bear a diagnosis of Lynch syndrome typically present with small intestine cancer in the seventh decade of life
C. Biologic therapy confers a protective benefit against development of adenocarcinoma in the small intestine among patients who have Crohn's disease
D. A diagnosis of Crohn's disease has been associated with increased risk of development of GISTs of the small intestine
E. There is an 11% to 13% incidence of small intestine malignancy in the setting of celiac disease, usually of B cell origin

126. A 27-year-old woman of Scandinavian descent presents to your clinic for evaluation of constipation, intermittent dark stools, and weight loss of 15 pounds over the last 2 months. She also has a diminished appetite due to a feeling of bloating or fullness. She denies nausea or vomiting. Her stools have become less frequent and smaller in caliber. She reports no medical history or use of daily medications. Aside from a maternal aunt with ulcerative colitis, the patient has no family history of GI disorders. She smokes 1 to 2 cigarettes socially, drinks 2 to 3 beers on the weekend, and has no history of drug use. She is sexually active with one male partner and uses contraception consistently. She experiences heavy periods once a month lasting for a week. On physical exam, vital signs are as follows:

Temperature	36.7° C
Heart rate	105 bpm
Blood pressure	92/64 mm Hg
Oxygen saturation	98% on room air

The patient has notable pallor, and she is mildly tachycardic on auscultation. Her abdomen is full but soft with mild epigastric tenderness. No rigidity, rebound, or guarding is present. Rectal exam demonstrates dark, melanotic appearing stools. Laboratory values are as follows:

WBC	8300/µL
Hemoglobin	10.3 g/dL
MCV	77 fL
Platelet count	217,000/µL
INR	0.87

The patient is evaluated further with a colonoscopy. No mucosal abnormalities are noted, but upon intubation of the terminal ileum, dark matter is seen passing from the proximal small bowel. Subsequently, an anterograde single balloon enteroscopy is performed with findings of nodular, polyploid, pigmented lesions 1 to 2 cm in size encountered in the jejunum (see figure). While awaiting pathology from biopsies of the lesions, what is the best next step in management?

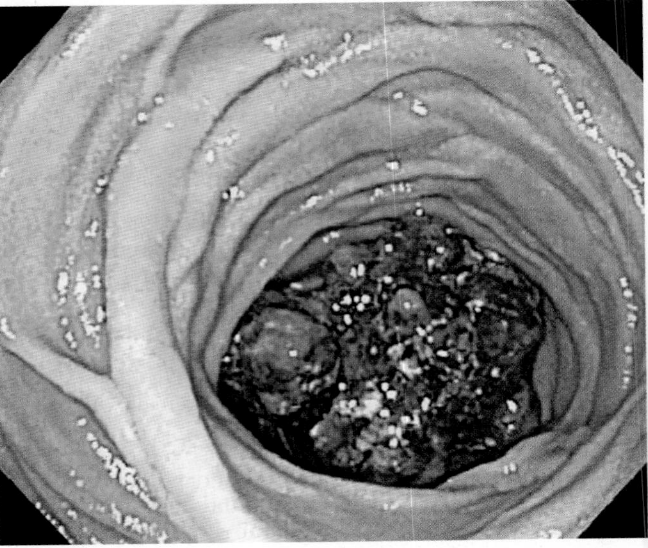

Figure for question 126.

- **A.** MR enterography
- **B.** C-reactive protein level, erthrocyte sedimentation rate level, and inflammatory bowel disease-7 serologies
- **C.** Transvaginal ultrasound and uterine biopsy
- **D.** CT angiography
- **E.** Dermatology evaluation

127. Which of the following is characteristic of primary small intestine lymphomas (PSILs)?
- **A.** PSILs are most commonly found in the duodenum
- **B.** PSILs rapidly progress extramurally
- **C.** PSILs commonly affect a large portion of intestine in a contiguous fashion
- **D.** Most PSILs are B-cell derived
- **E.** Patients with PSILs have palpable peripheral lymphadenopathy

128. Which of the following is correct regarding small intestinal tumors?
- **A.** Male gender, BMI, and age greater than 65 years are associated risk factors for small intestinal adenocarcinoma
- **B.** Point mutations in K-*ras* at codon 12 have been reported in up to half of all small intestinal tumors
- **C.** Type 1 neurofibromatosis is associated with multiple small intestinal GISTs
- **D.** *KIT* mutations are detected in most small intestinal carcinoid tumors
- **E.** DNA replication errors involving microsatellite instability (MSI) has been seen in up to 13% of small intestine carcinomas associated with Crohn's disease

129. Which of the following is a favorable prognostic factor in a patient with GIST?
- **A.** Tumor size of 3 cm
- **B.** Mitotic index of 1 per 50 high-powered fields
- **C.** Presence of *KIT* exon 11 deletion
- **D.** Tumor site of jejunum
- **E.** High cellularity of the tumor

130. A 75-year-old Caucasian man of Irish descent who was previously in good health presents to your office with 2 to 3 months of weight loss, decreased appetite, and diffuse abdominal cramps. Despite having no previous medical issues, the patient notes that he has always had a "sensitive stomach" with some bloating and diarrhea after meals, which has increased in severity more recently. He notes that his stool is malodorous and appears to float on top of the water in the toilet bowl at times. He has not seen any melena, hematochezia, or rectal bleeding. He has had night sweats with no fevers in the last 2 to 3 weeks. He reports mild nausea, although he has not had emesis. He has used 800 mg ibuprofen on a daily basis for the last year due to his osteoarthritis pain. Otherwise, he takes no daily medications. He drinks 2 to 3 glasses of wine daily and smoked half a pack of cigarettes daily for 20 years but quit 5 years ago. On exam, vital signs are as follows:

Temperature	37.8° C
Heart rate	112 bpm
Blood pressure	94/69 mm Hg
Oxygen saturation	97% on room air

He is a thin-appearing male in no acute distress. Exam is notable for dry mucous membranes and mild tachycardia. Abdominal exam reveals a soft abdomen with no distention but diffuse mild tenderness to palpation, which is greatest in severity over the umbilical area where he is noted to have a soft, 3 to 4 cm palpable mass. You obtained imaging with a small bowel follow-through, demonstrating an irregular mass in the distal jejunum with resulting partial luminal obstruction. Laparotomy is performed, and the involved segment of small intestine is sent to pathology. Which of the following is the most likely histologic finding?
- **A.** Diffuse growth of large lymphoma cells and Ig gene rearrangement
- **B.** Large cells with intense surrounding inflammation and adjacent atrophic mucosa, $CD103^+$ marker
- **C.** Medium-sized cells with many mitoses and chromosomal translocation involving *c-myc*
- **D.** Superficial plasma cells, α-heavy chain paraprotein
- **E.** Monotonous small cells with irregular nuclei, t(11:114)

131. A 61-year-old Caucasian man presents to your outpatient clinic for evaluation of iron deficiency anemia. He denies overt bleeding. Laboratory values are as follows:

Hemoglobin	9.2 g/dL
MCV	71 fL

He had an EGD and colonoscopy, which were normal. A capsule endoscopy is performed and shows a mass in the distal duodenum. A push enteroscopy shows a large friable mass in the fourth portion of the duodenum. Biopsy shows adenocarcinoma. CT scan of the abdomen and pelvis does not show metastatic spread. Which of the following is the treatment of choice in this patient?
- **A.** 5-Fluorouracil (5-FU) alone
- **B.** FOLFOX (5-FU, leucovorin, and oxaliplatin)
- **C.** Surgical resection
- **D.** Radiation therapy
- **E.** Bevacizumab

132. Which of the following is true regarding genetic polymorphisms of the *NOD2/CARD15* gene?
- **A.** They are associated with an older age of disease onset
- **B.** They are associated with higher likelihood of stricture formation
- **C.** They are association with colonic location of disease
- **D.** They are found in 75% of Crohn's disease patients
- **E.** They are associated with higher likelihood of extraintestinal manifestations

133. Which of the following best describes autophagy?
- **A.** It is a process that plays a role in cellular homeostasis by clearing abnormal proteins and apoptotic bodies
- **B.** It contributes directly to adaptive immunity by stimulating B cells
- **C.** It is an extracellular degradation process that works to clear Toll-like receptors
- **D.** It is an intracellular degradation process that involves transport through endocytic sorting pathways
- **E.** It directly up regulates the production of β-defensins

134. Which of the following is true regarding granulomas found in Crohn's disease?
- **A.** They are only found in isolated colonic Crohn's disease
- **B.** Interleukin (IL)-13 is the key cytokine in the formation of granulomas
- **C.** Noncaseating granulomas are a late finding in the disease course
- **D.** Crohn's disease–related granulomas have little or no central necrosis
- **E.** They are more commonly found in mucosal biopsies than surgical specimens

135. A 20-year-old female presents with 2 months history of intermittent low grade fevers up to 100.5° F associated with nonbloody watery diarrhea after returning from India. She notes mild lower abdominal crampy pain. An upper endoscopy reveals aphthous ulcers in the gastric antrum and duodenum. An ileocolonoscopy reveals scattered cratered ulcers in the terminal ileum and the colon. Biopsies show evidence of focally enhanced gastritis and chronic active inflammation with noncaseating granulomas in the duodenum, ileum, and colon. Which of the following is the most likely diagnosis?

A. Ulcerative colitis
B. Crohn's disease
C. Tuberculosis (TB)
D. Behçet's disease
E. NSAID-related GI damage

136. A 20-year-old Mexican male presents to the emergency department with 3 months history of epigastric abdominal pain with worsening nausea, vomiting, and diarrhea. He is a recent immigrant to the United States. He notes intermittent low-grade fevers and a weight loss of 25 pounds. On physical exam, he has a temperature of 101° F. He has no oral ulcers. There is mild upper abdominal tenderness to deep palpation. Upon admission to the hospital, an upper endoscopy and colonoscopy are performed. Upper endoscopy reveals a 3 cm stricture in the third portion of the duodenum, which could not be traversed. Ileocolonoscopy reveals normal colonic mucosa and normal ileal mucosa up to 10 cm from the ileocecal valve. A magnetic resonance enterography confirms the 3 cm duodenal stricture, but the remaining small bowel is normal. Biopsies of the stricture reveal granulomas. Biopsies from the ileum and colon were normal. Which of the following is the most likely diagnosis?

A. Tuberculosis
B. Crohn's disease
C. NSAID enteropathy
D. Sarcoidosis
E. Behçet's disease

137. A 55-year-old male is seen in clinic for follow-up of his 10-year history of Crohn's colitis. He was induced into remission with prednisone and has been on azathioprine 150 mg daily for 8 years. His most recent laboratory values are as follows:

Hemoglobin	12.4 g/dL
Platelet count	90,000/μL
Bilirubin	2.0 mg/dL
Alkaline phosphatase	250 U/L
AST	46 U/L
ALT	51 U/L

His liver biopsy reveals nodular regenerative hyperplasia (NRH). What is the most appropriate next step in management?

A. Decrease dose of azathioprine to 50 mg
B. Decrease dose of azathioprine to 50 mg and add allopurinol
C. Check 6-methylmercaptopurine (6-MMP) levels
D. Check 6-thioguanine (6-TG) nucleotide levels
E. Stop azathioprine

138. A 25-year-old female with ileocolonic Crohn's disease presents with worsening diarrhea and abdominal pain over 2 months. She has been on adalimumab 80 mg every 2 weeks for the past 4 months. She has not received any other biologic therapy in the past. On physical exam, she has a temperature of 97° F. Abdominal exam reveals mild periumbilical tenderness to deep palpation. Her laboratory values are notable for the following:

Albumin	3.1 g/dL
Hemoglobin	10.5 g/dL
C-reactive protein	15 mg/dL
Adalimumab levels	1.9 μg/mL (normal >5 μg/mL)
Drug antibody levels	>55 U/mL (normal <1 U/mL)

Stool studies are negative. A colonoscopy reveals active inflammation in the terminal ileum, ascending colon, and terminal ileum. Which of the following is the most appropriate next step in management?

A. Change to sulfasalazine
B. Add azathioprine 150 mg to her current adalimumab regimen
C. Increase adalimumab to 80 mg every 1 week
D. Change to vedolizumab
E. Change to infliximab

139. A 31-year-old female with ileocolonic Crohn's disease is seen in clinic for follow-up. She is currently asymptomatic. Her last flare of disease was 12 months ago, for which she was started on infliximab. Her last colonoscopy 6 months ago showed no active colitis or ileitis. She is interested in having children and asks you about the safety of infliximab and other anti–tumor necrosis factor (TNF) therapy during pregnancy. What is the pregnancy category for the anti-TNF agents?

A. A
B. B
C. C
D. D
E. X

140. Which of the following is true about hepatosplenic T-cell lymphoma (HSTCL)?

A. It is reported most often in young males
B. It is associated with the anti-TNF monotherapy
C. It is fatal in 60% of patients
D. Is associated with approximately a 1-year history of exposure to thiopurine
E. Reported most often in elderly patients on multiple immunosuppressants

141. A 40-year-old obese female is started on azathioprine 225 mg daily and adalimumab for treatment of ileocecal Crohn's disease. After 2 weeks of treatment, she presents to the emergency department with acute epigastric abdominal pain, nausea, and vomiting. On physical exam, vital signs are as follows:

Temperature	99° F
Heart rate	105 bpm

Abdominal exam reveals moderate epigastric and right upper quadrant tenderness to deep palpation. Her laboratory values are as follows:

Hemoglobin	12.4 g/dL
Platelet count	210,000/μL
Bilirubin	2.0 mg/dL
Direct bilirubin	0.8 mg/dL
Alkaline phosphatase	130 U/L
AST	36 U/L
ALT	41 U/L
Lipase	2250 U/L

A right upper quadrant ultrasound reveals a gallbladder wall of 3 mm and no gallstones. In addition to intravenous fluid resuscitation and analgesia, which of the following is an appropriate recommendation for this patient?
A. Switch azathioprine to 6-mercaptopurine
B. Lower dose of azathioprine to 50 mg
C. Stop adalimumab
D. Stop azathioprine
E. Continue current medications and refer for cholecystectomy

142. A 28-year-old female with colonic Crohn's disease is seen in clinic for follow-up. Over the last 14 days she developed a lesion on the lower abdomen (see figure). Which of the following is true regarding the lesion?

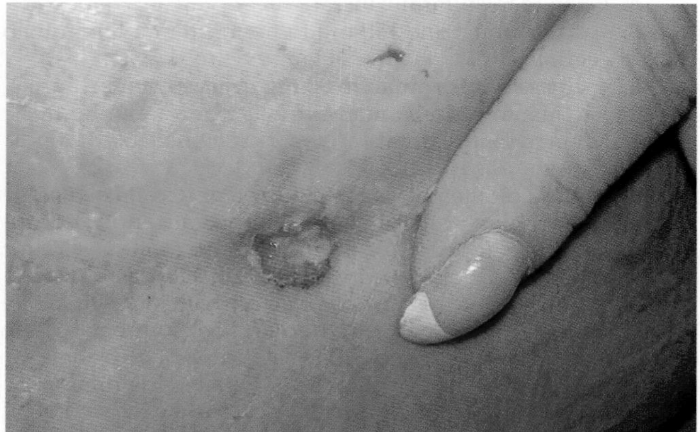

Figure for question 142.

A. It is solely found in patients with Crohn's disease
B. The condition often manifests during exacerbations of intestinal disease and tends to improve with treatment of the underlying disease
C. It usually heals with minimal scarring
D. It can develop at sites of minor trauma
E. It is associated with anti-OmpC antibodies

143. Which of the following cancers is associated with the use of thiopurines?
A. Colon cancer
B. Ovarian cancer
C. Nonmelanoma skin cancer
D. Lung cancer
E. Renal cancer

144. A 20-year old male presents with right lower quadrant abdominal pain and nonbloody diarrhea for the past 6 months. He notes joint swelling of his right knee and ankle. Laboratory values are as follows:

C-reactive protein	15.6 mg/dL
Hemoglobin	10.6 g/dL
Ferritin	3 ng/mL
Albumin	3.2 g/dL

An ileocolonoscopy reveals multiple cratered ulcerations in the distal 10 cm of terminal ileum. Biopsies show active inflammation with pyloric gland metaplasia in the ileum. A thiopurine methyltransferase (TPMT) level is normal. A purified protein derivative (PPD) is negative. Which of the following therapies is best to both induce and maintain remission in this patient?
A. Mesalamine 4.8 g daily
B. Azathioprine 150 mg daily
C. Methotrexate 25 mg subcutaneously (SC) weekly with daily folic acid
D. Prednisone 20 mg daily
E. Infliximab 5 mg/kg

145. A 55-year-old male with 6 months history of ileocecal Crohn's disease presents for his fifth infusion of infliximab. Within 30 minutes into the infusion, he develops chest tightness and shortness of breath. His blood pressure is 70/40 mm Hg, and his heart rate is 125 bpm. The nurse stops the infusion and treats him with an antihistamine and methylprednisolone. Which of the following is most likely seen on his laboratory tests?
A. Elevated antinuclear antibody (ANA) levels
B. Elevated human antichimeric antibodies
C. Positive interferon gamma release assay
D. Low hemoglobin levels
E. Normal 6-thioguanine levels

146. A 25-year-old male is seen in clinic with complaints of drainage from his perianal area. He reports lower abdominal pain and diarrhea for the past 6 months. A perianal examination reveals a 5 cm fluctuant tender area on the right buttock. A prominent firm perianal tag is noted. A magnetic resonance enterography reveals 20 cm of active inflammation in the terminal ileum. In addition, a 5 cm perirectal abscess is noted. Which of the following is the most appropriate treatment?
A. Oral antibiotics and surgical referral
B. Oral antibiotics and prednisone
C. Infliximab
D. Mesalamine
E. Methotrexate and folic acid

147. What is the mechanism of action of vedolizumab?
A. Anti IL–12/23 monoclonal antibody
B. Inhibitor of Janus kinase
C. Antibody to p40 subunit of IL-12/23
D. Nonselective antibody to $\alpha4\beta$ integrin
E. Antibody to $\alpha4\beta7$ integrin

148. A 31-year-old female presents with a 10-year history of moderate steroid-dependent colonic Crohn's disease. She was initially placed on infliximab and had a durable remission for 4 years and then subsequently stopped responding. Since then, she has been on adalimumab and then certolizumab in combination with azathioprine with no response. Her laboratory values are notable for the following:

Albumin	3.1 g/dL
Hemoglobin	9.8 g/dL
C-reactive protein	22.1 mg/dL

Her stool studies are negative. A repeat colonoscopy showed evidence of scattered cratered ulcerations extending from 20 cm from anal verge to the cecum and no strictures. The rectum was grossly uninvolved. Biopsies show chronic active colitis and no cytomegalovirus inclusions. What is the next step in management?
A. Place on antibiotics
B. Place on mesalamine
C. Obtain a hepatitis C antibody
D. Check for anti–John Cunningham virus (JCV) antibody
E. Check erythrocyte sedimentation rate (ESR)

149. A 28-year-old female with a 3-year history of moderate ileocolonic Crohn's disease managed with infliximab presents with complaints of increased right lower quadrant abdominal pain and diarrhea. Abdominal exam reveals a soft abdomen with no tenderness. Her laboratory values are as follows:

Albumin	3.5 g/dL
C-reactive protein	0.8 mg/dL
Hemoglobin	13.5 g/dL

Stool testing for enteric pathogens were negative. Her infliximab trough level was 8.5 μg/mL (therapeutic level > 4 μg/mL) and anti-chimeric antibody levels were undetectable. Which of the following is the most appropriate next step in management?

A. Perform an ileocolonoscopy
B. Check a thiopurine methyltransferase (TPMT) level
C. Switch infliximab to adalimumab
D. Switch infliximab to vedolizumab
E. Add methotrexate

150. An 18-year-old male presents with complaints of feculent discharge from a small skin opening in his right lower quadrant for the past 8 weeks. He underwent an appendectomy 4 months ago after presenting with acute right lower quadrant pain with fevers and CT scan evidence of appendicitis. Which of the following is the most likely diagnosis?

A. Behçet's disease
B. Crohn's disease
C. Common variable immunodeficiency disorder
D. Ulcerative colitis
E. Indeterminate colitis

151. A 45-year-old female presents to the emergency department with right lower quadrant pain and fevers to 102° F. A CT scan reveals a right lower quadrant 4.5 cm psoas abscess. The patient is admitted and undergoes drainage of the abscess. Upon further questioning she notes diarrhea for the past 6 months with a weight loss of 10 pounds. A magnetic resonance enterography reveals 12 cm of terminal ileal inflammation suggestive of Crohn's disease. After drainage of the abscess, she notes acute pain in her right hip and difficulty with ambulation. She continues to spike fevers to 101.8° F while in the hospital. Which of the following is the most likely diagnosis?

A. Deep vein thrombosis
B. Small bowel stricture
C. Septic arthritis
D. Ankylosing spondylitis
E. Sacroiliitis

152. A 64-year-old male is seen in clinic for follow-up after a recent hospitalization for an 8-month history of nonbloody diarrhea and weight loss of 20 pounds. He is diagnosed with moderate colonic Crohn's disease. He is placed on prednisone 40 mg daily with a taper. Upon further questioning, he notes an increase in urgency and looseness of bowel movements with decreasing his prednisone from 40 mg to 30 mg. His past medical history is notable for a history of renal cell cancer that was resected 8 years ago with subsequent scans that have been negative, class IV congestive heart failure with an ejection fraction of 25%, chronic obstructive pulmonary disease (COPD), latent tuberculosis (TB) diagnosed 3 years ago and treated with 9 months of isoniazid, and chronic tobacco use. Which of his comorbidities is an absolute contraindication to initiation of anti-TNF agent?

A. History of renal cell cancer
B. Class IV heart failure
C. COPD
D. Latent TB
E. Tobacco use

153. Which of the following inflammatory bowel disease medications can result in reversible male infertility?

A. Ciprofloxacin
B. Sulfasalazine
C. Mesalamine
D. Infliximab
E. Vedolizumab

154. A 45-year-old female is placed on prednisone 60 mg daily for treatment of moderate ileocecal Crohn's disease. Despite treatment she continues to suffer from diarrhea, low-grade temperatures, and intermittent right lower quadrant pain. A CT enterography shows evidence of an 8 cm segment of ileal wall thickening but no stricture or abscess. Her laboratory values are as follows:

Albumin	2.9 g/dL
Hemoglobin	8.8 g/dL
C-reactive protein	25.8 mg/dL
Stool studies	negative
TMPT level normal	

Which of the following is the most appropriate next step in management?

A. Increase prednisone to 60 mg orally twice daily
B. Start ciprofloxacin and metronidazole
C. Start sulfasalazine 4 g daily
D. Start mesalamine 4.8 g daily
E. Check PPD and hepatitis B serologies

155. Which of the following is the most frequent long-term toxicity of thalidomide?

A. Peripheral neuropathy
B. Leukopenia
C. Hepatotoxicity
D. Heart failure
E. Demyelinating disorder

156. A 38-year-old male with a history of Crohn's disease presents to the emergency department with a 2-hour history of severe groin and right flank pain. Her past history is significant for extensive small bowel resection due to recurrent episodes of obstruction. Urinalysis is positive for hematuria. An intravenous urogram shows two stones measuring 6 and 7 mm in the midportion of the right ureter, with no hydronephrosis. Which of the following is the most likely type of kidney stones in this patient?

A. Magnesium ammonium phosphate stones
B. Calcium phosphate stones
C. Calcium oxalate stones
D. Cystine stones
E. Struvite stones

157. Which of the following is true regarding family history and ulcerative colitis (UC)?

A. Familial associations generally occur more in second-degree relatives and offspring
B. Familial association is greater in persons of Jewish descent than non-Jewish patients
C. For all affected first-degree relatives within a family, there is a low concordance for type of disease (UC vs. Crohn's disease)
D. There is a consistent correlation with disease extent within families
E. Genetic factors are not major risk factors for development of UC

158. Which of the following is a side effect of cyclosporine?
A. Gingival hyperplasia
B. Low cholesterol
C. Psoriasis
D. Autoimmune pancreatitis
E. Congestive heart failure

159. A 41-year-old man with a 25-year history of ulcerative colitis presents for routine follow-up. He has been on mesalamine 2.4 g/day for many years. He has had one flare several years ago that required prednisone, but otherwise has done well. He notes recent alternating constipation with diarrhea but no blood in stool. His appetite is good, and his weight is stable. A colonoscopy is performed and shows a stricture in the midtransverse colon through which the colonoscope could not pass. Biopsies of the stricture are taken and reveal chronic active colitis. The more distal examined colon appears normal with no evidence of inflammation. A CT scan reveals a 5 cm long stricture in the midtransverse colon with no evidence of obstruction. Which of the following is the most appropriate next step in management?
A. Start infliximab
B. Start vedolizumab
C. Start prednisone
D. Increase mesalamine to 4.8 g/day
E. Refer to surgery

160. A 35-year-old woman with a 10-year history of ulcerative colitis is seen in clinic for complaints of joint discomfort in her fingers and wrists. She denies diarrhea or blood in the stool. Her last colonoscopy performed 3 months prior revealed normal mucosa with no inflammation seen on histology. She is on mesalamine 2.4 g/day. Her joints do not appear swollen. Her laboratory values, including hemoglobin, C-reactive protein, and albumin are normal. Which of the following is true regarding this patient's arthropathy?
A. It is often asymmetric and pauciarticular
B. Symptoms correlate well with disease activity
C. Fever is a common component
D. It most often affects the small joints
E. It is associated with HLA-B27

161. A 45-year-old man presents for follow-up of his pan-ulcerative colitis. He has been on maintenance infliximab 5 mg/kg every 8 weeks for 5 years. He complains of fatigue and mild pruritus. Physical exam reveals icteric sclera, soft nontender abdomen, and no organomegaly. He has no rashes. His laboratory values are as follows:

ALP	220 U/L
AST	55 U/L
ALT	46 U/L
Total bilirubin	3.8 mg/dL
Direct bilirubin	2.4 mg/dL

An MRI/magnetic resonance cholangiopancreatography (MRCP) reveals mild dilation of the left intrahepatic ducts but no cirrhosis or varices. He is referred for a liver biopsy. Which of the following findings would be most characteristic of the biopsy findings?
A. Concentric fibrosis around the small bile ducts
B. Prominent periportal lymphoplasmacytic infiltrate with interface hepatitis
C. Intracellular globules that stain positive with PAS
D. Steatosis with lobular and portal inflammation
E. Focal duct obliteration with granuloma formation

162. A 38-year-old woman with a 1-year history of panulcerative colitis presents to the emergency department. She notes worsening bloody diarrhea and a weight loss of 18 pounds over the past 8 weeks. She has been on 60 mg of prednisone during this time, along with mesalamine 4.8 g/day. Her vitals signs are as follows:

Temperature	101.5° F
Heart rate	120 bpm
Blood pressure	100/50 mm Hg

Her abdominal exam reveals mild tenderness to palpation in the left lower quadrant without rebound or guarding, hypoactive bowel sounds, and no hepatosplenomegaly. Her laboratory values are notable for the following:

Hemoglobin	6.8 g/dL
Albumin	1.6 g/dL
C-reactive protein	100.8 mg/dL

Which of the following is the most appropriate next step in management?
A. Start methylprednisolone 100 mg intravenously daily
B. Obtain plain film of abdomen
C. Start metronidazole
D. Start infliximab
E. Start cyclosporine

163. A 25-year-old woman presents with complaints of bloody diarrhea for the past 4 months. She notes 2 to 3 urgent bowel movements mixed with blood on a daily basis. She takes ibuprofen as needed for monthly menstrual pain. Abdominal exam reveals a soft, nontender abdomen with no organomegaly. An ileocolonoscopy is performed and shows erythema, friability, and loss of vascular markings extending from the rectum to the sigmoid colon. The transverse colon and ascending colon are grossly normal. There is erythema and a few erosions around the appendiceal orifice. The terminal ileum appears grossly normal. Biopsies of the rectosigmoid show chronic active inflammation with marked crypt architectural irregularity. Biopsies around the appendiceal orifice reveal the same. Biopsies of the transverse colon and ascending colon are normal. Which of the following is the most likely diagnosis?
A. Crohn's disease
B. Ulcerative colitis
C. Infectious colitis
D. NSAID-related colitis
E. Behçet's disease

164. A 48-year-old woman with newly diagnosed left-sided ulcerative colitis is seen in clinic for follow-up. She was started on mesalamine 2.4 g/day 4 months prior and is doing well. She passes two well-formed bowel movements per day with no blood. She has no abdominal pain. She is concerned about side effects. Which of the following laboratory values should be monitored while the patient is on mesalamine?
A. Total cholesterol
B. Vitamin B_{12}
C. Creatinine
D. Magnesium
E. Red blood cell (RBC) folate

165. Which of the following is the most common complication after ileal pouch anal anastomosis (IPAA) for treatment of UC?
A. Pouchitis
B. Small bowel obstruction
C. Anastomotic stricture

D. Abscess
E. Fistula

166. A 55-year-woman with a 15-year history of panulcerative colitis presents for surveillance colonoscopy. She is on azathioprine 150 mg daily. Her ileocolonoscopy reveals a normal terminal ileum and a normal colon with intact vascular markings and no visible inflammation. Surveillance biopsies are taken every 10 cm throughout the colon. All specimens were independently reviewed by two pathologists. The biopsy from the jar labeled "50 cm" is shown in the figure. Which of the following is the most appropriate next step in management?

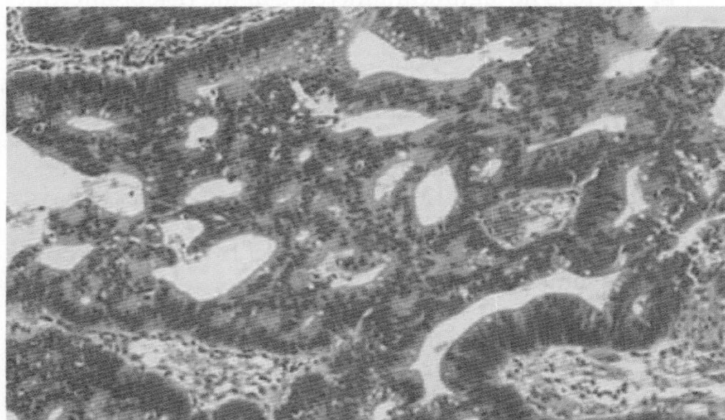

Figure for question 166.

A. Start mesalamine
B. Start prednisone
C. Start infliximab
D. Refer to surgery
E. Repeat colonoscopy in 2 years

167. A 28-year-old man presents for follow-up of his left-sided UC. He had recently been on prednisone 60 mg for a period of 3 months with an inability to taper past 40 mg daily. He was started on adalimumab and was able to successfully taper off the prednisone. He now notes one formed nonbloody bowel movement a day. Laboratory values are normal. A recent flexible sigmoidoscopy shows no gross active inflammation. He complains of pain and swelling of high right knee with inability to stand up for more than 10 minutes. Which of the following is the most likely diagnosis?
A. IBD-related peripheral arthropathy
B. Osteonecrosis of the right knee
C. Osteoporosis
D. Rheumatoid arthritis
E. Fibromyalgia

168. A 32-year-old woman with a 2-year history of severe panulcerative colitis presents to the emergency department. She notes severe bloody diarrhea and abdominal pain over the past 3 weeks. She has been noncomplicant with her mesalamine therapy, which she stopped 3 months ago. Physical examination reveals vital signs as follows:

Temperature	101° F
Heart rate	130 bpm
Blood pressure	110/50 mm Hg

There is periumblical tenderness to deep palpation without rebound or guarding. Her laboratory values are notable for the following:

Hemoglobin	7.8 g/dL
WBC	11,000/μL
Albumin	2.0 g/dL
C-reactive protein	110 mg/dL

Stool PCR is negative for *C. difficile.* A plain film of the abdomen is unremarkable. Intravenous methylprednisone was started at 30 mg twice daily, without improvement in her symptoms after 72 hours. A flexible sigmoidoscopy with limited insertion shows diffuse severe colitis starting from the rectum to the sigmoid colon. Biopsies are consistent with ulcerative colitis. You consider cyclosporin and infliximab therapy. Which of the following is true regarding cyclosporine and infliximab use in this setting?
A. Most adverse events related to cyclosporine use are idiosyncratic
B. Low cholesterol levels in the setting of cyclosporine use increases the risk of renal toxicity associated with the medication
C. Intravenous cyclosporine is as effective as infliximab in patients with severely active UC failing corticosteroids
D. A cyclosporine dose of 4 mg/kg is more effective than a dose of 2 mg/kg
E. In patients who fail cyclosporin, infliximab can be tried prior to referral for colectomy

169. A 25-year-old woman with a 5-year history of left-sided colitis presents with increased urgency and tenesmus for the past 3 weeks. She is having 3 to 4 loose bowel movements mixed with blood. She is maintained on mesalamine 2.4 g/day and was previously in clinical remission for the past 5 years on the medication. A sigmoidoscopy reveals erythema and erosions in the rectum and sigmoid colon. Which of the following is the most appropriate next step in management?
A. Obtain stool specimens to test for infection
B. Increase mesalamine to 4.8 g/day
C. Start mesalamine enemas
D. Start budesonide
E. Obtain a thiopurine methyltransferase level

170. A 22-year-old man presents with symptoms of abdominal pain, weight loss, and bloody bowel movements for the past 4 months. A colonoscopy to the cecum shows inflammation limited to the distal 20 cm of colon. The mucosa in this area exhibits loss of vascularity, erosions, and friability. He is placed on mesalamine enemas with no response in his symptoms. His laboratory values are as follows:

Hemoglobin	9.8 g/dL
MCV	68 fL
Ferritin	<10 ng/mL
C-reactive protein	28.2 mg/dL
Albumin	2.5 g/L
TMPT levels	normal
Interferon gamma release assay	negative

Which of the following is the most appropriate next step in management?
A. Start budesonide MMX
B. Start mesalamine 2.4 g/day
C. Start azathioprine 2.5 mg/kg/day
D. Obtain small bowel imaging
E. Refer to colorectal surgery

171. Which of the following medications consists of a 5-aminosalicylic acid (5-ASA) dimer?
A. Sulfasalazine
B. Olsalazine

C. Mesalamine (Pentasa brand)
D. Mesalamine (Asacol brand)
E. Balsalazide

172. A 48-year-old man with a history of ulcerative colitis and stapled ileal pouch-anal anastomosis is seen in clinic for follow-up. Over the last 2 weeks he developed increasing rectal urgency, tenesmus, and worsening diarrhea. He has no fevers, chills, joint pain, or skin rash. He works as a bartender and drinks alcohol on the weekends. Abdominal examination is soft with minimal hypogastric tenderness. An endoscopy is performed, which shows pouch erythema, edema, friability, and superficial ulcerations. Biopsy reveals acute inflammatory infiltrates, crypt abscesses, and ulcerations. Which of the following is the most appropriate treatment?
A. Metronidazole
B. Ciprofloxacin
C. Topical mesalamine
D. Oral steroids
E. VSL#3

173. A 25-year-old woman who is 28 weeks pregnant with ulcerative colitis is seen in clinic for follow-up. Her disease is in clinical remission. She is on infliximab therapy and plans to receive the last dose during pregnancy at week 33. Which of the following vaccines should be withheld in her baby during the first 6 months of life?
A. Diphtheria
B. Measles, mumps, rubella (MMR)
C. Pneumococcal conjugate vaccine (PCV)
D. Rotavirus
E. *Haemophilus influenzae* type b (Hib)

174. A 40-year-old man with a history of UC is seen in clinic for with abdominal pain of 2-day duration. One week ago, he underwent a total proctocolectomy with ileal pouch-anal anastomosis for refractory moderate to severe UC. He is currently taking prednisone 20 mg once daily as part of a dose taper over several weeks. Physical examination shows vital signs as follows:

Temperature	101° F
Heart rate	95 bpm
Blood pressure	120/60 mm Hg

His abdominal exam reveals a healing scar with no erythema. There is abdominal tenderness in the left lower quadrant. A CT scan was performed (see figure). Which of the following is the next best step in management?

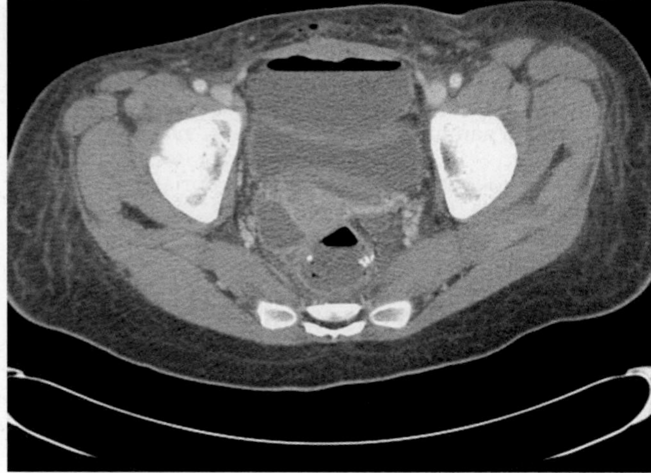

Figure for question 174.

A. Conservative management and repeat scan in 2 weeks
B. Broad-spectrum intravenous antibiotics and bowel rest
C. Diverting ileostomy
D. Laparotomy and drainage
E. CT-guided drainage

175. A 28-year-old woman with a history of UC is seen in clinic for follow-up. She has chronic UC that is refractory to medical therapies, including anti-TNF. She wants to discuss surgical options and is concerned regarding the effects on her fertility and pregnancy. Which of the following statements is true regarding surgical management of ulcerative colitis in this patient?
A. There is no significant increase in the risk of infertility after proctocolectomy and ileal pouch-anal anastomosis (IPAA)
B. Proctocolectomy and end-ileostomy increases her chances of having pregnancy and delivery related complications
C. In vitro fertilization (IVF) after IPAA is ineffective
D. If she receives a Kock pouch, she can expect to have a normal pregnancy
E. After an IPAA, she should expect to have 2 to 3 bowel movements during her pregnancy.

176. A 34-year-old woman with a 15-year history of ulcerative colitis is seen in clinic for follow-up. She has chronic left-sided ulcerative colitis that is refractory to medical therapies with prednisone and anti-TNF. Her last colonoscopy 1 month ago showed persistent moderately severe colitis extending from the rectum to the distal transverse colon. Biopsies show architectural distortion and crypt abscesses involving the left colon. Biopsies from the cecum, and ascending and proximal transverse colon, are normal. She wants to discuss surgical management of her ulcerative colitis. Which of the following statements is true regarding surgical management in this patient?
A. The recommended surgical treatment is left-sided colectomy
B. If she undergoes an ileal pouch-anal anastomosis (IPAA), she will need yearly endoscopic surveillance of the anal transition zone and pouch
C. There is no significant increase in the risk of infertility after proctocolectomy and IPAA
D. Her incidence of pouchitis post-IPAA decreases with time after surgery
E. There is a complication rate of 5% to 10% with IPAA

177. A 30-year-old man with a history of ulcerative colitis and stapled ileal pouch-anal anastomosis is seen in clinic for follow-up. Over the last 10 days, he developed increasing rectal urgency, tenesmus, and diarrhea. Four months ago, he had similar symptoms, and was diagnosed with acute pouchitis. He was treated with ciprofloxacin, and his symptoms resolved with treatment. Which of the following is the most appropriate therapy at this time?
A. Metronidazole 500 mg twice daily
B. Ciprofloxacin 500 mg twice daily
C. VSL#3
D. Mesalamine enemas
E. Prednisone 40 mg daily

178. Which of the following is the procedure of choice in patients with chronic ulcerative colitis who require colectomy?
A. Brooke ileostomy
B. Continent ileostomy (Kock pouch)
C. Ileal pouch-anal anastomosis (IPAA)
D. Ileorectal anastomosis
E. Loop ileostomy

179. A 62-year-old man presents to the emergency department with sudden onset epigastric pain that started 1 hour ago. He has a history of coronary artery disease and atrial fibrillation. On exam, the patient has pain with deep palpation and worse pain when the examiner suddenly removes his hand. CT angiography shows a rounded filling defect with nearly complete obstruction to flow in the proximal superior mesenteric artery (SMA). Which of the following is the most appropriate next step in management?

A. Exploratory laparotomy
B. Intravenous heparin
C. Endovascular therapy
D. Intravenous thrombolytic therapy
E. Angiography

180. A 65-year-old man presents to clinic with abdominal pain of 6 months duration. His pain is described as cramping that starts within 15 minutes, gradually increases in severity, and subsides over 2 to 3 hours. He is afraid to eat and reports a weight loss of 10 pounds. His past history is significant for hypertension and type 2 diabetes mellitus. He smokes 1 pack per day for the past 30 years. He reports moderate drinking of wine and beer at social gatherings. Physical exam shows vital signs as follows:

Temperature	100° F
Heart rate	75 bpm
Respiratory rate	12 breaths/min
Blood pressure	155/85 mm Hg

His abdomen is tender to palpation in the epigastrium. Laboratory values are as follows:

WBC	9,000/μL
Hematocrit	36%
Amylase	300 U/L
Creatinine	1.2 mg/dL
BUN	17 mg/dL

Which of the following findings is most likely to be found on further imaging and diagnostic workup?

A. Pancreatic interstitial edema
B. Malignancy
C. Gallstones
D. Prominent collaterals between the superior mesenteric artery and other splanchnic vessels
E. Inadequate filling of the SMA with no collaterals

181. A 45-year-old man with a history of hepatitis C cirrhosis and hypertension, presents with vague epigastric abdominal pain for the past week. Physical exam reveals mild epigastric tenderness to palpation without guarding or rebound tenderness. He has no ascites. He denies rectal bleeding. Laboratory values are as follows:

WBC	8000/μL
Hemoglobin	11.5 g/dL
Platelet count	120,000/μL
Bilirubin	1.3 mg/dL
Creatinine	1.1 mg/dL
INR	1.4

A right upper quadrant ultrasound with Doppler shows a nonocclusive portal vein thrombus with no collateral veins. An EGD performed 3 months ago showed no varices. Workup for factor V Leiden mutation and protein C, S deficiency is negative. Which of the following is the most appropriate next step in management?

A. Conservative management
B. 3 to 6 months of anticoagulation
C. Twelve months of anticoagulation
D. Lifelong anticoagulation
E. Repeat EGD

182. A 25-year-old man presents with a 1-month history of intermittent abdominal pain and diarrhea. He reports arthralgias and stiffness in his knees and shoulders. He smokes cigarettes daily. Review of systems is significant for decreased visual acuity and pain in both eyes, in addition to arthralgias and stiffness in the knees and shoulders. Physical exam reveals a thin male in no acute distress. There is erythema in both eyes with prominent superficial episcleral vessels. Ulcers are seen in the buccal mucosa. Abdominal exam reveals tenderness in the periumbilical area to deep palpation. There were a few small ulcerations on the penis and scrotum. Skin exam revealed tender erythematous subcutaneous nodules on the lower extremities. Which of the following is the most likely diagnosis?

A. Behçet's disease
B. Buerger's disease
C. Henoch-Schönlein purpura
D. Inflammatory bowel disease
E. Polyarteritis nodosa

183. A 53-year-old male with a history of gastroesophageal reflux disease and rheumatoid arthritis presents with complaints of abdominal cramping for the past few months. He states the cramping typically comes 30 minutes after eating and gradually increases in severity. It often resolves over 1 to 2 hours. He has limited the amount of food he eats due to the fear of having the pain and cramping return. CT scan showed an occlusive process of the splanchnic vessels with no other intraabdominal pathology. Angiography was completed, which showed occlusion of the superior mesenteric artery and inferior mesenteric artery. What is the next best step in management?

A. Coumadin
B. Observe
C. Surgical revascularization
D. Percutaneous transluminal mesenteric angioplasty (PTMA)
E. Exploratory laporatomy

184. A 70-year-old woman with a history of peripheral vascular disease, hypertension, and type 2 diabetes presents with an episode of light-headedness and dizziness. This was followed by left lower quadrant abdominal cramping and passage of bright red blood per rectum. Physical exam shows vital signs as follows:

Temperature	101° F
Heart rate	95 bpm
Respiratory rate	16 breaths/min
Blood pressure	105/55 mm Hg

Her abdomen is soft and tender to deep palpation in the periumbilical area. Laboratory values are as follows:

WBC	11,000/μL
Hematocrit	32%
Amylase	200 U/L
Creatinine	0.8 mg/dL
BUN	15 mg/dL

A colonoscopy was performed, and an image of her sigmoid colon is shown (see figure). A biopsy is pending. Which of the following is the most appropriate next step in management?

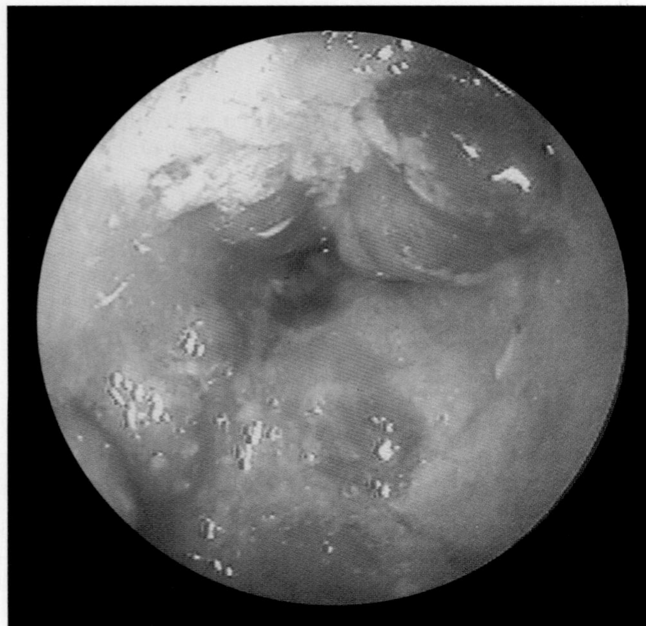

Figure for question 184.

A. Laparotomy
B. Intravenous methylprednisolone
C. CT scan of the abdomen and pelvis
D. Intravenous fluids and antibiotics
E. Barium enema

185. You are performing a colonoscopy on a 70-year-old man with abdominal pain and rectal bleeding. The colonoscopy reveals a single longitudinal ulcer in the sigmoid colon (see figure). There are few small sigmoid diverticula. The rest of the colon and the terminal ileum is normal. Which of the following is most likely diagnosis?

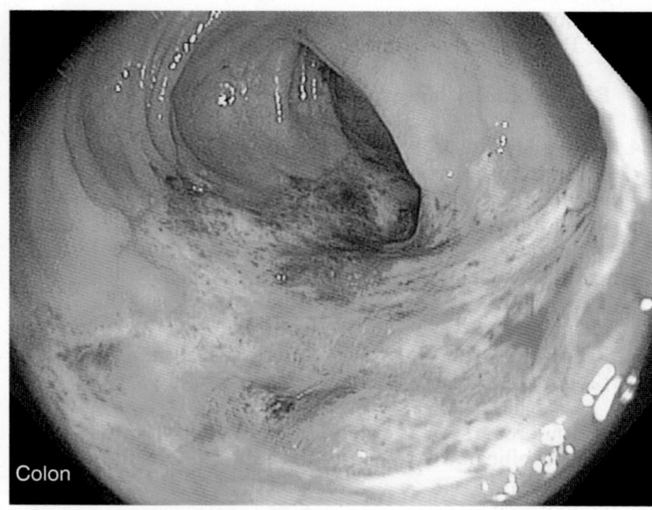

Figure for question 185.

A. Colon cancer
B. Crohn's disease
C. Acute infectious colitis
D. Colonic ischemia
E. Segmental colitis associated with diverticulosis

186. A 62-year-old woman presents with worsening exertional shortness of breath for the past 6 months. She denies any diarrhea, abdominal pain, or blood in her stool. She has lost 10 pounds in the last 2 months. Her past medical history includes a stroke for which she takes aspirin 325 mg daily. Laboratory values are as follows:

Hemoglobin	8.4 g/dL
Ferritin	6 ng/mL
Iron saturation	4%

Colonoscopy and upper endoscopy are performed and were normal. A capsule endoscopy is performed with results as follows:

Gastric passage time	0 h 10 m
Small bowel passage time	6 hr

Two hours into the study, there was an area with 3 small ulcerations (see figure, part A). There was an adjacent stricture that appeared short and concentric with thin septations (see figure, part B). The remainder of the small bowel mucosa appeared normal. What is the most likely etiology to the stricture?

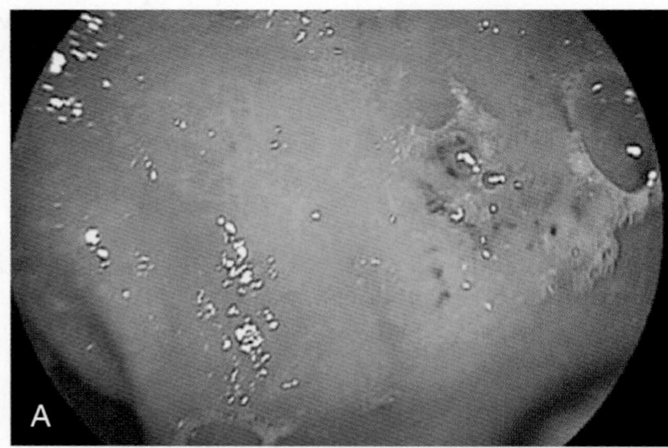

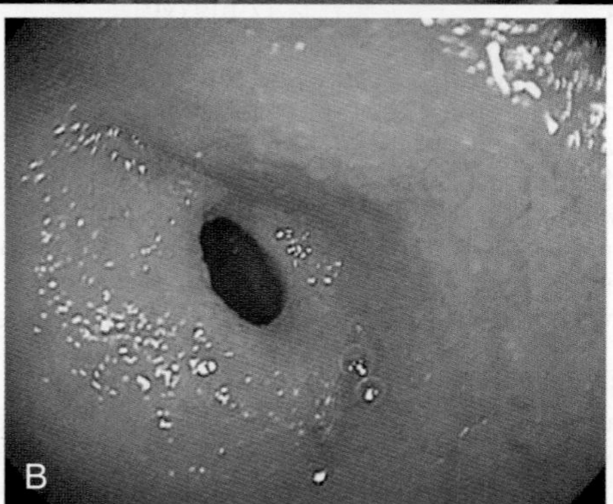

Figure for question 186.

A. Crohn's disease
B. NSAIDs
C. Idiopathic
D. Malignancy
E. Ischemia

187. Which of the following is the most common location for nonspecific or idiopathic small intestine ulcerations?
A. Duodenal bulb
B. Distal duodenum
C. Proximal jejunum
D. Distal jejunum
E. Ileum

188. A 50-year-old woman with history of well-controlled type 2 diabetes presents with worsening shortness of breath for the past 3 months. Her past medical history is significant for iron deficiency anemia diagnosed 8 months ago. She takes ferrous sulfate 325 mg orally 3 times a day, and metformin 500 mg orally once daily. Laboratory values reveal the following:

Hemoglobin	6 g/dL
Ferritin	10 μL/L

A diagnostic colonoscopy was performed with terminal ileal intubation. There were multiple small nonbleeding linear ulcers with overlying exudate and normal intervening mucosa noted in the terminal ileum. Biopsies were obtained, and the pathology revealed nonspecific inflammation without villous atrophy. There were no granulomas, eosinophils, or viral inclusions. The colonoscopy was repeated, and the ulcers were rebiopsied. Pathology revealed similar findings. Video capsule endoscopy was performed and showed the same ulcers confined to the distal ileum. The remainder of the small bowel mucosa appeared normal. Which of the following is the most appropriate next step in management?

A. Surgical resection
B. Prednisone
C. Refer to oncology
D. Add vitamin C
E. Repeat colonoscopy in 6 months

189. A 64-year-old man is seen in clinic for heme-positive stool. He denies weight loss, abdominal pain, and diarrhea. His medical history is significant for diabetes mellitus, osteoarthritis, and hypertension. He takes ibuprofen as needed, metformin 500 mg orally twice daily, and lisinopril 40 mg once daily. Physical examination reveals a soft abdomen with no tenderness. Colonoscopy is performed which shows 2 concentric strictures in the sigmoid colon with normal intervening mucosa. Biopsies of the strictures revealed ulcerated mucosa with submucosal fibrosis. What is the most likely etiology to his colonoscopic findings?

A. Drug-induced
B. Microscopic colitis
C. Inflammatory bowel disease
D. Idiopathic
E. Scarring from prior diverticulitis episodes

190. A 56-year-old woman presents with worsening shortness of breath for the past 3 months. Laboratory values show evidence of iron deficiency anemia. Initial EGD and colonoscopy do not reveal any source of bleeding. Capsule endoscopy was performed, which showed multiple small intestinal ulcerations at approximately 2 hours (gastric passage time was 15 minutes, small bowel passage time was 6 hours). Which of the following diagnostic test would provide the *lowest* diagnostic yield?

A. Push enteroscopy
B. Single balloon antegrade enteroscopy
C. Double balloon antegrade enteroscopy
D. Single balloon retrograde enteroscopy
E. Spiral enteroscopy

191. A 60-year-old African man with history of acquired immunodeficiency syndrome (AIDS) presents with intermittent fevers, night sweats, and anemia. He admits to passing dark, tarry stool intermittently for the past few months accompanied by a 10-pound weight loss. He denies having diarrhea. His CD4 count is 115 cells/mm^3. He had an EGD, which was unrevealing for a source of melena and anemia. Colonoscopy with terminal ileum intubation is performed. The mucosa in the terminal ileum shows thickening, nodularity, superficial ulcerations, and stricture formation. Which of the following findings will most likely be seen in biopsies of this abnormal area?

A. PAS-positive foamy macrophages with acid-fast bacilli
B. Noncaseating granulomas and crypt abscesses with lymphocyte infiltrate and architectural distortion
C. Villous atrophy with small sickle-shaped organisms on the surface epithelium
D. Atrophic villi with neutrophilic infiltrate and round, basophilic organisms
E. Owl's eye inclusion bodies

192. A 43-year-old woman with a history of congestive heart failure, hypertension, and peptic ulcer disease presents with recurrent melena. She presented to an outside hospital for evaluation. Upper endoscopy was nonrevealing. Her colonoscopy revealed melena throughout the right side of the colon. Subsequent capsule endoscopy showed active bleeding in the terminal ileum without an identifiable bleeding source. A single balloon retrograde enteroscopy was performed and showed an outpouching in the mucosa with associated overlying ulceration. What is the most likely etiology of the ulceration?

A. Medication effect
B. Idiopathic
C. Gastric acid hypersecretion
D. Malignancy
E. Ischemia

193. A 48-year-old woman presents to the emergency department with abdominal pain, nausea, and vomiting of 6 hours duration. The pain started in the middle abdominal region 6 hours prior to presentation and is now in the right lower quadrant of the abdomen. The pain is steady in nature and aggravated by coughing. She has no history of such symptoms in the past. Physical examination reveals vital signs as follows:

Temperature	100.4° F
Heart rate	110 bpm
Blood pressure	110/70 mm Hg

On exam, she has pain on palpation of the right lower quadrant without rebound tenderness or guarding. Laboratory values are as follows:

WBC	12,000/μL
Neutrophils	85%

Which of the following is the most likely diagnosis?

A. Acute pancreatitis
B. Acute appendicitis
C. Diverticulitis
D. Ovarian torsion
E. Crohn's disease

194. A 19-year-old man presents to the emergency department with right lower quadrant abdominal pain for the past 14 hours. Vital signs are as follows:

Temperature	100.0° F
Heart rate	80 bpm
Blood pressure	100/60 mm Hg

On physical examination, the abdomen is soft. There is tenderness to palpation and rebound tenderness in the right lower quadrant. On laboratory studies, WBC count is 7900/μL. Which of the following is the most appropriate next step in management?

A. Urgent CT scan of the abdomen
B. Emergent exploratory laparotomy
C. Intravenous fluids and serial abdominal exams
D. Administration of intravenous antibiotics
E. Ultrasonography of the abdomen

195. A patient presents with right lower quadrant pain of 6 hours duration. A CT scan of the abdomen is obtained which shows a dilated, inflamed appendix and a single periappendiceal abscess measuring 4 cm. What is the appropriate definitive management?
A. Percutaneous drainage under CT guidance
B. Operative drainage
C. Intravenous fluids and antibiotics
D. Colonoscopy
E. Right hemicolectomy

196. A 21-year-old man presents to the emergency department with abdominal pain, nausea, and vomiting of 8 hours duration. The pain started in the middle abdominal region 8 hours ago and is now in the located in the right lower quadrant of the abdomen. The pain is steady in nature and aggravated by coughing. The examiner elicits pain by internally and externally rotating the patient's flexed right hip. What is the name of this sign?
A. Psoas sign
B. Obturator sign
C. Rovsing's sign
D. McBurney's sign
E. Peritoneal sign

197. A 48-year-old man presents to the emergency department with sudden onset left lower quadrant abdominal pain and persistent emesis that woke him up from sleep. He is febrile to 38.6° C. Physical exam reveals localized tenderness in the left lower quadrant, without rebound tenderness or guarding. CT scan with intravenous contrast shows bowel wall thickening in the sigmoid colon with pericolonic fat stranding. What is the best antibiotic regimen for him?
A. Oral metronidazole
B. Oral levofloxacin + oral trimethoprim/sulfamethoxazole
C. Intravenous amoxicillin/clavulanate
D. Intravenous clindamycin + intravenous metronidazole
E. Intravenous metronidazole + intravenous vancomycin

198. A 54-year-old man presents with sudden left lower quadrant pain and fever. A CT scan performed in the emergency department reveals bowel wall thickening in the distal sigmoid and a 2 cm abscess confined to the colonic wall. What is the next best step in management?
A. Bowel rest and intravenous antibiotics
B. CT-guided percutaneous drainage
C. Surgical resection
D. Colonoscopy
E. Bowel rest and repeat imaging in 1 week

199. An 85-year-old man presents with left lower quadrant cramping pain, diarrhea, and rectal bleeding of 6 months duration. He underwent a colonoscopy that showed erythematous, friable mucosa in the sigmoid colon with multiple scattered sigmoid diverticula (see figure). Biopsies of the sigmoid colon reveal chronic lymphocytic infiltration and crypt abscesses. Which of the following is the most appropriate next step in management?

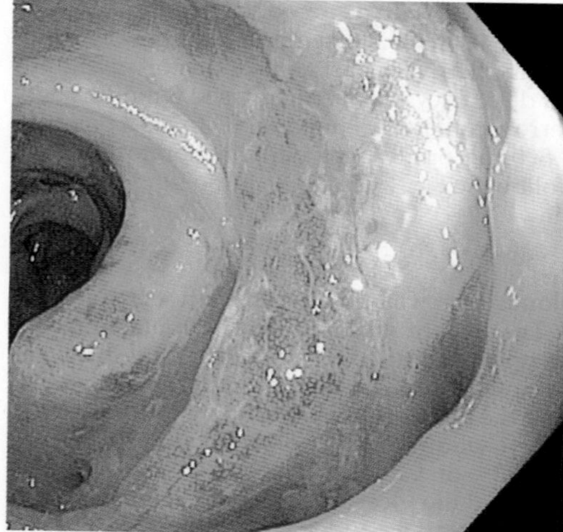

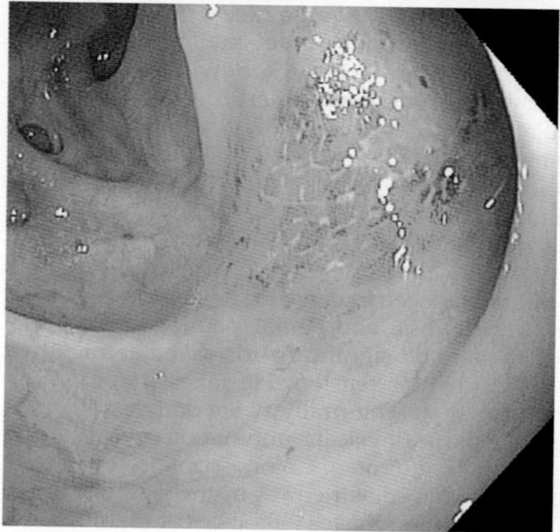

Figure for question 199.

A. Observation
B. Prednisone
C. Partial colectomy
D. Oral mesalamine
E. Infliximab

200. A 75-year-old man presents with severe acute hematochezia. He receives a nuclear medicine–tagged RBC scan, which is positive for an active bleeding in the sigmoid colon. He is sent immediately to angiography with embolization. At what rate can angiography detect rates of bleeding?
A. 0.1 mL/min
B. 0.25 mL/min
C. 0.5 mL/min
D. 1 mL/min
E. 5 mL/min

201. A 78-year-old woman is seen in the emergency department with abrupt, painless bright red blood per rectum that started 4 hours prior to presentation. She describes passing large amount of clots per rectum followed by light-headedness and dizziness. On physical exam, vital signs are as follows:

Blood pressure	80/60 mm Hg
Heart rate	120 bpm

She continues to pass bright red blood per rectum. An angiography of the superior mesenteric artery is shown (see figure). What is the next best step in management?

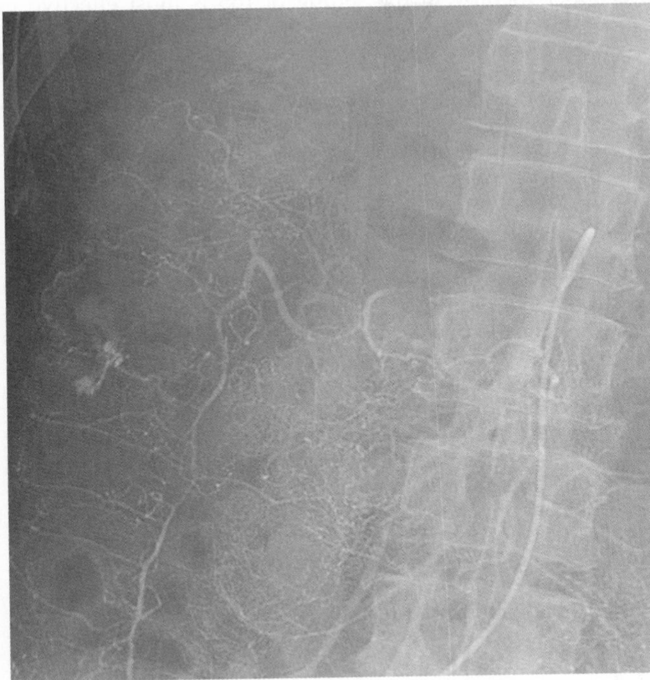

Figure for question 201.

A. Surgical consultation for segmental colectomy
B. Embolization
C. Colonoscopic evaluation
D. Admit to intensive care unit for resuscitation
E. Intravenous vasoconstrictors

202. A 62-year-old man presents to the emergency department with left lower quadrant pain of 2 days duration. He describes the pain as constant and sharp. He denies nausea, vomiting, or rectal bleeding. Vitals signs are as follows:

Temperature	101.5° F
Heart rate	105 bpm
Blood pressure	110/55 mm Hg
Respiratory rate	14 breaths/min

Abdominal exam reveals severe tenderness in the left lower quadrant without rebound tenderness or guarding. His laboratory values are as follows:

Hemoglobin	12.1 g/dL
Platelet count	220,000/μL
WBC	13,000/μL
Creatinine	1.1 mg/dL
ALT	20 U/L
AST	19 U/L
Alkaline phosphatase	120 U/L
Total bilirubin	2.2 mg/dL
INR	1.3

Which of the following is the most appropriate next step in management?

A. CT abdomen and pelvis with oral contrast
B. Abdominal ultrasound
C. Bowel prep and colonoscopy
D. Abdominal x-ray
E. MRI of the abdomen and pelvis

203. A 52-year-old woman presents to the emergency department with left lower quadrant abdominal pain and intermittent fevers for the past 2 weeks. She denies diarrhea or weight loss. Review of systems is significant for brownish discoloration of her urine with a sensation of passing air along with urine. She has no family history of inflammatory bowel disease. She does not smoke and denies excessive drinking. On physical examination, her vital signs are as follows:

Temperature	102° F
Heart rate	105 bpm
Respiratory rate	14 breaths/min
Blood pressure	110/50 mm Hg

Abdominal exam reveals tenderness to deep palpation in the left lower quadrant. Laboratory values are as follows:

Hemoglobin	11 g/dL
Platelet count	350,000/μL
WBC	12,000/μL
Urinalysis shows	3+ leukocyte esterase, nitrates, and urinary WBC >100/HPF
Urine culture pending	

Definitive management of this patient's underlying condition includes which of the following?

A. A 10-day course of oral trimethoprim/sulfamethoxazole
B. A double-stage operative resection with fistula closure and diverting colostomy
C. A single-stage operative resection with fistula closure and primary anastomosis
D. Bladder resection with bilateral nephrostomy tubes
E. Cystoscopy

204. Which of the following is the most common type of fistula associated with complicated diverticulitis?

A. Colovaginal
B. Colovesicular
C. Coloenteric
D. Coloureteral
E. Colouterine

205. Which of the following is the most common risk factor for irritable bowel syndrome (IBS)?

A. Celiac disease
B. Bacterial gastroenteritis
C. Antibiotic use
D. Low birth weight
E. Depression

206. A 27-year-old law student presents with a 10-month history of intermittent diffuse abdominal pain, associated with loose stool and bloating. His symptoms seem to be worse after eating. Therefore, he is concerned that he may have food allergies and asks you to test him for multiple food allergies. He denies seeing blood in his stool and his weight is stable. His physical exam is remarkable for mild diffuse abdominal tenderness. Which of the following tests would you order at this time?

A. Anti–tissue transglutaminase IgA antibody
B. Antigliadin antibody
C. Wheat IgE levels
D. Maize IgE levels
E. Soy IgE levels

207. Which of the following is the most effective psychological therapy for IBS?
A. Psychotherapy
B. Acupuncture
C. Biofeedback
D. Cognitive behavioral therapy (CBT)
E. Hypnotherapy

208. A 32-year-old woman who is 4 months pregnant presents with intermittent right lower quadrant crampy abdominal pain, gas, and bloating. Her stool is frequent and looks like "pudding." Usually her abdominal pain improves with defecation. These symptoms are similar to her irritable bowel flares. However, the stool is looser this time, and she also sees mucus. Which of the following tests would you recommend at this time?
A. Colonoscopy
B. Flexible sigmoidoscopy
C. Upper endoscopy with duodenal aspirate
D. Upper endoscopy with duodenal biopsies
E. Stool studies for ova, parasites, and *C. difficile*

209. A 25-year-old man presents with a 5-year history of postprandial abdominal pain associated with diarrhea and bloating. However, his symptoms have worsened in the past 8 months. He now has symptoms twice a week. He is a first-year medical student. He denies smoking or excessive alcohol intake. Physical examination reveals soft, nontender abdomen. Which of the following is the best recommendation for symptom control in this patient?
A. Trial of a 5-hydroxytryptamine 3 (5-HT3) receptor antagonist daily
B. Trial lubiprostone twice daily
C. Trial of an antispasmodic before meals
D. Trial of rifaximin three times daily
E. Trial of fiber supplementation twice day

210. A 60-year-old woman with a history hypertension and depression presents with a 7-month history of abdominal pain, bloating, distention, and constipation. She reports poor appetite and a 10-pound weight loss. Her symptoms are worse with eating. She denies rectal bleeding. She had a negative colonoscopy 1 year ago. Her examination is significant for mild abdominal distention and tenderness in the lower abdomen. Which of the following is the most appropriate next step in management?
A. Repeat the colonoscopy
B. CT scan of the abdomen and pelvis
C. Upper endoscopy
D. Gastric emptying study
E. No further workup and reassurance

211. A 33-year woman is referred to you for a 7-month history of abdominal pain, gas, bloating, and diarrhea. She gives a history of developing abdominal pain and diarrhea during a 10-day trip to Mexico 9 months ago. She was empirically treated with metronidazole for 5 days and slowly improved after 2 weeks. However, for the past few months she has had symptoms once per week. She has tried loperamide, which slows her diarrhea. However, she still has pain and urgency. She had a negative colonoscopy 3 months ago. What is the likely diagnosis?
A. Microscopic colitis
B. *C. difficile* infection
C. *Giardiasis* infection
D. Postinfectious irritable bowel syndrome
E. Antibiotic-induced colitis

212. Fiber therapy in the setting of IBS is most effective in which of the following scenarios?
A. Predominantly abdominal pain and diarrhea symptoms
B. Predominantly abdominal pain and constipation symptoms
C. Constipation only symptoms
D. Diarrhea only symptoms
E. Predominantly abdominal pain, constipation, and bloating symptoms

213. A 55-year-old business school professor presents with daily symptoms of abdominal pain, urgency, and diarrhea for the past 8 months. He has had several episodes of urgency while he was teaching with near fecal leakage. His anxiety of having an "accident" while lecturing has led to fear of teaching and a worsened cycle of symptoms. He had negative colonoscopy with mucosal biopsies 2 years ago for the same symptoms. What therapy would you advise at this time?
A. Trial of nortriptyline 10 mg every night
B. Trial of loperamide 2 to 16 mg/day
C. Trial of bismuth subsalicylate four times a day
D. Trial of alosetron and increase up to 1 mg twice daily
E. Trial of a probiotic daily

214. Which of the following correctly describes the mechanism of action of linaclotide?
A. Chloride channel agonist stimulating intestinal fluid secretion
B. Chloride channel antagonist stimulating intestinal fluid secretion
C. 5-HT4 agonist stimulating intestinal motility
D. Guanylate cyclase agonist stimulating intestinal fluid secretion
E. Guanylate cyclase antagonist stimulating intestinal fluid secretion

215. A 19-year-old college student presents with a 2-year history of intermittent abdominal pain, bloating, and constipation. His symptoms have been worse in the past month. Polyethylene glycol initially helped his constipation; however, it is no longer effective. He is concerned that he has Crohn's disease because his cousin has Crohn's disease and similar symptoms. He denies nausea, vomiting, and fever. His weight is stable. The physical examination is unremarkable. Which of the following is the most appropriate next step in management?
A. Schedule him for a colonoscopy
B. Schedule him for an abdominal CT
C. Schedule him for an abdominal ultrasound
D. Provide reassurance and no further testing
E. Order p-ANCA and anti–*Sachharomyces cerevisiae* antibody serologies

216. A 22-year-old-college students presents with a 2-year history of intermittent abdominal pain, bloating, and constipation. He denies nausea, vomiting, rectal bleeding, weight loss, and fever. His symptoms have been worse in the past 2 months. Polyethylene glycol initially helped his constipation; however, it is no longer effective. He has tried fiber in the past, which worsened his bloating. The physical examination is unremarkable.

Which of the following is the most appropriate treatment?
A. Trial of nortriptyline 10 mg every night
B. Trial of an antispasmodic as needed
C. Trial of linaclotide 290 μL daily
D. Trial of alosetron and increase up to 1 mg twice daily
E. Trial of a probiotic daily

217. A 25-year-old woman presents with a 10-year history of constipation and bloating. She has tried polyethylene glycol as well as lubiprostone in the past with minimal relief. She reports having a bowel movement once a week with the help of a stimulant laxative and an enema. She describes the need to strain and push on her left lower quadrant to have bowel movement. The bloating improves with defecation. What the most likely diagnosis?
A. Small bowel intussusception
B. Pelvic floor dysfunction
C. Constipation-predominant irritable bowel syndrome (IBS-C)
D. Functional constipation
E. Colon cancer

218. A 31-year-old woman presents for follow-up of a 2-year history of periumbilical abdominal pain 2 times per week. The pain is described as severe, crampy, and causing her to curl up in ball on the floor in the bathroom. She has diarrhea 3 to 4 times a day that is unpredictable and quite debilitating. She does not identify food or situational triggers. Her vital signs are within normal range but she looks in mild distress. Her weight is stable. Her abdomen is not distended and she has good bowel sounds. She has mild tenderness and rectal examination is unremarkable. She has had normal complete blood count, thyroid-stimulating hormone, comprehensive metabolic panel, and celiac serologies within the past year. She has tried fiber, antispasmodics, and a tricyclic antidepressant in the past. She got some relief with rifaximin several months ago. What would you recommend next?
A. Retreat with rifaximin 400 mg twice daily for 1 week
B. Increase fiber to three times daily
C. Add loperamide to the antispasmodic regimen
D. Start alosetron and increase up to 1 mg twice daily
E. Start a probiotic daily

219. Which of the following is a risk factor for postinfectious irritable bowel syndrome?
A. Alcohol use
B. Male sex
C. History of depression
D. Short duration of infection
E. Older age

220. A 41-year woman presents with a 1-year history of abdominal pain and erratic bowel patterns. She has loose stool with urgency for 1 week followed by 2 weeks of constipation. She denies rectal bleeding, weight loss, nausea, and vomiting. Her family history is significant for heart disease. Her physical examination is normal. What would you recommend for this patient?
A. Maintain a low fermentable oligosaccharides, disaccharides, monosaccharides and polyols (FODMAP) diet
B. Maintain a food/symptom diary
C. Start loperamide daily
D. Start alosetron and increase up to 1 mg twice daily
E. Start a linaclotide 145 μL daily

221. A 29-year-old man is seen in your office for a 3-month history of epigastric pain, fullness, and bloating. He has intermittent constipation; however, his pain is independent of bowel movements. What is the next step in management?
A. Trial of a 5-HT3 receptor antagonist daily
B. Trial of lubiprostone twice daily
C. Trial of an antispasmodic before meals
D. Trial of a proton-pump inhibitor
E. Trial of fiber supplementation twice daily

222. Which of the following factors is a poor prognostic indicator in patients diagnosed with irritable bowel syndrome (IBS)?
A. Longer duration of symptoms
B. History of lactose intolerance
C. Diarrhea-predominant IBS
D. Mixed-type IBS
E. Family history of IBS

223. Which of the factors below is most important in managing patients diagnosed with irritable bowel syndrome?
A. Extensive testing to rule out organic causes
B. Reassurance to the patient that there is nothing wrong
C. Advise food elimination
D. Provide education and validation
E. Refer to psychiatry

224. A 57-year-old woman presents to the emergency department with a 1-day history of nausea, vomiting, and crampy abdominal pain. Her past medical history is significant for diabetes mellitus, hypertension, and cervical osteoarthritis. Her surgical history is significant for a total abdominal hysterectomy. In the emergency department her abdomen is distended, bowel sounds are decreased, and her abdomen is diffusely tender. An abdominal plain film is shown (see figure). Which of the following is the most likely etiology of the patient's presentation?

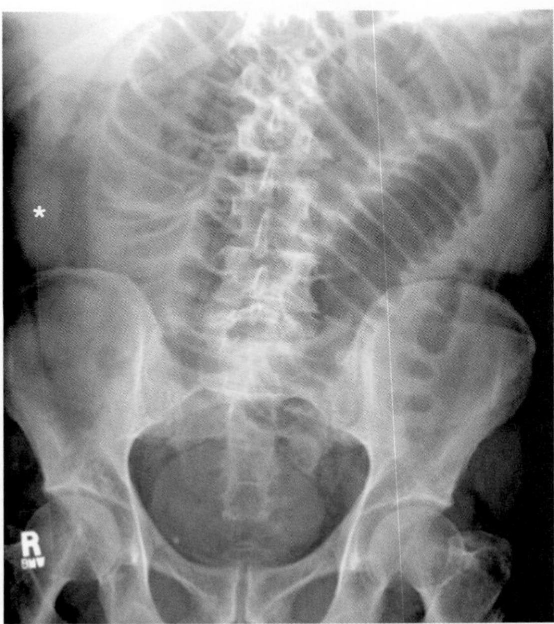

Figure for question 224.

A. Crohn's stricture
B. Intraabdominal adhesions

C. Narcotic-induced ileus
D. Bowel intussusception
E. Radiation-induced injury

225. A 79-year-old man presents with a 1-week history of dull periumbilical abdominal pain and intermittent nausea. He was seen by an urgent care office 3 days ago and was diagnosed with gastroenteritis. However, his symptoms have continued. On physical exam, his temperature is 101° F. His abdomen is mildly distended. An abdominal plain film reveals mildly distended loops of proximal small bowel and air in the biliary tree. CT scan reveals a biliary small bowel fistula. Which of the following is the most appropriate next step in management?
A. Nothing by mouth (NPO) and nasogastric tube on low intermittent suction
B. Intravenous fluids and observation
C. ERCP
D. Cholecystectomy
E. Emergent surgery

226. A 51-year-old woman with a history of hypertension and hypothyroidism presents to your office with a 3-day history of nausea, vomiting, and abdominal pain. She normally suffers from constipation, and she has not had a bowel movement in more than a week. She reports taking her levothyroxine and lisinopril regularly. She took her usual magnesium hydroxide for constipation, but it did not help. Her past medication history includes partial small bowel resection for a benign hamartoma. Her abdomen is distended, and a plain film is obtained (see figure). Which of the following is the most appropriate next step in management?

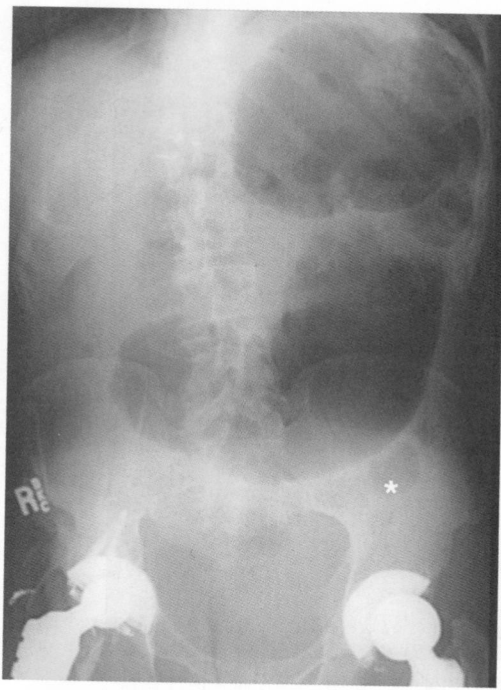

Figure for question 226.

A. Intravenous fluids and observation
B. Endoscopic colonic decompression
C. Right hemicolectomy with ileocolic anastomosis
D. NPO and nasogastric tube on low intermittent suction
E. Sigmoid resection with end colostomy

227. Which of the following is the most common cause of colonic obstruction?
A. Crohn's stricture
B. Diverticulitis
C. Intussusception
D. Ventral hernia
E. Adenocarcinoma

228. Which of the following is the most common anomaly associated with midgut volvulus?
A. Axial rotation of the midgut loop on it vascular pedicle
B. Axial rotation of the stomach
C. Inadequate rotation of the midgut loop around the celiac artery
D. Inadequate rotation of the midgut loop around the superior mesenteric artery
E. Failure of the small bowel to affix to the posterior body wall

229. A 72-year-old male develops nausea and vomiting 2 days after hip surgery. Initially, he was doing fairly well postoperatively, and he was able to start clear liquids. However, he now has not had a bowel movement or passed gas. His abdomen is distended, and he does not have bowel sounds. He is being given 2 mg of morphine every 4 hours for pain he is experiencing at the surgical wound site. What is the next step in the management of this patient?
A. Hold all narcotics
B. Colonoscopy for decompression
C. Nasogastric tube for decompression
D. Emergent colectomy
E. Neostigmine intravenously

230. A 21-year-old woman with a long-standing history of intermittent nausea, vomiting, abdominal distention, and constipation presents to your office for consultation. She has been managed with a prokinetic and antiemetic therapy for many years. However, her symptoms are worsening, and her nutritional status is poor. She is afebrile and vital signs are as follows:

Blood pressure	88/50 mm Hg
Heart rate	70 bpm
Respiratory rate	14 breaths/min
BMI	18 kg/m^2

She is a pale, thin woman, abdomen is distended and bowel sounds are decreased. Her past workup includes a negative upper endoscopy and colonoscopy, negative celiac, and thyroid blood work. Her C-reactive protein is negative. You suspect an enteric neuropathy or myopathy. Which test is most helpful in establishing a visceral neuromyopathy?
A. Small bowel scintigraphy
B. MRI
C. Laparoscopy with full thickness bowel biopsy
D. Blood serotonin level
E. Enteroscopy with random biopsy

231. A 50-year-old woman presents to your office with a 5-year history of systemic sclerosis and scleroderma. She complains of nausea, early satiety, and abdominal bloating and discomfort. She also reports a 15-pound weight loss. She reports diarrhea, which is unresponsive to over-the-counter treatments. However, the abdominal

distention is her most troubling symptom at this time. She has a gastric emptying study, suggesting gastroparesis documented in her chart. She is currently on lansoprazole 30 mg orally twice daily and metoclopramide 10 mg orally four times a day. One physical examination, exam the patient appears healthy. Her vital signs are as follows:

Temperature	98.4° F
Respiratory rate	16 breaths/min
Heart rate	102 bpm
Blood pressure	90/60 mm Hg

She has a pale conjunctiva. Her abdomen is mildly distended, with increased bowel sounds in all quadrants. There is no lower extremity edema. Skin examination shows telangiectasias on the nose and both cheeks, with taut skin on face and hands. Her abdominal x-ray is shown (see figure). What therapy will most likely improve her symptoms?

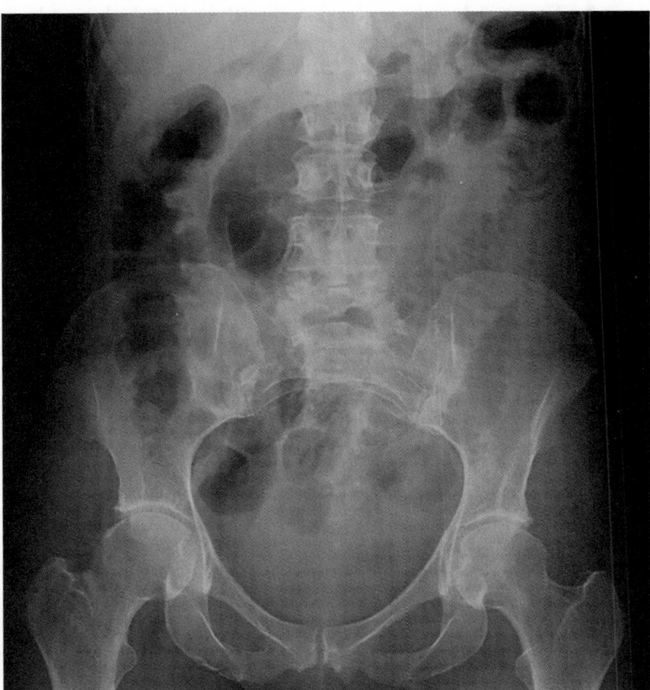

Figure for question 231.

A. An empiric trial of metronidazole
B. Increase metoclopramide
C. Start loperamide four times a day
D. Initiate a bile acid resin
E. Stop metoclopramide and add erythromycin

232. A 61-year-old woman with a history of hypertension, hypercholesterolemia, rheumatoid arthritis (RA), and unexplained liver enzyme elevation presents for evaluation of a 6-month history of diarrhea. She reports 5 to 6 loose stools per day that are unpredictable, and often she experiences stool incontinence. She denies abdominal pain, weight loss, or blood per rectum. Her exam is unremarkable. Her urine is positive for protein. You decide to perform a colonoscopy with random biopsy. The colonic mucosa has few superficial erosions. An image of her colonic biopsies is shown (see figure). What is the most likely diagnosis?

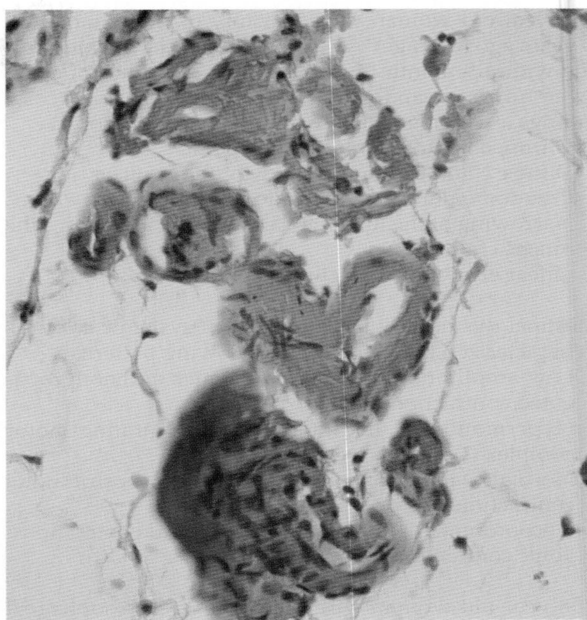

Figure for question 232.

A. Microscopic colitis
B. Systemic amyloidosis
C. Ischemic colitis
D. Crohn's colitis
E. Irritable bowel syndrome

233. You are asked to consult on a 73-year-old hospitalized man with abdominal distention with pain and decreased bowel sounds for the past 3 days. He is 4 days postcholecystectomy. Vital signs are as follows:

Temperature	37.3° C
Heart rate	84 bpm
Blood pressure	130/80 mm Hg

His abdominal exam reveals distension, sluggish bowel sounds, and mild diffuse tenderness. His abdominal x-ray shows diffuse colonic distension. Cecal diameter is 9 cm. Repeat x-ray after 3 days reveals a cecal diameter of 10 cm. Laboratory values are as follows:

Hemoglobin	12 g/dL
Platelet count	180,000/μL
Total bilirubin	1.3 mg/dL
Creatinine	1.5 mg/dL
INR	1.3
Magnesium	2 mEq/L
Potassium	3.4 mEq/L
Sodium	140 mEq/L

What would you recommend for this patient at this time?

A. Nasogastric tube insertion for decompression
B. Immediate surgery for segmental colonic resection
C. Bowel regimen with polyethylene glycol twice day
D. Emergent endoscopic decompression
E. Intravenous neostigmine over 3 to 5 minutes

234. Which of the following is the most common cause of acquired megacolon worldwide?

A. Poorly controlled diabetes mellitus
B. Hypothyroidism
C. *Trypanosoma cruzi* (Chagas' disease)
D. *C. difficile* colitis
E. Opioid-induced colonic dilation

235. A 55-year-old woman with a history of chemoradiation 10 years ago for Paget's disease of the perianal skin presents with a 9-month history of severe diarrhea and left lower quadrant abdominal discomfort. What mucosal findings are you most likely to find on colonoscopy?
A. Diffuse colonic ulceration and edema
B. Diffuse colonic erythema and aphthous ulceration
C. Pseudomembranes with profound mucous
D. Narrowing of the lumen, telangiectasia, atrophy of the mucosa folds
E. Linear erosions with active bleeding

236. Intestinal dysmotility in patients with systemic sclerosis is characterized by which of the following patterns?
A. Low-amplitude clusters of propagated and nonpropagated contractions
B. Hypermotility of the interdigestive migrating motor complex (MMC)
C. Normal amplitude but delayed postprandial contractions
D. Uncoordinated bursts of nonpropagated contractions
E. Tonic contractions at the pylorus

237. A 58-year-old woman with history of gastroesophageal reflux disease presents to a gastroenterologist office for a follow-up. She had a negative screening colonoscopy 5 years ago by the same physician. The report indicated excellent bowel preparation and a withdrawal time of 10 minutes. She denies any GI symptoms other than occasional heartburn, and she has no family history of colon cancer. The patient asks the gastroenterologist about her risk of having cancer or major findings if she repeats her colonoscopy at this time. What is the probability of finding an adenoma with advanced pathology (AAP) if her colonoscopy is repeated now?
A. 1% to 2%
B. 10%
C. 25%
B. 50%
C. 70%

238. The process of colon carcinogenesis has been considered to go through two general stages: the formation of the adenoma, termed *tumor initiation*, and the progression of the adenoma to carcinoma, termed *tumor progression*. Which genetic alteration is considered an important step in tumor initiation rather than a tumor progression?
A. Loss of *APC* gene function
B. Loss of function of DCC (deleted in colon cancer) genes
C. Mutations in DNA mismatch repair (MMR) genes
D. Allelic deletion of chromosome 17p at the locus that contains the *TP53* gene
E. K-*ras* gene mutations

239. A 63-year-old woman who has history of hypertension is seen in clinic for follow-up 1 month after a screening colonoscopy. During the exam, three small polyps were removed from the ascending colon, and histology reveals tubular adenomas. She asks about medications or other interventions to prevent future neoplasms in the colon. Which of the following statements is true?
A. Dietary changes (increased fiber and reduced fat) maintained over 2 years will significantly reduce the risk of adenomas
B. COX-2 inhibitors protect from adenomatous polyps, but this benefit was not seen with other NSAIDS
C. Hormone replacement therapy (HRT) is associated with 20% reduction in colon cancer and is recommended for this patient
D. Calcium supplements reduce adenoma recurrence
E. Moderate alcohol use could be protective from colon adenomas and cancer

240. An 81-year-old man presents to the emergency department with frequent mucous diarrhea of 1-month duration. He complains of generalized fatigue. Physical exam reveals dry skin. Abdomen is soft and nontender. Laboratory values show an elevated creatinine to 2.3 mg/dL. He is diagnosed with acute kidney injury and is admitted for further evaluation and treatment. The patient's weakness and renal function improves with intravenous hydration. Stool studies, including fecal leukocytes, cultures, *C. difficile* toxin, and ova and parasites, were all negative. A colonoscopy is performed which reveals a semicircumferential tumor in the rectum. Which os the following statement is true about his condition?
A. This syndrome is associated with both tubular and villous adenoma
B. Tumors that produce this syndrome are typically in the proximal colon
C. Tumors that produce this syndrome are typically larger than 3 to 4 cm in diameter
D. Diarrhea is related to a paraneoplastic hormonal secretion
E. Medical management with hydration is sufficient

241. A 64-year-old African-American man with a history of rectal bleeding undergoes a colonoscopy. A large 3 cm ulcerated pedunculated polyp is found in the rectum. Endoscopic polypectomy is performed by snare cautery on the stalk. Pathology report indicates the presence of villous adenoma with a focus of intramucosal adenocarcinoma. There is no invasion into the submucosa, and no tumor cells are seen in the polyp stalk. Which of the following is the most appropriate management of this patient?
A. CT of the abdomen and pelvis
B. Refer the patient for a surgical resection
C. Rectal ultrasound
D. Repeat colonoscopy in 2 months
E. Repeat colonoscopy in 3 years

242. Which of the following statements about quality measures in average-risk screening colonoscopy is true?
A. Adenoma detection rates should be at least 10% in women and 20% in men
B. Cecal intubation rates should be over 85% of screening colonoscopies
C. Colonoscopic withdrawal time should be at least 6 minutes
D. The use of narrow band imaging (NBI) is preferable over white-light endoscopy
E. The use of chromoendoscopy is preferable over white-light endoscopy

243. A 50-year-old asymptomatic woman with no family history of colon cancer undergoes a screening colonoscopy in an outpatient surgical center. Five small polyps are removed with the largest polyp measuring 8 mm. Two of the polyps are hyperplasic rectal polyps, and three are tubular adenomas in the descending colon. The reported bowel prep is good. When should the next surveillance colonoscopy be recommended?
A. 2 to 6 months
B. 1 year

C. 3 years
D. 5 to 10 years
E. 10 years

244. A 56-year-old Caucasian man with no family history of colon cancer undergoes a colonoscopy for intermittent rectal bleeding. His exam reveals large internal hemorrhoids and an 8 mm pedunculated polyp in the in the sigmoid colon that was completely resected. Pathology reveals sessile serrated adenoma with dysplasia. What is the molecular pathway that is involved in sessile serrated adenoma progression to colorectal cancer?
A. Increased CpG island methylation pathway (CIMP)
B. Loss of *APC* gene
C. Germline mutation in DNA mismatch repair Genes (MMR)
D. Germline mutations in base-excision repair (BER) genes
E. Germline mutations in the *LKB1* gene

245. A 56-year-old man with no family history of colon cancer undergoes a screening colonoscopy. His exam reveals an 8 mm pedunculated polyp in the sigmoid colon that was completely resected. Pathology reveals sessile serrated adenoma with dysplasia. When should the colonoscopy be repeated?
A. 2 to 6 months
B. 1 year
C. 3 years
D. 5 years
E. 10 years

246. A 17-year-old man presents with complains of intermittent rectal bleeding. He reports occasional prolapsed small mass during defecation. Flexible sigmoidoscopy reveals a 2 cm pedunculated polyp in the rectum. The polyp was biopsied, and the pathology reveals a juvenile polyp. Which of the following statements is correct regarding juvenile polyps?
A. They are mucosal tumors that consist primarily of an excess of lamina propria and dilated cystic glands
B. Juvenile polyps have malignant potential if they are single
C. Juvenile polyps tend to recur after resection
D. Removal of juvenile polyp is not recommended
E. They are frequently seen in the first year of life

247. A 21-year-old African-American man with a known history of familial adenomatous polyposis (FAP) presents to your office for follow-up. He underwent prophylactic proctocolectomy a year ago. His last EGD 1 year ago revealed no duodenal polyps. He is concerned about his risks of duodenal and gastric adenocarcinoma. Which statement is true about FAP patients' risks of upper GI tract cancers?
A. Most gastric polyps detected on EGD are adenomas
B. The lifetime risk of gastric cancer is 0.5%
C. A 60% lifetime incidence of duodenal cancer has been reported
D. Duodenal cancers are common before age 30 if patients have duodenal adenomas
E. Surveillance with EGD using a side-viewing endoscope is recommended annually in this patient population

248. An 18-year-old woman presents to your office with progressive vague abdominal pain and nausea over 3 months. She has history of familial adenomatous polyposis (FAP) that required prophylactic proctocolectomy at age 16 years. Abdominal CT shows a large 11 cm well-circumscribed soft tissue mass arising in the mesentery. Which of the following statements about her tumor is true?
A. It is associated with Turcot's variant of FAP
B. Previous abdominal surgery increases the risk for this disease
C. The absolute risk of these tumors in FAP patients has been estimated at 3/100 person-years
D. It is generally more prevalent in men
E. Radiotherapy is appropriate therapy for most cases of desmoid tumors

249. A 24-year-old woman with a recent diagnosis of familial adenomatous polyposis (FAP) is seen in clinic for follow-up. She initially presented to her primary care physician with hematochezia 2 months ago, and a colonoscopy revealed numerous adenomatous polyps throughout the colon. Genetic testing confirmed FAP. The patient wants to discuss her treatment options. Which of the following statements is true about treatment?
A. Total proctocolectomy is the only treatment option offered to patients with FAP
B. The risk of malignancy in the rectum if a patient undergoes subtotal colectomy is approximately 1% per year
C. Subtotal colectomy with ileorectal anastomosis has the same effect on fertility in women as ileal pouch-anal anastomosis (IPAA)
D. Subtotal colectomy with ileorectal anastomosis and restorative proctocolectomy with IPAA demonstrated comparable rates of sexual dysfunction and dietary restriction
E. The ileal pouch does not need to be monitored for future development of adenoma or adenocarcinoma

250. A 50-year-old Caucasian man with no significant past medical history undergoes a screening colonoscopy. He is found to have 13 different polyps throughout his colon. The largest one is a 3 cm sessile polyp in the descending colon, and it is not amenable to endoscopic resection so a biopsy is performed. The final pathology report indicates that 11 polyps are adenomas, one is a hyperplastic polyp, and the largest unresected polyp is an invasive adenocarcinoma. Genetic testing indicated the patient has the *Y179C* mutation in *MUTYH (MYH)* gene. Which of the following statements is true about this syndrome?
A. It is an autosomal-dominant disorder
B. Approximately 1% of the general population is heterozygous for *MUTYH* mutations
C. Among patients with 15 to 100 adenomas, only 5% have germline (usually biallelic) *MUTYH* mutations
D. Colonoscopic surveillance of patients with monoallelic *MUTYH* mutations is recommended every 2 years starting at age 18 to 20 years
E. Unlike familial adenomatous polyposis, risks of gastric cancer and duodenal adenoma are not increased

251. A 67 year-old Caucasian woman is seen in clinic for evaluation of a 6-month history of watery diarrhea and a 15-pound weight loss. She denies any recent travel. Her medical history is significant for hypothyroidism and osteoarthritis. Her father was diagnosed with colon cancer in his seventh decade of life. On physical examination, her abdomen is soft. She has significant hair loss, darkening of the skin on the palmar surfaces of her hands and extensor surfaces of elbows, and

fingernail dystrophic changes. Laboratory values are as follows:

Hemoglobin	12 g/dL
Platelet count	350,000/μL
WBC	7,000/μL
Total bilirubin	1.3 mg/dL
Creatinine	1.1 mg/dL
INR	1.3
Albumin	2.3 g/dL

Colonoscopy shows innumerable small erythmatous polyps throughout the colon and edematous mucosa. Histologically, lamina propria edema and inflammation is seen with cystically dilated glands. What is the most likely diagnosis?

A. Cronkhite-Canada syndrome
B. Serrated polyposis syndrome (SPS)
C. Cowden's disease
D. Bannayan-Ruvalcaba-Riley syndrome
E. Attenuated familial adenomatous polyposis

252. A 47-year-old asymptomatic woman underwent her first screening colonoscopy. Her mother had colon cancer at age of 55. Fourteen polyps are removed during colonoscopy ranging from 5 mm to 15 mm in size. Five of these polyps are found in the ascending colon and measure 12 to 15 mm in size. All polyps are completely resected endoscopically. Pathology results indicate four hyperplastic polyps, six sessile serrated adenoma without dysplasia, and four adenomas. All ascending colon polyps are sessile serrated adenomas/polyps. Which of the following statements is true about this syndrome?

A. A causative germline mutation has not yet been identified
B. 10% of patients with this syndrome have a family history of colorectal cancer
C. It is associated with multiple gastroduodenal polyps
D. Total proctocolectomy is recommended for treatment when the diagnosis is established
E. First-degree relatives of patients with this syndrome should begin their screening colonoscopy at age 20

253. Which of the following statements is true about current colorectal cancer (CRC) epidemiology in United States?

A. Overall death rates from CRC have been stable over the past 20 years
B. Incidence and mortality rates for CRC are higher in African Americans compared to Caucasians
C. CRC incidence rates are similar between men and women
D. The risk of CRC remains stable in populations that migrate from areas of low risk to areas of high risk
E. Rectal cancer incidence has increased, whereas cancers of the cecum and ascending colon have decreased in incidence

254. A 51-year-old African-American man is seen in clinic for a prescreening colonoscopy evaluation. He wants to know about the possible factors that can increase and decrease the risk of colon cancer. Which one of these factors is considered to be protective of colorectal cancer?

A. Sedentary lifestyle
B. Alcohol intake
C. High red meat consumption
D. Smoking
E. Aspirin and other NSAIDs

255. A 48-year-old man with iron deficiency anemia is referred for a colonoscopy. He has no family history of colon cancer. A 4 cm mass was seen in the ascending colon. Biopsies were obtained and confirmed the presence of invasive adenocarcinoma. Molecular testing confirms the presence of microsatellite instability (MSI-high), but it was negative for DNA MMR gene mutations. Which statement is true about this patient's tumor?

A. *BRAF* gene is often mutated in MSI-high tumors in Lynch syndrome
B. CPG island methylator phenotype (CIMP) is responsible for most cases of MSI-high tumors related to *hMLH1* inactivation
C. MSI-high tumors are associated with *18qLOH* and *TP53* mutations
D. Sporadic MSI-high cancers often arise through the tubular adenoma pathway
E. Inactivation of base excision repair genes is usually encountered in MSI-high tumors

256. A 40-year-old Caucasian man is referred for a screening colonoscopy. His mother was diagnosed with colon cancer at age 49, and his maternal grandmother had colon cancer at age 60. He is found to have a large mass in the ascending colon and a 1.5 cm sessile polyp in the transverse colon that was resected successfully during colonoscopy. Biopsies from the mass showed poorly differentiated adenocarcinoma, and the polyp was a villous adenoma with high-grade dysplasia. Which statement is true about his disease?

A. It is caused by germline mutations in the *APC* gene
B. The mean age of diagnosis of colon cancer is 35 years
C. It is an autosomal-recessive disorder
D. There is a risk of ~20% of synchronous colon cancer at the time of diagnosis
E. It tends to cause cancer in the distal colon

257. A 61-year-old man with iron deficiency anemia is referred for a colonoscopy. A large, 5 cm polypoid mass is found in the proximal transverse colon. Biopsies reveal invasive adenocarcinoma. The patient had surgical resection, and the tumor was found to be mucinous adenocarcinoma, invading the muscularis propria. One regional lymph node was positive for malignancy and microsatellite instability (MSI) was noted in the tumor. Which of the following factors is associated with a poorer prognosis in this patient?

A. Tumor size
B. Exophytic tumor compared to ulcerated infiltrating tumor
C. The presence of MSI
D. Mucinous histology
E. Age above 60 years

258. One of the hospital administrators has contacted you to discuss replacing guaiac-based fecal occult blood testing (gFOBT) with fecal immunochemical test (FIT) to screen for colorectal cancer. Which of the following statements about FIT is true?

A. Aspirin intake can result in false positive results
B. FIT detects the presence of heme in a fecal sample
C. FIT is more specific for lower GI bleeding than gFOBT
D. Diets high in vitamin C can cause false negative results
E. FIT is recommended by the U.S. Preventive Services Task Force (USPSTF) as an acceptable colorectal cancer screening test for both high-risk and average-risk individuals

259. A 61-year-old man is seen for the first time by a new primary care provider after he moved from a different state. He denies any gastrointestinal complaints. He states that he had a negative sigmoidoscopy approximately 4 years ago. He has also done three stool cards every year over the past 2 years for colon cancer screening and reports negative results. During this visit, the patient tests positive to in-office FOBT (Hemoccult II guaiac) on a specimen obtained by digital rectal examination. Which of the following is the most appropriate step in management?
- **A.** Disregard the result and no need for further workup at this time until the next annual physical examination
- **B.** Fecal immunochemical test (FIT)
- **C.** Repeat testing using Hemoccult SENSA
- **D.** Flexible sigmoidoscopy
- **E.** Colonoscopy

260. A 67-year-old man is seen in general medicine clinic for a routine annual visit. He has no gastrointestinal symptoms. He had a negative screening colonoscopy 12 years ago. His physician recommends repeating colonoscopy, but the patient is interested to know more about "virtual colonoscopy." Which of the following statements is true about CT colonography (CTC)?
- **A.** The Centers for Medicare and Medicaid Services (CMS) does not cover CTC screening
- **B.** CTC is comparable to colonoscopy in detecting small and large adenomas
- **C.** CTC requires sedation
- **D.** The radiation exposure of CTC is negligible
- **E.** CTC is not recommended by the American Cancer Society as a screening modality

261. A 76-year-old man presents for a screening colonoscopy at the ambulatory surgical center. He had a negative colonoscopy 15 years ago. His past medical history is significant for diabetes mellitus, stage III chronic kidney disease, chronic obstructive pulmonary disease, and stable coronary artery disease. His colonoscopy shows good bowel preparation and normal mucosa. What is the most appropriate option for his future colorectal cancer (CRC) screening?
- **A.** Stop CRC screening at this time
- **B.** Annual FIT testing starting next year
- **C.** Colonoscopy should be repeated in 10 years
- **D.** CT colonography every 5 years
- **E.** Double-contrast barium enema (DCBE) every 5 years

262. A 41-year-old Caucasian female presents with her 18-year-old son in the office of her gastroenterology for a consult. She has a history of iron deficiency anemia and is referred for a colonoscopy. Colonoscopy reveals a large mass in the ascending colon. Pathology report indicates adenocarcinoma. The patient undergoes right hemicolectomy. Molecular testing on the tumor confirms the presence of MSI, and it is positive for DNA MMR gene mutation. Genetic testing is offered to her 18-year-old son, and it is positive for the same mutation. Which of the following is the recommended colorectal cancer screening strategy in her son?
- **A.** Start screening at age 20 years using colonoscopy and repeat every 1 to 2 years
- **B.** Start screening at age 20 years using any cancer screening modality, and repeat every 1 year
- **C.** Start screening at age 20 years using colonoscopy and repeat every 5 years
- **D.** Start screening at age 31 years using colonoscopy and repeat every 1 to 2 years
- **E.** Start screening at age 40 years using colonoscopy and repeat every 5 years

263. A 63-year-old man presents to his gastroenterologist a week after a surveillance colonoscopy. He underwent curative resection of a descending colon adenocarcinoma 1 year ago. He denies any gastrointestinal symptoms today. One 8 mm polyp was removed from the rectum on the most recent colonoscopy, and it was a hyperplastic polyp. When should his colonoscopy be repeated for colorectal cancer surveillance?
- **A.** 1 year
- **B.** 2 years
- **C.** 3 years
- **D.** 5 years
- **E.** 10 years

264. A 71-year-old woman is seen in clinic for follow-up. She had a recent colonoscopy 10 days ago, which revealed a large 5 cm mass in the proximal ascending colon and an additional 2 cm sessile polyp in the descending colon. Biopsies of both lesions were consistent with invasive adenocarcinoma. Chest x-rays and CT scan of the abdomen and pelvis did not reveal any metastasis or lymphadenopathy. What is the next step in the management of this patient?
- **A.** Right hemicolectomy and endoscopic resection of the colon cancer in the descending colon
- **B.** Total proctocolectomy
- **C.** Subtotal colectomy
- **D.** Preoperative chemotherapy with radiotherapy then subtotal colectomy
- **E.** Chemotherapy

265. A 72-year-old woman is seen in the gastroenterology clinic for hematochezia of 2-month duration. Colonoscopy is performed, and a 2 cm sessile mass is seen 4 cm above the anal verge, and it involves 20% of the circumference. The lesion does not rise with submucosal saline injection. Biopsies are positive for invasive, well-differentiated adenocarcinoma. Staging by transrectal endoscopic ultrasound is consistent with a T1N0Mx lesion. Chest, abdomen, and pelvis CT do not reveal any metastases. What is the next step in the management of her rectal cancer?
- **A.** Endoscopic snare polypectomy
- **B.** Low anterior resection with primary reanastomosis
- **C.** Abdominoperineal resection
- **D.** Transanal excision
- **E.** Neoadjuvant therapy with chemotherapy and radiation prior to surgery

266. Which statement is true about the use of bevacizumab in the treatment of colorectal cancer?
- **A.** It is a chimeric antibody directed against epidermal growth factor receptor (EGFR)
- **B.** It is beneficial in patients whose tumors express wild-type K-*ras*, but not in those whose tumors express mutated K-*ras*
- **C.** It is currently approved for use in combination with intravenous 5-FU–based chemotherapy as first-line treatment of patients with stage III colorectal cancer
- **D.** It is associated with an increased risk of stroke and GI perforation
- **E.** It has no effect on wound healing, unlike other immunomodulators used for colon cancer

267. A 76-year-old Caucasian woman is seen in clinic with a 6-month history of diffuse abdominal cramps and watery diarrhea. She has 6 to 8 watery bowel movements per day with occasional stool incontinence. She has tried loperamide and fiber supplements without improvement. She denies weight loss, hematemesis, and rectal bleeding. She reports no chest pain or palpitations. Her past medical history is also significant for rheumatoid arthritis and a gastric peptic ulcer found on upper endoscopy 8 months ago. Current medications include daily lansoprazole, ibuprofen, and aspirin. She had a colonoscopy 3 years ago for polyp surveillance, which was negative with good bowel preparation. Physical examination reveals no rashes. The abdomen is soft and nontender. Serum IgA-tissue transglutaminase antibody is negative. Stool studies are negative for leukocytes, *C. difficile* toxin, and ova and parasites. Which of the following is the most appropriate next step in management?

A. Colonoscopy
B. CT scan of the abdomen and pelvis
C. Serum gastrin level, calcitonin, and somatostatin levels
D. Upper endoscopy and duodenal biopsy
E. 24-hour urine collection for 5-hydroxyindoleacetic acid

268. A 45-year-old man with a history of Crohn's disease is seen in clinic with a 2-month history of tenesmus and rectal bleeding. Six months ago, he underwent an emergent surgery for pelvic abscess and microperforation in his proximal sigmoid colon. The surgery included an end-colostomy with closure of the distal colon segment (Hartmann's procedure). He is currently only on oral mesalamine therapy. A flexible sigmoidoscopy of the rectal stump is performed (see figure). Biopsies showed lymphoid hyperplasia and mixed mononuclear and neutrophilic infiltration with few crypt abscesses. What is the most effective treatment for this condition?

A. 5 Aminosalicylate enemas
B. Hydrocortisone enemas
C. Short-chain fatty acids (SCFA) enemas
D. Surgical reanastomosis of the colon
E. Adding azathioprine 2 mg/kg to his oral mesalamine

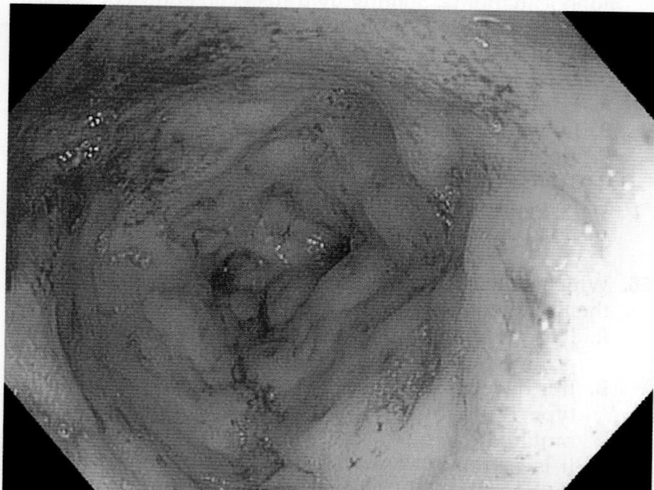

Figure for question 268.

269. A 60-year-old man is referred for colonoscopy for colorectal cancer screening. He has a history of chronic constipation that responds to over-the-counter laxatives. The endoscopic view of the colonic mucosa under white light is shown (see figure). Which statement is true about this finding?

A. This condition is associated with development of colonic neoplasms
B. Biopsies should be taken of any nonpigmented area of the colon
C. This condition is associated with the chronic use of osmotic laxatives
D. This condition is irreversible
E. This condition occurs due to the accumulation of melanin in the mucosa

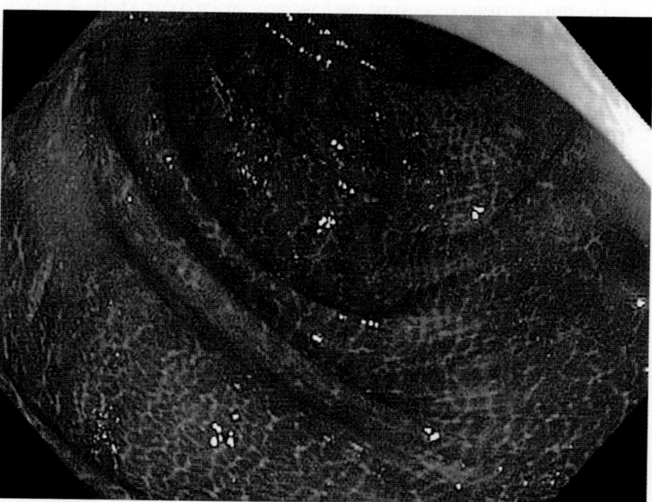

Figure for question 269.

270. A 50-year-old man underwent a colonoscopy for colorectal cancer screening. The exam did not reveal any polyps. The endoscopist reported a redundant colon, and there were few raised mucosal folds in the right and transverse colon. The patient was discharged home 1 hour after the procedure. He developed abdominal pain and distension 2 hours later, and returned to the hospital. Physical exam showed stable vital signs and a mildly distended and tympanic abdomen with positive bowel sounds. Abdominal x-ray did not reveal any free air, but there was mild distension in the transverse colon. His laboratory values were unremarkable with normal blood counts and electrolytes. The patient was admitted for observation on bowel rest and intravenous antibiotics. The next day he continued to have bloating and inability to have a bowel movement but was able to pass flatus. Abdominal CT was performed, and it showed gas-filled cysts in the wall of the ascending and transverse colon. Which of the following is the next best step in management?

A. Emergent surgery for resection
B. Colonoscopy
C. High-flow oxygen
D. Water enema to stimulate bowel movements
E. Discharge home

271. A 42-year-old woman presented the emergency department with rectal bleeding and left lower quadrant abdominal pain of 4 months duration. Her pain has worsened over the past 2 days. Physical exam revealed abdominal tenderness in the left lower quadrant. CT scan revealed thickening in the sigmoid colon. She was admitted to the hospital and treated with intravenous antibiotics. A colonoscopy was performed 6 weeks later, which revealed a 5 cm polypoid mass in the sigmoid colon. The surface of the polyp appeared ulcerated and inflamed. Biopsies indicated an inflammatory polyp with no evidence of malignancy. The patient underwent surgical resection of the sigmoid colon. Pathology of the surgical specimen showed mucin-filled cysts located in the submucosa, with no evidence of malignancy. Which of the following is the most likely diagnosis?

A. Juvenile polyp
B. Colitis cystic profunda
C. Solitary rectal ulcer syndrome
D. Rectal prolapse
E. Colonic carcinoid

272. Which statement is true about GI involvement in endometriosis?
A. It is usually symptomatic
B. Symptoms are always cyclical
C. Hematochezia is more common than abdominal pain
D. It could lead to small bowel obstruction
E. Diagnosis is usually made by mucosal biopsies

273. A 40-year-old man is seen in a clinic with a 1-year history of tenesmus, rectal bleeding, and constipation. He describes excessive straining and intermittent rectal prolapse. He uses over-the-counter laxatives with some benefit. He denies weight loss and abdominal pain. His abdominal examination is normal. Digital rectal examination reveals reduced anal sphincter tone, and an indurated area in distal rectum that was palpated on digital rectal exam. Flexible sigmoidoscopy reveals a large, 5 cm ulcer in the distal rectum 2 cm above the anal verge. Biopsies were obtained from the margins of the ulcer (see figure). What is the most likely diagnosis?
A. Stercoral ulcer
B. Inflammatory bowel disease
C. Rectal cancer
D. Medications side effect
E. Solitary rectal ulcer syndrome (SRUS)

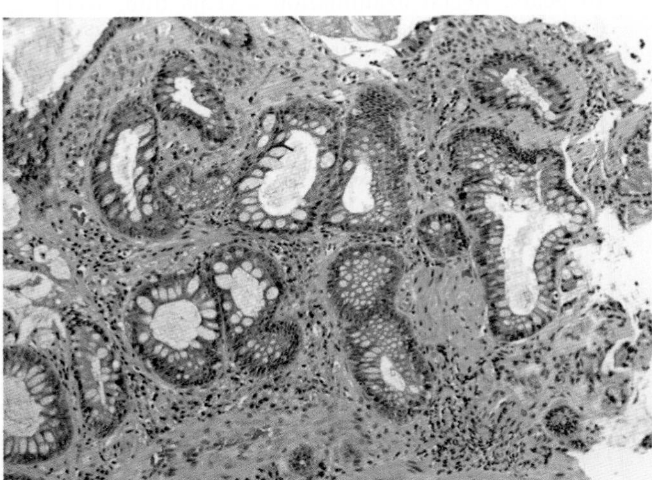
Figure for question 273.

274. A 42-year-old male presents to the office with a history of a hemorrhoidectomy 1 year ago. He had been well until 2 months ago when he began complaining of anal pain and drainage of a thick yellowish-white liquid from his anus. He tried topical antibiotics without resolution of his symptoms. On physical examination, there is one visible external opening in the left anterior perianal area. An internal opening is palpated below the dentate line. A conventional fistulogram and an MRI show a low intersphincteric fistula. Which of the following is the most appropriate treatment?
A. Seton placement followed by surgery
B. Anal plug to the area
C. Anal sphincterotomy
C. Immediate surgical repair
D. Fibrin glue

275. A 50-year-old man presents with perianal pain. Perianal exam shows the following lesion (see figure). Which of the following risk factors is associated with this lesion?

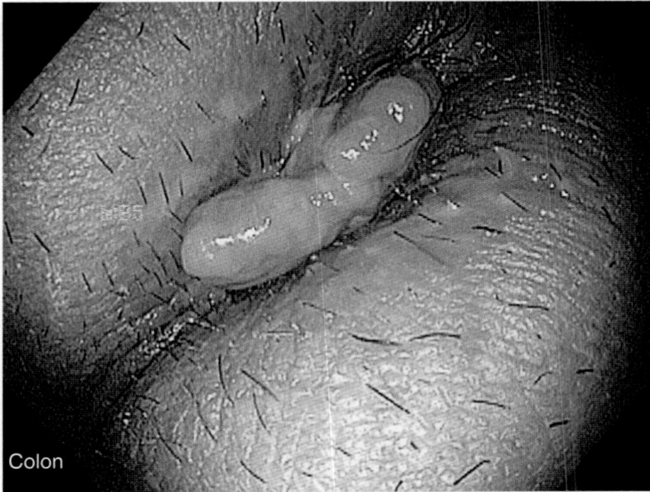

Figure for question 275.

A. Straining during defecation
B. Paget's disease
C. Men who have sex with men
D. Rectal cancer
E. Crohn's disease

276. A 52-year-old woman presents with a 6-month history of severe rectal pain. She reports that the pain usually wakes her from her sleep as a sharp, achy sensation in her rectum. She denies bowel urgency, rectal bleeding, or associated symptoms. The pain usually resolves after 20 minutes. She had a negative colonoscopy 1 year ago. Her physical examination, including rectal exam, is normal. What is the most likely cause of her symptoms?
A. Coccygodynia
B. Levator ani syndrome
C. Anal fissure
D. Internal hemorrhoids
E. Proctalgia fugax

277. A 54-year-old man presents to your office with a complaint of intermittent rectal bleeding with bowel movements. He does not strain, and his stool is not hard. The blood is seen on top of the stool and when he wipes his anus. He has no pain on defecation. His vitals are normal and physical exam, including digital rectal exam, is unremarkable. You perform a colonoscopy and find grade III internal hemorrhoids. He tries hydrocortisone suppositories and sitz baths for several weeks; his stool is always soft. However, he continues to have bleeding per rectum and experiences staining of his underwear with blood. Which of the following is the most appropriate recommendation for this patient?
A. Hemorrhoidectomy
B. Flexible sigmoidoscopy with band ligation
C. Hydrocortisone enemas and stool softeners
D. Infrared photocoagulation
E. Sclerotherapy

278. A 26-year-old woman presents with a 5-year history of constipation. She developed painful defecation and rectal bleeding 3 months ago. She reports that her stool is not hard and at times she does strain. Her abdominal exam is normal. Rectal exam revealed a linear tear in the posterior midline position 1 cm from her anus. Digital exam could not be performed due to severe patient discomfort. A trial of conservative therapy with steroid creams and sitz baths

provides no relief. Sigmoidoscopy revealed the same finding, and was otherwise normal. Which of the following is the most effective treatment for this patient's condition?
A. Hyoscyamine 0.125 mg orally twice a day
B. Topical nifedipine cream
C. Soluble fiber (35 mg/day)
D. Botulinum toxin injection to the anal sphincter
E. Lateral internal sphincterotomy

279. A 56-year-old woman presents to your office with a 2-day history of severe anal pain. On exam you observe the finding below (see figure). She is crying in your office with pain rated as 9/10. She has not been able to sit or sleep since the pain started. What should you recommend next?

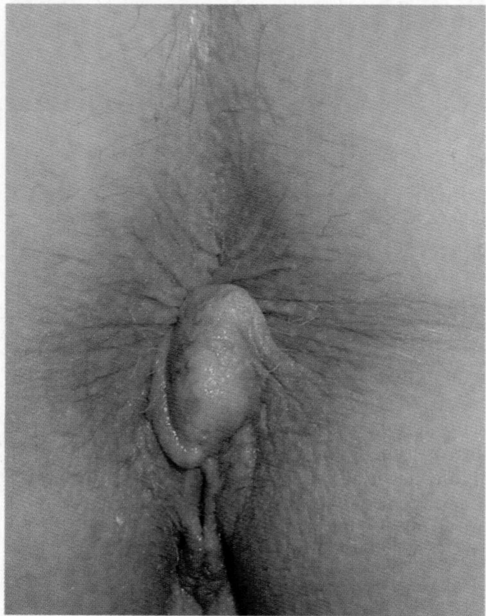

Figure for question 279.

A. Referral to colorectal surgeon for urgent excision
B. Hot sitz baths and acetaminophen
C. Topical steroids and high-fiber diet
D. Sigmoidoscopy with band ligation
E. Reassurance and follow-up in 2 weeks

280. A 55-year-old man presents with rectal bleeding of 3 months duration. Rectal exam reveals a painless, friable 5-cm mass at the anal canal. Biopsy reveals adenocarcinoma of the anal canal. CT scan of the abdomen and pelvis suggests nodal involvement. Which of the following is the most appropriate management strategy?
A. HIV and human pappilovirus (HPV) testing, followed by antiviral treatment
B. Endoscopic mucosal resection
C. Radiation therapy and cytotoxic chemotherapy
D. Abdominoperineal resection and chemoradiation
E. Proctectomy and permanent colostomy

281. A 39-year-old woman presents with 3-week history of worsening itching and burning around her anus. She denies rectal bleeding as well as constipation. She used over-the-counter steroid creams, which did not help. She has no other associated symptoms and has no other medical problems. Her only medication is an oral contraceptive, which she has taken for 10 years. Rectal examination reveals thin, weeping, excoriated perianal skin. Her examination is otherwise normal. Which of the following is the most likely diagnosis?
A. External hemorrhoids
B. Psoriasis
C. Condyloma acuminata
D. Anal herpes simplex
E. Pruritus ani

ANSWERS

1. E (S&F ch98)
The patient has intestinal perforation based on history, exam, and imaging showing air in the peritoneal space, which means that the perforated viscus is an intraperitoneal organ. Among all the mentioned options, the ascending colon is the only retroperitoneal organ, which its perforation would lead to the presence of retroperitoneal air. Other retroperitoneal organs include the first part of the duodenum, descending colon, and part of the rectum.

2. B (S&F ch98)
Brunner glands are specialized glands specific to the duodenum. They are located in the submucosa and function as a buffer for the acidic gastric chyme by producing bicarbonate-rich alkaline solution. Villi are leaf-like shaped in the duodenum, tongue-like shaped in the proximal jejunum, and finger-like shaped distal to the jejunum. Subtypes of enteroendocrine cells are found in both the duodenum and jejunum. The duodenum and jejunum have enterochromaffin cells. Goblet cells are found throughout the entire small and large intestine but are more pronounced in the distal ileum and colon.

3. C (S&F ch98)
Both anomalies are associated with elevated maternal levels of alpha-fetoprotein (AFP). Omphalocele occurs when the intestine fails to return to the abdomen after physiologic herniation. It is covered by a true avascular sac, whereas gastroschisis manifests as an extruded intestine left to the umbilical cord, and it lacks a sac. Omphalocele can present as a large visible sac or can be occult. The latter is difficult to detect at birth. Therefore, it is recommended to inspect the umbilical cord before clamping, and to clamp it at least 5 cm from the abdominal wall. Omphalocele is associated with other anomalies in 75% of the cases and has more extraintestinal manifestations than gastroschisis.

4. B (S&F ch98)
Duodenal atresia is the most common cause of congenital duodenal obstruction. It accounts for about 40% to 60% of the cases. Other causes are duodenal stenosis and intestinal webs. Duodenal atresia results from failure of

the solid stage of the duodenum to recanalize. Atresia in the remaining small bowel and colon is the result of ischemia. Duodenal stenosis, however, results from external compression from an annular pancreas. The most common location of duodenal atresia is just around or distal to the ampulla of Vater. It is detected on plain films by the classic double-bubble sign in which the large bubble corresponds to gastric air and the small bubble corresponds to duodenal air. In about 50% of the cases, there are other associated anomalies such as Down syndrome.

5. D (S&F ch98)
The diagnosis of Hirschsprung's disease (HD) is strongly suspected. HD results from the absence of the Meissner's and Auerbach's plexuses. When suspected, suction biopsy of the rectal mucosa is the most reliable diagnostic method, except in the ultrashort variant HD. The biopsy should be taken at least 2 cm above the mucocutaneous junction in infants, and 3 cm above the mucocutaneous junction in older children. The biopsies should be reviewed by an expert pathologist. Delaying the treatment of HD can be associated with serious complications such as enterocolitis, which is the most common cause of death in HD patients. Other methods of diagnosis include contrasted enemas on unprepared colons to avoid missing the transition zone in the rectosigmoid type of HD. Anal manometry is a good modality to detect HD, specifically, the ultrashort variant, but it is associated with a high false positive result in patients with constipation or mega colon. Flexible sigmoidoscopy, if performed as a complementary study, usually reveals a normal empty rectum and a dilated proximal colon if the scope is able to pass through the narrow area.

6. D (S&F ch99)
This patient is in good condition with no alarm symptoms or signs. She meets Rome III criteria for irritable bowel syndrome, likely correlating to her increased anxiety over her new and demanding job. In this patient with a functional disorder, the small intestinal motility experiences increased visceral sensitivity with heightened sensation and perception of pain as well as disordered motility (see table at the end of the chapter). The alternative scenarios describe connective tissue disorders, diabetes mellitus, intestinal obstruction, and myopathies.

7. E (S&F ch99)
Gap junctions are specialized areas of cell-to-cell contact between myocytes, which are visible by electron microscopy. A deep plexus (Schabadasch's plexus) does exist within the circular muscle, but it does not contain ganglia. Intrinsic sensory neurons synapse in the intramural plexuses with intrinsic motor neurons and interneurons where they induce excitation via release of acetylcholine and substance P. The myenteric interstitial cells of Cajal are distributed within the intermuscular space at the level of the myenteric plexus between the circular and longitudinal muscle layers and are the pacemaker cells of the small intestine. Intestinofugal neurons have cell bodies within the myenteric plexus but have projections out of the intestinal wall, via extrinsic nerve trunks, to prevertebral ganglia (PVG), which allow them to sense and receive information regarding intestinal distention.

8. C (S&F ch99)
This elderly nursing home resident appears to have acquired a urinary tract infection (UTI), resulting in mild renal insufficiency with the ensuing complication of anticholinergic toxicity due to multiple medications he takes, including diphenhydramine, benztropine, and nortriptyline. His presentation is consistent with anticholinergic toxicity (cutaneous vasodilation resulting in flushing, anhidrosis, nonreactive mydriasis, tachycardia, and delirium with hallucinations). The first step in evaluation is airway, breathing, and circulation, none of which are compromised for this patient. The next best step is immediate evaluation with a 12-lead ECG to rule out development of changes in QRS intervals or arrhythmias. As the patient has a primary acute illness, which resulted in his anticholinergic toxicity rather than acute ingestion leading to toxicity, physostigmine would not be a first choice for management. Conservative management would start with benzodiazepines for treating the patient's delirium and agitation. Although the patient will need to be evaluated for urosepsis, a rapid ECG should precede a lab draw for blood cultures. As the patient is alert, breathing at a normal rate, and has no evidence of hypoxemia, there is no role for elective intubation at this time. While the patient does have obstipation, this as well as his urinary retention are most likely secondary to his underlying illness of the UTI. Therefore, a CT of the abdomen and pelvis would not be an efficient use of time or resources and would not provide additional helpful information.

9. C (S&F ch99)
This patient with a long-standing history of poorly managed diabetes mellitus most likely has altered ICC function with disrupted neurotransmission and subsequent slow transit of the small bowel. From a practical and economic standpoint, the next best test would be a lactulose breath test, as this would be relatively easy to administer and inexpensive to assist in diagnosing increased orocecal transit time. A small bowel follow-through would elucidate if the patient had mucosal or mechanical structural abnormalities of the small bowel that directly were resulting in altered transit, but this is an unlikely scenario in this patient; therefore, the test would likely give low yield. There is no indication to perform a 6-hour gastric emptying study. Four hours is the acceptable gold standard, and as it was negative, particularly with no correlating symptoms, gastroparesis has already been ruled out for the patient. Small bowel manometry is a more expensive and less practical option for the patient. It also is more likely to be poorly tolerated. MRI offers higher resolution for imaging of the small bowel than standard fluoroscopy studies, but again, in this patient with little suggestion for a structural disruption of the small intestine, this would be an expensive and low-yield first diagnostic option for her.

10. A (S&F ch99)
Small intestinal contractions are the result of an electrical action potential (spike burst), which is superimposed on the slow wave. Not every slow wave results in a phasic contraction. Motor pattern of the small intestine is determined by the presence or absence of a significant amount of nutrient within the small intestine. Input of various stimuli may affect small intestinal motor activity. Hyperosmolar contents and pH changes are sensed by receptors in the mucosa, whereas luminal distention is perceived by receptors in the muscle. The small intestine exerts negative feedback control on the rate of gastric emptying through neural and humoral means, which indirectly results in longer small intestinal transit time.

11. A (S&F ch99)
This young woman has experienced complete resolution of her malignancy, but she is now experiencing the unfortunate complication of radiation enteritis with permanent fibrosis and subsequent small intestinal damage resulting in disordered transit, less mixing of intestinal contents, poor nutritional absorption, and steatorrhea. She needs to immediately initiate an alternative form of nutrition, but she is at risk for refeeding syndrome and needs to be closely monitored with inpatient hospitalization during slow initiation of CPN. In this patient with radiation enteritis, enteral feeds will not adequately supplement her nutrition and could worsen her symptoms. Therefore, she will be CPN dependent. There is no reason to obtain yet another imaging study as her symptoms are the same chronic symptoms for which she has undergone repeated imaging over the last year, rather than an acute change in condition. Repeated imaging is likely to be cost-ineffective, uncomfortable for the patient, and give low yield. There is no role for surgical management in this scenario. As the patient is suffering from radiation enteritis, examination of the upper and lower GI tract will provide little additional information to assist in her management and subjects her to unnecessary procedural and sedation risks.

12. C (S&F ch99)
A plain film of the abdomen would most likely confirm what this patient's presentation suggests, a paralytic ileus. Patients with myotonic dystrophy, particularly type 1, which more commonly manifests smooth muscle involvement, frequently have secondary gastrointestinal symptoms. These include dysphagia, colicky abdominal pain, constipation, diarrhea, and pseudo-obstruction. The patient is moving his bowels and has no vomiting; therefore he is not demonstrating true obstructive symptoms. He would not require surgical intervention. Unless a plain film specifically demonstrates that the patient has significant dilation of colonic loops of bowel, there is no role for empiric endoscopic decompression with a flexible sigmoidoscopy. Obtaining a CT of the abdomen is a more costly and unnecessary diagnostic modality unless the plain film is inconclusive. Additionally, the patient may be unable to tolerate oral contrast, which could lead to vomiting in a patient who is at higher risk than average for aspiration due to his underlying condition. The patient's last hospitalization was 2 months ago with little new risk factors for *C. difficile* in the last 2 weeks. Most likely, his intermittent diarrhea is actually the result of overflow due to slow colonic transit.

13. D (S&F ch99)
This patient is suffering from a common gastrointestinal complication of spinal cord injury, bowel dysfunction secondary to loss of afferent neurons with consequent loss of sensory information and transit failure. In addition to a diet that is higher in fiber intake with reduction of dairy products and fat content, the goal of management is to achieve predictable and timely bowel evacuation with a consistent regimen of oral bowel medications. She would also benefit from reduction of daily opioid use, which would further exacerbate delayed colonic transit. This patient has no alarm features, but rather is having difficulty managing significant bowel dysfunction with chronic constipation. Her KUB demonstrates evidence of fecal loading, but no other concerning findings are present. There is no role for endoscopic evaluation. Although the patient has family history for colorectal cancer, she would not be due for her first screening colonoscopy until age 50 years. The patient's KUB is noted to have fecal retention consistent with the history of chronic constipation in the setting of spinal cord injury. Her history and imaging do not suggest a clinical picture of small intestinal bacterial overgrowth. MR enterography is not required in this scenario as it would not add any relevant clinical information and would be cost-ineffective. There is no acute abdomen or impending surgical emergency.

14. E (S&F ch99)
This woman is undergoing a dermatologic evaluation for skin changes suggestive of a likely new diagnosis of scleroderma. In this setting, her symptoms of bloating and steatorrhea with noted macrocytic anemia due to a vitamin B_{12} deficiency raises the concern for small intestinal slowed transit predisposing her to small intestinal bacterial overgrowth (SIBO). Her elevated folate level further confirms this. The next step for confirmation would be breath testing using glucose as a substrate. This may also be performed using lactulose as a substrate. She has not been exposed to antibiotics in over a year, and infection with *C. difficile* would be unlikely. Despite a significant family history of Crohn's disease, the patient's symptoms are not suggestive of a new presentation of IBD, and her elevated inflammatory markers are nonspecific and could be seen in the setting of rheumatologic disease as well. Should her symptoms persist after either negative testing for SIBO or after successful therapy for SIBO, there may be a later role for invasive procedures with mucosal biopsies. However, given her clinical presentation, EGD and colonoscopy are unlikely to be high-yield diagnostic studies at this time. While the patient has traveled abroad recently, she has visited a highly developed metropolitan area with unlikely risk of exposure to traveler's diarrhea. Additionally, the timing of her symptoms far precedes her recent travel.

15. D (S&F ch99)
This patient's presentation is notable for diarrhea and heart failure, likely right sided, based upon his ascites and elevated JVP. This constellation of symptoms is concerning for systemic amyloidosis, which may result in diarrhea due to rapid bowel transit. This can also result in a restrictive cardiomyopathy. Obtaining a myocardial biopsy and submitting it for Congo red staining will assist with confirming a diagnosis. Video capsule enteroscopy will likely give low yield as minimal mucosal changes are seen in this cause of protein-losing enteropathy. An octreotide scan would allow localization of a hormone-secreting tumor, but the patient's gastrin, chromogranin A, 5-HIAA, and VIP levels are all normal, which renders a low pretest probability of positive findings from an octreotide scan. The patient's imaging has shown no abnormalities of the pancreas, and the patient has no history suggestive of chronic pancreatitis. Therefore, fecal elastase will be an unhelpful test and could be falsely positive in the setting of any form of diarrhea. The patient has already had unremarkable imaging, and more expensive, high-resolution imaging would not provide additional information.

16. B (S&F ch99)
This young female who is just entering the final trimester of her pregnancy could develop altered thyroid physiology as often seen in the pregnant state and should be screened for hypothyroidism. Should this be normal, she most likely is experiencing slow transit, which results

from decreased intestinal contractions during the state of pregnancy and may result in constipation. This should resolve postpartum, and the patient should be reassured and provided with a bowel regimen for relief of symptoms in the interim. There is no indication for a colonoscopy given the patient's lack of alarm symptoms, and colonoscopy should be avoided if at all possible during pregnancy to avoid mother and fetal adverse outcomes. Radiation should be avoided in the pregnancy, and a CT should not be pursued for this patient. Furthermore, CT is unlikely to provide additional information given the setting of her development of constipation. Fecal occult blood testing is only indicated for colorectal cancer screening, and it has no role in the management of this patient. She has no increased risk factors for colorectal cancer, which would prompt early screening. She has a single second-degree relative who developed colon cancer over the age of 60, which does not change the patient's risk profile.

17. D (S&F ch100)
ICC are a major target of neurotransmitters released from the axons of excitatory and inhibitory enteric motor neurons, acetylcholine and nitric oxide being two of them. ICC are nonneuronal in origin and are derived from progenitors of smooth muscle cells. ICC play a major role in the control of myogenic activity, in addition to amplifying the effects of motor neurons on the smooth muscles. They have no role in water and electrolyte secretion. Decreased numbers or volume of ICC (not increased) has been associated with normal aging, which correlates with decreased motility. ICC are recognized by their immunoreactivity for c-Kit *(CD117)*, not PDGFRα. Another cell type involved in control of colonic motility has been recently found in human colon that is a "fibroblast-like cell" and is identified by immunoreactivity for PDGFRα.

18. B (S&F ch100)
The GI system is well adept at responding to exercise, driven by the sympathetic nervous system. Option B is correct as the sympathetics from the spinal cord drive a powerful cholinergic drive. Answer A is incorrect because the sympathetic nervous system is responsible for this mechanism rather than the parasympathetic nervous system. Branches of the vagus nerve do reach the prevertebral ganglia as per option C, but their contribution to bowel activity is of a parasympathetic nature. In response to exercise, nerve fibers from prevertebral ganglia cause vasoconstriction of the mucosal and submucosal blood vessels, not vasodilation, making option D incorrect. Reflexive to exercise, axons act on the circuitry of the submucosal plexus to inhibit epithelial secretion, not promote it, making option E incorrect.

19. A (S&F ch100)
Option A is correct because phase III of the interdigestive motor cycle occurs every 90 to 120 minutes in the upper intestine during fasting and does not contribute to ileocecal transit because it rarely reaches the terminal ileum. Option B is incorrect because liquids empty more rapidly through the ascending colon and cecum than solids. Option C is incorrect because the ileocecal junction is composed of a specialized band of muscle from a low-pressure tonic sphincter. Option D is incorrect because studies have established that healthy control subjects have slow, retrograde movement from the transverse colon to the cecum before rapid forward propulsion to the descending colon, and short-extent retrograde propagating sequences occur in the distal colon and rectum, resulting in mixing of contents. Option E is incorrect because proximal colonic emptying depends on both increased wall tone and propagating contractions.

20. B (S&F ch100)
Lubiprostone is a type 2 chloride channel activator that increases intestinal chloride secretion and results in increased intraluminal fluid accumulation, which subsequently softens stool and accelerates intestinal transit in constipated patients. Ondansetron is a 5-HT3 receptor antagonist that, in addition to antiemetic effects, can blunt the gastrocolic response and delay colonic transit. Alosetron is another 5-HT3 receptor antagonist, which can slow down colonic transit. However, prucalopride is a highly selective 5-HT4 agonist that can increase stool frequency in patients with constipation. Bisacodyl acts as laxative through mucosal afferent nerve fibers, and its effect can be blocked by applying topical lidocaine to the mucosa.

21. C (S&F ch101)
The movement of chloride from the serosal to the luminal compartment is the principal driving force for fluid secretion in the intestines. Na^+ and water follow passively in response to electrical and osmotic gradients. There is a basal rate of Cl^- excretion that is maintained by cell volume and integrated paracrine, autocrine, luminal, and endocrine modulation. It is disruption of this balance that can lead to secretory diarrhea. Sodium channels are located on the basolateral membrane, not apical. The electrochemical gradient created by Cl^- and Na^+ transport helps to drive fluid secretion. Water is absorbed through passive diffusion across a channel protein.

22. E (S&F ch101)
This patient has a secretory diarrhea with stool osmolar gap ($290 - 2[Na^+ + K^+]$), which is less than 50. The patient's symptoms are suggestive of cholera, which through cAMP increases channel activity and the number of channels in apical membrane. The patient's stool did not demonstrate an osmotic gap, making an osmotic diarrhea incorrect. The patient has no fever or positive fecal leukocytes, making an infectious diarrhea less likely. Cholera does not inhibit expression of the *CFTR* gene nor inhibit reabsorption of the intestinal secretions.

23. C (S&F ch101)
The patient has typical features of diversion colitis. Short-chain fatty acids, including butyrate, propionate, and acetate are the main source of metabolic fuel for the colonocytes, and their deficiency is the main cause of colitis in the diverted segment of colon after end-colostomy.

24. A (S&F ch101)
In the small intestine, luminal negative potential difference drives the passive absorption of potassium, and in the colon, potassium is transported via active transport via luminal membrane H^+/K^+ ATPase and basolateral K^+/Cl^- cotransporters and potassium channels.

25. B (S&F ch101)
Butyrate and propionate are 2- to 4-carbon short-chain fatty acids that are the major source of metabolic fuel for colonocytes. They are the major luminal ion in the colon and enhance sodium and fluid reabsorption through linked transport mechanism and up-regulating expression of NHE3 and DRA on the apical membrane

of colonocytes. They are not absorbed in the jejunum or used as a major source of metabolic fuel for enterocytes. They are not the cause of osmotic diarrhea.

26. D (S&F ch102)
GLP-1 and GLP-2 are cosecreted by enteroendocrine cells in the small and large intestine in response to fat and carbohydrate. GLP-1 decreases appetite and slows gastric emptying. They are not high in a fasting state and do not decrease rapidly after nutrient digestion. They are not secreted in response to protein, but instead are released in response to fat and carbohydrate.

27. C (S&F ch102)
This patient likely has lactose intolerance or late-onset lactase deficiency. Lactase is a small intestinal brush-border enzyme that hydrolyzes lactose into glucose and galactose. The negative anti-tTG, antiendomysial antibodies in the setting of a normal total IgA make celiac disease less likely. The patient does not have a history of abdominal surgery, diabetes, or slow intestinal transit time, which makes small intestinal bacterial overgrowth unlikely. Pancreatic exocrine insufficiency is in the differential, but she has no history of pancreatitis in the past with a normal CT scan. Although IBD is a possibility, her diarrhea appears to be associated with eating certain foods and likely did not have dairy products while camping, suggesting an osmotic diarrhea.

28. A (S&F ch102)
Pancreatic lipase is less active at pH under 7.0. In conditions like ZES, hyperchlorhydria causes lower intraluminal pH that can lead in lipase deactivation and steatorrhea. PPI use, atrophic gastritis, and Billroth I surgery result in lower acid production in the stomach and they do not cause acidic intraluminal environment in the small intestine. Steatorrhea in patients with small intestinal bacterial overgrowth is mainly the result of deconjugation of bile acids by bacteria in the small intestine and, consequently, depletion of bile acid pool, leading to fat malabsorption.

29. A (S&F ch102)
Enterokinase is required to convert trypsinogen to its active form, trypsin. Trypsin then goes on to activate more trypsinogen and other proteolytic enzyme precursors. Chymotrypsin is not required to convert trypsinogen to its active form, but trypsin converts chymotrypsinogen to its active form chymotrypsin. Carboxypeptidase A cleaves aromatic amino acids, and carboxypeptidase B cleaves lysine or arginine from caboxy-terminal end of proteins.

30. B (S&F ch103)
This patient presents with anemia, paresthesia, and a possible surgery at some point in the past for her underlying Crohn's disease. These symptoms are suggestive of cobalamin deficiency, which is absorbed in the terminal ileum through a receptor-mediated endocytosis through binding to intrinsic factor. Although iron deficiency can cause anemia, it does not cause lower extremity paresthesia. Vitamin C deficiency typically presents with easy bruising, epistaxis, bleeding gums, and poor wound healing, which is not seen in this patient. Folic acid deficiency, in contrast to cobalamin deficiency, is rarely associated with neurologic abnormalities, and paresthesia is not a common feature of it. Although niacin deficiency is seen in patients with Crohn's disease, its deficiency leads to pellagra, which is characterized by dermatitis, dementia, and diarrhea.

31. D (S&F ch103)
This patient's history of a macrocytic anemia, alcohol abuse, and poor overall nutritional status suggests folate deficiency. These patients can also have thiamine deficiency. The macrocytic anemia makes both iron and copper deficiency less likely. He has no symptoms of GI bleeding or abdominal pain, making peptic ulcer disease unlikely.

32. C (S&F ch103)
This patient has clinical signs of thiamine deficiency and wet beriberi, which can cause congestive heart failure and lower extremity edema. Thiamine deficiency in developed countries is seen in alcoholics and in patients with diabetes mellitus, IBD, celiac disease, or chronic diuretic use. She has a mild normocytic anemia, which makes iron, cobalamin (vitamin B_{12}), and folate deficiency less likely. Copper deficiency is classically a microcytic anemia with leukopenia and normal iron studies.

33. D (S&F ch103)
Patients with history of Roux-en-Y gastric bypass have a gastrojejunostomy, which bypasses the duodenum, the primarily site of copper absorption. Copper deficiency can present with a microcytic anemia, normal iron studies, and a mild leukopenia. Folate or cobalamin deficiency causes a macrocytic anemia, and the patient does not have iron deficiency anemia. This patient does not have manifestations of thiamine deficiency that can include neuropathy (dry beriberi), cardiomyopathy (wet beriberi), or encephalopathy.

34. C (S&F ch103)
Vitamin D actually increases jejunal absorption of magnesium, whereas ileal absorption remains unaffected. Magnesium absorption at basal state is greater in the ileum than the duodenum or jejunum. This is in contrast to calcium, for which duodenum and proximal jejunum is the main site for absorption. While on normal dietary intake, overall efficiency of magnesium absorption is between 21% and 27%.

35. B (S&F ch104)
This patient has hepatomegaly, ascites, and a restrictive cardiomyopathy along with malabsorption. This is highly suggestive of amyloidosis. Diagnosis can be made by mucosal biopsy with amyloid deposits seen on 75% to 95% of gastric, 83% to 100% of duodenal, and 75% to 95% of colorectal biopsies. Pancreatic insufficiency, celiac disease, and small intestinal bacterial overgrowth can result in chronic diarrhea but cannot explain the cardiac findings of restrictive cardiomyopathy and thickened ventricular walls. Anorexia nervosa can lead to malnutrition but would not lead to severe steatorrhea and heart disease.

36. B (S&F ch104)
This patient has symptoms suggestive of systemic sclerosis. She has Raynaud's phenomenon, digital ulcers, and severe reflux. In addition, the disease causes atrophy of the muscle layers with increased depots of elastin and collagen in the intestinal wall, resulting in poor small bowel motility (delayed transit), malabsorption, and bacterial overgrowth. Having multiple duodenal and gastric ulcers is related to NSAIDS, *Helicobacter pylori*, or rarely Zollinger Ellison syndrome. These findings would not explain her clinical presentation. Having greater than 20 intraepithelial lymphocytes per 100 epithelial cells on colonic biopsies is suggestive of microscopic colitis, which could result in chronic nonfatty diarrhea. Architectural distortion and

chronic inflammation on colonic biopsy is compatible with inflammatory bowel disease, which results in chronic diarrhea (including fatty diarrhea with small bowel involvement). However, it does not explain the skin findings and the heartburn. Villous atrophy and increased intraepithelial lymphocytes on duodenal biopsy is suggestive of celiac disease. This results in steatorrhea, but does not lead to Raynaud's phenomenon, digital ulcers, or reflux. In addition, celiac disease is uncommon in African Americans. The patient's rash is nonspecific and is not consistent with dermatitis herpetiformis, which leads to severely pruritic papules and vesicles on extensor surfaces.

37. A (S&F ch104)
Markedly elevated serum homocysteine levels can be seen in folate or vitamin B_{12} deficiency. On the other hand, serum methylmalonic acid levels can be markedly increased in vitamin B_{12} deficiency (not folic acid deficiency). Serum citruline level may be decreased in small intestinal resection or mucosal destruction.

38. B (S&F ch104)
This patient's presentations of bloating and chronic diarrhea in the setting of previous abdominal surgeries, and also jejunal diverticula found in the small bowel series, is very suggestive of small intestinal bacterial overgrowth. In patients with small intestinal bacterial overgrowth, elevated serum folate is commonly seen due to synthesis of folate by the gut flora. Also, vitamin K is made by the gut bacteria, which can potentially decrease the INR level. The bacteria consume vitamin B_{12}, thiamine, and nicotinamide, and the serum levels could be decreased.

39. C (S&F ch104)
Patients with CVID can present with adult-onset mild immunodeficiency and signs of malabsorption. The small bowel biopsy may show the typical findings of celiac disease, but absence of plasma cells suggests CVID. Folate and vitamin B_{12} deficiency are commonly seen in these patients. Small intestinal bacterial overgrowth may present with similar manifestation. However, folate level is usually elevated as the result of synthesis by the bacteria. ZES is unlikely in this patient, given lack of peptic ulcer disease seen during endoscopy. Lactose malabsorption does not explain the anemia and folate/vitamin B_{12} deficiency.

40. B (S&F ch104)
Consuming whole milk or chocolate milk rather than skim milk prolongs gastric emptying time and can diminish the symptoms of lactose intolerance. Lactase deficiency is seen in 60% to 100% of Asians and people from Middle East or Mediterranean ethnicity. It is less common in Northern Europeans (2% to 30%). In patients with lactose intolerance/malabsorption, even after being on lactose-free diet, symptoms may persist due to metabolism of dietary fiber by colonic bacteria or incomplete absorption of carbohydrates other than lactose. In patients with lactase deficiency, symptoms usually begin to manifest in adulthood. There has not been any clear relation found between the amount of lactose ingestion and the severity of the symptoms in patients with lactose malabsorption.

41. B (S&F ch105)
Luminal competition by the bacteria in small intestinal bacterial overgrowth will lead to various vitamin deficiencies. Mucosal injury by the bacteria will result in a decrease in brush-border enzymes and an increase in intestinal permeability, hence, the carbohydrate malabsorption and protein-losing enteropathy. Diarrhea in small intestinal bacterial overgrowth can be caused by the effect of deconjugated bile salts on the colon, not the small bowel. Synthesis of acetaldehyde by bacteria may cause liver injury, not diarrhea.

42. B (S&F ch105)
Folic acid is synthesized as part of the bacterial metabolism in the small intestine, and high serum folate levels are seen in small intestinal bacterial overgrowth. The same is true about vitamin K, which can interfere with dosing of warfarin by decreasing the INR levels. Vitamin B_{12}, thiamine, and nicotinamide are consumed by the bacteria and might have lower-than-normal levels in patients with small intestinal bacterial overgrowth.

43. D (S&F ch105)
Among all the above options, diabetes carries the highest risk for developing small intestinal bacterial overgrowth (SIBO) by affecting intestinal motility. Advanced age is linked to SIBO. Ileal diverticula are usually single and small and, unlike jejunal diverticula, which are usually multiple and large, are not commonly associated with SIBO. Hysterectomy is not a risk factor for SIBO as there is no anatomic alteration to the digestive system. Hypochlorhydria, associated with PPI use, has been described as a potential risk factor for SIBO, but not antacids use.

44. D (S&F ch105)
Recent food ingestion can lead to an exaggeration of the test results, and patients are instructed to fast for 12 hours prior to the test. Patients are also advised to avoid smoking and exercise, as they can be associated with false negative results. Gastroparesis can lead to a longer transit time and more false positive results. The first peak in the hydrogen breath test is related to the hydrogen production by the small intestinal bacteria; this can be misinterpreted when there is contamination with oral flora. Methanogenic bacteria, when present, can convert hydrogen to methane, which can lead to false negative results.

45. D (S&F ch105)
Breath tests are usually cheaper, easier, and less invasive than jejunal aspirates. Histologic examination of small intestinal biopsies in patients with small intestinal bacterial overgrowth (SIBO) is unremarkable in over half of the patients. In areas where there are higher levels of bacterial contamination, such as the tropics, the diagnosis of SIBO requires greater than 10^7 CFU/mL in jejunal aspirates, instead of greater than 10^5 CFU/mL, which is the number used in the United States. A positive LHBT is characterized by a double peak in which the first one is related to hydrogen production from small intestinal bacteria, and the second peak results from hydrogen production by colonic bacteria. Contamination with oral flora can lead to confusion regarding the first peak. Fecal calprotectin is usually normal in patients with SIBO.

46. D (S&F ch105)
Synthesis of acetaldehyde by bacteria can potentially be the cause of liver injury, including florid nonalcoholic steatohepatitis in patients with small intestinal bacterial overgrowth. Other possible mechanisms include inflammatory cytokines generated during inflammatory response and also synthesis of alcohol by intestinal bacterial metabolism. Deconjugation of primary bile acids may lead to diarrhea from irritation of the colon by bile acids. Luminal competition with the host and consumption of

dietary proteins by the bacteria can result in hypoproteinemia and edema. Fermentation of unabsorbed carbohydrates may cause bloating and flatulence in patients suffering from small intestinal bacterial overgrowth.

47. D (S&F ch105)
Ileocecal valve resection with possible reflux of colonic bacteria to small bowel has been linked to small intestinal bacterial overgrowth (SIBO). Hysterectomy does not alter the anatomy of the gut and is not associated with SIBO. Intestinal dysmotility from hypothyroidism (not hyperthyroidism) can contribute to SIBO. Small bowel, not colonic, diverticulosis has been linked to SIBO. Symptoms and complications related to SIBO have been reported more commonly in jejunal than ileal diverticulosis. Recirculation of intestinal contents resulting from strictures and fistulas in Crohn's disease (not ulcerative colitis) may predispose these patients to SIBO.

48. B (S&F ch106)
This patient has short bowel syndrome and thus is at risk for developing oxalate kidney stones. Normally, oxalate binds to calcium and is excreted in the feces as calcium oxalate. However, when there is malabsorption in short bowel syndrome, unabsorbed long-chain fatty acids bind to calcium, leaving free oxalate, which is absorbed by the colon and excreted in the kidney (enteric hyperoxaluria). This is prevented with a low oxalate diet. Limiting simple sugars and providing complex carbohydrates is important to prevent D-lactic acidosis. Low fat diet, low calcium diet, and cholestyramine do not prevent oxalate kidney stones.

49. C (S&F ch106)
This patient has short bowel syndrome with intact colon, and is presenting with features of D-lactic acidosis due to increased fermentation of simple carbohydrates. The patient has recently increased her intake of simple carbohydrates, which increases delivery of glucose and other carbohydrates to the colon. These get fermented by colonic bacteria into D-lactic acid, which is absorbed into the circulation but poorly metabolized. Symptoms are mainly neurologic, including ataxia, slurred speech, and confusion. Regular tests for lactic acid measures L-lactate, which is normal in these cases, thus the lab should be notified to quantify D-lactic acid. Salicylate overdose results in tinnitus, vertigo, early respiratory alkalosis, and later anion gap metabolic acidosis. Dehydration resulting in renal failure does not explain the neurologic symptoms. Thiamine deficiency may result in similar neurologic symptoms but does not lead to anion gap acidosis. Alcohol intoxication is unlikely in this patient and does not lead to anion gap metabolic acidosis.

50. D (S&F ch106)
The patient is presenting with signs and symptoms of heart failure, and should raise the suspicion of selenium deficiency. Selenium is an essential component of the enzyme glutathione peroxidase that plays an important role in the metabolism of different tissues and organs. Patients with short bowel syndrome who are not compliant with TPN, or who receive TPN without multivitamins and trace elements, are prone to develop selenium and other trace element deficiencies. Copper, vitamin D, chromium, and manganese deficiency do not lead to heart failure.

51. E (S&F ch106)
This patient has intestinal failure–associated liver disease and now has an elevated bilirubin, suggesting impaired hepatic function. In this setting, manganese, which is one of the trace elements provided in TPN, which is normally secreted in bile, can accumulate, resulting in toxicity that results in Parkinson-like neurologic symptoms along with confusion, ataxia, tremor, and dystonia. Although thiamine deficiency can present with difficulty with standing (dry beriberi) and confusion (Wernicke's), it does not lead to dystonia and tremor. The patient's symptoms are not related to B_{12} deficiency (leads to anemia and neuropathy), selenium toxicity (leads to neuropathy, skin rash), or copper deficiency (anemia, neuropathy, skin pigmentation).

52. E (S&F ch106)
This patient has exit-site infection. The recommendation is to empirically initiate treatment for methicillin-resistant *Staphylococcus aureus* (MRSA) (vancomycin or linezolid) after sending the culture, and then adjust antibiotics according to culture and sensitivity results. If the infection resolves, there is no need to remove the catheter (see figure).

53. D (S&F ch106)
The patient underwent an ileal resection and most likely had less than 100 cm of ileum resected. This leads to mild bile acid malabsorption that is delivered to the colon, leading to irritation and diarrhea (choleretic "secretory" diarrhea). When greater than 100 cm of ileum is resected, there is severe malabsorption of bile salts, and once the bile acid pool is depleted, insufficient micellar solubilization of lipids occurs, causing steatorrhea and fat malabsorption. The diarrhea is not from carbohydrate malabsorption because these are absorbed in the proximal small intestine and should not be affected with ileal resection. Fecal fat <7 grams/day is considered normal.

54. A (S&F ch106)
This patient most likely has recurrence of thrombotic occlusion of the catheter. In this case, empiric treatment with tPA followed by aspiration through the catheter in 60 minutes is the recommended approach. If these steps are unsuccessful, then radiologic contrast study or eventually replacing the catheter is indicated. This patient does not have any evidence of infection, and antibiotics are not indicated (see figure).

55. B (S&F ch106)
Teduglutide is a synthetic analog of GLP-2, which is an intestinotrophic enteric hormone. It has been approved by the U.S. Food and Drug Administration for use in patients with short bowel syndrome for up to 24 weeks. Administration of teduglutide is shown to be associated with increased height of villus and increased water absorption, which results in less chronic dehydration and less chance of nephropathy in patients with TPN. The use of this medication has been linked with increased plasma levels of citrulline (likely due to increased functional mucosal surface in small bowel). The use of teduglutide has been linked with more significant improvement in fluid absorption compared to nitrogen absorption.

56. B (S&F ch106)
This patient has developed progressive liver disease in the setting of short bowel syndrome (SBS) and chronic TPN dependence. Combined small intestine–liver transplantation is the best long-term option in patients with SBS who develop end-stage liver disease.

57. A (S&F ch106)
The patient likely underwent a significant small intestinal resection, resulting in malabsorption. Symptoms of

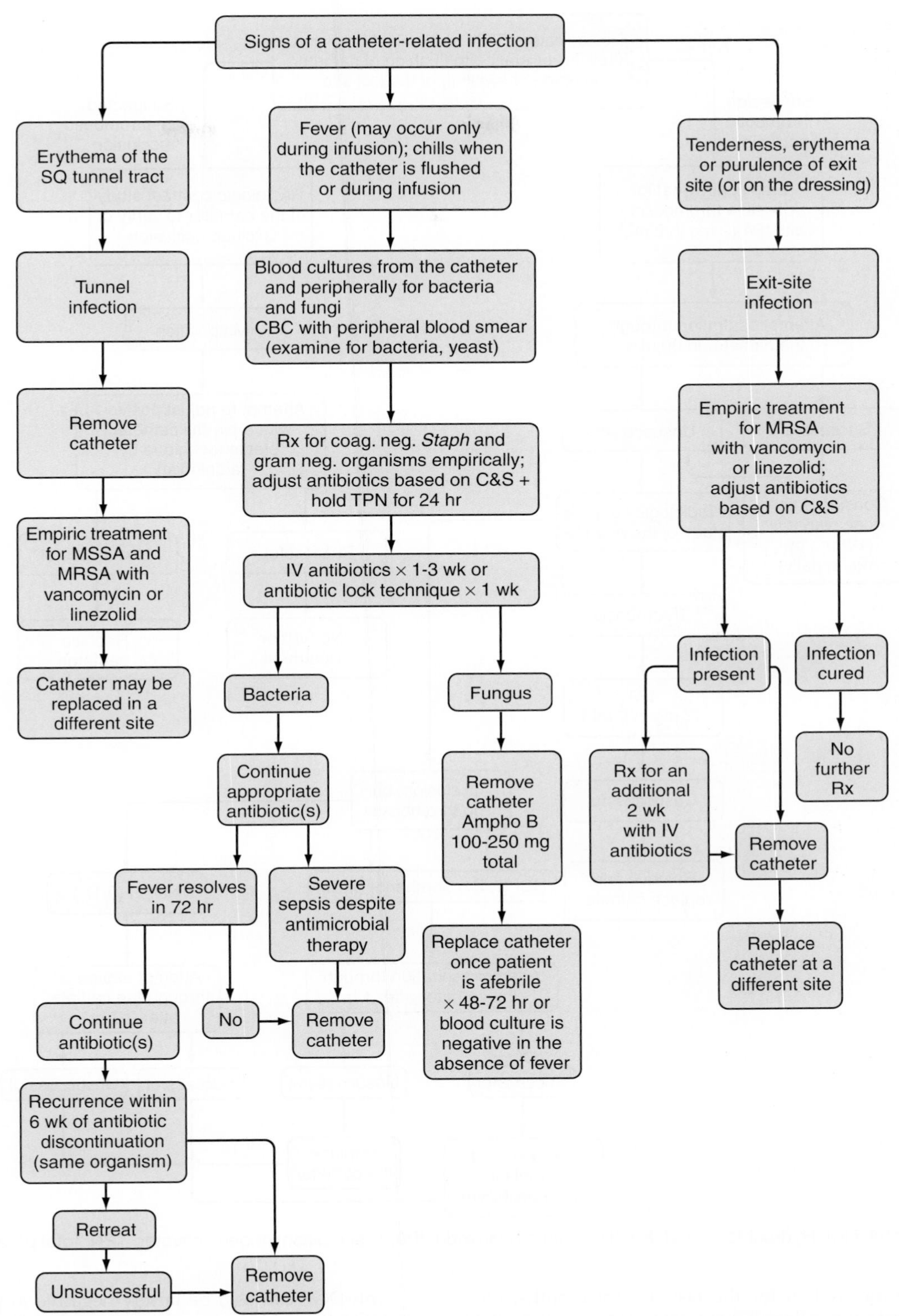

Figure for answer 52. Ampho B, Amphotericin B; CBC, complete blood count; coag. neg., coagulation negative; C&S, culture and susceptibility; IV, intravenous; MRSA, methicillin-resistant *Staphylococcus aureus;* MSSA, methicillin susceptible *Staphylococcus aureus;* Rx, treatment; SQ, subcutaneous; Staph., *Staphylococcus;* TPN, total parenteral nutritiion.

night blindness and dry eyes are suggestive of vitamin A deficiency due to fat malabsorption. The patient has no signs of vitamin B_{12} deficiency (anemia and peripheral neuropathy), folate deficiency (anemia), or niacin deficiency (dermatitis, dementia). Fermentation of unabsorbed carbohydrates by colonic bacteria may lead to D-lactic acidosis (altered mentation, nystagmus, ataxia), which the patient does not have.

58. C (S&F ch107)
This patient has moderate to high probability of having celiac disease. However, because she has been on the

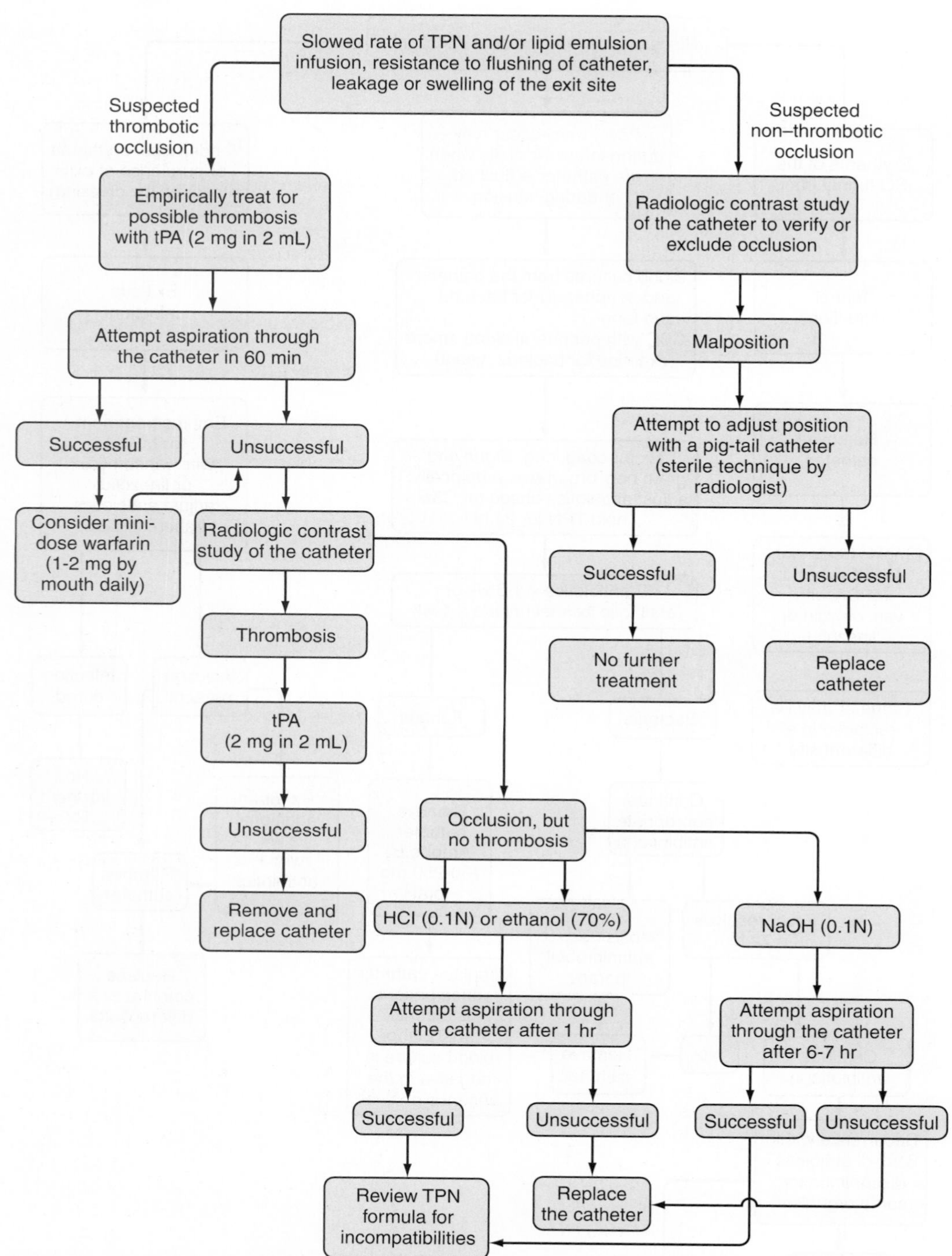

Figure for answer 54. HCl, Hydrochloric acid; NaOH, sodium hydroxide; tPA, tissue plasminogen activator; TPN, total parenteral nutrition.

gluten free diet (GFD) for the last several months, the standard tests for celiac disease, including small bowel biopsy and IgA anti-tTG antibody could be falsely negative. To confirm the diagnosis of celiac disease in this case, she needs to agree with discontinuation of GFD for about 4 weeks, followed by celiac serology and small bowel biopsy. As she is not willing to discontinue GFD, the best option for her is genetic testing for HLA-DQ2/DQ8. If this test is negative, celiac disease can be reliably ruled out. However, a positive test does not confirm the diagnosis of celiac disease as it can be seen in normal populations. IgG anti-DGP can also be falsely negative in patients on the GFD. Its main use is to diagnosis celiac disease in patients with concomitant IgA deficiency. Option E is incorrect, as improvement of symptoms on the GDF cannot differentiate celiac disease from nonceliac gluten sensitivity.

59. **A** (S&F ch107)
Celiac disease primarily affects the mucosa, whereas the submucosa, muscularis propria, and serosa are not involved in the disease process. When examining a small intestinal specimen of patients with untreated

celiac disease, the enterocytes might lose their columnar shape and become cuboidal or squamous; their cytoplasm is basophilic from the high content of RNA. Due to the increased numbers of undifferentiated crypt cells in patients with untreated celiac disease, the crypt's length will increase. Also, the lamina propria will be infiltrated with plasma cells and intraepithelial lymphocytes (IEL), not neutrophils. The increased IELs are suggestive of celiac disease, but by no means diagnostic because they can be found in other conditions, including NSAID use, small intestinal bacterial overgrowth and *H. pylori* infection.

60. C (S&F ch107)
Barley, wheat, and rye belong to the prolamins storage form of wheat proteins. Prolamins are water-insoluble proteins responsible for grains sensitivity in celiac disease. Rice, corn, sorghum, and millet do not activate celiac disease. It is important to mention that oats are tolerated by most patients with celiac disease despite the fact that they belong to the prolamins group. This is due to the smaller proportion of toxic prolamin moiety.

61. B (S&F ch107)
Tissue transglutaminase IgA has a high sensitivity and specificity for celiac disease. If it is positive, it is likely that the patient has celiac, despite negative biopsies. This is the definition of latent celiac disease. Given the patient's history of infertility and bloating, a trial of gluten free diet is warranted. However, positive celiac serologies need to be followed by positive small bowel biopsies to confirm the diagnosis of celiac disease before the patient be instructed to remain on lifelong gluten free diet. There is no advantage to adding genetic testing to positive celiac disease serologies because positive serologies usually indicate the diagnosis of celiac disease. Antigliadin antibodies are nonspecific and are not generally used to diagnose celiac disease. Because IgA tTG antibodies are positive, there is no benefit in checking serum IgA level.

62. E (S&F ch107)
This patient has high probability to have celiac disease given the small bowel biopsy results. However, due to concomitant IgA deficiency (which is seen more in patients with celiac disease), IgA tTG and IgA endomysial antibodies were negative. IgG DGP (deamidated gliadin peptides) assays are very sensitive and commonly used in these scenarios with positive small bowel biopsies for celiac disease and IgA deficiency syndrome. IgG and IgM tTG assays can also be used in these cases, but they are less sensitive than IgG DGP assays. Genetic HLA testing for HLA-DQ2/DQ8 is indicated in 2 scenarios: (1) Patients who are already on gluten free diet and have negative celiac serologies. If the HLA-DQ2/DQ8 is negative, celiac disease is excluded, and the need for gluten challenge is obviated. (2) When small bowel biopsies are consistent with celiac enteropathy, but IgA tTG, endomysial antibody and IgG DGP assays are all negative. IgA and IgG antigliadin antibodies are not specific and should not be used in the diagnosis of celiac disease.

63. D (S&F ch107)
The patient has probable celiac disease. It is important to differentiate between celiac disease and nonceliac gluten sensitivity. For this reason, this patient should undergo a gluten challenge to confirm or exclude the diagnosis. Optimally, the challenge should continue for 6 to 8 weeks. Serologies and small bowel biopsies are checked at the end of the challenge to confirm or exclude the diagnosis; those tests can be done as early as 2 weeks if the patient cannot tolerate gluten challenge. Also, if serologies are negative by the end of the challenge, they should be repeated after 4 weeks. Reassuring the patient at this stage is not ideal as she could possibly have celiac disease. Repeating IgA tTG or obtaining a barium study will not be helpful. HLA-DQ2 and -DQ8 might be helpful in this case if they were negative, but positive results are neither specific nor sensitive for celiac disease.

64. C (S&F ch107)
Dermatitis herpetiformis is a gluten sensitivity disorder and should be treated with a gluten free diet regardless of the presence or absence of celiac disease. Skin lesions in most of the patients with dermatitis her DH resolves after 6 to 12 months of gluten free diet. However, patients need to stay on dapsone during this time to prevent extreme pruritus. The addition of steroids is not necessary in this patient as he is responding to the dapsone. Checking HLA-DQ2/DQ8 in this patient will not change the management plan in any way.

65. B (S&F ch107)
It is important at the beginning of therapy to avoid dairy products because there might be a concomitant lactase deficiency due to epithelial damage, which can improve after implementing gluten free diet. Beer and fermented beverages can contain gluten, but not distilled beverages like wine. Management of celiac disease should include a multidisciplinary approach with education about the disease and diet recommendations. Moderate amounts of oats are usually safe. Generally speaking, grains that should be avoided in celiac disease include wheat, barley, and rye. Identification of nutritional and vitamin deficiencies is important in the treatment of celiac disease as gluten free diet can lack iron, vitamin D, B vitamins, and calcium. Therefore, supplementations and nutritional counseling are important. Patients with celiac disease should be diligent about reading product labels, including vitamins and medications as they can contain gluten.

66. A (S&F ch107)
The most likely etiology for persistent symptoms in celiac disease patients is continued ingestion of gluten, intentionally or unintentionally. This is proven by the patient's persistently elevated tissue transglutaminase antibodies. The patient does have celiac disease, based on serologies, which have a high sensitivity and specificity. Microscopic colitis is more common in celiac patients but is much less likely in this case given the persistently elevated tissue transglutaminase antibodies. Refractory celiac and ulcerative jejunoileitis are rare complications of the disease and present with severe symptoms of abdominal pain, diarrhea, and weight loss despite a strict gluten free diet.

67. C (S&F ch107)
EATL accounts for more than half of the malignancies complicating celiac disease. It carries a poor prognosis with 1-year and 5-year survival rates of 31% and 11%, respectively. EATL, as the name implies, is of T cell origin. Unlike celiac disease, EATL does not respond to gluten withdrawal. Generally, patients with celiac disease have increased risks of multiple GI malignancies with variable rates in different studies. However, recent studies have shown that the risk of all malignancies, including EATL, declines to that of the general population after 5 years of strict gluten free diet.

68. D (S&F ch107)
The patient does not have celiac disease. She had normal small bowel biopsies and celiac serologies before starting a gluten free diet. She probably has nonceliac gluten intolerance given the resolution of her symptoms with avoiding gluten. Her anemia could be related to other etiologies, but with a normal MCV and no celiac disease, B_{12} supplementation is not indicated.

69 E. (S&F ch107)
This patient has typical presentations of ulcerative jejunoileitis, which is a rare complication of celiac disease. The small bowel barium study shows a segmental area of fixed narrowing with associated mucosal ulcerations in the jejunum that is characteristic of this condition. These patients rarely respond to gluten free diet. Surgical excision of the affected segment of small bowel is the most effective treatment. There is increased risk of enteropathy-associated T-cell lymphoma in these patients. However, it can be seen without any evidence of malignancy as well. The prognosis is very poor and 5-year survival rate is less than 50%. In localized cases, glucocorticoids or azathioprine can play a role in the treatment of ulcerative jejunoileitis.

70. D (S&F ch108)
Enterotoxin-producing *E. coli* (ETEC) is the most common cause of traveler's diarrhea. Geography can provide clues about the offending pathogens. ETEC is more common in Mexico and South America; *Vibrio cholerae* in India; *Giardia lamblia* and *Cryptosporidium* in southern Central Asia; and *Campylobacter jejuni* in Southeast Asia.

71. A (S&F ch108)
Western visitors are usually affected by tropical sprue, but local residents and expatriates returning to Western developed countries can also be affected. Adults are affected with epidemic and sporadic tropical sprue more frequently than children. Tropical sprue epidemics are rarely, if ever, reported these days. However, sporadic tropical sprue continues to be a common cause of adult malabsorption in South Asia. If a tropical sprue epidemic occurs, patients are usually protected against a second wave.

72. D (S&F ch108)
Patients with tropical sprue have reduced acid secretion, which can ultimately lead to atrophic gastritis. Villus atrophy and increased intraepithelial lymphocytes can be observed with tropical sprue but are not diagnostic as they can be seen with other diseases like celiac disease. Villus atrophy can also lead to scalloping of the duodenal mucosa on gross examination. This finding can be seen in both celiac disease and tropical sprue. The villus to crypts ratio in tropical sprue is usually 2:1 or 1:1, and the villus atrophy is usually incomplete unlike what can be seen with celiac disease.

73. E (S&F ch108)
A high calorie, high protein, fat-restricted diet is usually recommended in tropical sprue patients. Restriction of long-chain fatty acids and using medium-chain fatty acids is particularly helpful in reducing steatorrhea.

74. D (S&F ch108)
Ogilvie syndrome, or colonic pseudo-obstruction, can rarely occur in the setting of tropical sprue. Initial treatment should be conservative, especially if the patient is hemodynamically stable. After correction of electrolytes, which are typically abnormal given the malabsorption related to the sprue, colonic decompression, not surgery, should be considered first. There is no reason to suspect malignancy in a 38-year-old with no family history of colon cancer. There is only anecdotal experience with using antibiotics, other than tetracycline, in the treatment of tropical sprue.

75. D (S&F ch108)
Tropical enteropathy, tropical sprue, and celiac disease share very similar small bowel histologic features. Celiac disease is ruled out with negative serology and lack of iron deficiency anemia. Given the lack of symptoms in this patient, tropical sprue is less likely. The mucosa of the small bowel in residents of the tropical area is structurally different from that of residents of other regions. This has been referred to as "tropical enteropathy" or "subclinical tropical malabsorption," which in contrast to tropical sprue is asymptomatic. The biopsy findings and clinical presentation are not consistent with Whipple's disease or CVID, respectively.

76. C (S&F ch108)
Colonoscopy with examination of terminal ileum and possible biopsy is the best next step to diagnose possible intestinal tuberculosis (TB) in this patient. Intestinal TB is common in tropical countries. Although, the ulcerative variety of TB presents with diarrhea and malabsorption, the hypertrophic variety causes abdominal pain and obstruction without malabsorptive symptoms. The diagnosis is made by a combination of histology, culture, and PCR. Crohn's disease is less likely in this patient, and should not be treated empirically without histologic evidence of the disease. Abdominal MRI would not add significant information to help the management of this patient at this time.

77. D (S&F ch109)
Whipple's disease is primarily seen in adults with an average age of 56 years in recent studies. No cases were reported in children or young adults. It is more common in men (about 75%), and whites. It is caused by *T. whipplei*, which is a gram-positive bacteria that has a very slow doubling time (28 hours to 4 days). Symptomatic CNS manifestations are seen in 10% to 40% of patients.

78. B (S&F ch109)
Patients with intestinal Whipple's disease have inflammatory cell infiltration of the mucosa of the small intestine, which leads to malabsorption manifested by low serum carotene level, low serum iron, low serum proteins, anemia, high fecal fat content, and proteinuria. Also, the C-reactive protein and erythrocyte sedimentation rate are usually elevated due to systemic inflammation.

79. C (S&F ch109)
The clinical presentation is not consistent with Whipple's disease. Whipple's disease typically causes abdominal pain, weight loss, diarrhea with malabsorption, in addition to multiple other extraintestinal manifestations. Asymptomatic carrier state, though rare, has been reported in the literature. The lack of the typical manifestations of the disease argues against Whipple's disease, hence, no need for treatment. Small bowel biopsy is the diagnostic modality of choice in patients with intestinal manifestations. The yield of an enteroscopy in a patient without typical manifestations and with negative

abdominal imaging is low. *T. whipplei* involves the small bowel, not the colon, and short duration of treatment is not adequate in Whipple's disease.

80. E (S&F ch109)
It used to be believed that Whipple's disease is a disorder of fat metabolism, but with the discovery of the PAS stain, it is now known that the reaction reflects the glycoprotein content of bacterial cell wall. The infiltration pattern of positive PAS cells in the small intestine is usually diffuse, and tends to gradually become patchy with treatment, after which some macrophages might still harbor a small amount of PAS-positive material (type 3 macrophages). During electron microscopy examination of the small intestine in patients with Whipple's disease, structurally intact bacteria are usually extracellular. On the other hand, degraded bacteria are usually intracellular inside macrophages. Positive PAS stain in extraintestinal tissue is not specific, as it can be seen with other conditions like *Mycobacterium avium* complex.

81. E (S&F ch109)
The patient has immune reconstitution inflammatory syndrome (IRIS). This syndrome typically occurs in patients who have received immunosuppression prior to the initiation of treatment of Whipple's disease and results in deterioration of the clinical status days to months after initiation of antibiotic treatment. It responds to steroid therapy. Trimethoprim/sulfamethoxazole (TMP-SMX) is superior to tetracycline in the management of Whipple's disease because it crosses the blood-brain barrier and has a lower risk of central nervous system relapses. Adding another antibiotic is not a treatment modality for IRIS.

82. E (S&F ch109)
A 2-week course of parenteral antibiotics followed by long-term oral antibiotics has been associated with the lowest risk of CNS relapse. Trimethoprin/sulfamethoxazole is associated with a lower number of CNS relapses compared to tetracycline. Tetracycline does not cross the blood-brain barrier, hence the higher risk of CNS relapse in patients treated with tetracycline. CNS relapses have a poor prognosis, regardless of the initial treatment choice.

83. C (S&F ch109)
When selecting an antibiotic to treat Whipple's disease, it is important for the antibiotic to be able to cross the blood-brain barrier to avoid CNS relapse, which is challenging to treat because it is often refractory to the treatment and has a poor prognosis. Oral antibiotics, such as TMP-SMX and cefixime, can be used to treat Whipple's disease. The usual treatment started involves an induction course for 14 days, followed by long-term oral treatment (usually TMP-SMX) for at least 1 year. *T. whipplei* is a gram-positive bacteria.

84. C (S&F ch110)
This patient has been infected with *V. cholerae*, which is often seen in natural disasters. Stool output can exceed 1 L/hr with daily fecal outputs of 15 L to 20 L if parenteral fluid replacement keeps up with losses. Choice C is correct because the cholera toxin acts on intestinal epithelial cells to increase adenylate cyclase activity with resultant elevated levels of cAMP, which causes increased intestinal secretion in the small intestine. Choice A is incorrect because for every clinical case of cholera, there are approximately 400 asymptomatic people who have had contact with the organism. Choice B is incorrect because cholera does not invade the mucosal surface, and a biopsy specimen taken from the mucosa during acute cholera largely shows normal architecture. Choice D is incorrect because in addition to administration of bicarbonate and potassium via oral rehydration solutions, antimicrobial agents are useful ancillary measures to treat cholera because they reduce stool output, duration of diarrhea, fluid requirements, and *Vibrio* excretion. The CDC recommends doxycycline as a single oral dose of 300 mg for nonpregnant adults and 2 to 4 mg/kg for children. A single oral dose of azithromycin 1 g is recommended for pregnant women. Choice E is incorrect because *Vibrio* predominantly affects the small bowel.

85. C (S&F ch110)
This patient is infected with *Vibrio vulnificus.* Choice C is correct because those with underlying liver disease are warned to avoid eating raw seafood because *V. vulnificus* can be fatal. Choice A is incorrect because *V. vulnificus* is gram-negative motile, rod-shaped bacteria that appear like commas. There is an increased severity of illness in those with underlying liver disease, diabetes mellitus, or other compromising conditions, making choice B incorrect. Choice D is incorrect because recommended treatment for severe infection is a tetracycline plus a third-generation cephalosporin or a fluoroquinolone in conjunction with local debridement of infected tissue and supportive therapy for septicemia. Choice E is incorrect because septicemia due to *V. vulnificus* actually exceeds 50% mortality.

86. B (S&F ch110)
The patient is presenting with anemia, thrombocytopenia, leukocytosis, and evidence of acute renal failure with bloody diarrhea. This is most concerning for possible hemolytic-uremic syndrome (HUS) caused by *Shiga* toxin–producing *E. coli* O157:H7.

87. B (S&F ch110)
Y. enterocolitica has most intense radiologic findings in the terminal ileum and can resemble those of Crohn's disease, although most have normal findings on endoscopy, intestinal biopsy, and barium studies. Other pathogens that can involve terminal ileum include *M. tuberculosis, Salmonella* spp, and less commonly *Shigella dysenteriae.*

88. A (S&F ch110)
The clinical presentation is consistent with intestinal tuberculosis. The micrograph shows granulomas of the mucosa and submucosa. Crohn's disease is possible but less likely. There are no architectural changes in the crypts in the surgical specimen. The clinical presentation is not consistent with the other answer choices.

89. B (S&F ch110)
Answer B is correct because dairy products in acute diarrhea may not be well tolerated due to the potential for secondary lactase deficiency. Option A is incorrect because reduced-osmolarity ORS has been studied to result in a significant reduction in stool output and incidence of vomiting compared with standard World Health Organization (WHO)-ORS. The risk of hyponatremia with reduced-osmolarity ORS is not increased, based on available data in studied populations that exceed 50,000 adults or children. Choice C is incorrect because enteral intake should be encouraged as soon as the patient is able to accept oral intake. Even in patients who are vomiting, ORS can be used in small doses effectively. Choice

D is incorrect because parenteral repletion can always be used if the patient does not tolerate oral intake. Choice E is incorrect because glucose in ORS is given to enhance sodium absorption (not calorie intake) in the small intestine, even in the presence of secretory losses caused by infections.

90. B (S&F ch110)
Norovirus, originally discovered as the Norwalk agent in Norwalk, Ohio, in 1968, is the most common cause of community-acquired diarrhea, gastroenteritis outbreaks, and foodborne disease in the United States and globally. Answer B is correct because viral shedding peaks at 1 to 3 days of disease, and the viral antigen is detected in stool for a median of 7 days, so ill individuals are to be excluded from work for 48 to 72 hours post illness, and individual rooms are recommended to prevent nosocomial infections. Answer A is incorrect because soap-and-water hand hygiene (washing for 20 seconds) is recommended because the virus is relatively resistant to alcohol-based hand sanitizers. Answer C is incorrect because most individuals of all ages are susceptible to norovirus infections, which occur year-round, although outbreaks may be more frequent in winter. Answer D is incorrect because 70% of those who acquire norovirus infection are symptomatic, and 30% are asymptomatic. Ten percent of individuals are not susceptible to norovirus infection. Answer E is incorrect because there is no specific therapy available for norovirus infections and maintenance of hydration is the cornerstone of care. A very small study suggested activity of nitazoxanide against norovirus, similar to rotavirus, but this has not been recommended as standard of care.

91. A (S&F ch110)
This patient with iron overload has developed *Y. enterocolitica* enteral infection and bacteremia, so answer A is correct. Although several clinical syndromes have been described with *Yersinia*, adults typically present with fever, abdominal pain, profuse watery diarrhea, and vomiting lasting 1 to 3 weeks. It is often acquired from contaminated food, and pigs are believed to be the major animal reservoir. *Yersinia* bacteremia is a relatively uncommon condition that is seen in patients with underlying diseases, such as malignancy, diabetes mellitus, anemia, liver disease, iron overload (or treatment with an iron chelator), and blood transfusions. Metastatic foci can occur in bones, joints, and lungs. Radiologic findings in *Yersinia* are most intense in the terminal ileum, and most patients with *Yersinia* have normal findings on endoscopy and intestinal biopsy, both of which are found in this patient. *V. cholerae* is a gram-negative rod but often presents with large volume diarrhea up to 20 L/day in an epidemic pattern. Choice B is incorrect because *V. cholerae* is rarely found de novo in the United States with only two such cases reported in 2011. *S. enterica* is a gram-negative bacilli, and bloodstream invasion typically occurs in patients with hemolytic anemias, immunosuppression such as HIV and glucocorticoid use, or neoplastic disease, including use of chemotherapy and radiation, but not iron overload, making answer C incorrect. Answer D is incorrect because *M. tuberculosis* is impervious to Gram stain and is detected as TB bacilli in an acid-fast stain. *S. dysenteriae* causes diarrheal illness, is a gram-negative rod, transmitted through person-to-person transmission and contaminated food transmission. *S. dysenteriae* accounts for less than 1% of cases of shigellosis in the United States compared with *S. sonnei* (80%) and rarely invades the bloodstream except for malnourished children and immunocompromised hosts, making answer E less likely. Furthermore, colonoscopy in shigellosis would typically demonstrate focal ulcers and mucosal inflammation with edema, formation of microabscesses, loss of goblet cells, and loss of tissue architecture on biopsy.

92. D (S&F ch110)
This patient recently was infected with *C. jejuni* and is now suffering from Guillain-Barré syndrome. Answer D is correct because *C. jejuni* is a motile, comma-shaped gram-negative rod with a polar flagellum. Answer A is incorrect because *C. jejuni* is not associated with sexual transmission like shigellosis. Answer B is incorrect because *C. jejuni* is not associated with cellulitis, although *V. vulnificus* and *Vibrio alginolyticus* are. Answer C is incorrect because *C. jejuni* is not commonly associated with toxic megacolon, but *Shigella* spp., *C. difficile*, and *Salmonella* are. Answer E is incorrect because *C. jejuni* is one of the most common causes of foodborne bacterial illness and is transmitted to humans most commonly from infected animals and their food products.

93. A (S&F ch110)
The patient is suffering from invasive salmonellosis resulting in aortitis. Patients with sickle cell anemia are predisposed to invasive salmonellosis, making answer A correct. Answer B is incorrect because *S. enterica* is not known to cause HUS through the release of Shiga toxin, as is the case of Shiga toxin–producing *E. coli*. Answer C is incorrect because *S. enterica* attacks the ileum and, to a lesser extent the colon, causing mild mucosal ulcerations. Answer D is incorrect because the vast majority of salmonellosis is due to foodborne infections from poultry, shell eggs, amphibian and reptile pets, raw vegetables, raw fruits, peanut butter, ground beef, dog food, and even pet hedgehogs. Answer E is incorrect because enteritis and diarrhea need not precede *Salmonella* bacteremia, but bacteremia complicates approximately 5% of cases of enteritis with an attributable mortality of 1% to 5%.

94. E (S&F ch110)
Shigella can be transmitted during sex and especially homosexual men are at increased risk of infection. Meningismus and seizures can occur with shigellosis, particularly in children. However, there is no direct involvement of the CNS, and it may be related to fever, metabolic derangements, and/or the effects of circulating toxins for *S. dysenteriae*. Chronic carriers of *Shigella* are rare but have been identified and can pass the organism in their feces for a year or more. Such carriers are distinctly uncommon and usually stop shedding the organism spontaneously. In contrast to *Salmonella* carriers who very rarely become recurrently symptomatic with the strain they carry, *Shigella* carriers are prone to intermittent attacks of the disease. Risk of HUS with *S. dysenteriae* infection seems to be less when appropriate antibiotics are given within the first 4 days of symptoms. HUS is fairly uncommon and, on average, 13% of infections result in HUS. Answer C is incorrect as careful hand washing and stool precautions are the main measures to prevent dissemination of the disease because shigellosis is highly contagious and no vaccine is currently available.

95. B (S&F ch110)
This patient has been infected with *Salmonella typhi* and has typhoid fever. During the first week of infection, high fever, headache, and abdominal pain are common. The pulse is often slower than what would be expected for the degree of fever, a finding referred to as Faget's sign, which this patient exhibits. Abdominal pain is localized to the right lower quadrant in most cases but can be diffuse. Near the end of the first week, enlargement of the spleen is noticeable, and an evanescent classic rash (rose spots) becomes manifested, most commonly on the chest.

96. A (S&F ch110)
The patient has developed *V. parahaemolyticus* and her recent exposure to seafood and seawater in the Gulf of Mexico are key clues. Foodborne outbreaks of *V. parahaemolyticus* in the United States are characterized by diarrhea with associated cramping, nausea, and vomiting, and outbreaks are most common between April and October. Cases tend to be clustered along coastal states where shellfish consumption and seawater exposure are common, as seen in this patient. The median reported duration of illness is 2.4 days. Choice B is incorrect because although *S. enterica* can cause watery diarrhea, it is typically acquired from livestock in the United States. Furthermore, it is often invasive and can present with bloody diarrhea due to dysentery. *E. coli* infection is not associated with the coast or seafood consumption, but more commonly with hamburger meat, fresh-pressed apple cider, produce, and unpasteurized milk. *E. coli* presents similarly to *V. parahaemolyticus* with watery, nonbloody diarrhea but often progresses to frankly bloody stool. *C. jejuni* is one of the most common causes of foodborne bacterial illnesses in the United States, it occurs through infected animals, including cattle, sheep, swine, birds (poultry and others), and dogs, but not typically seafood. Unpasteurized dairy products and drinking water are other common vehicles for *C. jejuni* outbreaks. *C. jejuni* presents with diarrhea, but unlike this patient, 65% to 90% of cases present with fever and half have bloody stools. *Y. enterocolitica* typically presents with fever in addition to the abdominal pain, diarrhea, and vomiting. Symptoms last 1 to 3 weeks, which is significantly longer than this patient's presentation.

97. B (S&F ch110)
Chemoprophylaxis is indicated in only a selected group of travelers, which include patients with IBD, severe liver, kidney or heart diseases, achlorhydria, or patients on immunosuppressive medications. Also, it can be considered in patients with important business plans during the trip. Possible prophylactic agents include rifaximin, fluoroquinolones, or bismuth subsalicylate. Bismuth subsalicylate should be avoided in patients taking warfarin or salicylates. Azithromycin can be used for treatment of traveler's diarrhea but is not indicated for prophylaxis. Loperamide may be used for symptomatic relief, but there is no prophylactic role for it in traveler's diarrhea.

98. E (S&F ch111)
PPI use deliberately suppresses acid production thereby decreasing the effectiveness of gastric acidity as a natural barrier against gastrointestinal infection. Foodborne disease from *C. jejuni* is more common in the spring and fall. The majority of laboratory-confirmed cases of foodborne illness are outbreaks secondary to *Salmonella* and *Campylobacter*. *Shigella* is also common, but less so. The incidence of vibriosis has tripled over the last 2 decades, presumably due to warming of coastal waters. Both incidence and mortality rate of foodborne illness with *V. vulnificus* is significantly higher in patients with liver disease compared to those of adults with normal liver.

99. E (S&F ch111)
The clinical presentation of this infant is concerning for botulism. Although he initially had symptoms of general gastroenteritis, he eventually became constipated with lethargy and evidence of peripheral muscle weakness and ensuing respiratory compromise. Additionally, his mother notes a recent history of the baby's ingestion of vegetables harvested and stored at home, raising the concern of improper storage, which could lead to the presence of *Clostridium botulinum* in the vegetables. In this setting, the clinical concern for botulism is high enough that the infant should receive immediate administration of antitoxin to avoid progression of illness. In this critically ill infant, the usefulness of the antitoxin has a limited window of time, and its administration should not be delayed by diagnostic testing for confirmation of botulism, although, testing is still necessary, as confirmation should raise concern for exposure of the baby's family to *C. botulinum* and the need for testing of their food stores. Although an emergent neurologic evaluation could be obtained, arranging for immediate administration of antitoxin should be the first step taken. Although the patient's brother recently had a reported case of the flu, the patient's history and clinical presentation are not consistent with that of influenza. Although the infant ingested scrambled eggs, his symptoms are not limited to a gastroenteritis typically expected of *Salmonella,* and the imminent fatal potential of botulism should prompt immediate empiric therapy for this infant with a clinical presentation consistent with botulism.

100. A (S&F ch111)
This patient has recently spent time in the water and eaten indigenous foods around the Chesapeake Bay area that has a high incidence of *V. vulnificus.* This history with clinical findings of fever, shock, and bullous cutaneous manifestations should raise suspicion for *V. vulnificus* septicemia either due to a wound with exposure to local water or through direct ingestion while eating undercooked seafood. This should prompt immediate aggressive management in a critical care setting. The patient's history of morbid obesity and alcohol abuse are risk factors for possible chronic liver disease, which portends an increased likelihood of a fatal outcome up to 200 times greater than those without chronic liver disease. Demonstration of thrombocytopenia, abnormal liver function tests, hypoalbuminemia, and coagulopathy would be concerning for chronic liver disease and greater risk of mortality. Chest x-ray and noncontrast CT of the head are not indicated as part of this patient's initial assessment, and would not add prognostic value. Although blood cultures would be essential to confirming the diagnosis, they would not change the patient's prognosis nor delay empiric management. A skin biopsy is not required for diagnosis as this may be confirmed from blood cultures and would not provide additional prognostic information.

101. D (S&F ch111)
The patient's presentation is secondary to infection with *Clostridium perfringens* in the setting of consumption of poorly cooked meat that was prepared in bulk and underwent insufficient heating to kill the spores. The patient, who appears stable, is likely manifesting type A infection. The diarrhea occurs due to a heat-labile enterotoxin (secretory cytotoxin) that has maximum activity in the ileum. The main factor for infection is ingestion of improperly cooked meat rather than inhalation or cutaneous exposure to spores, which is characteristic of *Bacillus anthracis*. As stated, diarrhea with *C. perfringens* is the result of an enterotoxin that causes changes in membrane ion permeability rather than changes in the intracellular calcium. *C. perfringens* type A infection is rarely fatal and is generally a short-term infection limited to gastrointestinal symptoms, as opposed to *Listeria* infections, which have high rates of hospitalization and death with possible CNS involvement. *C. perfringens* ingestion is the result of improperly prepared meat, as opposed to food handler involvement that is common in *Staphylococcus aureus*.

102. C (S&F ch111)
The patient is manifesting scombroid poisoning that occurs in the setting of poorly stored fish, particularly, mackerel, tuna, and bonito. The bacteria present in the fish proliferate in these circumstances, resulting in decarboxylation of histidine in the muscle of the fish, resulting in high levels of histamine. Consumption of the contaminated fish leads to flushing, an erythematous rash, tachycardia, and pruritus. This reaction usually resolves within 12 hours, and management is largely supportive with administration of antihistamines. Although occasional cases may involve facial and lingual swelling with respiratory distress, this patient is not manifesting such signs and is already several hours post-ingestion (time of onset of symptoms is typically 1 hour). Thus, there is no indication to prophylactically intubate her. There is no role for blood cultures or stool cultures as the patient's presentation is consistent with scombroid poisoning, which is a result of excessive histamine consumption. The diagnosis is a clinical one. If laboratory values were to be drawn, histamine levels would be the most helpful in aiding diagnosis confirmation. This patient is having a histamine-mediated reaction, but it is due to bacterial production of histamines in contaminated food rather than a food allergy. Further, the patient has had exposure to peanuts within the last 24 hours with no reaction, which does not support a new onset of peanut allergy. There is no role for botulism antitoxin as the patient's presentation is not suggestive botulism.

103. B (S&F ch111)
The patient presents with sudden onset vomiting without diarrhea after eating fried rice, which is typical of vomiting syndrome due to *Bacillus cereus* food poisoning. The vomiting syndrome is nearly always secondary to consumption of fried rice, not poultry or meat. Onset of illness is rapid, but the course is self-limited and mild. Food poisoning with *S. aureus* has also a short incubation period of about 3 hours. However, it usually occurs after eating foods with high sugar content, such as custard and cream. It starts with vomiting and abdominal pain and then followed by diarrhea. The incubation periods for *C. perfringens*, *S. typhi*, and *Campylobacter* are 12 hours, 24 hours, and 48 hours, respectively.

104. C (S&F ch111)
The patient presents with significant neurologic abnormalities, cardiac arrhythmia, and hypotension after recent ingestion of sushi in Japan, where puffer fish is found as a sushi delicacy. His clinical condition is concerning for tetrodotoxin poisoning from consumption of puffer fish improperly prepared rather than being prepared by a specially appointed chef. Mortality may approach 50%, but those who survive recover entirely. The patient's presentation is less consistent with shellfish poisoning given lack of gastrointestinal symptoms and less likely to have been secondary to oyster consumption due to the oysters being fried. Tetrodotoxin (TdT) is a heat-stable, water-soluble neurotoxin. Although the action of TdT is upon nerve tissue with prevention of depolarization and propagation, the action is upon the sodium channels. The next step of management is aggressive supportive care in an intensive care setting. There is a lack of evidence to support effective management of TdT poisoning with charcoal lavage. It may be tried given the high mortality with only supportive care; however, its most effective window is typically within the first hour of symptom onset.

105. B (S&F ch111)
S. aureus has five distinct enterotoxins (A, B, C, D, and E). It is infection with *C. perfringens* type C that results in intestinal necrosis with up to 40% mortality due to perforation, sepsis, and hemorrhage. It is *B. anthracis* that results in endotoxin complexes that lead to systemic toxemia with 50% mortality as a consequence of perforation, shock, and hemorrhage. Scombroid poisoning is generally mild and self-limited. Ciguatera poisoning can result in chronic effects from 1 month up to a year later with fatigue, myalgias, and headaches. Symptoms may be aggravated by caffeine or alcohol.

106. C (S&F ch112)
This elderly female is high risk for development of *C. difficile* colitis as a nursing home resident with recent exposure to a fluoroquinolone. Her presentation is notable for evidence of sepsis and early end-organ damage. Imaging demonstrates toxic megacolon. This patient requires an emergent evaluation by a surgical team for subtotal colectomy for her *severe C. difficile* infection. Given the severity of her disease with complication of toxic megacolon, the patient requires immediate intervention and would not benefit from delayed management with initiation of antibiotics. In this critically ill patient, invasive procedures should not be undertaken and would not change management. Due to the severity and progression of her *C. difficile* infection, the patient is not a safe candidate for FMT. The patient is not exhibiting an allergic reaction to levofloxacin, which has already been completed, and there is no role for antihistamines or epinephrine.

107. C (S&F ch112)
Patients suffering from antibiotic-associated diarrhea typically have a previous history of diarrhea in the setting of antibiotic use, which differs from *C. difficile* infection where the patients often have no history of adverse events during antibiotic use. Antiperistaltic medications are helpful in management of antibiotic-associated diarrhea (AAD). AAD does not usually manifest abnormal findings on imaging or colonoscopy. The course of illness is mild and self-limited for most cases of AAD. Withdrawal of the implicated antibiotic generally leads

to prompt resolution of symptoms in the case of AAD as opposed to *C. difficile* infection where illness may persist or even progress in severity despite discontinuation of the original antibiotics.

108. D (S&F ch112)
As this is the patient's third discrete episode of *C. difficile* infection (second recurrence), she requires pulsed or tapered vancomycin for therapy (see box at the end of the chapter). A limited course of scheduled vancomycin is indicated for severe first or second infections with *C. difficile.* Metronidazole is a good choice for a first or second uncomplicated infection with *C. difficile.* FMT is not indicated for this patient, who is only experiencing her second recurrence. Additionally, administration via nasogastric tube is higher risk than colonic or rectal administration due to potential for aspiration. Teicoplanin is difficult to obtain and expensive, and it is not available in oral form in the United States. It would not be a first-line agent for a second recurrence of *C. difficile.*

109. B (S&F ch112)
High concentrations of IgG antitoxin A serum antibody are associated with protection against *C. difficile*–associated diarrhea and colitis, whereas low serum antibody levels have been associated with recurrent *C. difficile* infection (see figure). Although colonization rates of *C. difficile* infection may be elevated among young children, they rarely manifest gastrointestinal disease. Aminoglycosides and tetracyclines are rarely associated with *C. difficile* infection. Commonly implicated antibiotics are clindamycin, ampicillin, amoxicillin, cephalosporins, and fluoroquinolones (see table at the end of the chapter). PPI use was initially found to have a dose-dependent association with risk for *C. difficile*-associated disease (CDAD). However, subsequent studies have questioned the strength of this relationship. Patients receiving chemotherapy are at risk for developing *C. difficile* infection even in the absence of antibiotic use due to alteration of the colonic microbiota and reduced resistance to *C. difficile* colonization.

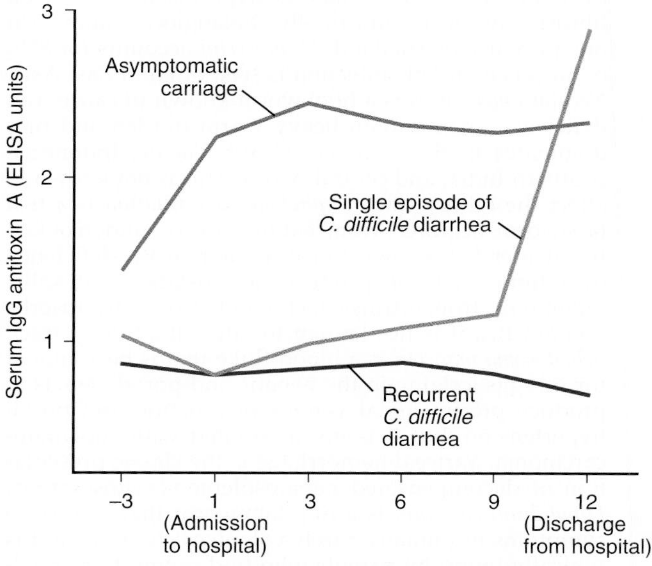

Figure for answer 109.

110. A (S&F ch112)
This elderly female is a vasculopath who presents in septic shock likely secondary to pneumonia. Her prolonged period of shock followed by cardiac arrest for several minutes would have resulted in significant end-organ hypoperfusion. This is seen in her superimposed acute kidney injury over her chronic renal insufficiency. Her colonoscopic evaluation demonstrates evidence of ischemic colitis in the region of the splenic flexure, a common watershed area. A pseudomembranous appearance is not limited to *C. difficile* colitis infection and may be seen in limited segments of ischemic colitis. If biopsies had been obtained, histologic changes may still be difficult to distinguish from *C. difficile* infection. In this scenario, however, the clinical presentation is key to making a diagnosis. FMT is not indicated for this patient who does not manifest evidence of a severe *C. difficile* infection. Similarly, empiric broad antibiotic coverage is not indicated in this case. The patient has had a small drop in her hemoglobin, but no active bleeding is seen at the time of exam, and the most likely source for her earlier bleeding was the ischemic colitis. CT angiography is not indicated, and further, it may pose further adverse consequences for her renal function. There is no evidence of an acute surgical abdomen on external abdominal exam, and the endoscopic evaluation demonstrates no evidence of necrosis with high risk for perforation or bacterial translocation. There is no indication for emergent surgical intervention.

111. D (S&F ch112)
This patient is overall well, and he has a negative PCR study for demonstration of *C. difficile* infection. Additionally, his symptoms are minimal and appear to fluctuate throughout the week. His clinical presentation is consistent with postinfectious IBS. Given lack of any alarm features, there is no role to proceed to invasive testing at this time. The alternating pattern to the patient's bowel habits is not consistent for small intestinal bacterial overgrowth. MR enterography will not demonstrate any abnormalities and is an expensive diagnostic modality. There is no reason to suspect a falsely negative PCR study in a patient who lacks clinically significant symptoms to strongly support a diagnosis of *C. difficile* colitis.

112. E (S&F ch112)
Treatment of asymptomatic carriers of *C. difficile* is not indicated and may, in fact, prolong the carrier state. Asymptomatic patients without diarrhea do not need to be checked for *C. difficile* toxin. Washing hands with soap and water after going to bathroom and before preparing food is the best recommendation for both the patient and her husband.

113. E (S&F ch113)
This patient presents with a history of drinking well water in a rural area of a locale endemic to *Entamoeba histolytica.* Her presentation with dysentery is that of invasive amebic colitis. Stool specimen shows *E. histolytica* trophozoite. Infection with *Giardia, Isospora, Cryptosporidium,* and *Cyclospora* usually does not cause dysentery.

114. A (S&F ch113)
This patient is presenting with fatigue, abdominal cramps with bloating, and watery diarrhea consistent with *Giardia intestinalis,* most likely acquired from her child who attends day care. As the diagnosis can be made accurately by molecular stool studies, including ELISA,

there is no role for invasive evaluation involving endoscopy to confirm diagnosis. As cysts and trophozoites are only present intermittently in the stool, even with multiple specimens, the sensitivity of ova and parasite exam is only around 50%.

115. A (S&F ch113)
This patient presents with a history and stool studies suggestive of infection with *Cryptosporidium*, likely acquired during his visits to the public swimming pool. The patient also has a history of intravenous drug use, a risk factor for acquiring HIV and should be tested for HIV given concern of his general presentation being consistent with early HIV infection. The only available therapy is nitazoxanide, although this may be less effective should this patient be found to be immunosuppressed. Although *Cryptosporidium* may occasionally be seen on an intestinal biopsy, the patient's history and stool studies already suggest the diagnosis. Further, this may be confirmed with the FDA-approved PCR detection test, rendering an invasive procedure unnecessary. Imaging may reveal changes of the gastrointestinal tract secondary to cryptosporidiosis; however, it will render a specific diagnosis. Duodenal aspirate will confirm a diagnosis of infection with *Giardia* for which the treatment of choice would be metronidazole. This patient is not manifesting evidence of infection secondary to *Salmonella*.

116. C (S&F ch113)
This patient's concerning presentation is consistent with infection with *T. cruzi* (Chagas' disease). The barium enema reveals megarectum and megasigmoid in this patient. The most commonly involved system is the cardiovascular system, with manifestations of arrhythmias and congestive heart failure. Given the patient's presentation of bradycardia on exam, she is likely to have abnormal tracings. Although chronic Chagas' disease may require assistance from the CDC for detection of serum antibodies to *T. cruzi*, this patient is manifesting acute Chagas' disease, which is diagnosed by demonstration of trypanosome forms on blood smears. Neostigmine will not be helpful with this patient who has an irreversible underlying cause of her megacolon. Moreover, her current cardiac condition is a contraindication for receiving neostigmine. She would benefit from surgical evaluation to determine if she needs resection of the affected bowel. Although her presentation may mimic myxedema, the patient is suffering from complications of Chagas' disease. She will not improve with treatment for hypothyroidism. The patient's sister notes that prior to sudden onset of symptoms, the patient was in good health and had the stamina to perform arduous physical labor, which does not suggest missed coronary artery disease but rather acute cardiac decompensation secondary to her infection.

117. D (S&F ch113)
Although treatment of *Blastocystis* results in improvement in symptoms in up to 50% of those treated, it is thought that this may actually result from treatment of other unidentified organisms. One study showed that in 84% of patients with *B. hominis* infection, at least one other pathogen was found in their stool. The burden of parasites does not correlate with the severity of symptoms. There is a suggestion of an association of *Blastocystis* with IBS not IBD. Infection burden is greatest in the tropics, but it is found worldwide.

118. B (S&F ch114)
Patients with *S. stercoralis* infection may have occult disease until treatment with glucocorticoids causes fulminant disease, as is the case with this patient. His previous eosinophilia suggests an occult undiagnosed infection, and his parasite burden had been balanced in a setting of asymptomatic, chronic infestation. Glucocorticoids administration upset this balance, inducing fulminant strongyloidiasis that presents with polymicrobial sepsis with enteric organisms due to intestinal injury from filariform larvae and pneumonitis from larvae migrating through the lungs. Endocarditis, meningitis, and appearance of worms in the brain can occur and fulminant strongyloidiasis is often fatal. *E. vermicularis* typically presents with pruritus ani and restless sleeping and rarely causes eosinophilia. *A. duodenale* typically causes iron deficiency only with moderate to heavy hookworm infestation. *T. trichiura* is typically asymptomatic but known to cause rectal prolapse with a high worm burden. *Trichuris* dysentery syndrome can cause mucoid diarrhea with bleeding. *T. saginata* is a beef tapeworm that is typically asymptomatic but can cause vague symptoms of abdominal discomfort, loss of appetite, or change in stool pattern. Rarely, acute biliary or pancreatic duct obstruction can occur if proglottids migrate into these sites. *T. saginata* is not associated with cysticercosis, which is due to *T. solium*.

119. C (S&F ch114)
This patient has developed hilar cholangiocarcinoma as evidenced by the radiographic, endoscopic, and laboratory values. Most infections with the liver fluke *Clonorchis sinensis* are asymptomatic, but heavy exposures can cause fever, malaise, hepatic tenderness, and eosinophilia that initially improves as the worms mature and begin laying eggs in the bile ducts. A minority of infected patients can develop relapsing cholangitis, fibrotic and adenomatous reactions that can cause localized obstruction and hepatic abscess formation, and pancreatitis due to migration into the pancreatic duct. The most important complication of chronic infection with *C. sinensis* or *O. viverrini* is cholangiocarcinoma from cellular desquamation of the bile duct, followed by hyperplasia, adenomatous hyperplasia, periductal fibrosis, dysplasia, and finally cholangiocarcinoma. (In one province in Thailand, *O. viverrini* accounts for 85% of all cancers). This infection is seen often in East Asia. *Necator americanus* is a hookworm known to cause iron deficiency anemia with heavy worm burden and predominates in the Americas, South Pacific, Indonesia, southern India, and central Africa. This is not known to affect the biliary tract. *Diphyllobothrium latum* is a fish tapeworm acquired from eating raw or undercooked freshwater fish known to cause vitamin B_{12} deficiency over time. *D. latum* produces a substance that splits vitamin B_{12} from intrinsic factor and also avidly absorbs vitamin B_{12}; it is not known to affect the biliary tract. *Schistosoma mansoni* is a blood fluke that is best known for its eggs lodging in the hepatic and portal vessels to produce presinusoidal venous obstruction and portal hypertension, but it is not associated with cholangiocarcinoma. Variceal hemorrhage is the classic presentation of decompensated hepatosplenic schistosomiasis. *Dipylidium caninum* is a dog tapeworm that causes no symptoms in humans, rarely colonizes children, and is typically found by parents who find proglottids crawling in their child's diaper.

120. D (S&F ch114)
This patient has developed variceal hemorrhage due to decompensated hepatosplenic schistosomiasis, which is a classic presentation of the disease. *S. mansoni* is a blood fluke acquired through contact with contaminated water, affecting 200 million people worldwide including Africa, the Middle East, Puerto Rico, the Dominican Republic, Central America, and South America. Dermal invasion and migration through swimming in infected water can cause swimmer's itch, but the schistosome eggs can cause intestinal inflammation leading to tenesmus, sigmoid colon tenderness, bloody diarrhea, or colitis with inflammatory pseudopolyps resembling IBD. Eggs not passed out of the body get lodged in the liver via portal flow with resultant presinusoidal venous obstruction and portal hypertension. Patients typically have an enlarged left hepatic lobe, splenomegaly, and thrombocytopenia due to platelet sequestration with normal hepatocellular function. Patients may have normal serum aminotransferase levels and mildly elevated serum levels of alkaline phosphatase. None of the other options are known to cause noncirrhotic portal hypertension. *Ascaris lumbricoides* is a nematode that is typically asymptomatic, but a heavy worm burden can cause pulmonary ascariasis presenting as pneumonia; intestinal ascariasis presenting with abdominal pain, distention, nausea, vomiting, and even small bowel obstruction, with fatality from obstruction, intussusception, or volvulus; and hepatobiliary ascariasis causing biliary colic, obstructive jaundice, ascending cholangitis, acalculous cholecystitis, or acute pancreatitis. *T. saginata* is a beef tapeworm that is typically asymptomatic but can cause vague symptoms of abdominal discomfort, loss of appetite, or change in stool pattern. Rarely, acute biliary or pancreatic duct obstruction can occur if proglottids migrate into these sites. *T. saginata* is not associated with cysticercosis, which is due to *T. solium*. *Ancylostoma ceylonicum* is a hookworm that can cause iron deficiency anemia, with heavy infections typically affecting animals or in humans, often in coinfection with another hookworm. *S. stercoralis* can cause nausea, abdominal pain, occult GI blood loss, or colonic inflammation resembling ulcerative colitis, but is right-sided and eosinophilic. Rarely it can cause fulminant disease manifesting with polymicrobial sepsis, endocarditis, meningitis, or pneumonitis, and is often fatal.

121. A (S&F ch114)
The patient has B_{12} deficiency anemia, which has been caused by the fish tapeworm *D. latum*. This is the largest parasite of humans, reaching lengths up to 40 feet and is acquired by eating raw or undercooked freshwater fish. It is endemic in northern Europe, Russia, and Alaska but has been reported worldwide. Fish tapeworm is not invasive and has no direct symptoms. It produces a substance that splits B_{12} from intrinsic factor in the intestine, thereby preventing host absorption of the vitamin, and also avidly absorbs B_{12}. It can rarely cause enough deficiency to result in megaloblastic anemia and neurologic symptoms. The other organisms are not known to cause vitamin B_{12} anemia. *T. solium* is one of the pork tapeworms and is mostly asymptomatic except for those that have mild abdominal discomfort, loss of appetite, or change in stool pattern. *T. solium* can cause the dreaded cysticercosis if its eggs are consumed and can cause cysticerci with localized inflammation in the brain, spinal cord, eye, and heart, with dire consequences. *Hymenolepis nana* is the dwarf tapeworm and is the smallest but most common tapeworm that colonizes people. Colonization can be asymptomatic, but heavy infestations can result in anorexia, abdominal pain, and diarrhea. *C. sinensis* is a liver fluke that is usually asymptomatic, but a minority of patients can develop relapsing cholangitis and even cholangiocarcinoma. *Schistosoma japonicum* is a blood fluke endemic in China, Indonesia, the Philippines, and Thailand that can acutely present with Katayama's fever, marked by fever, malaise, arthralgia, myalgia, cough, diarrhea, and marked eosinophilia. In a chronic manner, *S. japonicum* can involve the portal venous system causing portal hypertension through presinusoidal venous obstruction.

122. E (S&F ch114)
This patient is presenting with iron deficiency anemia from hookworm *A. duodenale*. It is acquired by skin contact with contaminated soil and is common in North Africa, the Middle East, Europe, Pakistan, and northern India. Light infestations are asymptomatic, but moderate to heavy hookworm infestation causes iron deficiency anemia by feeding on intestinal epithelial cells and blood. The other organisms are not known to cause iron deficiency anemia. *T. solium* is one of the pork tapeworms and is mostly asymptomatic except for those that have mild abdominal discomfort, loss of appetite, or change in stool pattern. *T. solium* can cause the dreaded cysticercosis if its eggs are consumed, resulting in cysticerci with localized inflammation in the brain, spinal cord, eye, and heart, with dire consequences. *O. viverrini* is a liver fluke endemic to Russia and the Ukraine that migrates into the biliary tree and can cause relapsing cholangitis and cholangiocarcinoma. *Enterobius vermicularis*, commonly called pinworm, typically presents with pruritus ani and restless sleeping and rarely causes eosinophilia.

123. D (S&F ch125)
This elderly male is presenting with a partial bowel obstruction picture in the setting of a new onset microcytic anemia and weight loss. Given his normal upper and lower GI exams within the last year, there should be concern for small bowel pathology contributing to his presentation, particularly adenocarcinoma. CT enterography would provide high resolution imaging of the small bowel to assist with diagnosis. FOBT is indicated for colorectal cancer screening in the outpatient setting, which has no role in this patient's case. Repeating the patient's endoscopic procedures would be unlikely to provide new diagnostic information given the recent history of normal exams. Additionally, the patient is presenting with a significant obstruction of the bowel and would not be safe to undergo bowel preparation or invasive procedures. Given the acute clinical presentation of bowel obstruction, gastric dysmotility would be unlikely to explain the patient's symptoms. Cirrhosis of the liver would not contribute to the patient's acute presentation. Further, although he has mild elevation of his ALT (likely due to fatty liver disease given his obesity), the remainder of the patient's liver function tests are within normal limits.

124. B (S&F ch125)
Almost all GISTs express KIT or CD117. Generally, GISTs are 3 to 4 times more likely to exhibit benign behavior. They rarely express S100. Most prognostic indicators for GISTs are not consistently helpful. However, the most useful indicators of survival and risk of metastases are

the size of the tumor at presentation and the mitotic index. Chemotherapy and radiation are highly ineffective for treatment of advanced GIST.

125. A (S&F ch125)
Periampullary duodenal carcinoma is the most common extracolonic malignant tumor in patients with familial adenomatous polyposis for which these patients require periodic endoscopic screening. Patients with Lynch syndrome who develop small intestine tumors typically present 10 to 20 years earlier than the general population, and in the fourth or fifth decade of life. There is a protective effect of ileal resection and prolonged salicylate may confer a protection against development of small intestine adenocarcinomas in the setting of Crohn's disease. An increased incidence of adenocarcinoma and lymphoma of the small bowel has been reported to occur in the setting of Crohn's disease. There is an 11% to 13% incidence of small intestine malignancy associated with celiac disease, mostly enteropathy-associated T-cell lymphomas.

126. E (S&F ch125)
This young female of a high-risk ethnic background patient presents with endoscopic findings concerning for possible metastatic melanoma. Given the high suspicion on exam, dermatology evaluation is warranted even while awaiting histologic confirmation. An MR enterography, inflammatory markers, and IBD serologies would be helpful for evaluating a patient with concerning findings for inflammatory bowel disease, but this is not consistent with this patient's presentation. The patient has a history of heavy menstruation, but she has not experienced any changes in regularity to raise alarm for uterine cancer. There is dark matter passing through the GI tract due to the metastases from the melanoma, but there is no active gastrointestinal bleeding warranting intervention.

127. D (S&F ch125)
With the exception of enteropathy-associated T-cell lymphomas, most PSILs are B-cell derived. Most PSILs are found in the ileum and have a prolonged period of intramural containment. They do not have palpable peripheral lymphadenopathy. PSILs affect an isolated segment of bowel rather than diffuse disease in a contiguous fashion, which is characteristic of immunoproliferative small intestinal disease.

128. C (S&F ch125)
Type 1 neurofibromatosis has been associated with multiple small intestinal GISTs. Age older than 65 years is an associated risk factor for small bowel adenocarcinoma. However, male gender and BMI are associated risk factors for malignant carcinoids, not adenocarcinomas. Point mutations in K-*ras* at codon 12 is present in up to half of small intestinal adenocarcinomas, not all small intestinal tumors. *KIT* mutations are present in 75% t80% of GISTs. DNA replication errors characterized by microsatellite instability are seen in up to 13% of sporadic small intestine carcinomas.

129. B (S&F ch125)
The size and mitotic index are the most important indicators of survival and the risk of metastasis. Mitotic index of 0 to 1 per 50 high-powered fields and tumor size of smaller than 2 cm are associated with lower risk of malignancy. Tumors with exon 11 *KIT* deletion, jejunal tumors, and tumors with high cellularity are usually associated with poor prognosis (see table at the end of the chapter).

130. B (S&F ch125)
This elderly male of northwestern Europe descent has most likely has undiagnosed celiac disease in which his presentation is concerning for an enteropathy-associated T-cell lymphoma (EATL), the most commonly associated primary small intestine lymphoma with celiac disease. The remaining findings are representative of various B-cell lymphomas: diffuse large B-cell lymphoma, Burkitt's lymphoma, immunoproliferative small intestinal disease, and mantle cell lymphoma (see table at the end of the chapter).

131. C (S&F ch125)
Small intestine adenocarcinoma typically manifests when disease is advanced, with over half of patients being diagnosed at stage III and IV. Treatment of choice remains surgical resection. There is no evidence at this time to support adjuvant chemotherapy or radiation therapy. However, if a patient has a small intestine adenocarcinoma that is deemed unresectable, it may be reasonable to consider chemotherapy as an alternative first-line choice of treatment. Bevacizumab, a vascular endothelial growth factor (VEGF) receptor inhibitor, has had success in case reports, but thus far, there is not a role for molecular targeted agents in management of small intestine adenocarcinoma.

132. B (S&F ch115)
Genetic polymorphisms of the *NOD2/CARD15* gene are associated with a higher likelihood of stricture formation. They are also associated with younger age of disease onset and ileal location of disease. Up to 30% of Crohn's disease patients bear an abnormal *NOD2/CARD15* gene. There is no association between extraintestinal manifestations and polymorphisms of the *NOD2/CARD15* gene.

133. A (S&F ch115)
Autophagy is a unique process that plays a role in cellular homeostasis by clearing abnormal proteins and apoptotic bodies. It contributes directly to innate immunity through direct killing of pathogens, activation of Toll-like receptors, and NOD-like receptors. The intracellular process delivers segments of cytoplasm isolated within a membrane to lysosomes through mechanisms that do not involve transport through endocytic or vacuolar sorting pathways. Autophagy does not play a role in production of β-defensins.

134. D (S&F ch115)
Unlike granulomas of TB, there is little or no central necrosis in Crohn's disease–related granulomas. They may involve any portion of the intestine as well as outside the GI tract. TNF is the key cytokine in the formation of granulomas. Noncaseating granulomas are an early finding in the disease course. They are more commonly found in surgical specimens than mucosal biopsies.

135. B (S&F ch115)
The patient's presentation and histologic findings are consistent with Crohn's disease. Granulomas related to tuberculosis are caseating. In addition, AFB stains and mycobacterial cultures are positive in tuberculosis (not mentioned in the question). Patients with Behçet's disease have a history of oral ulcers and present with colitis/ileitis and ischemic changes without granulomas. Patients with NSAID enteropathy usually have scattered aphthous ulcers, inflammation, or diaphragmatic strictures. However, noncaseating granulomas are not seen in this condition.

136. A (S&F ch115)
The finding of an isolated duodenal stricture characterized by granulomas in a recent immigrant from Mexico is suspicious for intestinal tuberculosis. Although similar findings may be seen with Crohn's disease, the lack of involvement of the more distal small bowel and colon makes the diagnosis of Crohn's less likely. Granulomas are not present in NSAID enteropathy, which can present with diaphragm-like strictures. Isolated duodenal involvement with sarcoidosis is rare. Behçet's disease presents with oral ulcers, uveitis, and genital involvement, which were not reported with this patient's case.

137. E (S&F ch115)
Nodular regenerative hyperplasia (NRH) is a rare condition in which the liver is transformed into nodules of 1 to 3 mm in size. It can lead to severe portal hypertension. NRH has been linked to chronic treatment with azathioprine, 6-MMP, and possibly methotrexate. Patients who develop NRH due to azathioprine should stop the medication. Decreasing the dose of azathioprine and adding allopurinol may be beneficial in the subset of patients with elevated 6-MMP : 6-TG ratios. Elevated 6-MMP levels are associated with elevated transaminases, not cholestasis. 6-TG nucleotide levels are not associated with cholestasis.

138. E (S&F ch115)
The patient has lost response to adalimumab due to the development of drug antibodies. Switching to another medication within the same class (anti-TNF) is recommended prior to switching to another class of medications. Sulfasalazine is not recommended in patients with ileocolonic Crohn's disease failing biologic therapy. Low titers of antibodies may clear with the addition of azathioprine; however, this patient has high levels of antibodies that are unlikely to clear. Increasing the dose of adalimumab may be beneficial in patients with low adalimumab levels and undetectable or low antibody levels. This patient is already on a high dose of adalimumab. Switching to a medication with a different mechanism of action, such as vedolizumab (antiintegrin) is recommended in patients with continued colitis despite therapeutic levels of anti-TNF medication.

139. B (S&F ch115)
The anti-TNF agents including infliximab, adalimumab, and certolizumab are category B in pregnancy, and they are considered safe in pregnancy. The rate of birth defects is not elevated in pregnancies in which the mother is receiving anti-TNF.

140. A (S&F ch115)
HSTCL is a rare type of lymphoma associated with Crohn's disease treatment with thiopurine alone or in combination with anti-TNF. It is mostly reported in young males. It is universally fatal. The risk of HSTCL does not begin until approximately 2 years of thiopurine exposure.

141. D (S&F ch115)
The patient is presenting with drug-induced pancreatitis secondary to azathioprine. The medication should be stopped, and further treatment with thiopurines is contraindicated. There is a slow suspicion of gallstone pancreatitis in this patient; therefore cholecystectomy should be deferred. Adalimumab is not known to be associated with acute pancreatitis. The development of pancreatitis is a contraindication to further treatment with thiopurines.

142. D (S&F ch115)
The lesion is pyoderma gangrenosum (PG). A characteristic feature of PG is its development at the site of trauma (pathergy phenomenon). The condition may be found in other conditions such as ulcerative colitis and rheumatoid arthritis. In Crohn's disease, PG often occurs without an associated flare of intestinal symptoms. It usually heals, forming a significant cribriform scar. It is not associated with any specific autoantibodies.

143. C (S&F ch115)
Thiopurine use is associated with a risk of nonmelanoma skin cancer. No other solid tumors have been found to be associated with thiopurine use in inflammatory bowel disease.

144. E (S&F ch115)
The patient has moderate ileal Crohn's disease, which requires both induction and maintenance of long-term remission. Infliximab has the ability to maintain and induce remission. Mesalamine has not been found to be effective for achieving remission in patients with moderate Crohn's disease. Azathioprine may take several weeks to take effect, so the medication is not ideal to induce remission. The value of methotrexate in inducing remission is not clear. Prednisone is used to induce remission but is ineffective in maintaining remission, and it is associated with significant side effects when used for a prolonged period of time.

145. B (S&F ch115)
The patient is presenting with an acute infusion reaction, which is associated with human antichimeric antibodies in some patients. Elevated ANA levels can be seen in patients on infliximab after 2 years of therapy; however, drug-induced lupus is rare. Positive interferon gamma release assay and anemia are not associated with infusion reactions. The use of a concomitant thiopurine may help to prevent such reactions.

146. A (S&F ch115)
The patient has a pyogenic complication related to Crohn's disease. Antibiotic treatment and adequate drainage must be performed prior to initiating therapy for Crohn's disease.

147. E (S&F ch115)
Vedolizumab is antiintegrin molecule that selectively targets the intestine-specific $\alpha4\beta7$ integrin. It is FDA approved for the treatment of Crohn's disease and ulcerative colitis. Natalizumab is a nonselective antiintegrin molecule that targets both $\alpha4\beta1$ (present in brain) and $\alpha4\beta7$. Ustekinumab is a human monoclonal antibody to IL-12/23. Tofacitinib is an oral Janus kinase inhibitor. Ustekinumab and tofacitnib are still experimental in inflammatory bowel disease.

148. D (S&F ch115)
The patient has moderate colonic Crohn's disease, which has not responded to anti-TNF agents. The patient may be a candidate for an antiintegrin agent such as natalizumab or vedolizumab. Prior to starting the patient on natalizumab, anti-JCV antibody should be checked, given the risk of progressive multifocal leukoencephalopathy (PML) associated with natalizumab. If anti-JCV

antibody is negative, then the risk of PML is close to zero, and treatment with natalizumab may be considered. Antibiotics and mesalamine have little role in management of this patient's moderate Crohn's disease. Laboratory values for hepatitis C antibody and ESR are unlikely to provide useful additional clinical information.

149. A (S&F ch115)
The patient has clinical symptoms of active disease but has normal lab values, including adequate drug level. An objective evaluation with the use of ileocolonoscopy should be performed to assess for endoscopic disease activity prior to attempting to optimize treatment for Crohn's disease.

150. B (S&F ch115)
The patient is presenting with an enterocutaneous fistula after an appendectomy. This presentation is highly suggestive of Crohn's disease. The other conditions are unlikely to present with an enterocutaneous fistula.

151. C (S&F ch115)
The findings of fever, hip pain, and difficulty with ambulation in the setting of a recent psoas abscess are suspicious for a septic hip joint. Deep vein thrombosis does not present with localized hip pain or high-grade temperatures. The acute nature of the patient's pain and associated fever make ankylosing spondylitis and sacroiliitis less likely.

152. B (S&F ch115)
Decompensated heart failure is a contraindication to treatment with an anti-TNF agent as it can increase mortality. Remote history of cancer that is treated, COPD, and tobacco use are not absolute contraindications to treatment with an anti-TNF agent. The patient has been treated for latent tuberculosis so it would not be considered a contraindication to initiation of anti-TNF agent.

153. B (S&F ch115)
Sulfasalazine can result in reversible male infertility. Other notable side effects with sulfasalazine include agranulocytosis, neutropenia, and folate deficiency. The remaining medications have no effect on male fertility.

154. E (S&F ch115)
The patient has moderate steroid refractory Crohn's disease. Increasing the dose of prednisone above 60 mg is unlikely to add therapeutic benefit and may increase the risk of complications, most notably infections. The use of antibiotics, sulfasalazine, and mesalamine have little role in steroid-refractory Crohn's disease. The patient would be a candidate for anti-TNF treatment; however, latent tuberculosis and chronic hepatitis B must be ruled out prior to initiation of treatment.

155. A (S&F ch115)
The most frequent long-term toxicity of thalidomide is peripheral neuropathy, which is often reversible. It is also teratogenic, and concomitant contraception is needed.

156. C (S&F ch115)
In the setting of fat malabsorption resulting from intestinal resection, malabsorbed free fatty acids bind luminal calcium, thereby decreasing the amount of calcium available to bind oxalate. This results in an excess of oxalate that binds to sodium. Sodium oxalate is easily absorbed in the colon, resulting in hyperoxaluria and calcium oxalate stone formation.

157. B (S&F ch116)
Familial association is threefold higher among first-degree relatives of Jewish patients compared with relatives on non-Jewish patients. Familial associations generally occur in first-degree relatives. Epidemiologic studies in families with multiple affected members have demonstrated disease-type concordance rates of 75%. In UC, no consistent correlation has been observed in studies that examined disease extent. Family history is one of the most important risk factors for development of disease.

158. A (S&F ch116)
The side effects of cyclosporine limit its use in many hospitals. Side effects include gingival hyperplasia, infections, hypertension, renal insufficiency, and seizers. Low cholesterol levels are associated with increased risk of seizures in the setting of cyclosporine use; however, they are not a side effect of cyclosporine. The other side effects have not been associated with cyclosporine use.

159. E (S&F ch116)
There should be a high index of suspicion of malignancy in patients with colonic strictures, especially in the setting of long-standing disease. In addition, strictures that are located proximal to the splenic flexure are more likely to harbor malignancy. Carcinoma may not be detected on mucosal biopsies; therefore surgical resection of the stricture is advised.

160. D (S&F ch116)
This patient has type 2 peripheral arthropathy, which affects the small joints. It is symmetric and polyarticular. It runs a course independent of disease activity. Fever is not a common component of this peripheral arthropathy. HLA-B27 positivity is found in most patients with ankylosing spondylitis but is not associated with peripheral arthropathy. Of note, type 1 peripheral arthropathy is pauciarticular, affects large joints, and parallels intestinal disease activity.

161. A (S&F ch116)
The patient is presenting with signs of primary sclerosing cholangitis (PSC). The characteristic histologic finding is the onion-skin pattern with concentric fibrosis around the small bile ducts with eventual obliteration. The findings in option B is characteristic of autoimmune hepatitis, option C is consistent with α1-antritrypsin deficiency, option D is suggestive of nonalcoholic liver disease, and option E is suggestive of primary biliary cirrhosis.

162. B (S&F ch116)
The patient is presenting with severe symptoms related to her history of ulcerative colitis and is at risk of toxic megacolon and perforation. Plain films should be ordered to evaluate for these complications. The use of high-dose glucocorticoids may mask signs of peritonitis.

163. B (S&F ch116)
The chronicity of the patient's symptoms along with the endoscopic and histologic findings are consistent with a diagnosis of IBD. Up to 75% of patients with left-sided ulcerative colitis may have periappendiceal inflammation. Despite the "skip pattern" of this type of

inflammation, the diagnosis remains ulcerative colitis. Such findings are a common reason for mislabeling UC as Crohn's disease. The histologic findings and clinical presentation is not consistent with Behçet's disease, NSAID, or infectious colitis.

164. C (S&F ch116)
Oral mesalamine therapy may place patients at slightly increased risk of reversible acute kidney injury. Routine measurements of serum creatinine level are recommended for patients on mesalamine. Mesalamine does not affect the other lab parameters.

165. A (S&F ch116)
Pouchitis is the most common complication of ileal pouch-anal anastomosis. It is seen in up to 70% of patients at 20 years post surgery. The other complications are less common and occur at the following rates: small bowel obstruction (42% by 20 years), anastomotic stricture (39% by 20 years), abscess (16% by 20 years), and fistula (14% by 20 years).

166. D (S&F ch116)
The histologic findings are characteristic of high-grade dysplasia. The nuclei are stratified to the surface and there is marked increase in nuclear pleomorphism. The finding of high-grade dysplasia is an indication for surgery due to the high risk of concurrent colonic malignancy or development of colonic malignancy.

167. B (S&F ch116).
The patient has been on high-dose steroids for an extended period of time and is at risk for osteonecrosis. Most cases involve the hips, but knees and shoulders may be affected as well. IBD-related arthropathy would be less likely given that his IBD appears to be in remission. Osteoporosis does not cause swelling or pain. The presentation is not typical for rheumatoid arthritis or fibromyalgia.

168. C (S&F ch116)
An open-label, randomized multicenter trial comparing infliximab to cyclosporine in acute severe UC showed similar clinical response in 1 week (85.4% with cyclosporine arm vs. 85.7% with infliximab) and similar response in 3 months (18% with cyclosporine vs. 21% with infliximab). Therefore, the choice between infliximab and cyclosporine should be individualized and based on local expertise. Most adverse events related to cyclosporine are dose-dependent, and doses less than 4 mg/kg are desirable. Low cholesterol levels in the setting of cyclosporine use can increase the risk of seizures. Doses of 2 mg/kg are as effective as 4 mg/kg in clinical response rates, time to response, and short-term colectomy rates. Patients who fail either cyclosporin or infliximab should undergo colectomy and not receive the other drug, as this sequential therapy is associated with increased risk of adverse events.

169. A (S&F ch116)
UC patients with documented clinical remission may develop acute infectious colitis. Such patients may present with symptoms that mimic a UC flare. Endoscopic appearance alone does not distinguish infectious proctosigmoiditis from active UC, with the exception of pseudomembranes that are associated with *C. difficile* infection. Stool tests for infections should be ordered in patients with symptoms of UC flare.

170. D (S&F ch116)
The patient's symptoms, which include abdominal pain and weight loss, and the abnormal blood work suggest that there is additional disease elsewhere in the GI tract that has yet to be identified. The colonoscopic examination was limited to the colon, and no ileal findings were reported. The concern for Crohn's disease exists, therefore imaging of the small bowel should be performed to evaluate for small bowel Crohn's disease.

171. B (S&F ch116)
Olsalazine is a 5-ASA dimer linked by an azo bond. Balsalazide consists of a 5-ASA monomer linked to an inactive molecule. Sulfasalazine consists of 5-ASA linked to a sulfapyridine ring. Mesalamine preparations contain 5-ASA monomers (see figure).

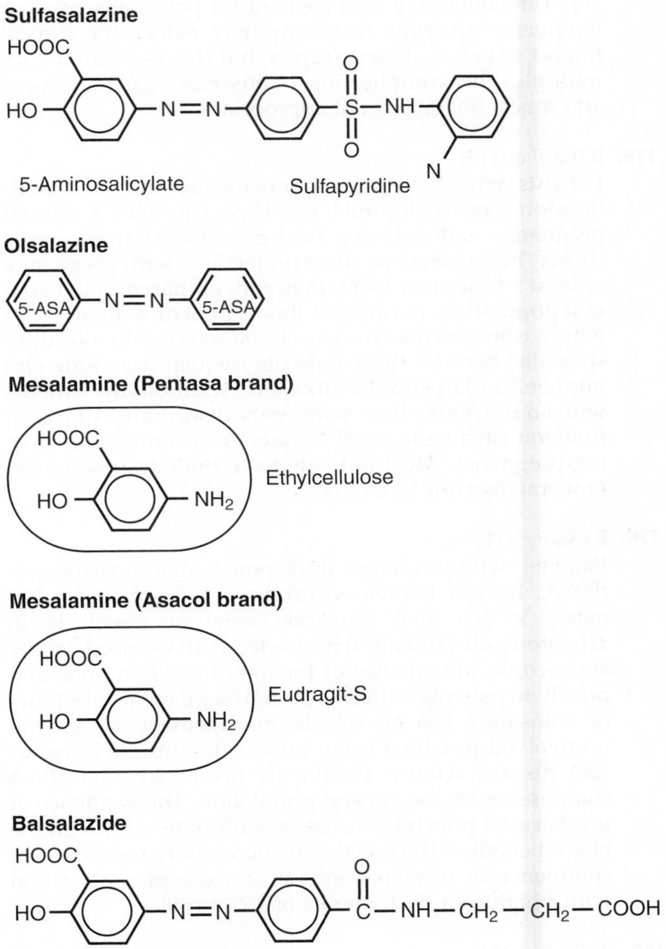

Sulfasalazine
HOOC
HO
N=N
O
S—NH
O
N
5-Aminosalicylate
Sulfapyridine

Olsalazine
5-ASA —N=N— 5-ASA

Mesalamine (Pentasa brand)
HOOC
HO
NH_2
Ethylcellulose

Mesalamine (Asacol brand)
HOOC
HO
NH_2
Eudragit-S

Balsalazide
HOOC
HO—N=N—C(=O)—NH—CH_2—CH_2—COOH

Figure for answer 171.

172. B (S&F ch116)
The patient has typical features of acute pouchitis. Antibiotics are the first-line treatment. Ciprofloxacin and metronidazole are both treatment options; however, ciprofloxacin is more appropriate in this patient who drinks alcohol and will likely not tolerate metronidazole. Topical and oral mesalamine are second-line options for acute pouchitis. VSL#3 is a probiotic that was shown to decrease the recurrence of pouchitis.

173. D (S&F ch116)
Infants born to women who received infliximab during pregnancy have detectable levels of anti-TNF. Therefore, all live vaccines should be withheld during the first 6 months of life. The only live vaccine given routinely to infants during this age period is rotavirus. All the other vaccines listed (diphtheria, MMR, PCV, Hib) are inactivated vaccines. Of note, BCG (bacille Calmette-Guérin) is another live vaccine that is selectively given to special high-risk groups, and should be avoided.

174. E (S&F ch117)
The CT scan shows a postsurgical peripouch abscess. This would best be managed by attempted placement of a CT-guided percutaneous drain. If not feasible, laparotomy and drainage would be the next step in management. Intravenous antibiotics and bowel rest should be the initial management in a patient with a phlegmon, but is not the definitive management for pelvic abscesses. A temporary diverting ileostomy may reduce the clinical impact of pelvic abscess/sepsis, but it is associated with multiple other complications. Conservative management and repeat imaging is not appropriate.

175. D (S&F ch117)
Patients who have had a proctocolectomy and end-ileostomy or Kock pouch can expect to have a normal pregnancy and delivery. Ileal pouch-anal anastomosis (IPAA) has a negative effect on fertility, with pregnancy at least 5 times less likely to occur compared to the general population. Because of this, a patient with an IPAA who wishes to conceive should be referred to a fertility specialist because these patients frequently require clomiphene and in vitro fertilization. Additionally, patients with an IPAA may have temporary disturbance of pouch function (increased stool frequency, incontinence) during pregnancy. Most patients have three to nine bowel movements after IPAA.

176. B (S&F ch117)
Patients who undergo ileal pouch-anal anastomosis (IPAA) have a known occurrence of dysplasia/malignancy in the anal transition zone or pouch itself. Therefore, all patients who undergo IPAA need yearly endoscopic surveillance of the anal transition zone and pouch. In patients with UC, partial/segmental colectomy or colostomy has no role in management, as leaving uninvolved proximal colon intact often results in recurrent disease activity. Fertility is decreased after IPAA compared with the general population. The incidence of postsurgical pouchitis increases with time. Although the major benefit of IPAA is that it successfully restores fecal continence in most patients, it is a complex operation with a high complication rate of 25% to 30%.

177. B (S&F ch117)
Recurrence of pouchitis after treatment of the first episode is treated with a second course of the same therapy that was used for initial treatment. Metronidazole is another treatment option for acute pouchitis. However, because the patient responded initially to ciprofloxacin, there is no need to switch to metronidazole. In addition, ciprofloxacin is more tolerated than metronidazole. VSL#3 is recommended for the prevention of recurrent pouchitis, rather than treatment of the acute episode. Treatment with prednisone or mesalamine enemas should be tried if symptoms do not respond to antibiotic therapy.

178. C (S&F ch117)
There has been increasing experience with the ileal pouch-anal anastomosis (IPAA) over the last 3 decades. This procedure removes the entire colonic and rectal mucosa, while preserving a functional anal sphincter. IPAA has excellent outcomes when performed by experienced surgeons. Brooke ileostomy (conventional end ileostomy) or continent ileostomy are alternative surgical options. Ileorectal anastomosis is less preferred because it leaves potentially diseased mucosa in situ, resulting in poor anastomotic healing. It could be considered in patients who do not wish to undergo an IPAA, or in patients with Crohn's disease and minimal or no rectal inflammation. Loop ileostomy is used to provide temporary fecal diversion but is not a main treatment option for ulcerative colitis.

179. A. (S&F ch118)
Superior mesenteric artery embolus (SMAE) is responsible for 30% of acute mesenteric ischemia (AMI) episodes. Emboli often arise from a left atrial or ventricular mural thrombus. CT angiography reveals a filling defect with nearly complete obstruction of flow. This patient has an embolus, in the proximal SMA, which is classified as major emboli (proximal to the origin of the ileocolic artery). Given that this patient has peritoneal signs and a major embolus exploratory laparotomy is mandatory. Thrombolytic therapy or anticoagulation with heparin is used in the management of mesenteric vein thrombosis, or minor arterial occlusion or embolus, but is not indicated for major embolus with signs of peritonitis. Repeat angiogram can be performed after an intervention is done but would not be the first step in management of SMAE. Endovascular therapy is not appropriate in patients with signs of peritonitis.

180. D. (S&F ch118)
The patient's history of postprandial abdominal pain and weight loss is common for chronic mesenteric ischemia. Patients with this condition also often have a history of coronary, cerebrovascular, or peripheral arterial insufficiency. Prominent collaterals between the SMA and other major splanchnic vessels indicate chronic SMA occlusion. Inadequate filling of the SMA with no collaterals in patients with acute abdominal pain indicates an acute arterial occlusion. Pancreatic interstitial edema is seen in acute pancreatitis, which would present with acute onset epigastric abdominal pain accompanied by nausea and vomiting. Nonspecific elevations of amylase are seen in nonpancreatic disorders. Although malignancy or gallstones cannot be completely excluded, the patient's risk factors and symptoms of sitophobia make chronic mesenteric ischemia more likely.

181. B (S&F ch118)
Current recommendations for the duration of anticoagulation in acute mesenteric vein thrombosis are based on practice rather than evidence-based data. The general recommendation is lifelong treatment with warfarin if the patient has an underlying hypercoagulable state. However, if no underlying thrombophilic state is documented, a 3 to 6 months course of therapy is adequate. If the patient had a history of GI bleeding, an argument could be made to withhold anticoagulation. There is no need to repeat the EGD in this patient.

182. A (S&F ch118)
Behçet's disease is characterized by recurrent oral and genital ulcers, ocular involvement, (recurrent iritis, chorioretinitis, uveitis, episcleritis) and skin lesions, such as erythema

nodosum. GI disease is present in 50% of patients. The most common GI symptoms are abdominal pain, diarrhea, and bleeding. Inflammatory bowel disease can manifest as in the case presented in the question, except for genital ulcers, which are not associated with IBD. Buerger's disease (thromboangiitis obliterans) involves medium-sized and small peripheral arteries and veins. Patients commonly present with foot claudication that can progress to severe ischemia. Henoch-Schönlein purpura is a result of immunoglobulin immune complexes deposited within the small vessels of the skin, GI tract, joints, and kidneys and is often preceded by an upper respiratory infection. The classic triad consists of palpable purpura, arthritis, and abdominal pain. Polyarteritis nodosa is a necrotizing vasculitis of medium-sized and small arteries with aneurysm formation at branch points. Abdominal symptoms, most commonly abdominal pain, are reported in up to half of the patients.

183. C (S&F ch118)
This patient presents with typical symptoms of chronic mesenteric ischemia (CMI) and unexplained weight loss. Angiography shows occlusive involvement of at least 2 of the 3 major arteries, which necessitates revascularization. Surgical revascularization has been the traditional method of therapy for patients with CMI, but PTMA alone or with stent insertion can be used as primary or secondary therapy as well. However, it is recommended that patients with CMI who are young and otherwise healthy should undergo surgical intervention given the decreased frequency of restenosis and better long-term patency rates.

184. D (S&F ch118)
The colonoscopic image shows subepithelial hemorrhage and edema. This finding, combined with the clinical presentation of acute abdominal pain and rectal bleeding, is highly suspicious for colonic ischemia (CI). An algorithm for management of CI is shown (see figure). After CI is diagnosed and other etiologies excluded (e.g., *C. difficile*), the patient is initially managed conservatively with intravenous fluids, antibiotics, and kept NPO for 48 to 72 hours. This clinically stable patient is not demonstrating signs of peritonitis; therefore, there is no indication for surgery at this time. Clinical deterioration and/or development of signs of peritonitis require emergent surgical intervention. Intravenous methylprednisolone is not helpful in colonic ischemia, and there is low suspicion for Crohn's disease, for which this treatment would be beneficial. CT scan may confirm the diagnosis and show the extent of involvement, but it is not required and is not the next best step in management. There is no added yield of a barium enema, and it should be avoided in severe cases of colonic ischemia.

185. D (S&F ch118)
The image shows the "single stripe sign," which refers to the finding of a single linear ulceration or erythema oriented along the longitudinal axis of the colon. This finding combined with the clinical presentation of abdominal pain and bleeding is highly suggestive of ischemic colitis as the underlying etiology. Colon cancer usually presents with a mass rather than a longitudinal linear ulcer. Acute infectious colitis and Crohn's disease are possible, although endoscopic appearance is usually of a more circumferential bowel involvement. Segmental colitis associated with diverticulitis presents with circumferential erythema with or without ulcerations in areas adjacent to diverticulosis. There is no diverticulosis in the figure.

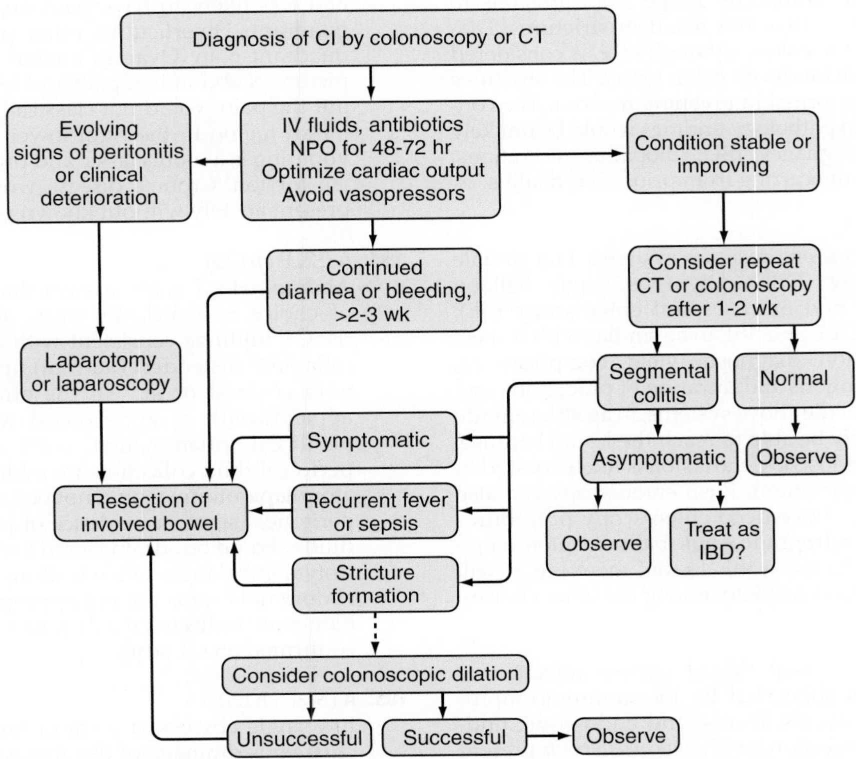

Figure for answer 184. IBD, Inflammatory bowel disease; IV, intravenous; NPO, nothing by mouth.

186. B (S&F ch119)
A concentric stricture with a thin septae is consistent with NSAID-induced diaphragm disease. Crohn's disease is on the differential of small bowel ulcerations and strictures; however, Crohn's disease typically affects the distal ileum, and this patient denied chronic symptoms of diarrhea or abdominal pain. Although her age and comorbidities put her at risk for mesenteric ischemia resulting in ulcerations, an ischemic small bowel ulceration would not present as a focal ulceration with a diaphragm. Additionally, a malignant ulceration would not have this classic appearance of diaphragm formation on capsule endoscopy.

187. E (S&F ch119)
The ileum is the most common location of nonspecific ulcerations (78% in a series of 59 patients from the Mayo Clinic). Perforation of these lesions occurs more commonly in the jejunum.

188. A (S&F ch119)
This patient most likely has nonspecific or idiopathic small intestinal ulcerations because she does not have clinical and pathologic features suggestive of inflammatory bowel disease. She is not on NSAIDs, which could cause small intestinal ulcerations. Due to the symptomatic nature of these ulcers, the next step would be segmental intestinal resection. Prednisone has not been used for treatment of idiopathic or nonspecific ulcerations. Adding vitamin C is unlikely to improve her anemia significantly and would not address the cause of chronic occult blood loss. Referral to oncology is not indicated because there is no evidence of malignancy based on pathology. Given that the patient is symptomatic, it would not be appropriate to monitor with repeat colonoscopy.

189. A (S&F ch119)
Findings in NSAID colopathy range from erosions to ulcers, which may or may not result in strictures. Diaphragm disease of the colon, although rare, is considered diagnostic for NSAID-induced colon injury. The strictures are concentric with normal intervening mucosa. The concentric strictures and pathology findings would be unlikely to be found in malignancy, IBD, idiopathic ulcerations, microscopic colitis, or scarring from prior diverticulitis.

190. D (S&F ch119)
There are three deep enteroscopy systems: Fuji double balloon enteroscopy (DBE), Olympus single balloon enteroscopy (SBE) and Spirus spiral enteroscopy (SE). One review found DBE and SBE to be similar with respect to depth of insertion, diagnostic yield, complications, therapeutic interventions and duration of procedure, and sedation. All three of the above systems, in an anterograde fashion, would likely be able to reach the lesion because, based on capsule endoscopy, the lesion is likely located in the proximal or midjejunum. Push enteroscopy can also be attempted if the above deep enteroscopy procedures are not available. A retrograde single balloon enteroscopy would not be able to reach this lesion; therefore, it will have the lowest diagnostic yield among the other choices.

191. A (S&F ch119)
This patient presents with *Mycobacterium* infection of the small bowel as suggested by his immunocompromised state, night sweats, fevers, and endoscopic findings. Small bowel infections with *Mycobacterium* present with nodular, thickened folds along with ulceration. Pathology reveals villous atrophy, increased epithelial lymphocytes, PAS (+) foamy macrophages, and acid-fast bacilli. It is highly unlikely that this patient presents with active Crohn's disease (noncaseating granulomas, crypt abscesses, and lymphocyte infiltrate with architectural distortion), given his marked immunocompromised state. Additionally, *Giardia* infection (villous atrophy with small sickle-shaped organisms on the surface epithelium) would not cause this endoscopic appearance or clinical presentation. *Cryptosporidium* infection (atrophic villi with neutrophilic infiltrate and round, basophilic organisms) can cause ulcerative enteritis but would clinically present with severe diarrhea. Cytomegalovirus ulcers (owl's eye inclusions) could cause melena, though it would more likely have a classic endoscopic appearance of deep serpiginous ulcers.

192. C (S&F ch119)
The patient's presentation is consistent with Meckel's diverticulum. Gastric acid hypersecretion (from ectopic gastric mucosa) is thought to play a role in mucosal ulcerations often seen with Meckel's diverticulum. No known medication, idiopathic ulceration, malignancy, or ischemic ulcer will be associated with an endoscopically visualized mucosal outpouching.

193. B (S&F ch120)
Most patients with simple appendicitis have a temperature below 100.5° F. Fevers above 100.5° F are most often associated with perforated or gangrenous appendicitis. Right lower quadrant tenderness, both voluntary and involuntary, are common findings. A variety of maneuvers exist to elicit localized right lower quadrant peritonitis, including the cough sign (presence of point tenderness with a cough), percussion tenderness, and formal elicitation of rebound tenderness. Acute pancreatitis presents with epigastric pain radiating to the back and less likely to have pain migrate to the right lower quadrant. Diverticulitis often presents with left lower quadrant pain. Ovarian torsion could present with this picture of abdominal pain and fevers in a female patient, but the pain would not classically migrate from periumbilical region to the right lower quadrant. Additionally, vomiting is a more classic and prominent feature of ovarian torsion. Crohn's disease would be less likely to be present acutely without known prior signs or symptoms.

194. A (S&F ch120)
Abdominal CT scans are considered the imaging study of choice in nonclassic cases of suspected appendicitis. CT findings consistent with appendicitis include an inflamed, distended (>6 mm) appendix that fails to fill with contrast or air. This is often accompanied by an appendicolith or appendiceal wall thickening. Periappendiceal inflammation, cecal apical thickening, and pericecal fluid collection are additional findings. Exploratory laparotomy would not be indicated unless there are peritoneal signs or evidence of perforation. Intravenous fluids should be administered to correct any fluid or electrolyte imbalances while waiting for emergent CT. Serial abdominal exams are not appropriate. Intravenous antibiotics are indicated if a diagnosis of acute appendicitis is confirmed on CT scan.

195. A (S&F ch120)
If a single abscess of 3 cm or larger is discovered, percutaneous drainage of the abscess under CT guidance is indicated. If multiple abscesses are found or the patient does not improve within 24 to 48 hours of conservative

therapy, operative drainage is recommended. Intravenous fluids and antibiotics should be initiated, but given the size of the abscess, percutaneous drainage is the definitive management. Colonoscopy may be indicated in the future once the acute issues resolve to assess for Crohn's disease, but endoscopy has no role in the acute management of a periappendiceal abscess. Finally, a right hemicolectomy would not be indicated for management of a periappendiceal abscess.

196. B (S&F ch120)
This patient has features suggestive of acute appendicitis. The obturator sign is elicited by internally and externally rotating the flexed right hip. Pain is thought to arise when the inflamed pelvic appendix irritates the adjacent obturator internus muscle. The psoas sign is elicited by having a supine patient actively flex the right hip against resistance or by the examiner flexing and extending the patient's right hip with the patient in the left lateral decubitus position. Pain with these maneuvers is thought to result from irritation of the underlying psoas muscle by an inflamed retroperitoneal appendix. Rovsing's sign is the finding of right lower quadrant pain during palpation of the left side of the abdomen or when left-sided rebound tenderness is elicited. McBurney's point is the point of the abdomen that is one third of the distance from the anterior superior iliac spine to the umbilicus. Deep tenderness at McBurney's point is known as McBurney's sign.

197. C (S&F ch121)
An important initial consideration in the management of diverticulitis is the decision to initiate management as an outpatient or inpatient basis. Hospitalization should be considered if the patient is unable to tolerate oral intake, has signs of peritonitis, fevers, or has failed outpatient therapy. Antibiotic therapy should be directed at colonic bacteria, especially gram-negative rods and anaerobic bacteria. Given this patient's inability to tolerate oral intake, intravenous antibiotics should be used initially in addition to bowel rest. Commonly used antibiotic regimens include a quinolone or sulfa agent in combination with metronidazole (or clindamycin if the patient is intolerant to metronidazole), or amoxicillin/clavulanate as a single agent, for approximately 10 days.

198. A (S&F ch121)
Hinchey classification (see table at the end of the chapter) is a grading system that reflects the severity of perforation and is useful to guide patient management. Small pericolic abscesses (Hinchey stage 1) can be managed with broad-spectrum antibiotics and bowel rest as abscesses less than 3 cm often resolve with antibiotics alone. CT-guided percutaneous drainage can be complementary to surgery. If the abscess is multiloculated, anatomically inaccessible, or not resolving with percutaneous drainage, urgent surgery is indicated. This patient has a small abscess that can be conservatively managed with antibiotics and bowel rest. If the patient is unstable or clinically worsens, CT-guided drainage or surgical management may be warranted. Colonoscopy is contraindicated in the setting of acute diverticulitis with concern for perforation or abscess. Repeat imaging after antibiotics is considered on a case-by-case basis, but is not done routinely.

199. D (S&F ch121)
This patient presents with segmental colitis associated with diverticulosis (SCAD). SCAD often affects the sigmoid colon due to high incidence of diverticulosis in this area. It can mimic the clinical presentation of IBD with symptoms of left lower quadrant cramping pain, diarrhea, and rectal bleeding. Endoscopically, the sigmoid colonic mucosa shows variable degrees of erythema, friability, and erosions within the segment of diverticular disease. Biopsies may show chronic lymphocytic infiltration, cryptitis, crypt abscesses, and granulomas, making it histologically indistinguishable from IBD and ischemic colitis. Patients with SCAD generally are responsive to 5-ASA compounds. The age of this patient would be atypical for newly diagnosed IBD and, therefore, prednisone or infliximab therapy would not be indicated. In most cases, SCAD tends to be self-limited, but for patients with uncontrolled bleeding or stricture complications, sigmoid colectomy has been required. This patient is symptomatic; therefore, observation alone is not appropriate management.

200. C (S&F ch121)
Angiography is not as sensitive as nuclear scintigraphy for lower gastrointestinal bleeding (LGIB) because it detects bleeding in the rate above 0.5 mL/min. Nuclear scintigraphy (tagged RBC scan) can detect bleeding rates as low as 0.1 mL/min.

201. B (S&F ch121)
The primary advantage of angiography is accurate identification of the bleed site to direct segmental surgical resection or angiographic embolization via superselective embolization (see figures). If superselective embolization is unsuccessful and bleeding continues, a segmental colectomy should be considered. Given the patient's hemodynamic instability and the fact that her colon is not prepped, a colonoscopy would not be the next best step in management. She will likely need admission to the intensive care unit, but an embolization attempt should be made once bleeding is identified. In addition to blood transfusions, intravenous vasoconstrictors may be needed in patients who are critically ill and remain hypotensive in the intensive care unit.

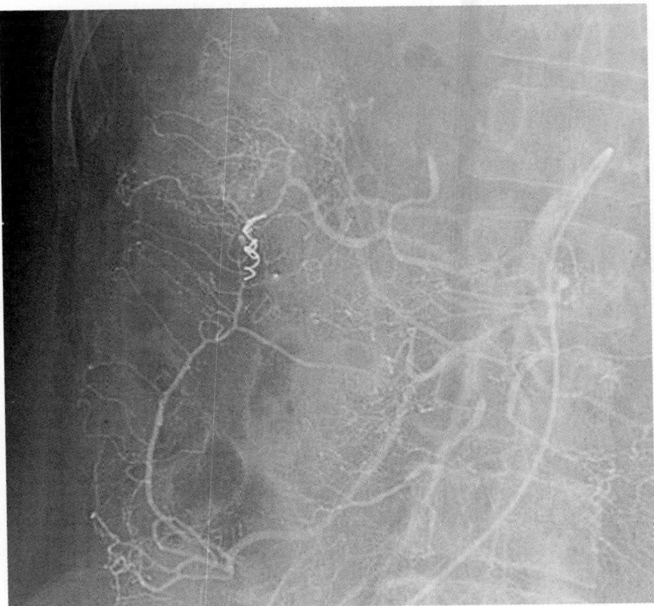

Figure for answer 201.

202. A (S&F ch121)
This patient is most likely suffering from diverticulitis. Patients with uncomplicated diverticulitis typically present with left lower quadrant abdominal pain, reflecting the propensity for this disorder to occur in the sigmoid colon. Anorexia, nausea, vomiting, and fevers also can occur. CT scan is the radiologic test of choice in patients with suspected diverticulitis. Colonoscopy should be avoided in patients with suspected acute diverticulitis due to perforation risk but should be performed 1 to 3 months after an acute episode to exclude colorectal cancer. Ultrasound and abdominal x-ray is not a good test for diverticulitis. MRI is less preferred because it is more expensive and time-consuming that CT scan.

203. C (S&F ch121)
This patient is presenting with complicated diverticulitis with colovesicular fistula, for which fecaluria is pathognomonic. CT scan would show fistula formation between the inflamed sigmoid colon and bladder resulting from extension of a diverticular phlegmon or abscess. Cystoscopy, cystography, or barium enema can also be useful in establishing a diagnosis but have no role in treatment of this pathology. The definitive management is a single-stage operative resection with primary anastomosis. Antibiotics alone would not be sufficient to treat fistula formation.

204. B (S&F ch121)
Colovesicular fistulae are the most common type of fistula in complicated diverticulitis. Colovaginal fistulae are the second most common. The other fistulae are much less common.

205. B (S&F ch122)
Bacterial gastroenteritis is the most significant risk factor for irritable bowel syndrome. This risk is enhanced in young, female patients as well as in individuals with depression. The other choices are associated with IBS, however, to a lesser degree than bacterial gastroenteritis.

206. A (S&F ch122)
There is a fourfold increased odds of celiac disease in patients presenting with irritable bowel symptoms. Therefore, serologic testing for celiac disease in a patient with abdominal pain, distention, bloating, and diarrhea is reasonable. If serology suggests celiac disease, duodenal biopsies should be performed. Antigliadin antibody should not be used as a screening test for celiac disease due to the high false positivity rates. The other IgE blood tests are not helpful for investigating the patient's symptoms.

207. D (S&F ch122)
Cognitive behavioral therapy (CBT) has been shown to lead to very good efficacy results in patients with IBS, particularly in patients with a shorter duration of symptoms. Hypnotherapy has been shown to improve symptoms in patients with diarrhea, but the data are inconsistent. Symptoms do not necessarily improve with psychological treatments, but rather patients are better able to cope with their symptoms.

208. E (S&F ch122)
The symptoms are typical of the patient's IBS flares and mucus in the stool is not uncommon in IBS. The patient has no true alarm symptoms; therefore, invasive testing is not indicated at this time whether she was pregnant or not. Stool for ova, parasites, and *C. difficile* are reasonable at this time. However, if the stool studies are negative, her symptoms persist or worsen, and she experiences bloody diarrhea, lower endoscopy may be warranted.

209. C (S&F ch122)
This patient has diarrhea-predominant irritable bowel syndrome (IBS) that is triggered by eating. Therefore, he may respond to an antispasmodic taken 30 minutes before eating to reduce intestinal peristalsis and its resulting abdominal cramping and diarrhea. Lubiprostone is approved for IBS-C and fiber can often worsen bloating symptoms. Rifaximin has been shown to be superior to placebo in nonconstipated IBS patients; however, it is second-line therapy.

210. B (S&F ch122)
This is an older woman with new onset symptoms. Therefore, the threshold for an IBS diagnosis should be high compared to a younger patient with long-standing symptoms. This woman is experiencing visible as well as palpable distention; therefore intraabdominal/pelvic pathology such as ovarian cancer should be considered. Computerized tomography is a sensitive test for evaluating for mass lesions. The utility of repeat colonoscopy is low. The patient does not have significant upper gastrointestinal symptoms. Therefore, an upper endoscopy and a gastric emptying study have little value in this setting. It would be inappropriate to do no further workup.

211. D (S&F ch122)
This patient had gastrointestinal symptoms for 2 weeks after a bacterial gastroenteritis 7 months ago. She is a young woman, which puts her a greater risk for developing postinfectious irritable bowel syndrome. Furthermore, her current symptoms are classic for IBS. She is not likely to have a *C. difficile* or *Giardiasis* infection because she was treated with metronidazole previously. Microscopic colitis is uncommon in patients younger than 40 years.

212. C (S&F ch122)
Soluble fiber starting at low dose has been shown to improve symptoms in patients with IBS compared to placebo in a meta-analysis of randomized controlled trials. However, insoluble fiber is no better than placebo. It is important to note that fiber helps with constipation in some patients, but it is not helpful for abdominal pain. In fact, it can exacerbate abdominal pain and bloating due to fermentation by intestinal microbiota and excess gas production. Fiber can be helpful for diarrhea, however, to a lesser extent than constipation symptoms.

213. A (S&F ch122)
Tricyclic antidepressants (TCAs) such a desipramine or nortriptyline have been shown to improve IBS symptoms compared to placebo. However, TCAs are constipating and, therefore, tend to be more efficacious and better tolerated in patients with diarrhea-predominant IBS. The anticholinergic affects of TCAs have been found to reduce intestinal transit and urgency symptoms. Additionally, they may reduce visceral hypersensitivity associated with abdominal pain in these patients. Loperamide and bismuth may improve the diarrhea, but they do not improve abdominal pain in patients with IBS.

214. D (S&F ch122)
Linaclotide acts on the guanylate cyclase receptors on the intestinal enterocyte thereby stimulating intestinal fluid secretion and enhancing stool passage. In randomized controlled tirals, the higher dose of 290 μL daily has been shown to reduce abdominal pain experienced by patients with IBS-C. Lubiprostone acts on intestinal chloride channel receptors to stimulate intestinal fluid secretion as well. 5-HT4 agonists (e.g., prucalopride) have been shown to be beneficial in patients with chronic constipation. However, they are not currently available for use the United States.

215. D (S&F ch122)
This is a young patient with classic IBS-C symptoms and no alarm features. Therefore, additional testing will give low yield. In fact, extensive testing to exclude the usual diseases is expensive and may yield clinically insignificant findings and reinforce abnormal illness behaviors. Furthermore, this patient has chronic symptoms (greater than 6 months) without significant risk for organic disease.

216. C (S&F ch122)
This patient meets the ROME III criteria for IBS-C. He has failed fiber as well as polyethylene glycol in the past, and his symptoms are quite troublesome. Therefore additional pharmacologic therapy is appropriate. Linaclotide acts on the guanylate cyclase receptors on the intestinal enterocyte, stimulating intestinal fluid secretion and stool movement. In randomized controlled trials, the higher dose of 290 μL daily has been shown to reduce abdominal pain and bloating experienced by patients with IBS-C. Alosetron is contraindicated in patients with constipation. Moreover, tricyclic antidepressants and antispasmodics will worsen constipation.

217. B (S&F ch122)
This patient may have slow transit constipation; however, she also exhibits symptoms of pelvic floor dysfunction (straining, pressure on lower abdomen, and relief with an enema). It is common for patients to have concomitant IBS as well as pelvic floor dysfunction. It is important to identify this from the patient history and the rectal examination. Indeed, the treatment of pelvic floor dysfunction involves pelvic floor retraining, and constipated patients may not respond to the use of laxative only. The patient has abdominal bloating but pain is not a significant complaint. Therefore, she does not have IBS-C. She does not have symptoms or risk factors for colon cancer.

218. D (S&F ch122)
This patient has severe IBS symptoms, which are refractory to first- and second-line agents. Alosetron is a 5-HT3 antagonist, which has been shown to be effective in women with severe IBS symptoms. It is available through a restricted prescribing program due to concerns for ischemic colitis. Alosetron is contraindicated in patients with constipation. Fiber will not help her symptoms. In fact, it may worsen the abdominal pain due to bloating. There is insufficient data to recommend retreatment with rifaximin or probiotic in this setting.

219. C (S&F ch122)
History of depression is a risk factor for postinfectious IBS in patients that experience bacterial enteritis. Other risk factors include smoking, female sex, and younger age. Additionally, if the illness lasts more than 3 weeks or the organism is toxigenic, the risk of developing postinfectious IBS increases. Alcohol use is not a known risk factor for postinfectious IBS.

220. B (S&F ch122)
This patient has IBS-mixed type in which patients have alternating diarrhea and constipation. This is the most challenging form of IBS to treat. However, some patients are able to correlate IBS symptoms with specific food triggers. A low FODMAP diet is beneficial in some patients; however, it is difficult to adhere to consistently. Therefore, a food/symptom diary is usually the best way to begin life style modification. Exercise helps to prevent worsening of symptoms as well.

221. D (S&F ch122)
This patient has dyspeptic symptoms; therefore, a trial a proton-pump inhibitor would be reasonable in this patient. He does not meet the ROME III criteria for irritable bowel syndrome based on duration of symptoms, nor are his symptoms associated with change in bowel habits. Therefore the other therapies listed are not indicated. Fiber would likely make his fullness and bloating worse. The 5-HT3 antagonist is indicated for women with severe diarrhea-predominant IBS.

222. A (S&F ch122)
Long duration of gastrointestinal complaints and presence of severe psychological distress or anxiety is associated with a poorer prognosis in IBS patients. However, there is no evidence of increased mortality in IBS. Additionally, the diagnosis is durable at long-term follow-up studies.

223. D (S&F ch122)
The establishment of a strong physician-patient relationship is crucial to providing good care to patients suffering with IBS. A relationship of trust and acknowledgment can improve clinical outcomes in these patients. Many patients go from "doctor shopping" seeking medical care because some health care providers are not comfortable making the diagnosis of IBS and/or are unable to explain the diagnosis to patients. This leads to frustration and dissatisfaction on the part of the physician as well as the patient. Education has been shown to be beneficial in patients with IBS in randomized controlled trials.

224. B (S&F ch123)
The patient's clinical presentation is consistent with acute small bowel obstruction (SBO). Findings on plain film in a patient with SBO include air-filled distended loops of small bowel and a decompressed colon. Intraabdominal adhesions from previous abdominal surgery are the most common cause of SBO. In fact, there is a 90% chance that patients will develop adhesions after abdominal surgery, particularly lower abdominal or pelvic surgeries. This patient had a hysterectomy. Crohn's disease stricture, intussusception, and radiation-induced injury can lead to mechanical small bowel obstruction but are less common than intraabdominal adhesions.

225. E (S&F ch123)
This patient has a small bowel obstruction due to a gallstone (gallstone ileus). Gallstone ileus may be difficult to diagnose due to the movement of the stone within the small bowel. It is particularly difficult to diagnose in the elderly, although it is more common in this population. Pneumobilia is one the most common radiographic

findings due to the presence of a biliary-enteric fistula leading to the stone entering the small bowel. Treatment is emergent enterolithotomy. Cholecystectomy should be performed electively after the stone is removed.

226. C (S&F ch123)
This patient's clinical symptoms and radiographic findings are consistent with a cecal volvulus. Patients typically are younger than patients with sigmoid volvulus and have a history of constipation and previous abdominal surgery. The plain film reveals the cecum in the left upper quadrant. Treatment is right hemicolectomy with primary ileocolic anastomosis. Endoscopic decompression or sigmoid resection in the setting of strangulation is the treatment for sigmoid volvulus.

227. E (S&F ch123)
Over half of all cases of colonic obstruction are due to adenocarcinoma of the colon. Most of the obstructing lesions are distal to the splenic flexure due to smaller luminal diameter and the need for solid stool passage. Volvulus (sigmoid or cecal) and benign stricturing (<10%) from diverticulitis are also common causes of colonic obstruction.

228. D (S&F ch123)
Midgut volvulus is caused by the inadequate counterclockwise rotation of the midgut loop around the superior mesenteric artery. This results in the small bowel being located to the right of the midline, and the colon is located in the left abdomen. Most cases (90%) are detected in the first year of life. Patients present with clinical signs of obstruction and often, ischemia. The mortality is high; therefore, early recognition and surgical intervention is key.

229. C (S&F ch124)
This patient has classic postoperative ileus likely from the combination of anesthesia, opiates, and immobility. The best treatment is decompression with a nasogastric tube to alleviate symptoms until intestinal motility recovers. If possible, it may be necessary to reduce the frequency and dose of the opiates the patient is receiving. However, it is not usually feasible to hold opiates completely. Neither colectomy nor colonoscopy is indicated in postoperative ileus. Intravenous neostigmine is indicated for cases of acute colonic pseudoobstruction that do not respond to conservative therapy.

230. C (S&F ch124)
This patient has signs and symptoms of intestinal pseudo-obstruction. She does not have evidence of an autoimmune or metabolic disorder. The most definitive way to diagnose visceral neuromyopathies is by full thickness tissue biopsy. These are characterized by an intense infiltration of CD3-positive, CD4, and CD8 lymphocytes in the myenteric plexus. Enteroscopy will be nondiagnostic due to the superficial nature of the biopsies. The imaging modalities listed will not yield a specific etiology of the intestinal dysmotility.

231. A (S&F ch124)
This patient has a scleroderma, which is a systemic autoimmune disease that commonly affects the gastrointestinal system. This patient has symptoms suggesting gastric, small bowel as well as colonic involvement. She most likely has small bowel dysmotility causing intestinal dilation and small intestinal bacterial overgrowth (SIBO). A breath test can be done to document SIBO, however, and empiric trial of metronidazole is also reasonable. The patient is already on a maximum dose of metoclopramide, and increasing the dose beyond 10 mg four times daily is unsafe and will not improve her symptoms. Loperamide may help with the patient's diarrhea, but it will not address the other symptoms of nausea and bloating. Bile acid resin is helpful in cases of mild bile acid malabsorption resulting in chronic diarrhea but will not improve diarrhea and bloating in this case. Switching from metoclopramide to erythromycin will not improve her diffuse intestinal dysmotility and symptoms resulting from suspected SIBO.

232. B (S&F ch124)
The biopsy reveals the classic appearance of amyloid seen in patients with secondary amyloidosis. Using the Congo red stain, this amorphous material appears reddish brown under white light examination. Amyloidosis is present in 7% to 21% of individuals with rheumatoid arthritis. The treatment for this patient is to manage the underlying disease, but also, antidiarrheal medications may help reduce episodes and improve quality of life. The patient does not have abdominal pain; thus she does not meet the clinical criteria for irritable bowel syndrome. The colon biopsies are not consistent with the other choices.

233. E (S&F ch124)
Acute pseudoobstruction is characterized by diffuse colonic dilation, typically more severe on the right side. The risks for developing acute pseudo-obstruction include hospitalized and institutionalized patients, surgery, the presence of multiple comorbidities, and certain medications. Neostigmine has been shown in randomized controlled trials to have an initial response rate of 60% to 90% in patients with acute pseudoobstruction and should be tried before endoscopic decompression. Nasogastric tube decompression will not be helpful as the dilation is in the colon. This patient does not have significant amounts of stool in the colon; therefore, a bowel regimen is not likely to improve dilation.

234. C (S&F ch124)
Chagas' disease is caused by the parasite *T. cruzi*. It has an acute phase resulting in fever, lymphadenopathy, and other systemic manifestations. The chronic phase of the disease mainly results in cardiomegaly and gastrointestinal involvement. Chagas' disease is the most common cause of acquired megacolon worldwide, although most cases are described in South America. Diabetes mellitus is increasingly common in the United States; however, it does not commonly cause megacolon. Megacolon is a complication of *C. difficile*; however, most patients respond to a 10- to 14-day course of antibiotics, and it is not commonly found in developing areas around the world.

235. D (S&F ch124)
This patient is at risk for chronic radiation changes given the history of radiation treatment 10 years ago. The more typical endoscopic findings include atrophy and scarring of the smooth muscle resulting in luminal narrowing and the development of telangiectasias. The other choices imply a more acute inflammatory process.

236. A (S&F ch124)
Systemic sclerosis is a systemic disorder that results in increased deposition of collagen and other connective

tissue components, leading to thickening and fibrosis of the intestinal mucosa. Gastrointestinal motility is affected in many ways, including absence or hypomotility of the interdigestive MMC, low-amplitude clusters of propagated and nonpropagated contractions, and a prolonged MMC phase. Normal amplitude but delayed postprandial contractions, and uncoordinated bursts of nonpropagated contractions are motility alterations that occur as a result of diabetic gastropathy and enteropathy.

237. A (S&F ch126)
In average-risk patients, asymptomatic persons with no adenomas at baseline colonoscopy, repeat colonoscopy within 5 years detects an adenoma in approximately 16% to 27% and an AAP in approximately 1% to 2.4%. Patients who had one or two tubular adenomas smaller than 10 mm were no more likely to have advanced neoplasia than patients with negative baseline colonoscopies. This risk is lower than that in healthy patients aged 50 years or older undergoing their first screening colonoscopy. Approximately 27% to 32% of such individuals will have an adenoma, and 6% to 10% will have an AAP.

238. A (S&F ch126)
It is believed that most adenomas arise from an initial loss of *APC* gene function, and for that to happen, epithelial cells must lose the function of both *APC* alleles (2 hits). Mutations in DNA MMR genes result in microsatellite instability (MSI), which is seen in approximately 85% of Lynch syndrome colon cancers and 15% of sporadic colon cancers. Mutations in K-*ras*, loss of function of DCC, and allelic deletion of chromosome 17p, (at the locus that contains the *TP53* gene), contribute to later steps in colon cancer carcinogenesis.

239. D (S&F ch126)
Calcium supplements have been shown in 2 randomized placebo-controlled phase III studies to reduce adenoma recurrence by approximately 19% to 34%. Even though diet high in fiber has been shown to be protective in epidemiologic studies, prospective studies failed to demonstrate this protective effect. Four classes of chemopreventive compounds have been shown to be protective against colon adenomas or cancers: NSAIDs, calcium, HRT, and selenium. Of these, NSAIDs, including aspirin, are the most well established. The adverse side effects of HRT outweigh the beneficial chemopreventive effects of these agents, and they are not routinely recommended. Smoking and moderate to heavy alcohol use were found to increase the risk of colon adenomas in asymptomatic male veteran population undergoing screening colonoscopy.

240. C (S&F ch126)
A syndrome of secretory diarrhea combined with water and electrolyte depletion has occasionally been observed in patients with villous adenomas. These tumors are usually larger than 3 to 4 cm in diameter and are almost always located in the distal colon. Secretory villous adenomas have a net secretion of water and sodium and an exaggerated secretion of potassium. The diarrhea is not related to paraneoplastic hormonal secretion.

241. E (S&F ch126)
Complete endoscopic removal of an adenoma with noninvasive carcinoma is curative. Both colorectal carcinoma in situ and intramucosal carcinoma are noninvasive lesions without metastatic potential. This is due to the fact that lymphatics are not present in the colonic mucosa above the level of the muscularis mucosae. Follow-up examination in 3 years is appropriate. Rectal ultrasound and CT scan are indicated for staging invasive adenocarcinoma of the rectum. Repeat colonoscopy in 2 months is appropriate after piecemeal endoscopic resection of large sessile polyps to ensure complete resection.

242. C (S&F ch126)
Important measures of high-quality colonoscopy include adequacy of bowel preparation, cecal intubation rate, withdrawal time, and adenoma detection rate. A large study showed that adenoma detection rate was 28.3% among endoscopists with a withdrawal time of 6 or more minutes compared with 11.8% when the withdrawal time was less than 6 minutes. A withdrawal time of ≥6 minutes is recommended to maximize detection of adenomas. Current guidelines suggest that cecal intubation rates should be over 90% for all colonoscopies and over 95% in screening colonoscopies. The recommended adenoma detection rates are ≥15% in women and ≥25% in men. Advanced imaging modalities, such as NBI and chromoendoscopy, are not recommended for colonoscopic screening in an average-risk population.

243. C (S&F ch126)
A summary of a recent consensus statement for postpolypectomy surveillance guidelines is shown in the table at the end of the chapter. In this patient, the surveillance is determined by the presence of tubular adenomas. Current guidelines suggest 3-year follow-up if 3 or more adenomas are found.

244. A (S&F ch126)
Sessile serrated polyps/adenoma progress to colorectal cancer via a separate molecular pathway that involves increased methylation of CpG islands. This hypermethylation results in decreased expression of DNA mismatch repair genes, which can lead to microsatellite instability (MSI). Mutations or loss of the *APC* gene lead to colonic adenomas in patients with familial adenomatous polyposis, as well as in sporadic adenomas. Germline mutations in DNA mismatch repair genes (MMR) is seen in Lynch syndrome. Inheritance of a mutated BER gene (e.g., *MUTYH*, also known as *MYH*) is responsible for a type of attenuated adenomatous polyposis. Germline mutations of the *STK11/LKB1*, a serine-threonine kinase gene on chromosome 19, are associated with Peutz-Jeghers syndrome.

245. C (S&F ch126)
The recommended surveillance colonoscopy postresection of sessile serrated polyp(s) less than 10 mm with no dysplasia is 5 years, whereas it is 3 years if there is dysplasia, size greater than 10 mm, or if it is a traditional serrated adenoma. If the patient is found to have serrated polyposis syndrome then the recommended surveillance colonoscopy is 1 year (see table at the end of the chapter).

246. A (S&F ch126)
Juvenile polyps are hamartomatous mucosal tumors that consist of an excess lamina propria and dilated cystic glands. Single juvenile polyps have no malignant potential and do not recur after resection. Multiple juvenile polyps in the setting of juvenile polyposis syndrome are associated with increased risk of colon cancer. Rectal juvenile polyps can prolapse during defecation and can lead to rectal bleeding. Therefore, removal of these polyps is recommended.

247. B (S&F ch126)
The development of gastric adenocarcinoma in patients with familial adenomatous polyposis (FAP) is estimated to be 0.5%. Most of gastric polyps in FAP are fundic gland polyps. Gastric adenomas occur in approximately 5% of FAP patients. There is a 4% to 12% lifetime incidence of duodenal cancer (mostly periampullary). Development of duodenal carcinoma is rare in patients younger than 30 years old. Patients with low polyp burden are at a lower risk of duodenal cancer, and EGD could be repeated every 3 to 5 years.

248. B (S&F ch126)
This case describes a serious complication of the adenomatous polyposis syndromes, namely, the development desmoid tumors. Risk factors for developing desmoid tumors include a family history of desmoid tumors, abdominal surgery, and *APC* mutation site (distal to codon 1444). It is not particularly associated with the Turcot variant of familial adenomatous polyposis (FAP). Desmoid tumors seem to occur more often in women than men. The absolute risk of desmoid tumors in FAP patients is around 2.5/1000 person-years. Radiotherapy is appropriate for patients with small and accessible tumors; however, most tumors involve the mesentery, which makes radiotherapy impractical in most patients.

249. B (S&F ch126)
Although surgery is the only reasonable option for colonic polyposis in familial adenomatous polyposis, the timing and extent of surgery are important clinical considerations. Any rectal mucosa that is not resected is at risk for developing carcinoma (approximately 1% per year). Young women are advised about the risk of decreased fecundity following proctocolectomy and ileal pouch-anal anastomosis (IPAA), and they may elect to undergo primary subtotal colectomy with ileorectal anastomosis (which is not associated with decreased fecundity), with plans to convert to IPAA after they are finished with child-bearing. After restorative proctocolectomy and IPAA, the ileal pouch needs to be monitored for the future development of adenomas and, very rarely, carcinoma.

250. B (S&F ch126)
Mutations of the *MUTYH* (also called *MYH*) gene are a common cause of the multiple colorectal adenoma phenotype. Around 1% of the general population is heterozygous for an *MUTYH* mutation. *MUTYH*-associated polyposis is an autosomal-recessive disorder. In patients with 15 to 100 adenomas, up to 30% have germline *MUTYH* mutations. Risks of gastric cancer and duodenal adenomas appear to be increased in patients with *MUTYH* mutations. It is recommended that patients with biallelic *MUTYH* mutations undergo a colonoscopy every 2 years, starting at age 18 to 20 years. Monoallelic mutations are not associated with increased risk of colon cancer.

251. A (S&F ch126)
Cronkhite-Canada syndrome is an acquired nonfamilial syndrome characterized by the GI hamartomatous polyposis, skin pigmentation, alopecia, and nail dystrophy. Patients may present with chronic diarrhea, weight loss, abdominal pain, and complications of malnutrition. GI polyps are found in 52% to 96% of patients. Histologically, they show hamartomatous changes similar to the juvenile (retention) polyps. However, unlike juvenile polyposis, the mucosa between polyps is histologically abnormal, with edema, congestion, and inflammation. Serrated polyposis syndrome (SPS) is characterized by multiple colonic serrated polyps and increased risk for colon cancer. Cowden's disease is associated with GI hamartomatous polyps associated with extraintestinal manifestations, such as orocutaneous hamartomas, fibrocystic disease and cancer of the breast, nontoxic goiter, and thyroid cancer. GI symptoms are uncommon. Bannayan-Ruvalcaba-Riley syndrome is a rare autosomal-dominant syndrome of hamartomatous GI polyposis, macrocephaly, developmental delay, and pigmented spots on the penis. Attenuated familial adenomatous polyposis (FAP) is associated with fewer adenomatous polyps compared to classic FAP. It is not associated with hamartomatous polyposis or skin and nail changes.

252. A (S&F ch126)
This patient has serrated polyposis syndrome (SPS), which is associated with multiple serrated polyps in the colon. The World Health Organization definces SPS as follows: (1) at least 5 serrated polyps proximal to the sigmoid colon, with at least 2 larger than 10 mm; or (2) any number of serrated polyps occurring proximal to the sigmoid colon in a patient with a first-degree relative with SPS; or (3) more than 20 serrated polyps of any size distributed throughout the colon. Some features of this syndrome (younger age of onset, family history of colorectal cancer) are suggestive of an inherited syndrome; however, a causative germline mutation has not yet been identified. Around 50% of patients have a family history of colon cancer. SPS is not associated with gastroduodenal polyps. Surgery (segmental colectomy) is recommended when colorectal cancer is diagnosed. It is recommended that first-degree relatives of SPS patients begin their screening colonoscopy at age 40, or 10 years younger than the youngest affected relative.

253. B (S&F ch127)
African Americans have higher incidence and mortality rates for colorectal cancer (CRC) compared to Caucasians. CRC incidence and mortality have declined since 1985 at an average annual rate of 1.6% and 1.8%, respectively. Overall death rates from CRC declined between 1990 and 2004 by almost 30% in men and 25% in women. The incidence of CRC is higher in men than in women. Studies have shown that incidence rates have increased for cancers of the cecum, ascending colon, and sigmoid colon, and have decreased for cancers of the rectum. Many studies have demonstrated that the risk of CRC increases in populations that migrate from areas of low risk to areas of high risk. This is likely the result of changing dietary patterns, and increased obesity and smoking.

254. E (S&F ch127)
There is strong evidence that shows aspirin and other NSAIDS are protective against colon cancer. Alcohol intake is associated with increased colorectal cancer risk, especially among men. Studies of different designs have suggested that red meat consumption, smoking, and alcohol intake are associated with increased risk of colon cancer, whereas dietary fiber, calcium, and physical exercise are associated with decreased risk of colon cancer (see box at the end of the chapter).

255. B (S&F ch126 and 127)
This case represents a sporadic microsatellite unstable (MSI-high) colon cancer without mutations in the known MMR genes. These tumors arise through epigenetic mechanisms (hypermethylation of the *hMLH1* promoter) through a hypermethylator phenotype (CPG island methylator phenotype [CIMP]). This leads to the inactivation

of the *hMLH1* gene, resulting in microsatellite instability (MSI), and has been reported of 70% of sporadic MSI-high tumors. The *BRAF* gene is often mutated in sporadic MSI-high tumors, but not in tumors from patients with Lynch syndrome. MSI-high tumors are not associated with 18qLOH or *TP53* mutations. Sporadic MSI-high cancers often arise through the serrated neoplasia pathway. The other mechanism of MSI-high tumors is through germline genetic mutations in DNA MMR genes *hMLH1, hPMS1, hPMS2, hMSH2, hMSH3,* and *hMSH6.* These mutations lead to Lynch syndrome. Mutations in the base excision repair genes *(MUTYH)* is a cause of attenuated familial adenomatous polyposis.

256. D (S&F ch137)
This patient's presentation is suggestive of Lynch syndrome, also called hereditary nonpolyposis colorectal cancer (HNPCC). Synchronous tumors occur in 18% of cases, and metachronous tumors arise in 24%. HNPCC is an autosomal-dominant disorder with high penetrance. HNPCC tumors have a tendency to involve the proximal colon. Mean age of colorectal cancer diagnosis in HNPCC is 45 years. HNPCC is caused by germline mutation in mismatch repair genes (*hMLH1, hPMS1, hPMS2, hMSH2, hMSH3,* and *hMSH6*).

257. D (S&F ch127)
Mucinous colon carcinomas are biologically more aggressive and associated with worse prognosis. The size of the primary tumor in colorectal cancer does not correlate with prognosis. Exophytic or polypoid tumors are associated with a better prognosis than ulcerating tumors. Tumors that demonstrate MSI appear to have a better prognosis irrespective of age.

258. C (S&F ch126&127)
FIT uses specific antibodies to detect human globin. Because globin is degraded by digestive enzymes in the upper gastrointestinal tract, FIT detects only globin originating from the lower gastrointestinal tract; therefore, it is specific for lower gastrointestinal bleeding. FIT is not affected by diet or drugs. gFOBT (not FIT) detects heme in a fecal sample through a peroxidase reaction. This heme can originate from an upper or lower GI bleeding. Unlike gFOBT, FIT is not subject to false-negative results in the presence of high-dose vitamin C supplements, which block the peroxidase reaction. FIT is endorsed by the U.S. Preventive Services Task Force as an acceptable colorectal cancer screening test for average risk individuals; however, colonoscopy remains the method of choice for high-risk individuals (e.g., familial adenomatous polyposis, Lynch syndrome).

259. E (S&F ch127)
A colonoscopy is the best test to further evaluate a positive gFOBT. The other choices are appropriate for screening in average risk persons but not for follow-up on a positive gFOBT. U.S. Preventive Services Task Force (USPSTF) guidelines for colon cancer screening recommend against the use of in-office gFOBT on stool obtained by digital rectal examination because of low sensitivity. However, almost a third of primary care physicians report the use of in-office method of gFOBT. Nonetheless, a positive FOBT needs to be addressed, and colonoscopy is the best method for evaluation. Sigmoidoscopy is not appropriate to use after a positive FOBT. Hemoccult SENSA is more accurate than the traditional gFOBT but is not appropriate as a follow-up test of a positive gFOBT.

260. A (S&F chs126 and 27)
The Centers for Medicare and Medicaid Services (CMS) does not cover CTC screening for colorectal cancer. This is mostly due to the exclusion of CTC from the recommended tests of colon cancer screening by the USPSTF. Other societies such as the American Cancer Society and the American College of Gastroenterology, include CTC in their guidelines. CTC has lower sensitivity for polyps smaller than 10 mm compared to colonoscopy. CTC is noninvasive and does not require sedation. There is a concern about the radiation exposure from CTC.

261. A (S&F ch127)
This patient has a normal, good quality colonoscopy. Theoretically, the colonoscopy could be repeated in 10 years if there is a mortality benefit at that time and life expectance of greater than 7 years. However, given that his age would be 86 at that time, and with his multiple medical problems, a colonoscopy is unlikely to be beneficial. Routine screening is not recommended for adults 76 to 85 years of age, and it is generally recommended to stop screening in patients older than 85 years. Because colonoscopy was used as a screening modality and it was negative in this patient, there is no indication to use the other screening modalities during the next 10 years.

262. A (S&F ch126)
The mother has Lynch syndrome with confirmed MMR germline mutation. Her son also has the same mutation. In these patients, colonoscopy screening should begin at age 20 to 25, or 10 years before the youngest case in the immediate family, and repeated every 1 to 2 years. Colonoscopy is the recommended screening tool in these high-risk patients. Other screening modalities are not recommended.

263. C (S&F ch127)
Patients with colorectal cancer who have had a colon cancer resected should have colonoscopy performed 1 year after surgery. If the examination performed at 1 year is normal, then the interval before the next colonoscopy should be performed in 3 years. If that examination is normal, colonoscopy should be repeated in 5 years.

264. C (S&F ch127)
Surgical resection is the treatment of choice in patients with invasive nonmetastatic colorectal cancer (CRC). In this patient, both cancers will require wide resection, and subtotal colectomy will be needed. Total proctocolectomy could be used in some familial polyposis syndromes, but it is not appropriate in this case. Because there is no evidence of metastatic disease or locally advanced disease at this time, chemotherapy is not recommended. Preoperative chemotherapy with radiotherapy has a role in management of locally advanced rectal cancer but has no role in colon cancer.

265. D (S&F ch127)
The approach toward rectal cancers depends on the location of the lesion. Transanal excision can be performed for selected T1, N0 early-stage cancers with small (<3 cm) tumors located within 8 cm of the anal verge. More advanced lesions should be treated with transabdominal resection and total mesorectal excision. Because surgical resection is the treatment of choice for patients with invasive nonmetastatic colorectal cancer, endoscopic resection is not advised at this point, especially that this is not a pedunculated polypoid lesion. A combination of radiation

and chemotherapy is used in locally advanced rectal cancer, but this patient has a superficial T1 disease without lymph node involvement; therefore it is not indicated.

266. D. (S&F ch127)
Bevacizumab is associated with an increased risk of stroke, GI perforation, and decreased wound healing. An interval of at least 6 weeks between the last dose of bevacizumab and elective surgery is recommended. Bevacizumab is a recombinant humanized monoclonal immunoglobulin IgG1 antibody against vascular endothelial growth factor-A (VEGF-A). Bevacizumab is approved for use in combination with intravenous 5-FU–based chemotherapy as first-line treatment of patients with metastatic colorectal cancer. It is not approved for nonmetastatic colon cancer. Bevacizumab provides clinical benefits for patients with metastatic colorectal cancer, regardless of K-*ras* status. This is in contrast to cetuximab (chimeric antibody directed against epidermal growth factor receptor), which was found to be of benefit in patients with wild-type K-*ras* tumors, and not in those whose tumors expressed mutated K-*ras*.

267. A (S&F ch128)
This patient with chronic diarrhea and negative initial stool studies and celiac serology should have a colonoscopy and biopsy for further evaluation. The main indication for colonoscopy is to rule out microscopic colitis. She takes lansoprazole and NSAIDs, which have been associated with microscopic colitis. Diarrhea due to paraneoplastic syndrome is rare, and this workup should be deferred at this time. A negative serum Iga tTG is sufficient to exclude celiac disease in this patient. A duodenal biopsy could be considered if there is a very strong suspicion for celiac disease; however, other causes of diarrhea have not been ruled out yet. A CT scan is not an appropriate next step in workup and is unlikely to show an etiology for her symptoms. Urine collection for 5-hydroxyindoleacetic acid is done when there is a suspicion of carcinoid syndrome, which is less common and unlikely in this case given absent symptoms, such as flushing and palpitations.

268. D (S&F ch128)
This patient has diversion colitis based on history and biopsy findings. Diversion colitis occurs in isolated colonic segments that are not exposed to the fecal stream. The absence of fecal material results in lack of bacterial fermentation, which deprives the colonic epithelium from important fermentation metabolites (short-chain fatty acids [SCFA]). This results in mucosal inflammation, and the preferred treatment is surgical restoration of colonic continuity. SCFA enemas, 5-aminosalicylate, and hydrocortisone retention enemas could be used if symptoms are moderate to severe and if reanastomosis is not feasible. The clinical presentation is not consistent with Crohn's disease recurrence, and adding azathioprine to his current treatment regimen is not required.

269. B (S&F ch128)
This patient has pseudomelanosis coli, or what is commonly known as melanosis coli. This refers to the dark discoloration of the colonic mucosa caused by the accumulation of pigment (lipofuscin, not melanin) in macrophages within the lamina propria due to the chronic use of anthraquinone laxatives. Because there are no pigment-containing macrophages in colonic neoplasms, they are identified more easily in patients with *pseudomelansosis coli*, and biopsies should be taken from any nonpigmented area of the colon. The condition is not associated with colonic neoplasia, and it resolves within a year of stopping laxatives.

270. C (S&F ch128)
This patient has *pneumatosis coli*, which is also called *pneumatosis cystoid intestinalis* (PCI). This uncommon disorder is characterized by multiple gas-filled cysts located in the submucosa and subserosa of the intestine. Symptomatic patients (such as the one in this case) are treated with breathing high-flow oxygen for several days. Hyperbaric oxygen can be used in resistant cases. This high-flow oxygen therapy replaces hydrogen by oxygen inside the cysts and leads to reduction in their size. Surgical treatment with colonic resection is reserved for patients with complications such as intestinal obstruction and massive bleeding. It is important to distinguish PCI from pneumatosis linearis, which refers to the presence of bands of gas within the bowel wall. Pneumatosis linearis is associated with intestinal ischemia and loss of bowel viability, and prompts urgent surgery. Colonoscopy is not needed in this case because it was just performed, and the CT scan findings were typical of PCI. Discharging the patient is not appropriate because he is symptomatic. There is no role for enemas in the treatment of this condition.

271. B (S&F ch128)
This patient has colitis cystica profunda (CCP). CCP is a rare disorder characterized by the presence of mucin-filled cysts beneath the muscularis mucosa. Most cases involve the submucosa, but cases have been described where cysts are in the muscularis propria or subserosa. CCP is associated with several disorders that predispose to mucosal ulceration and inflammation, including UC, Crohn's disease, and infectious colitis. Symptoms include rectal bleeding, mucus discharge, diarrhea, abdominal pain, and rectal pain. Rarely, the patient may present with intestinal obstruction, as in the case in this question. Histologically, the submucosa is thickened by the presence of the mucus-filled cysts. Histologic examination of a juvenile polyp would show distended, mucous-filled glands, with inflammation in the lamina propria. Although rectal prolapse and solitary rectal ulcer syndrome have been associated with colitis cystica profunda, they are not associated with lesions in the sigmoid colon as seen in this case. A carcinoid tumor would have monomorphic neuroendocrine cells on histology, rather than mucin-filled cysts.

272. D (S&F ch128)
Penetration of endometrial tissue into the bowel wall could lead to partial or complete obstruction. Most women with endometrial GI endometriosis are asymptomatic. Patients with serosal implants may complain of localized tenderness, low back pain, or abdominal pain. Hematochezia is uncommon and occurs when endometrial implants penetrate to the mucosa. Mucosal biopsies are rarely helpful, and the definitive diagnosis is obtained by laparoscopy or laparotomy. Symptoms of GI involvement in endometriosis are not always cyclic and may not fluctuate with hormonal levels.

273. E (S&F ch128)
The biopsy shows disorganized crypts, reactive epithelium, and hyperplasia of the muscularis mucosa seen as smooth muscle fibers (pink) in the mucosa. The patient's clinical presentation and endoscopic and histologic

findings are typical of SRUS. This is seen in patients with chronic constipation and straining. Common symptoms include passage of mucus and blood with stool and tenesmus. Stercoral ulcers result from pressure necrosis due to impaction of hard stool. They are usually located in the proximal rectum or sigmoid colon, and histology reveals necrotic mucosa with inflammation. The clinical and histologic features in this case do not support inflammatory bowel disease or malignancy.

274. A (S&F ch129)
Fistula-in-ano is often associated with IBD. However, it may arise spontaneously. The treatment is surgical, specifically fistulotomy; however, if pus is present, seton placement helps drain the tract prior to surgery to prevent postoperative pus accumulation. Anal plugs and fibrin glue may be an option in patients who are poor surgical candidates or in whom surgery has failed.

275. C (S&F ch129)
Anal warts are seen more commonly in men who have sex with men because of the transmission of the causative agent human papilloma virus (HPV). Other risks for developing anal warts includes immunocompromised states (HIV) as well as increased number of sexual partners. Rectal cancer affects columnar mucosa, whereas HPV infects squamous mucosa. Paget disease manifests as an eczematoid plaque. Straining during defecation is a risk factor for rectal prolapse. Crohn's disease is associated with perianal fissures and fistulas.

276. B (S&F ch129)
The patient exhibits typical symptoms of levator ani syndrome (LAS). This is a functional disorder. The examination is often normal, and there is no diagnostic test for this disorder. However, the classic presentation is severe pain that last seconds to minutes occurring at night and spontaneously resolves. Coccygodynia is aching in the coccyx. LAS pain persists longer, and there is tenderness along the puborectalis muscle on rectal examination.

277. B (S&F ch129)
The patient has grade III internal hemorrhoids, which can usually be treated without surgery (65%). Band ligation is the common treatment modality at this time. The band facilitates scar formation and affixes the hemorrhoid to the underlying tissues. The patient's stool is already soft and he has failed medical management. Infrared phototherapy and sclerotherapy is indicated for patients with grade I or II hemorrhoids.

278. E (S&F ch129)
This patient has had a poorly healing anal fissure for several months. She has failed medical therapy; therefore, lateral internal sphincterotomy is the treatment of choice in this patient. First-line therapy of a chronic anal fissure, including sitz baths, fiber, and stool softeners, have led to healing rates of up to 35%. Topical agents such as nitrates and calcium channel blockers lead to healing rates of approximately 80%. However, the literature reports healing after lateral sphincterotomy of 90% to 100%, with less than 10% experiencing minor postsurgical incontinence. Healing rates after botulinum toxin injections to the anal sphincter are reported to be 80% to 90%.

279. A (S&F ch129)
Excision of the clot in this patient with severe pain and a thrombosed external hemorrhoid is indicated. The symptoms have been present for less than 3 days; therefore, excision at this point can significantly reduce her symptoms and quality of life. Symptoms typically subside in 4 to 7 days and can be treated conservatively in patients with milder symptoms. Band ligation is indicated for internal hemorrhoids.

280. D (S&F ch129)
Adenocarcinoma of the anal canal is managed similarly to rectal cancers. The appropriate treatment for large adenocarcinomas of the anal canal or those with nodal involvement is abdominoperineal resection with chemoradiation therapy. Contrary to squamous cell cancers, adenocarcinomas are not related to infection with human papillomavirus. Proctectomy by itself is not sufficient in this patient with lymph node involvement.

281. E (S&F ch129)
Pruritus ani occurs in approximately 5% of the U.S. population, and its etiology is unknown. However, other systemic and dermatologic diseases, malignancy, and medication-induced causes must be ruled out. This patient has the classic anal findings seen in this condition. This patient has no evidence of wartlike growth (condyloma acuminata), or clusters of blisters seen with herpes simplex.

BOX FOR ANSWER 108 Treatment of *Clostridium difficile* Infection

Minimize use of concomitant antibiotics
Discontinue all other antimicrobial drugs whenever possible
If additional antimicrobials are required, change to those least likely to exacerbate *C. difficile* infection

Initial Episode
Mild to Moderate Infection
Metronidazole (500 mg orally 3 times daily for 10 to 14 days)

Severe Infection or Unresponsiveness to or Intolerance of Metronidazole
Vancomycin (125 mg orally 4 times daily for 10 to 14 days)

Other Approved Therapy
Fidaxomicin (200 mg orally 2 times daily for 10 days)*

First Recurrence
Treat as for initial episode (see above)*

Second Recurrence†
Vancomycin in tapered and pulsed doses:
- 125 mg daily 4 times daily for 14 days
- 125 mg daily 2 times daily for 7 days
- 125 mg once daily for 7 days
- 125 mg once every 2 days for 8 days (4 doses)
- 125 mg once every 3 days for 15 days (5 doses)

Fidaxomicin (200 mg orally 2 times daily for 10 days)*

Third Recurrence
Vancomycin in tapered and pulsed doses (see above)
Fidaxomicin (200 mg orally 2 times daily for 10 days)*
Vancomycin (125 mg orally 4 times daily for 14 days), followed by rifaximin (400 mg orally 3 times daily for 20 days)

Other Options for Recurrent Infection
Fecal microbiota transplantation‡
Intravenous immune globulin (400 mg/kg of body weight every 3 weeks for a total of 2 or 3 doses)

*Fidaxomicin therapy is followed by fewer recurrences compared with vancomycin, both for an initial episode and for a first recurrence. The efficacy of fidaxomicin in second or subsequent recurrences is not yet known.
†A *Lactobacillus*-containing probiotic or *Saccharomyces boulardii* may be added during the final 2 weeks of the vancomycin regimen and for 4 to 8 weeks thereafter. However, the efficacy of probiotics in preventing recurrent *C. difficile* infection is unclear.
‡Fecal microbial transplantation appears to be highly effective in preventing further episodes in patients with multiple recurrences.

BOX FOR ANSWER 254 Factors That May Influence Carcinogenesis in the Colon and Rectum

Probably Causative
- High-fat and low-fiber diet (adjusted for energy intake)*
- Red meat consumption

Possibly Causative
- Beer and ale consumption (especially for rectal cancer)
- Cigarette smoking
- Diabetes mellitus
- Environmental carcinogens and mutagens
- Heterocyclic amines (from charbroiled and fried meat and fish)
- Low dietary selenium
- Microbial dysbiosis

Probably Protective
- Aspirin, NSAIDs, and COX-2 inhibitors
- Calcium
- Hormone replacement therapy (estrogen)
- Low body mass
- Vigorous physical activity

Possibly Protective†
- Carotene-rich foods
- High-fiber diet
- Vitamins C and E
- Vitamin D
- Yellow-green cruciferous vegetables
- Fish oil (omega-3 fatty acids)
- Statins
- Selenium

*Dietary fats and fiber are heterogeneous in composition, and not all fats or fiber components play a role in cause or protection.
†Based on limited data.
COX-2, Cyclooxygenase-2; NSAIDs, nonsteroidal antiinflammatory drugs.

TABLE FOR ANSWER 6 Disorders Associated with Abnormal Small Intestinal Motility

Disorder	Smooth Muscle Abnormalities	Neural Abnormalities	Sensory Abnormalities	Potential Outcomes
IBS	*NaV1.5* mutation causes loss of function and increased reporting of pain	Postinfection and inflammatory changes (subset of patients)	Altered afferent function Increased visceral sensitivity	Heightened sensation Disordered motility
Acute severe illness	Decreased strength of contractions	Altered neurotransmission (related to metabolic or electrolyte disturbances?)	Heightened sensitivity to neurohumoral feedback loops	Delayed transit Ileus Decreased intestinal absorption
Pregnancy	Decreased strength of contractions	None identified	None identified	Slowed transit
Diabetes mellitus	Altered ICC function	Altered neurotransmission	Enhanced perception of GI stimuli	Abnormal patterning of contractions Slow or rapid transit
Metabolic disturbances*	Possible decreased strength of contractions	Altered neurotransmission	Nausea Altered sensory perception	Abnormal patterning of contractions Slow or rapid transit
Drugs†	Possible decreased strength of contractions	Altered neurotransmission	None identified	Ileus Slow or rapid transit Disordered contractions
Intestinal obstruction	Hypertrophy, if chronic	None identified	None identified	High-amplitude forceful contractions
Pseudoobstruction syndromes	Myopathy of hollow viscera	Multiple neural abnormalities: neuron loss, plexus abnormalities, altered distribution of neurotransmitters	None identified	Feeble contractions Absent phase III of the IDMC Slow or failed transit
Scleroderma and other connective tissue disorders	Ischemia and fibrosis	Nerve loss in intestinal wall Extrinsic neural supply may also be damaged by vasculitis	None identified	Feeble contractions Thickening of bowel wall Slow transit
Neurologic syndromes‡	N/A	Neural absence or loss	Loss of afferent neurons with consequent loss of sensory information for reflux control	Disorganized IDMC Failure to convert to fed pattern Transit failure
Rare myopathies	Myocyte and mitochondrial abnormalities; inadequate contractile force	N/A	*NaV1.7* mutation leading to rectal pain	Insufficient force for transit and mixing
Radiation enteritis	Fibrosis (possibly related to ischemia)	Increased muscarinic 3 receptors	None identified	Less mixing, disordered transit Stasis, bacterial overgrowth, diarrhea
Acromegaly	None identified	Postulated autonomic nerve dysfunction	None identified	Delayed orocecal transit time SIBO

*Examples include disturbances of potassium, calcium and magnesium homeostasis, and renal and hepatic failure.
†Examples include antidepressants, calcium channel blockers, and beta-blockers.
‡Examples include dysautonomia and Parkinson's disease.
IBS, Irritable bowel syndrome; ICC, interstitial cells of Cajal; IDMC, interdigestive motor cycle; N/A, not applicable; SIBO, small intestinal bacterial overgrowth.

TABLE FOR ANSWER 109 Antimicrobial Agents That Predispose to *Clostridium difficile* Infection

Frequently	Sometimes	Rarely
Amoxicillin Ampicillin Cephalosporins Clindamycin Fluoroquinolones	Macrolides Other penicillins Sulfonamides Trimethoprim Trimethoprim ± Sulfamethoxazole	Aminoglycosides Bacitracin Carbapenems Chloramphenicol Daptomycin Metronidazole Rifampin Rifaximin Teicoplanin Tetracyclines Tigecycline

TABLE FOR ANSWER 129 Gastrointestinal Stromal Tumors: Prognostic Factors*

	Risk of Malignancy	
Factor	**Low**	**High**
Size	<2 cm	>5 cm
Mitosis	0-1 per 30-50/high-powered fields	>5 per 10-50/high-powered fields
Cellularity	Low	High
Necrosis	Absent	Present
KIT exon 11 deletion*	Absent	Present
Anatomic site	Rectum	Jejunum
Infiltration into lamina propria†	Absent	Present
Cystic spaces†	Absent	Present
Irregular borders†	Absent	Present

*Size and mitosis are the only consistently reported prognostic factors. Clinical variables negatively associated with outcome in gastrointestinal stromal tumors include tumor rupture and performance status. Patients whose tumors contain exon 11 *KIT* mutations are more likely to respond to imatinib mesylate compared to those with *KIT* exon 9 mutations or wild-type *KIT*.

†Endoscopic ultrasound criteria.

TABLE FOR ANSWER 130 Features of the Major Small Intestinal Lymphomas

Type	Histopathology	Immunohistochemistry	Genotype
Diffuse large B-cell lymphoma	Diffuse growth of large lymphoma cells, often with necrosis	B cell markers (B1), $^{+}$sIG	Ig gene rearranged
Burkitt lymphoma	Medium-sized cells with many mitoses; "starry sky" appearance from histiocytes	B cell markers, $^{+}$sIG, CD10^{+}	Chromosomal translocation involving *c-myc*
Follicular lymphoma Marginal B cell (MALT) lymphoma	Small cleaved lymphocytes or centrocytes with admixture of large cells Centrocyte-like cells with formation of lymphoepithelial lesions	B cell markers, sIG^{+}, CD10^{+}, bcl2^{+}, CD5^{-}, cyclin D1^{-} B markers, CD5^{-}, CD10-CD23^{-}, cyclin D1^{-}	t(14:18) t(11:18), t(14:18), t(1:14), t(3:14) possible
Mantle cell lymphoma (multiple lymphoid polyposis)	Monotonous small cells with irregular nuclei; epithelial invasion uncommon	B cell markers, CD5^{+}, CD23^{-}, cyclin D1^{+}, often IgM^{+} IgD^{+}	t(11:114) Translocation with implication of *bcl-1* oncogene
T-cell lymphoma (predominantly enteropathy-associated T-cell lymphoma)	Large cells with intense surrounding inflammation; adjacent atrophic mucosa	T cell markers, CD103^{+}, HML-1, CD4^{-}, CD8^{-}	T cell receptor genes rearranged
IPSID (alpha chain disease)	Early: superficial plasma cells Late: atypical large lymphoma cells with bowel wall invasion	B cell markers, KB61^{+}, α–heavy chain paraprotein	

IPSID, Immunoproliferative small intestinal disease; MALT, mucosa-associated lymphoid tissue; sIG, secretory immunoglobulin.

TABLE FOR ANSWER 198 Hinchey Classification of Colonic Diverticular Perforation

Stage	Definition
I	Confined pericolic abscess
II	Distant abscess (retroperitoneal or pelvic)
III	Generalized peritonitis caused by rupture of a pericolic or pelvic abscess (not communicating with the colonic lumen because of inflammatory obliteration of the diverticular neck)
IV	Fecal peritonitis caused by free perforation of a diverticulum (communicating with the colonic lumen)

TABLE FOR ANSWER 243 Surveillance Recommendations after Polypectomy

Findings on Colonoscopy	Next Colonoscopy (Years)
No polyps	10
Small (<10 mm) hyperplastic polyps in rectum or sigmoid	10
1-2 small (<10 mm) tubular adenomas	5-10
3-10 tubular adenomas	3
1 or more tubular adenomas >10 mm	3
1 or more villous adenomas	3
Adenoma with HGD	1
>10 adenomas	<3
Serrated Lesions	
Sessile serrated polyp(s) <10 mm with no dysplasia	5
Sessile serrated polyp(s) >10 mm	3
Sessile serrated polyp with dysplasia	3
Traditional serrated adenoma	3
Serrated polyposis syndrome	1

CHAPTER

11

Additional Treatments for Patients with Gastrointestinal and Liver Disease

Emad Qayed and Lauren M. Shea

QUESTIONS

1. Which of the following probiotics is effective in preventing the first episode of pouchitis after ileal pouch anal anastomosis (IPAA)?
   A. *Lactobacillus rhamnosus* GG
   B. *Bifidobacterium lactis*
   C. *Saccharomyces boulardi*
   D. VSL#3
   E. *Saccharomyces cerevisiae*

2. Which of the following probiotic strains have the strongest evidence for efficacy in the prevention of antibiotic-associated diarrhea?
   A. *Saccharomyces boulardii* and *Lactobacillus rhamnosus* GG
   B. *Escherichia coli* Nissle strain 1917 and VSL#3
   C. *Bifidobacterium* spp. and *Streptococcus* spp.
   D. *Lactobacillus bulgaricus* and *Lactobacillus casei*
   E. *Lactobacillus acidophilus* and *Lactobacillus plantarum*

3. A 13-year-old boy is seen in clinic for acute diarrhea and abdominal pain. For the past 2 days, he has been passing loose brown stool several times per day. He complains of midabdominal crampy pain associated with nausea. He is able to maintain oral intake. On physical examination, he is afebrile with a blood pressure of 105/65 mm Hg and a heart rate of 70 bpm. He appears healthy and in no distress. There is mild middle abdominal tenderness to deep palpation. Based on this presentation, you suspect self-limited acute infectious diarrhea and recommend oral hydration therapy without antibiotics. His mother asks you about the benefit of probiotics as a treatment for her son. Which of the following is a true regarding probiotics in the treatment of diarrheal diseases?
   A. Probiotics decrease the rate of hospitalization in acute diarrhea
   B. Probiotics decrease the occurrence of fever in acute diarrhea
   C. Probiotics shorten the duration of diarrhea by an average of 1 day
   D. Probiotics decrease the occurrence of extraintestinal complications
   E. Probiotics improve symptoms of nausea and vomiting in acute diarrhea

4. The 64-year-old patient is admitted to the hospital with worsening abdominal pain and severe watery diarrhea of 2-day duration. She reports four previous episodes of *Clostridium difficile* infection over the past 8 months. She was treated with metronidazole for the first two episodes and oral vancomycin for the last two flares. Her last treatment with oral vancomycin was 4 weeks ago. Other significant history include a long-standing history of rheumatoid arthritis, for which she takes weekly methotrexate (20 mg/week). Physical exam reveals a soft abdomen with middle abdominal tenderness. Laboratory studies are remarkable for a leukocytosis with a white blood count (WBC) of 21,000/μL. Stool testing for *C. difficile* by polymerase chain reaction (PCR) is positive. She is interested in fecal microbiota transplantation (FMT) as a treatment for her recurrent *C. difficile* infection. Which of the following statements about this treatment is true?
   A. FMT has an overall cure rate of 70%
   B. FMT is safe regardless of the route of administration
   C. FMT is ineffective against the *C. difficile* NAP1/B1/027 strain
   D. FMT has higher complication rates in immunosuppressed patients
   E. FMT is contraindicated in severe complicated *C. difficile* infection

5. A 53-year-old woman with symptomatic gallstones undergoes laparoscopic cholecystectomy. Postoperatively, she is recovering well but complains of persistent nausea. She is able to ingest liquids and is prepared for discharge. She is prescribed oral ondansetron as needed for nausea and vomiting. However, she is interested in an herbal supplement for her nausea, rather than a medication. Which of the following herbal supplements was shown to be effective in the treatment of postoperative nausea and vomiting?
   A. Capsaicin *(Capsicum annuum)*
   B. Ginger *(Zingiber officinale)*
   C. Celandine *(Chelidonium majus)*
   D. Peppermint *(Mentha piperita)*
   E. Caraway *(Carum carvi)*

6. Which of the following herbal supplements treats functional dyspepsia by inhibiting C-type pain fibers?
   A. Capsaicin *(Capsicum annuum)*
   B. Banana *(Musa sapientum)*

C. Celandine *(Chelidonium majus)*
D. Peppermint *(Mentha piperita)*
E. Caraway *(Carum carvi)*

7. Which of the following herbal supplements increases the risk of bleeding in patients on warfarin or antiplatelet agents?
   A. Oregon grape *(Berberis vulgaris)*
   B. Psyllium *(Plantago isphagula)*
   C. Ginger *(Zingiber officinale)*
   D. Peppermint *(Mentha piperita)*
   E. Caraway *(Carum carvi)*

8. A 55-year-old man with compensated alcoholic cirrhosis presents to clinic for follow-up. He quit alcohol 1 year ago. He has no ascites or encephalopathy. He had an endoscopy that showed no esophageal or gastric varices. His laboratory values are as follows:

ALT	128 U/L
AST	175 U/L
Bilirubin	2.8 mg/dL

His Model for End-Stage Liver Disease (MELD) score is 12. His friend suggested he uses milk thistle to treat his cirrhosis. Which of the following is true about the effects of milk thistle in chronic alcoholic liver disease?
   A. It improves overall survival
   B. It improves symptoms of ascites
   C. It decreases the incidence of hepatocellular carcinoma
   D. It improves liver enzymes
   E. It improves fibrosis on liver biopsy

9. A 35-year-old woman presents to clinic for follow-up of her irritable bowel disease symptoms. She has had long-standing history of abdominal pain and "sensitive stomach." Her abdominal pain is located in the hypogastric area and is relieved by defecation. She frequently has bothersome bloating. She mentions that she is interested in complementary and alternative medical therapies for her symptoms. Her friend suggested she tries Ayurvedic medicine. Which of the following correctly describes this alternative medical therapy?
   A. A deeply relaxed state in which therapeutic suggestions are made to alter behavior and alleviate symptoms
   B. Indian medicine that provides diet, herbal, and lifestyle recommendations to improve health
   C. A process of reflection, contemplation, and focused thinking to alleviate symptoms
   D. Massage and pressure over specific areas to improve symptoms
   E. A system of alternative medicine based on the belief that a disease can be cured by a substance that can cause illness in a healthy individual

10. A 42-year-old woman is seen in clinic for follow-up of irritable bowel disease. She has had long-standing history of hypogastric abdominal pain, intermittent diarrhea, and bloating. She is interested in nonpharmacologic treatment to ameliorate her symptoms. Which of the following is a useful nonpharmacologic therapy for irritable bowel syndrome (IBS)?
   A. Mindfulness training
   B. Biodynamic psychotherapy
   C. Interpersonal therapy
   D. Psychodynamic therapy
   E. Cognitive-analytic therapy

11. A 45-year-old Chinese patient with chronic hepatitis B is seen in clinic for follow-up. He recently visited his family in China and started taking TJ-9 (xiao-chai-hu-tang), one of many Chinese herbal medicines (CHM) for the treatment of hepatitis B. Which of the following statements regarding CHM and treatment of chronic viral hepatitis is true?
   A. CHM was shown to decrease the occurrence of hepatocellular carcinoma in patients with chronic hepatitis B
   B. The mechanism of action of CHM includes activation of stellate cells
   C. There is strong evidence that CHM increases seroconversion rate for hepatitis B surface antigen (HBsAg) and hepatitis B early antigen (HBeAg)
   D. Randomized trials showed that CHM is effective in the treatment of hepatitis C virus
   E. Hepatotoxicity and autoimmune hepatitis are potential adverse effects

12. A 32-year-old man is seen in clinic for follow-up of dyspepsia. He complains of postprandial abdominal burning pain associated with a bothersome sensation of "stomach fullness." A trial of omeprazole for 4 weeks was ineffective in relieving his symptoms. An upper endoscopy was unremarkable. Gastric biopsies were negative for *Helicobacter pylori* infection. Two weeks ago, he started taking the herbal supplement STW 5 (Iberogast), with some improvement in symptoms. Which of the following is true about this herbal supplement?
   A. It is composed of two active ingredients: chamomile and peppermint
   B. Randomized controlled trials show efficacy in the treatment of functional dyspepsia
   C. It causes gastric smooth muscle contraction
   D. It increases gastric emptying
   E. Insomnia is a common side effect

13. A 30-year-old woman with a long-standing history of Crohn's disease is seen in clinic for follow-up. She has no diarrhea or rectal bleeding. Her disease seems to be well controlled on infliximab every 8 hours. She tells you that she wants to start the herbal supplement fenugreek to promote her colonic health. Which of the following is a side effect of fenugreek?
   A. Lethargy
   B. Hypermagnesemia
   C. Bloating
   D. Galactorrhea
   E. Oligomenorrhea

14. A 70-year-old man is admitted to the hospital with abdominal pain and nausea. He has a history of small bowel adenocarcinoma that was resected. He has diffuse metastasis in his spine and extremities and is currently under hospice care. His pain is treated with oral oxycodone as needed and long-acting oral morphine formulation. He passes small amounts of hard stool every 2 days. On physical examination, he is debilitated but not in pain. His abdomen is mildly distended. There are active bowel sounds and no tenderness to palpation. Digital rectal exam does not reveal any hard stool in the rectum. Due to his inability to maintain adequate oral hydration, he is given intravenous (IV) fluid. Which of the following is the *least* preferred treatment for this patient's constipation?
   A. Psyllium
   B. Docusate sodium
   C. Lactulose
   D. Bisacodyl
   E. Lubiprostone

15. In the United States, patients qualify for hospice care if their expected life span is which of the following durations?
   A. ≤6 weeks
   B. ≤3 months
   C. ≤6 months
   D. ≤8 months
   E. ≤1 year

16. A 55-year-old woman with decompensated cirrhosis secondary to hepatitis C and alcoholism presents to clinic for follow-up. She was previously admitted with encephalopathy, for which she takes lactulose. She has an INR of 1.6, bilirubin of 2 mg/dL, and creatinine of 1.5 mg/dL. Her prognostic MELD is 18, which predicts a 3-month mortality of 8%. She is currently listed for liver transplantation. She is interested in palliative and hospice care. According to the Medicare Hospice Benefit, which of the following precludes acceptance of this patient into a hospice program?
   A. Continued active drinking
   B. The patient wishes to be admitted to the hospital in case of future complications
   C. The patient wishes to receive hospice care in an assisted-living facility
   D. The patient wishes to remain full code and receive cardiopulmonary resuscitation
   E. The patients is listed for liver transplantation

17. A 59-year-old man with stage IV pancreatic cancer is admitted to the hospital with abdominal pain and nausea. His wife reports that he has not had a bowel movement in 4 days. His pain is treated with oxycodone as needed, and long-acting morphine formulation. His abdomen is mildly distended, with hypoactive bowel sounds. There is no tenderness to palpation. He is started on a regimen of senna, docusate, and magnesium citrate with no improvement in his constipation. Which of the following medications is U.S. Food and Drug Administration (FDA) approved for opioid-induced constipation?
   A. Lactulose
   B. Polyethylene glycol
   C. Lubiprostone
   D. Methylnaltrexone
   E. Linaclotide

18. A 60-year-old woman with hepatitis C cirrhosis is seen in clinic for follow-up. Over the past 6 months, she developed worsening ascites, and her renal function has deteriorated. Her diuretics were stopped, and she required large-volume paracentesis with albumin infusion. Appropriate tests are ordered, and hepatorenal syndrome (HRS) type 2 is diagnosed. The patient's husband is concerned and asks about his wife's prognosis. Which of the following is the median survival of a patient with HRS type 2?
   A. 2 weeks
   B. 1 to 2 months
   C. 4 to 6 months
   D. 6 to 12 months
   E. 12 to 18 months

19. A 79-year-old man with a history of metastatic pancreatic cancer on palliative chemotherapy presents to your office for follow up. His daughter is concerned about anorexia and weight loss. She read about the appetite stimulant Megestrol and is requesting that you prescribe it for her father. Which of the following facts about appetite stimulants in the setting of malignancy is true?
   A. Indications for starting an appetite stimulant include a prognosis of longer than 4 months and the patient's interest in improving his or her appetite
   B. Multiple studies have shown that appetite stimulants improve quality of life
   C. There are no significant side effects to the use of Megestrol
   D. Megestrol results in weight gain of adipose tissue and not muscle mass
   E. Megestrol prolongs survival in patients with advanced cancer

ANSWERS

1. D (S&F ch130)
   Studies have shown that patients treated with VSL#3 had lower incidence of pouchitis compared to placebo in the first year after surgery. This product contains eight strains of bacteria (*Streptococcus salivarius* subsp., *Bifidobacterium* sp., and *Lactobacillus* sp.). The other probiotics were not shown to prevent pouchitis.

2. A (S&F ch130)
   Saccharomyces boulardii and *Lactobacillus rhamnosus* GG have very good evidence in the form of meta-analysis and randomized trials for their efficacy in the prevention of antibiotic-associated diarrhea in children and adults. The other probiotics do not have evidence for efficacy for this indication.

3. C (S&F ch130)
   A Cochrane review of probiotics therapy in acute infectious diarrhea showed that probiotics shorten the duration of diarrhea by an average of 1 day. Probiotics do not influence the rate of hospitalization in acute diarrhea. They do not improve fever, nausea, or vomiting and do not affect the development of extraintestinal complications.

4. B (S&F ch1)
   FMT appears to be equally effective and safe, regardless of the route of administration (oral vs. colonic). The overall cure rate is around 90% in most studies or case series. FMT is effective even in patients with *C. difficile* NAP1/B1/027 strain. FMT appears to be safe and effective in immunosuppressed patients and in those with severe, complicated *C. difficile* infection.

5. B (S&F ch131)
   Ginger was shown in randomized controlled trials to be effective in postoperative and chemotherapy-induced nausea and vomiting. It also improves symptoms of seasickness and morning sickness of pregnancy. Capsaicin, celandine, peppermint, and caraway are used to treat functional dyspepsia. They improve symptoms of epigastric pain, bloating, and nausea.

6. A (S&F ch131)
   Capsaicin selectively impairs the activity of nociceptive C-type pain fibers in the central nervous system. Bananas *(Musa sapientum)* are thought to increase gastric mucous secretion, therefore preventing ulcer formation. Celandine

has spasmolytic activity on intestinal smooth muscle. Peppermint and caraway inhibit gastric smooth muscle contractions.

7. **C** (S&F ch131)
Ginger inhibits platelet aggregation by inhibiting thromboxane synthase, thereby increasing the risk of bleeding in susceptible patients. Other supplements that increase the risk of bleeding are chamomile, papaya, and fenugreek. The other supplements mentioned in the question (Oregon grape, psyllium, peppermint, and caraway) do not increase the risk of bleeding.

8. **D** (S&F ch130)
Studies of milk thistle in chronic liver disease are difficult to interpret due to their heterogeneity in etiology of liver disease, methodology, sample size, and duration. The positive outcome most frequently seen in these studies is minor decrease in liver enzymes (mostly ALT). There is no evidence to suggest any improvement in mortality, morbidity, liver fibrosis, or hepatocellular carcinoma prevention.

9. **B** (S&F ch131)
Ayurvedic medicine (Ayurveda) is a holistic system of medicine that originated in India more than 3000 years ago. It provides diet and lifestyle recommendations to improve health. Hypnosis induces a deeply relaxed state in which therapeutic suggestions are made to alter behavior and improve symptoms. Meditation is a process of reflection, contemplation, and focused thinking to alleviate symptoms. Reflexology uses massage and pressure at specific areas to alleviate symptoms. Homeopathy is based on the belief that a disease can be cured by a substance that can cause illness in a healthy individual.

10. **A** (S&F ch131)
Mindfulness training is practice of attention to the present moment or experience without judgment, and being fully aware of that moment, including its sensations, perceptions, and emotions. In a prospective randomized controlled trial, mindfulness training was found to improve the symptoms of IBS. The other therapies mentioned in the questions are not used to treat IBS.

11. **E** (S&F ch131)
Hepatotoxicity, autoimmune hepatitis, interstitial pneumonitis, and immune thrombocytopenic purpura are potential adverse effects of Chinese herbal medicine (CHM). There is no evidence to suggest that CHM decreases the incidence of hepatocellular carcinoma. The suggested mechanism of action for CHM is inhibition of stellate cells and inhibition of HBV DNA polymerase. The research performed on CHM in chronic hepatitis B suffers from many methodologic flaws. Small, low-quality studies suggest that CHM might increase seroconversion rate for HBsAg and HBeAg, especially when given in conjunction with interferon. Randomized trials revealed no benefit of CHM in HCV. Overall, due to lack of high quality studies, CHM cannot be recommended for the treatment of chronic hepatitis B.

12. **B** (S&F ch131)
Multiple randomized controlled trials showed that Iberogast is more effective than placebo in treating dyspepsia. This agent is composed of nine plant extracts, including chamomile, peppermint, caraway, licorice, bitter candytuft, lemon leaves, celandine, angelica root, and milk thistle. Iberogast causes smooth muscle relaxation, not contraction. It has no effect on gastric emptying. Iberogast has not been associated with any adverse effects. However, individual components are known to cause hepatotoxicity, increased bleeding risk, and potentiation of anxiolytics and sedatives. It is not associated with insomnia.

13. **D** (S&F ch131)
Fenugreek is an herbal supplement that is taken for various gastrointestinal symptoms (anorexia, dyspepsia, constipation), although without clear evidence of efficacy. Galactorrhea is a side effect that occurs due to interaction at dopamine receptors. This supplement is also given to lactating women to promote milk production.

14. **A** (S&F ch132)
Fiber supplements can lead to worsening constipation in patients who are unable to drink adequate amounts of fluid. They are generally not recommended for palliative care and hospice patients. Docusate sodium is a stool softener. It is ineffective when used as a sole treatment for constipation. However, it does not worsen constipation as do fiber supplementations. Lactulose, bisacodyl, and lubiprostone are all effective agents in the treatment of constipation (see table at end of chapter).

15. **C** (S&F ch132)
In the United States, a prognosis of 6 months or less is required for patients to qualify for hospice care.

16. **E** (S&F ch132)
Patients referred to hospice should not be pursuing curative treatment. Therefore, patients listed for liver transplantation are not eligible for hospice care. Continued active alcoholism is not a contraindication to hospice care. The Medicare Hospice Benefit does not require the patient to relinquish heroic life-saving measures or future hospitalizations. Patients can remain full code if this is their wish. Hospice care can be provided in the patient's home, hospice unit, or assisted-living facility.

17. **D** (S&F ch132)
Methylnaltrexone is the only medication approved by the FDA for opioid-induced constipation. It does not cross the blood-brain barrier and therefore does not reverse the central analgesic effects of opioids. Lactulose, polyethylene glycol, lubiprostone, and linaclotide are used to treat constipation but are not specific nor approved for opioid induced constipation.

18. **C** (S&F ch132)
HRS refers to functional renal failure that develops in the setting of end-stage liver disease and portal hypertension. Type 1 HRS exhibits a rapidly progressive renal failure with high mortality, and has a median survival of 2 weeks. Patients with type 2 HRS develop slowly progressive renal failure and have a median survival of 4 to 6 months.

19. **D** (S&F ch132)
Megestrol results in weight gain of adipose tissue, not muscle mass. Appetite stimulants have a limited role in patients with advanced cancer. Indications for starting an appetite stimulant include a prognosis of greater than 4 weeks and the patient's interest in improving his or her appetite. Megestrol has important side effects including edema and thromboembolic events. No appetite stimulant has shown efficacy in prolonging survival or improving quality of life in population-based research.

TABLE FOR ANSWER 14 Laxatives in Palliative Care

Class	Laxative(s)	Side Effects	Relevance to Palliative Care
Bulk-forming agents	Bran, psyllium, calcium polycarbophil, methyl cellulose	Impaction above strictures, bloating	Patients with serious illnesses are often unable to consume a large amount of fiber Because these patients often eat and drink little, fiber supplements can worsen constipation
Emollient, softener	Docusate sodium	Rash	Constipation in a palliative care setting is multifactorial, and emollients per se are often ineffective in reversing the underlying malfunction
Osmolar agents	Sorbitol, lactulose	Abdominal bloating, flatulence	Many patients dislike the sickly sweet taste, which can exacerbate their nausea
	Polyethylene glycol	Nausea, bloating, cramping	Patients might be unable to drink large volumes of the constituted solution
	Magnesium citrate, magnesium sulfate	Magnesium toxicity (with renal insufficiency)	Unpleasant taste can exacerbate nausea
Stimulant agents	Bisacodyl, senna	Colicky pain	First-line laxatives in all patients taking opioids
Chloride channel activator	Lubiprostone	Nausea	Easy to swallow, small capsule, well tolerated

ILLUSTRATION CREDITS

All figures and tables are original to the Sleisenger and Fordtran companion text except for those noted here.

Table for Answer 31, Chapter 2, Data from American Psychiatric Association. Diagnostic and statistical manual of mental disorders, 5th ed (DSM-5). Arlington, VA, American Psychiatric Association, 2013.

Figure for Question 56, Chapter 3, Courtesy Emad Qayed, MD, Atlanta, Georgia.

Figure for Question 61, Chapter 3, Courtesy Emad Qayed, MD, Atlanta, Georgia.

Figure for Answer 61, Chapter 3, Courtesy Emad Qayed, MD, Atlanta, Georgia.

Figure for Answer 69, Chapter 3, From Drossman DA. Functional abdominal pain syndrome. Clin Gastroenterol Hepatol 2004;2:353-65.

Figures for Questions 5 through 8, Chapter 4, Courtesy M.A. Rosenbach, MD, Department of Dermatology, University of Pennsylvania, Philadelphia, Pennsylvania.

Figure for Question 39, Chapter 4, Courtesy Edward Lee, MD, Washington, D.C.

Figure for Question 55, Chapter 4, Courtesy Brian P. Rubin, MD, Cleveland, Ohio.

Figure for Question 119, Chapter 4, From Frumovitz MM, eMedicine. com, Inc., 2004.

Figure for Question 134, Chapter 4, Courtesy Lawrence J. Brandt, MD, Bronx, New York.

Figures for Answers 26 and 29, Chapter 6, From Schubert ML, Peura DA. Control of gastric acid secretion in health and disease. Gastroenterology 2008;134:1842-60.

Figure for Question 55, Chapter 6, Courtesy Pamela Jensen, MD, Dallas, Texas.

Table for Answer 77, Chapter 6, Modified from Laine L, Peterson WL. Bleeding peptic ulcer. N Engl J Med 1994;331:717-27.

Figure for Answer 68, Chapter 6, Modified from Talley NJ. American Gastroenterological Association medical position statement: evaluation of dyspepsia. Gastroenterology 2005;129:1753-5.

Figure for Question 90, Chapter 6, Courtesy Rhonda K. Yantiss, MD, Boston, Massachusetts.

Table for Answer 81, Chapter 6, Data from Age-Adjusted SEER Incidence and US Death Rates and 5-Year Relative Survival Rates. National Cancer Institute, 2012. Available at http://seer.cancer.gov/statfacts/html/stomach.html.

Table for Answers 88, 89, and 94, Chapter 6, From Edge S, et al (eds). AJCC cancer staging manual, 7th ed. New York, Springer, 2010.

Figure for Question 53, Chapter 7, Courtesy Emad Qayed, MD, Emory University School of Medicine, Atlanta, Georgia.

Figure for Question 66, Chapter 7, Courtesy Saurabh Chawla, MD, Atlanta, Georgia.

Figure for Question 4, Chapter 8, From Kocoshis SA, Riely CA, Burrell M, Gryboski JD. Cholangitis in a child due to biliary tract anomalies. Dig Dis Sci 1980;25:59-65.

Figure for Question 27, Chapter 8, Courtesy Julie Champine, MD, Dallas, Texas.

Figure for Question 63, Chapter 8, Courtesy Matthew Yeh, MD, PhD, Seattle, Washington.

Figure for Question 64, Chapter 8, Courtesy Emad Qayed, MD, Atlanta, Georgia.

Figure for Answer 64, Chapter 8, Modified from Blechacz BR, Komuta M, Roskams T, Gores GJ. Clinical diagnosis and staging of cholangiocarcinoma. Nat Rev Gastroenterol Hepatol 2011;8:512-22.

Figure for Answer 74, Chapter 8, Modified from Misra S, Chaturvedi A, Misra NC, Sharma ID. Carcinoma of the gallbladder. Lancet Oncol 2003;4:167-76.

Figure for Questions 80 and 89, Chapter 8, Courtesy Emad Qayed, MD, Atlanta, Georgia.

Figure for Question 82, Chapter 8, Courtesy Saurabh Chawla, MD, Atlanta, Georgia.

Figure for Question 91, Chapter 9, From Lucas SB. Other viral and infectious diseases and HIV-related liver disease. In Burt AD, Portmann BC, Ferrell LD (eds). Pathology of the Liver, 5th ed. London, Churchill Livingstone, 2007, p 446.

Figure for Answer 103, Chapter 9, From Gitlin N, Strauss R. Atlas of Clinical Hepatology. Philadelphia, WB Saunders, 1995, p 72.

Figure for Question 137, Chapter 9, Courtesy Mukesh Harisinghani, MD, Boston, Massachusetts.

Table for Answer 161, Chapter 9, Modified from Alvarez F, Berg PA, Bianchi FB, et al. International Autoimmune Hepatitis Group report: review of criteria for diagnosis of autoimmune hepatitis. J Hepatol 1999;31:929-38. Used with permission from Elsevier BV.

Box for Answer 108, Chapter 10, Modified from Kelly CP, Lamont JT. *Clostridium difficile*—more difficult than ever. N Engl J Med 2008;18:1932-40.

Table for Answer 109, Chapter 10, Modified from Kelly C, Lamont J. Treatment of *Clostridium difficile* diarrhea and colitis. In Wolfe MM (ed). Gastrointestinal Pharmacotherapy. Philadelphia, WB Saunders, 1993, p 199.

Figure for Question 142, Chapter 10, Courtesy Tanvi Dhere, MD, Atlanta, Georgia.

Figure for Question 166, Chapter 10, Courtesy Feldman M, Boland CR (eds). Slide Atlas of Gastroenterology and Hepatology. Philadelphia, Current Medicine, 1996.

Figure for Answer 184, Chapter 10, Modified from Brandt LJ, Boley SJ. AGA technical review on intestinal ischemia: American Gastrointestinal Association. Gastroenterology 2000;118:954.

Figure for Question 185, Chapter 10, Courtesy Emad Qayed, MD, Atlanta, Georgia.

Figure for Question 199, Chapter 10, Courtesy Jennifer Christie, MD, Atlanta, Georgia.

Figures for Questions 231 and 232, Chapter 10, Courtesy Emad Qayed, MD, Atlanta, Georgia.

Table for Answer 243, Chapter 10, Modified from Lieberman DA, Rex DK, Winawer SJ, et al. Guidelines for colonoscopy surveillance after screening and polypectomy: a consensus update by the US Multi-Society Task Force on Colorectal Cancer. Gastroenterology. 2012;143:844-57.

Figure for Question 268, Chapter 10, Courtesy Emad Qayed, MD, Atlanta, Georgia.

Figure for Question 269, Chapter 10, Courtesy Emad Qayed, MD, Atlanta, Georgia.

Figure for Question 273, Chapter 10, Courtesy Marie E. Robert, MD, New Haven, Connecticut.

Figure for Question 275, Chapter 10, Courtesy Emad Qayed, MD, Atlanta, Georgia.

Table for Answer 14, Chapter 11, From Periyakoil VS. Opioid conversion. Stanford palliative care online curriculum 2008. [cited 2009 June 23] Available at http://endoflife.stanford.edu.